T0383783

Global Maternal and Child Health

Medical, Anthropological, and Public Health Perspectives

Series Editor

David A. Schwartz, Atlanta, GA, USA

Global Maternal and Child Health: Medical, Anthropological, and Public Health Perspectives is a series of books that will provide the most comprehensive and current sources of information on a wide range of topics related to global maternal and child health, written by a collection of international experts.

The health of pregnant women and their children are among the most significant public health, medical, and humanitarian problems in the world today. Because in developing countries many people are poor, and young women are the poorest of the poor, persistent poverty exacerbates maternal and child morbidity and mortality and gender-based challenges to such basic human rights as education and access to health care and reproductive choices. Women and their children remain the most vulnerable members of our society and, as a result, are the most impacted individuals by many of the threats that are prevalent, and, in some cases, increasing throughout the world. These include emerging and re-emerging infectious diseases, natural and man-made disasters, armed conflict, religious and political turmoil, relocation as refugees, malnutrition, and, in some cases, starvation. The status of indigenous women and children is especially precarious in many regions because of ethnic, cultural, and language differences, resulting in stigmatization, poor obstetrical and neonatal outcomes, limitations of women's reproductive rights, and lack of access to family planning and education that restrict choices regarding their own futures. Because of the inaccessibility of women to contraception and elective pregnancy termination, unsafe abortion continues to result in maternal deaths, morbidity, and reproductive complications. Unfortunately, maternal deaths remain at unacceptably high levels in the majority of developing countries, as well as in some developed ones. Stillbirths and premature deliveries result in millions of deaths annually. Gender inequality persists globally as evidenced by the occurrence of female genital mutilation, obstetrical violence, human trafficking, and other forms of sexual discrimination directed at women. Many children are routinely exposed to physical, sexual, and psychological violence. Childhood and teen marriages remain at undesirably high levels in many developing countries.

Global Maternal and Child Health: Medical, Anthropological, and Public Health Perspectives is unique in combining the opinions and expertise of public health specialists, physicians, anthropologists and social scientists, epidemiologists, nurses, midwives, and representatives of governmental and non governmental agencies to comprehensively explore the increasing challenges and potential solutions to global maternal and child health issues.

Series Editorial Advisory Board

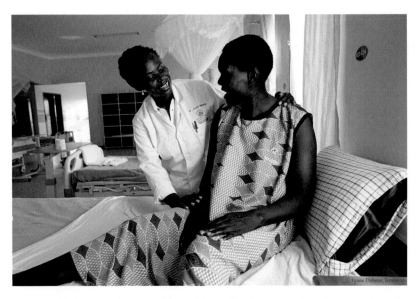

An obstetric fistula patient consulting with her fistula surgeon, Dr. Namugenyi, at the Terrewode Women's Community Hospital in Soroti, Uganda. Photo by: Lynne Dobson, Terrewode Women's Fund

Laura Briggs Drew · Bonnie Ruder
David A. Schwartz

Editors

A Multidisciplinary Approach to Obstetric Fistula in Africa

Public Health, Anthropological, and Medical Perspectives

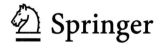

Editors
Laura Briggs Drew
Office of the Senior Vice
President and Provost
University of Maryland
College Park, MD, USA

David A. Schwartz
Perinatal Pathology Consulting
Atlanta, GA, USA

Bonnie Ruder
Terrewode Women's Fund
Eugene, OR, USA

International Fistula Alliance
Sydney, Australia

ISSN 2522-8382   ISSN 2522-8390   (electronic)
Global Maternal and Child Health

ISBN 978-3-031-06313-8   ISBN 978-3-031-06314-5   (eBook)
https://doi.org/10.1007/978-3-031-06314-5

This Springer imprint is published by the registered company Springer Nature Switzerland AG
The registered company address is: Gewerbestrasse 11, 6330 Cham, Switzerland

This book is dedicated to the women and girls in Africa who have suffered from the physical, psychological, and social distress caused by obstetric fistula. Obstetric fistulas are both preventable and treatable. Their continued presence among the world's poorest women is a human rights tragedy. The purpose of this book is to bring greater awareness, resources, and collaboration to the collective efforts to finally end fistula and the suffering it causes.

The editors and authors of this book also wish to dedicate this collection to the organizations and individuals who are providing fistula treatment and reintegration services to women and girls who have suffered from fistula. International and local nongovernmental organizations (NGOs) have served a tremendous role in providing surgical care for victims of obstetric fistula. NGOs have been at the forefront of making a wide range of services available including rehabilitation, psychological and family counseling, physical therapy, education and vocational training, and assisting women and girls so they successfully reintegrate back into society post-surgical repair.

A special dedication of this book is extended to Catherine Hamlin, AC, FRCS, FRANZCOG, FRCOG. Dr. Catherine Hamlin was a pioneer in fistula surgery and an advocate for women and girls who suffered from obstetric fistula. With her husband, Reginald Hamlin, Dr. Hamlin cofounded the Addis Ababa Fistula hospital, which has provided free obstetric fistula repair surgery to thousands of women and girls in Ethiopia. Her lifelong dedication to the prevention and treatment of obstetric fistula brought global awareness to this preventable childbirth injury. Without her work, the eradication of obstetric fistula in our lifetimes would not be as achievable. Dr. Hamlin's dream of eradicating obstetric fistula through over 60 years of service is highlighted in Chapter 2 of this book.

Foreword

This book is about obstetric fistula—a preventable and tragic condition that continues to be an important cause of morbidity and mortality throughout Africa as well as in many other parts of the world. It is a terribly debilitating sequelae of childbirth that can be considered to be a disease of poverty and neglect, ruining the lives of countless women and their families. I have spent a good part of my life working to improve conditions for women with diseases such as fistula and pioneered the campaign to abolish female genital mutilation, and I would like to relate a little of my history and how I became involved with the health of women.

I was born in 1937 in Hargeisa, British Somaliland, the daughter of a prominent Somali medical doctor. Because girls were not routinely educated in Somaliland, my father arranged for me to be tutored to learn to read and write. In those times, pregnancy and childbirth were dangerous, and in my family, two of my siblings died at delivery. From an early age, I worked alongside my father in his hospital. I'd go in and help him during the school holidays, or whenever he needed an extra pair of hands. There were no bandages, so one of my jobs would be to cut bedsheets into strips, boil them, iron them, and then roll them up. If he had to go away, he'd leave me notes—make sure they feed this child properly or remove those sutures. I would listen to his frustrations too, about the lack of materials and poor facilities. I promised myself that one day I would create the kind of hospital my father would have loved to work in.

After I attended school in Djibouti in French Somaliland, I then traveled to the United Kingdom where I was trained as a nurse and a midwife in the 1950s at the Borough Polytechnic, now London South Bank University, at the West London Hospital, the Hammersmith Hospital, and at the Lewisham Hospital. Midwifery was not my first choice of specialization, as I really wanted to specialize in surgery. It was the one time I remember my father really questioning one of my decisions. He said, "Yes, surgery is great. But what are you going to do for the women back home in Somaliland who need you at the most vulnerable time in their lives?" And I thought, after all the opportunities I've had and the freedom I've enjoyed, I should think about giving something back, so I signed up for midwifery. There was never any question in my mind that I would come back to Somaliland. I was very clear that the knowledge and experience I was gaining in England was for the benefit of the people here. When I came back, there was a definite air of optimism. The British had left, and Somaliland was independent. Still, the infrastructure was virtually nonexistent, and no one knew what to do with a female nurse/midwife, nor how to pay one—I worked for 22 months without a salary. I also believed that I could use my training as a nurse to return to my homeland and abolish the traumatic practice of genital mutilation and other injuries to young women. Two years after I returned, I was married in 1963 to Mohamed Haji Ibrahim Egal, who became Leader of the Opposition and later became the first Prime Minister of the Somali Republic in 1967, making me the nation's First Lady.

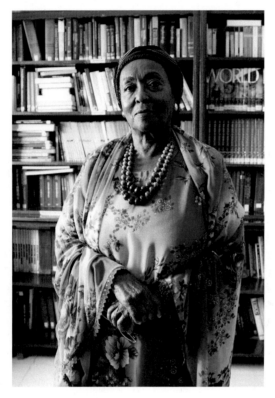

Hon. Edna Adan Ismail

I began to fulfill my dream of building a hospital in Mogadishu for the care of women starting in 1980, but with the start of the Somali civil war in 1981 I had to leave the country—that hospital fell into the hands of the warlords during the civil war. I returned to Somaliland after the civil war in 1991 and found that the entire health infrastructure had, for all intents and purposes, been destroyed by the conflict. At that time, the rates of maternal death and infant mortality were among the highest in the world.

How do you build a hospital in a country with no infrastructure? You just get up and do it. I began to build my maternity hospital in Hargeisa in 1998, on a plot of land donated to us by the government that had once been a killing ground and a garbage dump! Finding that the region lacked trained nurses to staff the hospital, I recruited more than 30 candidates and began training them, while the hospital was still under construction. With the help of financial and material donations from concerned persons, international organizations, businesses, and my own United Nations pension, our hospital opened on March 9th, 2002.

It was when we opened the hospital that we discovered more and more women coming to us with obstetric fistula and I became a bigger advocate for women suffering from maternal morbidities. Obstetrical fistula dehumanizes women— the smell of the feces and urine that leaks out of their bodies stains their clothes but also damages their morale—it totally destroys women affected. The woman becomes rejected. She is put in a hut outside the house because they—her family, relatives, husband, children, the people around her—cannot tolerate the smell of urine which is constant. Many of them commit suicide when they become rejected. And we can all understand how morally destroying it is for a woman— who was once pretty, who was loved, who was a member of that community, a mother to children, a wife to a husband—to suddenly become somebody who is sent out of the house as an outcast simply because she smells bad.

Returning home gave me an opportunity to be a role model. I started training auxiliaries in the hospital to take better care of the women. From there, I started inviting girls who'd been my pupils back when I was a schoolteacher to come in and help me. Their families didn't want them to get involved with the patients. However, very slowly, they began to get interested and excited by the possibilities. Of that first group, five received scholarships to study in England, and three came back to work here. That's really how nursing in this country got started. Later, I held various roles within the World Health Organization (WHO) and started training midwives for Libya from 1965 to 1967, and from 1986 to 1991, became the WHO Regional Technical Officer for Mother and Child Health, having the responsibility for working to end harmful traditional practices which affect the health of women and children (such as female genital mutilation), and for training midwives and traditional birth attendants in the 22 countries of the Eastern Mediterranean Region. During the last six years of my career with WHO, I became their Representative in the Republic of Djibouti from 1991 to 1997 when I retired and then went home to build my hospital in Hargeisa, Somaliland.

Although I was soon appointed the Minister of Family Welfare and Social Development of Somaliland and became Somaliland's Foreign Minister from 2003 to 2006, I continued to work on improving the quality of healthcare training to prevent maternal mortality and morbidity and increase the quality and coverage of health care throughout the country. We are now proud to have 7 midwifery training schools in Somaliland. The Edna Adan University Hospital now has over 200 staff members, 2 operating rooms, fully equipped laboratory, library, computer facilities, and a complete wing dedicated to the education of nurses and midwives. Our community midwives typically each assist with from 150 to 200 births per year, while some may deliver as many as 400 babies a year if they work in a major regional hospital.

As a result of improved midwifery, the women who suffer from obstetrical fistula are becoming fewer. However, there is still much to do here and elsewhere and in the remote rural locations and beyond. Many girls and women travel for days to come to us. Many have to walk from their towns and villages to arrive here and reach us, weak, anemic, and at times in a state of near collapse. Many have bruises, wounds, and ulcers on the soles of their feet that we have to take care of in addition to their fistula. Their morale is destroyed; their hope in life is lost. And many have doubts that the surgery that we are offering will really take care and solve their problem. Many cry when they become healed, when they become dry, and when they no longer smell.

Having the surgical skills to repair obstetrical fistula is important, of course. But the prevention of obstetrical fistula is the most important action that we can take because however skilled the surgeon is, sometimes the damage that happens to the pelvic organs of the woman is so bad that they cannot be fixed. Once again, prevention is the best strategy. And to get there we need to improve and expand the training of the midwives who deliver these women. We cannot rest on our accomplishments and need to increase training because there are still locations, especially within Africa, where there are no trained midwives. Poverty exacerbates girl's and women's lack of access to education and quality health care. Furthermore, the lacerations that occur during childbirth can become greatly exacerbated for women who have genital cuts and mutilations. Living in villages without access to running water to clean themselves, women with fistula become social pariahs, shunned and ostracized, facing a lifetime of rejection and shame. I know of one young woman who was almost murdered by her husband because he found her so repulsive to be near.

In a normal delivery—in a hospital with appropriate equipment—under the care of a trained health professional, a baby with a large head would be identified long before the birth and would be delivered instead by cesarean section. Or, if it was delivered vaginally and became stuck in the birth canal, it would be helped out with forceps, vacuum extraction, or other medical interventions that prevent extensive pelvic floor lacerations from happening. A nomadic mother in Africa giving birth out in the bush who has never had prenatal care and is unassisted or being delivered by traditional attendant would have no such help and—if she has been infibulated—then she and her baby are at even a higher risk.

The best way to overcome obstetric fistula is through the education of girls and women, through improved training of health professionals, and through better equipment and coordination of health facilities. This book, *A Multidisciplinary Approach to Obstetric Fistula in Africa: Public Health, Anthropological, and Medical Perspectives*, highlights such strategies as solutions to prevent and treat obstetric fistula. Within this text are the opinions and experiences from a wide range of experts with differing educational backgrounds—anthropologists, nurses, physicians, midwives, epidemiologists, public health specialists, maternal and child health specialists, and others. The authors come from not only Africa but around the world, writing on the physical, psychological, medical, and societal effects of obstetric fistula throughout the continent of Africa.

I am honored to have been asked to write this Foreword. I am thrilled that a multidisciplinary approach is being explored by the editors—Laura, Bonnie, and David—who themselves represent a variety of specialties. These perspectives will help find solutions and help ensure that one day obstetric fistula surgeries in hospitals like mine will become unnecessary and obsolete.

Edna Adan Ismail
Edna Adan Maternity Hospital
Hargeisa, Somalia

Edna Adan University
Hargeisa, Somalia

Acknowledgments

We, the editors, would like to acknowledge each of the dedicated individuals who contributed to this book's content. We appreciate the time the authors took to develop their respective chapters and their ongoing efforts to provide treatment to women and girls who have suffered from obstetric fistula as well as their work towards obstetric fistula prevention. We also extend our appreciation to the women and girls who have endured obstetric fistula. Their stories and experiences highlight the urgent need to address this preventable childbirth injury. Without their advocacy in communities and their participation in obstetric fistula research studies, we would not know how to best prioritize efforts so we can achieve the goal of obstetric fistula eradication. We also thank our families, friends, and colleagues, who throughout the years have continuously supported our work on this collaborative effort.

Contents

Editors and Contributors

About the Editors

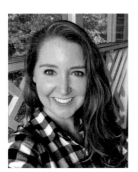 **Laura Briggs Drew, PhD, MPH** received her PhD in Maternal and Child Health from the University of Maryland (UMD) School of Public Health in College Park. She was appointed as a Maternal and Child Health Student Fellow with the American Public Health Association in 2016–2017. Laura completed her Master of Public Health in Epidemiology and Interdisciplinary Specialization in Global Health at the Ohio State University. Prior to UMD, she worked with University of North Carolina Project-Malawi on various research studies that aimed to improve the quality of life for women with obstetric fistula at the Freedom from Fistula Foundation's Fistula Repair Centre at Bwaila Hospital in Lilongwe, Malawi. Laura's primary research interests focus on the intersection of human rights and reproductive, maternal, and child health outcomes. Her research focuses on birth outcomes, intimate partner violence, female genital cutting, sexual health, infertility, infectious diseases, and gender inequality. Laura's research has been published in numerous public health journals, including *Women's Reproductive Health, BMC Pregnancy and Childbirth, American Journal of Preventive Medicine, PLOS Neglected Tropical Diseases,* and *Journal of Women's Health.* Laura's work has received support and recognition from multiple institutions, including the Maryland Population Research Center and the Delta Omega Honorary Society in Public Health.

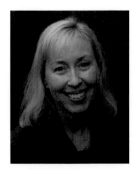

Bonnie Ruder, PhD, MPH, CPM holds a PhD in Applied Medical Anthropology and a Master's in Public Health in International Health from Oregon State University. She is the cofounder and Executive Director of Terrewode Women's Fund, a US-based nonprofit organization; a senior research consultant with the International Fistula Alliance; and sits on the Board of Governors for Terrewode Women's Community Hospital. She conducts research on maternal health and obstetric fistula and has worked on projects in Uganda, Somalia, The Gambia, Zimbabwe, and the USA. Her research focuses on obstetric fistula, residual incontinence post-fistula repair, maternal and infant health, reproductive justice, traditional birth attendants, social justice and systems of oppression, and community-engaged research. Bonnie is a licensed midwife with over 20 years' experience, working primarily in the USA. She has also attended births in Haiti after the 2010 earthquake and at a referral hospital in Soroti, Uganda. Her current research examines the COVID-19 pandemic's impact on gender and maternal health in Uganda.

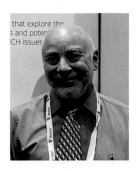

David A. Schwartz, MD, MS Hyg, FCAP has an educational background in Anthropology, Medicine, Emerging Infections, Maternal Health, and Medical Epidemiology and Public Health. He has professional and research interests in reproductive health, diseases of pregnancy, and maternal and infant morbidity and mortality in both resource-rich and resource-poor countries. In the field of Medicine, his subspecialties include Obstetric, Placental and Perinatal Pathology as well as Emerging Infections. An experienced author, editor, investigator, and consultant, Dr. Schwartz has long experience investigating the anthropological, biomedical, and epidemiologic aspects of pregnancy and its complications as they affect society, in particular among indigenous populations and when they involve emerging infections. Dr. Schwartz has been a recipient of many grants, was a Pediatric AIDS Foundation Scholar, and has organized and directed national and international projects involving maternal health, perinatal infectious diseases, and placental pathology for such agencies as the US Centers for Disease Control and Prevention, National Institutes of Health, and the United States Agency for International Development, as well as for the governments of other nations. He has published 3 previous books on pregnancy-related morbidity and mortality, the first in 2015 entitled *Maternal Mortality: Risk Factors, Anthropological Perspectives, Prevalence in Developing Countries and Preventive Strategies for Pregnancy-Related Deaths*; a book published in 2018 entitled *Maternal Death and Pregnancy-Related Morbidity Among Indigenous Women of Mexico and Central America: An Anthropological, Epidemiological and Biomedical Approach*; and in 2019 a book entitled *Pregnant in the Time of Ebola. Women and Their Children in the 2013-2015 West African Epidemic.* Dr. Schwartz is the editor of the Springer book series *Global Maternal and Child Health: Medical, Anthropological and Public Health Perspectives,* of which this book is a volume. He has been involved with maternal, fetal, and neonatal aspects of such epidemic infections as HIV, Zika, and Ebola viruses, and is currently researching these issues with the COVID-19 pandemic. Dr. Schwartz serves on the Editorial Boards of several international journals and was formerly Clinical Professor of Pathology at the Medical College of Georgia of Augusta University in Augusta, Georgia.

Contributors

Mulat Adefris, MD, MPH Department of Obstetrics and Gynecology, University of Gondar, Gondar, Ethiopia

Alice Abokai Agana, RN, RM, MPhil Nursing and Midwifery Training College, Yeji, Bono East Region, Ghana

Saifuddin Ahmed, MBBS, PhD Department of Population, Family, and Reproductive Health, Johns Hopkins University Bloomberg School of Public Health, Baltimore, Maryland, USA

Robert Andrianne, MD, MMed Urology, PhD Department of Urology, University Hospital, University of Liège, Liège, Belgium

Aduragbemi Banke-Thomas, MD, PhD, MPH School of Human Sciences, University of Greenwich, London, UK

Justus K. Barageine, MBChB, MMed, PhD, FCOG (ECSA) Department of Obstetrics and Gynaecology, Makerere University College of Health Sciences, Kampala, Uganda

Meghan Beddow, MD Southcentral Foundation, Alaska Native Medical Center, Anchorage, AK, USA

Laurence Bernard, MD, MPH University of Ottawa, Ottawa, ON, Canada

Priscilla N. Boakye, RN, Mphil, PhD. (Cand.) Lawrence S. Bloomberg Faculty of Nursing, University of Toronto, Toronto, ON, Canada

Andrew Browning, AM, MBBS, FRCOG FRANZCOG (Hon) Maternity Africa, Arusha, Tanzania

Barbara May Foundation, Bowral, NSW, Australia

Bahir Dar Fistula Centre, Bahir Dar, Ethiopia

Ennet Banda Chipungu, MBBS, FCOG Freedom from Fistula Foundation, Freetown, Sierra Leone

Jacques Corcos, MSC, MD, FRCS(S) Department of Surgery (Division of Urology), McGill University, Jewish General Hospital, Montréal, QC, Canada

Karen D. Cowgill, PhD, MSc University of Washington Tacoma, Tacoma, WA, USA

University of Washington, Seattle, WA, USA

Alexandre Delamou, MD, MSc, MPH, PhD Department of Public Health & Africa Center of Excellence (CEA-PCMT), University Gamal Abdel Nasser of Conakry, Conakry, Guinea

Julie Désalliers, MD, MSc Espace Santé Nun's Island Clinical, Hôpital de LaSalle, Montréal, QC, Canada

Laura Briggs Drew, PhD, MPH Office of the Senior Vice President and Provost, University of Maryland, College Park, MD, USA

Alison M. El Ayadi, ScD, MPH Department of Obstetrics, Gynecology and Reproductive Sciences, University of California San Francisco, San Francisco, CA, USA

Alice Emasu, MBA, MSW TERREWODE and Terrewode Women's Community Hospital, Soroti, Uganda

Kathomi Gatwiri, PhD, M Couns Psych, BASW Faculty of Health, Centre for Children & Young People, Southern Cross University, Gold Coast, Australia

René Génadry, MD, FRCS (C) Department of Obstetrics & Gynecology, University of Iowa, Iowa City, IA, USA

Judith Goh, MBBS (Qld), FRANZCOG, PhD, AO Griffith University, Gold Coast, QLD, Australia

Greenslopes Hospital, QEII Hospital, Brisbane, QLD, Australia

Laura Jacobson, MPH, Doctoral Student Oregon Health & Science University-Portland State University, School of Public Health, Portland, OR, USA

Kimberly Jarvis, PhD, R.N Faculty of Nursing, Memorial University, St. John's, NL, Canada

University of Alberta, Edmonton Clinic Health Academy, Edmonton, AB, Canada

Caroline Johnson, MPH Independent Contributor, Washington, DC, USA

Jean-Baptiste S. Z. Kakoma, MD, MMed OG, PhD, AESM Department of Gynecology and Obstetrics, University of Lubumbashi, Lubumbashi, Democratic Republic of the Congo

University of Rwanda, Kigali, Republic of Rwanda

Prosper L. Kakudji, MD, MMed OG, PhD Department of Gynecology and Obstetrics, University of Lubumbashi, Lubumbashi, Democratic Republic of the Congo

Ivy Kalama Freedom from Fistula Foundation, Freetown, Sierra Leone

Weston Khisa, PhD Reproductive Health Department, Kenyatta National Hospital, Nairobi, Kenya

Xavier K. Kinenkinda, MD, MMed OG, PhD Department of Gynecology and Obstetrics, University of Lubumbashi, Lubumbashi, Democratic Republic of the Congo

Salam Kouraogo, MA Department of Sociology, Université de Ouagadougou, Ouagadougou, Burkina Faso

Hannah G. Krause, MBBS, FRANZCOG, AO Greenslopes Hospital, QEII Hospital, Brisbane, QLD, Australia

Ann E. Kurth, PhD, MSN, MPH Yale University School of Nursing, New Haven, CT, USA

Epidemiology of Microbial Diseases, Yale School of Public Health, New Haven, CT, USA

Tina Lavender, DBE, PhD Department of International Public Health, Liverpool School of Tropical Medicine, Liverpool, Great Britain

Jordann Loehr, MD, MPH, FACOG University of Gondar, Gondar, Ethiopia

Heather Lytle, MD, MSPH, FACOG Department of Obstetrics and Gynecology, University of Utah Health, Salt Lake City, UT, USA

Marielle E. Meurice, MD Department of Obstetrics & Gynecology, University of California, Irvine, CA, USA

Stella Masala Mpanda, MSc, BNS Childbirth Survival International, Dar es Salaam, Tanzania

Lilian Teddy Mselle, PhD, Mphil, BA, RNM Department of Clinical Nursing, Muhimbili University of Health and Allied Sciences, Dar es Salaam, Tanzania

Olivier Mukuku, MD Department of Maternal and Child Health, High Institute of Medical Techniques of Lubumbashi, Lubumbashi, Democratic Republic of the Congo

Prudence Mwini-Nyaledzigbor, RN, RM, PhD Catholic University College, Fiapre, Sunyani, Ghana

Rahel Nardos, MD, MCR, FPMRS Division of Female Pelvic Medicine and Reconstructive Surgery, Department of Ob/Gyn & Women's Health, Center for Global Health and Social Responsibility, University of Minnesota, Minneapolis, MN, USA

Joseph B. Nsambi, MD, MMed OG, PhD Department of Gynecology and Obstetrics, University of Lubumbashi, Lubumbashi, Democratic Republic of the Congo

Dorothy N. Ononokpono Department of Sociology and Anthropology, University of Uyo, Uyo, Nigeria

Marie-Eve Paré, PhD Department of Anthropology, College Professor at Cégep Edouard-Montpetit, Longueuil, QC, Canada

Beth S. Phillips, MPH Institute for Global Health Sciences, University of California San Francisco, San Francisco, CA, USA

F. Beryl Pilkington, RN, PhD School of Nursing, Faculty of Health, York University, Toronto, ON, Canada

Rachel Pope, MD, MPH University Hospital, Cleveland Medical Center, Urology Institute, Cleveland, OH, USA

Fistula Care Center, Lilongwe, Malawi

Solina Richter, MCur, DCur, RN College of Nursing, University of Saskatchewan, Saskatoon, SK, Canada

Bonnie Ruder, PhD, MPH, CPM Terrewode Women's Fund, Eugene, OR, USA

International Fistula Alliance, Sydney, Australia

Nessa Ryan, PhD, MPH, MSCI New York University School of Global Public Health, New York, NY, USA

Susan and Henry Samueli College of Health Sciences, Irvine, CA, USA

David A. Schwartz, MD, MS Hyg, FCAP Perinatal Pathology Consulting, Atlanta, GA, USA

Gillian Slinger, RN, RM, BSc, MSc Fistula Surgery Training Initiative, FIGO, London, UK

Theresa Spitznagle, PT, DPT, MHS, WCS Program in Physical Therapy, Department of Obstetrics and Gynecology, Washington University School of Medicine in St. Louis, St. Louis, MO, USA

Global Women's Health Initiative, Millis, MA, USA

Worldwide Fistula Fund, Schaumburg, IL, USA

Pooja Sripad, PhD, MPH Social Behavioral Science Research, Population Council, Washington, DC, USA

Mary J. Stokes, MD Department of Global Women's Health, Obstetrics and Gynecology, Baylor College of Medicine, Houston, TX, USA

Lilli Trautvetter, BA, MSc Fistula Surgery Training Initiative, FIGO, London, UK

Vandana Tripathi, PhD, MPH Fistula Care Plus, EngenderHealth, New York, NY, USA

Helen Vallianatos, PhD Department of Anthropology, University of Alberta, Edmonton, AB, Canada

Sabina Wakasiaka, PhD College of Health Sciences, University of Nairobi, Nairobi, Kenya

L. Lewis Wall, MD, DPhil Departments of Anthropology and Obstetrics & Gynecology, Washington University in St. Louis, St. Louis, MO, USA

Charlotte E. Warren, PhD, MEd, RSCN, RN, ON Social Behavioral Science Research, Population Council, Washington, DC, USA

Introduction to Obstetric Fistula: A Multidisciplinary Approach to a Preventable Childbirth Tragedy

Bonnie Ruder, Laura Briggs Drew, and David A. Schwartz

This book discusses an ancient and catastrophic complication of childbirth which remains a modern-day public health tragedy—obstetric fistula. Tragically, this debilitating condition, which is entirely preventable, has continued to occur among hundreds of thousands of the world's poorest women even into the third decade of the twenty-first century. Its continued existence is the result of the low status of women and the unjust and unethical allocation of healthcare resources in the parts of the world where obstetric fistula remains endemic, and an inexcusable failure of political will. This book utilizes a team of expert authors from countries where fistula continues to occur, as well as experts from other parts of the world, to address factors that contribute to obstetric fistula development, including pathophysiological aspects and social determinants of health. Additionally, we bring attention to how an obstetric fistula can negatively impact the quality of life for a woman and her family, as well as efforts to improve fistula prevention, diagnosis, medical treatment, and continuing support for women when they reintegrate into their communities after fistula repair.

An obstetric fistula is caused by unrelieved obstructed labor, which damages tissues in the birth canal and leads to unremitting urinary and/or fecal incontinence. Considered the most severe and debilitating of all maternal morbidities, women with obstetric fistula experience severe physical, psychological, social, and economic consequences. Although individual experiences are unique to each woman, in the worst cases women are ostracized and abandoned by their husbands, families, and communities.

Obstetric fistula rarely occurs in wealthy countries in the Global North where pregnant women have access to high-quality maternal health care. Their prevalence in low-resource countries is a clear indication that healthcare systems are failing to meet the needs of childbearing women. Women and girls in countries across sub-Saharan Africa, referred to as the "fistula belt," experience unacceptably high rates of fistula, a result of the intersection of chronically underfunded and poor-quality healthcare systems, gender discrimination, systems of inequity, and poverty—and its accompanying conse-

B. Ruder (✉)
Terrewode Women's Fund, Eugene, OR, USA

International Fistula Alliance, Sydney, Australia

L. B. Drew
Office of the Senior Vice President and Provost, University of Maryland, College Park, MD, USA

D. A. Schwartz
Perinatal Pathology Consulting, Atlanta, GA, USA

quences for women and girls, including child marriage and low education attainment. The occurrence of obstetric fistula is internationally recognized as a gross violation of women's human rights.

The exact prevalence of obstetric fistula is difficult to determine for several reasons. First, obstetric fistula occurs in a small proportion of obstructed labors, and a clinical diagnosis is needed to confirm the presence of obstetric fistula. Public health surveillance systems in the endemic countries are often underfunded and ineffective; as a result, affected women may be difficult to identify. Many women affected by fistula live in rural and remote areas and are outside of the reach of poorly provisioned local healthcare systems. Furthermore, because of the shame and stigma connected to this condition, women with fistula often self-isolate and may be unaware of the cause of their problem or treatment options. Thus, prevalence estimates often rely on hospital data based on the number of patients receiving treatment for fistula or physician's estimates; others are based on countries' rapid needs assessments rather than robust epidemiological studies (Adler et al., 2013; Stanton et al., 2007).

As interest and services for obstetric fistula have intensified in recent years, many countries that participate in the Demographic and Health Surveys (DHS) program have added fistula symptom-related questions to their surveys as a proxy for fistula prevalence. While this is an encouraging development and will assist in estimations of prevalence when combined with diagnostic algorithms (Tunçalp et al., 2014), prevalence rates based primarily on self-reported data are likely to vastly overestimate prevalence, as incontinence secondary to childbirth may be caused by factors such as pelvic organ prolapse and not solely obstetric fistula. To accurately estimate fistula prevalence, reports of symptoms must be followed up with a clinical examination to confirm causation of incontinence, which adds significant complexity and cost.

Results from two recent large-scale, community-based studies that confirmed self-reported fistula symptoms with clinical diagnosis provide insight here. Both studies, one conducted in rural Ethiopia (Ballard et al., 2016) and another in Bangladesh (MEASURE Evaluation, 2018), found that only one-third of women reporting fistula symptoms received a positive diagnosis following clinical examination. The authors of both studies conclude that fistula prevalence based on self-reported symptoms is likely to vastly overestimate the magnitude of the problem (Ballard et al., 2016; MEASURE Evaluation, 2018). Furthermore, both studies found actual prevalence was significantly lower than previous estimates from these countries where clinical diagnosis was not confirmed, 0.06% in Ethiopia versus the previously reported 1% and 0.037% in Bangladesh versus the previously reported 1.21%. Ballard and colleagues point to improvements in the provision of maternal health services as a contributing factor to the overall decline in obstetric fistula.

The United Nations' recent report, *"Intensifying Efforts to End Fistula Within a Decade,"* recently released a new estimate of global fistula prevalence, stating that 500,000 women currently live with fistula, with additional cases occurring annually (2020). This is a significant reduction from previous estimates (which are reflected throughout this book as this latest figure was released as the book was going to press) and is based on modeled data from 55 countries, developed by Johns Hopkins Bloomberg School of Public Health in collaboration with UNFPA and WHO (UN, 2020). This reduction from previous prevalence estimates reflects a more nuanced understanding of the magnitude of fistula burden along with the significant achievements made in the collective efforts to identify and treat women with fistula and prevent the injury from occurring in the first place. Years of dedicated work by practitioners across disciplines to identify and treat women with fistula have had a positive impact, as have efforts to improve the access and provision of maternal healthcare services.

However, the fact that a half-million women continue to endure lives of suffering due to obstetric fistula, a completely preventable and treatable injury, is a stark reminder of the work that remains. In 2018, the UN General Assembly made the call to end fistula by 2030. This is an ambitious and exciting goal, one that requires an all hands on deck approach. In order to truly end fistula within a decade, increased and sustained funding is critical and should be directed to both proven and well-targeted programs and creative, community-appropriate innovations desperately needed for progress. Collaboration, sharing of best practices, and coordinated efforts will help ensure resources are put to their greatest use to increase awareness and provide comprehensive, high-quality fistula services. Additionally, if we truly hope to end fistula, we must prevent new cases from occurring. Access to family planning information and services; improved sexual, reproductive, and maternal healthcare services with a focus on quality; and training of thousands of additional healthcare workers is essential.

This book provides a unique and timely contribution in our efforts to meet this goal and end fistula by 2030. The detailed chapters encompass a historical and broad understanding of obstetric fistula and the structural factors that disproportionly expose vulnerable women to this fate. They also reveal the tremendous breadth and depth of work that is being done to end fistula—from FIGO's fistula surgeons' training program, to clinical advancements in treatment, including greater attention to residual incontinence post-repair, to women's needs beyond surgery, including holistic reintegration and mental health services. The multidisciplinary nature of this volume provides a range of expertise and diverse perspectives to explore the complexity of obstetric fistula and potential solutions. The authors highlight targeted interventions, best practices, and key challenges, with the collective goal of moving toward the eradication of fistula and alleviating the suffering of hundreds of thousands of women. The editors of this book and its team of authors hope that this text will raise awareness of the continuing tragedy of obstetric fistula as an avoidable childbirth injury and galvanize efforts among the global public health, governmental, health care, and policymaking communities to take aggressive action to eliminate this debilitating condition.

References

Adler, A., Ronsmans, C., Calvert, C., & Filippi, V. (2013). Estimating the prevalence of obstetric fistula: A systematic review and meta-analysis. *BMC Pregnancy and Childbirth, 13*(1), 246.

Ballard, K., Ayenachew, F., Wright, J., & Atnafu, H. (2016). Prevalence of obstetric fistula and symptomatic pelvic organ prolapse in rural Ethiopia. *International Urogynecology Journal, 27*(7), 1063–1067.

MEASURE Evaluation, i., b, The Maternal & Child Health Integrated Program, fistula care plus, and Johns Hopkins University. (2018). Prevalence of obstetric fistula and pelvic organ prolapse in Bangladesh: Summary of the 2016 National Estimates. https://www.measureevaluation.org/resources/publications/fs-18-290. Accessed 9 2019.

Stanton, C., Holtz, S., & Ahmed, S. (2007). Challenges in measuring obstetric fistula. *International Journal of Gynecology & Obstetrics, 99*, S4–S9.

Tunçalp, Ö., Tripathi, V., Landry, E., Stanton, C. K., & Ahmed, S. (2014). Measuring the incidence and prevalence of obstetric fistula: Approaches, needs and recommendations. *Bulletin of the World Health Organization, 93*, 60–62.

United Nations (2020). Intensifying efforts to end obstetric fistula within a decade. https://documents-dds-ny.un.org/doc/UNDOC/GEN/N18/445/45/PDF/N1844545.pdf?OpenElement. Accessed November 2020.

A Human Rights Approach Toward Eradicating Obstetric Fistula: Expanding Data Collection, Prevention, Treatment, and Continuing Support for Women and Girls Who Have Been Neglected

Laura Briggs Drew

2.1 Geographic Disparities in Maternal Health Outcomes: Unequal Prioritization of Women's Health and Human Rights Across the Globe

In the twentieth and twenty-first centuries, we have achieved great improvements in maternal health, including access to health care, nutrition, and hygiene. However, pregnancy and childbirth continue to be dangerous periods for women and their babies, particularly in resource-limited settings. In 2017, an estimated 295,000 women across the globe died during pregnancy or childbirth, and most of these deaths were preventable. Although this metric was a 35% reduction in global maternal mortality from 2000 (United Nations Population Fund et al., 2019), indicators of poor maternal health remain far too high. Maternal health disparities also elucidate significant inequities across the globe, with 94% of maternal deaths occurring in low and lower-middle-income countries (World Health Organization, 2019). In countries where access to family planning resources may be limited, the average number of pregnancies per woman is higher than it is in other settings, which further increases the lifetime risk of death and disability due to pregnancy (World Health Organization, 2019). Although reductions in maternal mortality have traditionally been used as indicators of progress in maternal health, maternal mortality estimates are dwarfed in comparison to the global burden of maternal morbidities. For every maternal death, an additional 20–30 women endure maternal morbidities, including life-threatening complications, infections, disabilities, and injuries, like obstetric fistula, which can negatively affect their quality of life (United Nations Population Fund, 2020).

Among the many factors that can lead to death from pregnancy, the primary direct causes of maternal mortality in Africa include hemorrhage (33.9%), sepsis/infections (9.7%), hypertensive disorders (9.1%), complications from unsafe abortion (3.9%), and obstructed labor (4.1%) (Khan et al., 2006). Although obstructed labor can be alleviated via a cesarean section, many women labor outside of healthcare facilities and they do not have access to emergency obstetric care. In addition to being a

L. B. Drew (✉)
Office of the Senior Vice President and Provost,
University of Maryland, College Park, MD, USA
e-mail: lbdrew@umd.edu

© Springer Nature Switzerland AG 2022
L. B. Drew et al. (eds.), *A Multidisciplinary Approach to Obstetric Fistula in Africa*, Global Maternal and Child Health, https://doi.org/10.1007/978-3-031-06314-5_2

leading cause of maternal mortality, obstructed labor is a major cause of neonatal morbidity and mortality, and it can also lead to devastating maternal complications and morbidities (Dolea & AbouZahr, 2000). One of the most severe and debilitating long-term complications of obstructed labor is obstetric fistula: a hole that forms when tissues in the vaginal wall are damaged during prolonged, obstructed labor, which leads to chronic incontinence of urine and/or feces.

The true number of maternal morbidity cases across the globe is not known. However, maternal deaths are often referred to as the tip of the iceberg with maternal morbidity its base (Firoz et al., 2013). Additionally, estimates suggest the global burden of severe maternal morbidity (SMM), which is defined as an unintended outcome of labor and delivery that leads to significant short-term and long-term consequences to a woman's health, is increasing over time, with sub-Saharan Africa having the highest burden of SMM at 198 per 1000 live births (American College of Obstetricians and Gynecologists, 2016; Geller et al., 2018). Estimating the prevalence and incidence of maternal morbidities is challenging because in some contexts the majority of births and subsequent maternal morbidities occur outside hospital settings, and for women in these areas who successfully access healthcare facilities, there is often poor record-keeping.

Until the early 1900s, when advancements in obstetric care to prevent and treat obstructed labor were achieved in America and Europe, obstructed labor was one of the leading causes of both maternal mortality and morbidity across the globe (EngenderHealth, 2015), but today it rarely contributes to maternal deaths in developed countries (Khan et al., 2006). As access to safe delivery care improved and the need for obstetric fistula repair became unnecessary, the first obstetric fistula hospital in the United States closed its doors, and the site became the Waldorf Astoria Hotel in New York City (EngenderHealth, 2015). Continuing advancements in modern obstetric care have almost universally eliminated obstetric fistula in settings with adequate access to these services. However, an estimated 500,000 women and girls are currently enduring untold suffering from obstetric fistula (Ahmed, 2020; United Nations General Assembly, 2020), and almost all of these cases are within the "fistula belt," which extends across countries in the northern half of sub-Saharan Africa (Tebeu et al., 2012). In addition to poor healthcare access and quality, other factors that contribute to the prevalence of unrepaired obstetric fistula in this region include a shortage of trained providers for fistula repair, limited awareness about repair possibilities, poor integration of services, and the marginalization of women (Cook et al., 2004).

Geographic disparities in the prevalence of obstetric fistula elucidate injustices and human rights violations that affect women who are young, poor, and in resource-limited settings with inadequate access to skilled emergency obstetric care. In low and lower-middle income countries, obstetric fistula cases occur due to early marriage and childbearing before a girl's pelvis is fully developed, as well as inadequate prenatal and obstetric care access, which stems from poverty and living in remote and rural areas (Cook et al., 2004). Social determinants of health, including inadequate nutrition, limited education, and low health literacy additionally contribute to obstetric fistula development, and many of these factors are tied to gender inequality. Although a number of proximal and distal factors influence why obstetric fistula continues to occur in these settings, it would be remiss to fail to recognize how lack of political will also contributes, including failure to prioritize healthcare services and neglecting the sexual and reproductive health and rights (SRHR) of women and girls. The consequences of these failures are profound, particularly in developing regions. Each year, more than 30 million women give birth outside of a healthcare facility, more than 45 million women receive no or inadequate antenatal care, and more than 200 million women who want to avoid pregnancy are not using modern contraception (Starrs et al., 2018).

Although obstetric fistula is almost completely preventable, it persists due to gross societal and institutional neglect of women and girls, which is an issue of rights and equity (Donnay & Weil, 2004). Collectively, the continuing occurrence of obstetric fistula, inadequate provision of timely repair, as well as the suffering and stigma that result from obstetric fistula, illuminate gross violations of human rights, which are intended to protect women's dignity (Cook et al., 2004). Therefore, if we are to achieve the United Nations' goal to eradicate obstetric fistula by 2030 (United Nations General Assembly, 2020), we must utilize an approach that prioritizes the SRHR of women and girls across the globe. From a human rights perspective, these efforts should focus on expanding data collection to accurately monitor progress, implementing programs to promote safe motherhood and prevent obstetric fistula development, increasing access to skilled obstetric fistula repair, and strengthening reintegration programs to address the totality of obstetric fistula consequences, including outcomes that pertain to SRHR.

2.2 Obstetric Fistula Development and Risk Factors

Obstetric fistula primarily occurs due to prolonged, obstructed labor without skilled care, and most women who develop an obstetric fistula labor at home between 2.5 and 4 days (Tebeu et al., 2012). During this extended period of time, the baby's head puts increasing pressure on tissues in the birth canal, which blocks blood supply to the surrounding tissues and leads to ischemia and necrosis. Consequently, a hole develops in the tissues that separate the vagina and the bladder (vesicovaginal fistula) and/or the vagina and the rectum (rectovaginal fistula). Once the obstetric fistula develops, the woman experiences chronic incontinence of urine and/or feces. In addition to this physical suffering, the prolonged, obstructed labor impacts the health of the baby; stillbirths occur in 90% of pregnancies in which the woman develops an obstetric fistula (Saifuddin Ahmed et al., 2016). Therefore, when the painful and prolonged labor ends, women are left uncertain of the cause of their incontinence and why their baby died.

Although prolonged, obstructed labor is the primary direct cause of obstetric fistula, a number of indirect factors contribute to maternal mortality and morbidity in resource-limited settings, including gender inequality, poverty, distance to healthcare facilities, lack of information, low education attainment, inadequate services, and cultural practices. These contributing factors reflect inequities in access to healthcare services and highlight the gap in maternal health outcomes between the rich and the poor (World Health Organization, 2019). In some countries where obstetric fistula is more common, fewer than one in three births are assisted by a skilled professional attendant, such as a midwife, nurse, or physician, and in rural areas, the rate of cesarean deliveries is often less than 2% (Velez et al., 2007). The international healthcare community has recommended the ideal rate for cesarean sections to be 10–15% since research has shown maternal and newborn deaths decrease when the cesarean section rate rises toward 10% (World Health Organization & Human Reproduction Programme, 2015); however, regional disparities, particularly within the "fistula belt," reveal gross inequities in access to this life-saving emergency obstetric care.

In some cases, there may be access to emergency obstetric care, but a number of factors contribute to why women may not receive it. The "Three Delays" model specifically attributes maternal mortality to delays in deciding to seek medical help for an obstetric emergency, delays in reaching an appropriate obstetric facility, and delays in receiving adequate care when an individual has reached the facility (Barnes-Josiah et al., 1998). Although this model was developed for maternal mortality, the framework can also be applied to maternal morbidities (Pacagnella et al., 2012), particularly obstetric fistula.

A cesarean section can relieve prolonged, obstructed labor and prevent an obstetric fistula from developing; however, for many women in resource-limited settings, this emergency obstetric service is often unavailable, unreachable, or unaffordable. Additionally, when women labor outside healthcare facilities, women, their families, and traditional birth attendants (TBAs) may not recognize the signs of prolonged, obstructed labor and/or know that an emergency cesarean section is necessary.

Fig. 2.1 Women in rural Malawi return to their homes after a community meeting to promote safe motherhood, which announced construction of a nearby maternal waiting home and encouraged women with obstetric fistula to seek repair services at the Obstetric Fistula Repair Centre at Bwaila Maternity Hospital in Lilongwe, Malawi. (Photograph credit: Laura Briggs Drew)

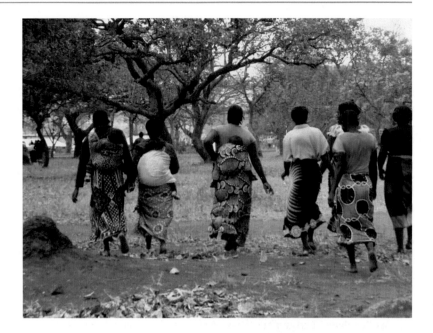

When women try to labor at home but are unsuccessful, they are also more likely to reach a healthcare facility at a late stage, and this can be further delayed by lack of transportation, poor roads, heavy rains, great distances, and cost barriers (Tebeu et al., 2012). Therefore, obstetric fistula results from obstructed labor *and* obstructed transportation; the patient is often unable to access a hospital for delivery when labor stops progressing normally or the decision to seek a facility is made too late. For these reasons, key strategies to improve maternal health in rural and resource-limited settings include implementing community outreach programs that promote safe motherhood, increasing skilled attendance at birth, and constructing maternal waiting homes (Fig. 2.1).

In addition to limited access to skilled emergency obstetric care, many of the other risk factors for obstetric fistula development are tied to gender inequality, particularly poor nutrition for girls as well as marriage and childbearing at a young age. To begin, women who develop obstetric fistula are often small, short, and young. Characteristics of fistula patients reveal 40–80% of obstetric fistula occurs in women less than 150 cm tall (Tebeu et al., 2012; Wall et al., 2004), and a study in Nigeria found being less than 150 cm tall nearly doubles the risk of obstetric fistula occurrence (Ampofo et al., 1990). In many patriarchal societies, women and girls often eat their meals after men, and this can lead to chronic under-nutrition and ill health (Babiker, 2017). Additionally, poor nutrition is associated with small stature, pelvic immaturity, and chronic malnutrition, which can limit pelvic growth in young women (Zabin & Kiragu, 1998). Although growth in height stops or slows with the onset of menarche, the pelvis continues to grow through late adolescence and the birth canal is smaller the first 3 years after the onset of menarche than it is at age 18 (Moerman, 1982).

Although delaying pregnancy until pelvic structures have matured and grown to their full adult size can decrease the risk of cephalopelvic disproportion, early marriage and pregnancy are common among many cultures in sub-Saharan Africa. In 2018, West and Central Africa, which are within the "fistula belt," had the highest regional adolescent birth rate in the world, with 115 births per 1000 girls aged 15–19 (UNICEF, 2019). Although adolescent birth rates have been decreasing across the globe, pregnancy at a young age is particularly dangerous, and adolescent mothers are less likely to receive skilled assistance during delivery or postnatal care compared to older mothers (UNICEF, 2019). Therefore, the risk of obstructed labor is greater in areas where both marriage and childbearing commonly occur at a young age (Wall, 2006), thereby increasing the risk of obstetric fistula development.

2.3   Long-Term Consequences and Quality of Life After Obstetric Fistula Development

When a woman or girl develops an obstetric fistula, her life is dramatically changed. She often does not know the cause of the incontinence, what contributed to the stillbirth, or that her condition can be resolved via surgery. In 1996, Arrowsmith and colleagues presented the "obstructed labor injury complex" to describe the multitude of factors that lead to obstructed labor, and consequently obstetric fistula development, as well as the physical and social injuries that result from obstetric fistula (Arrowsmith et al., 1996). In addition to obstetric fistula formation, obstructed labor can lead to fetal death, complex urologic injuries, vaginal scarring and stenosis, secondary infertility, musculoskeletal injury, and foot drop (Arrowsmith et al., 1996). For women who have obstetric fistula, nearly 80% will develop skin abrasions due to their urinary incontinence (Ahmed & Holtz, 2007).

In addition to the physical suffering of chronic incontinence, obstetric fistula is often a lifelong maternal morbidity that can impact a woman's quality of life socially, psychologically, and economically. Because women with obstetric fistula are unable to manage their chronic incontinence and its subsequent odor, they are often stigmatized and shunned from their partners, families, and communities, which can negatively impact their quality of life in many ways. They may be unable to care for their family, share meals with their family, attend religious services, travel, and work because they are seen as "unclean" and unable to control their incontinence (Drew et al., 2016). Additionally, their social roles as women, wives, and mothers can be impacted; sexual dysfunction as well as fears and uncertainty about their ability to achieve a future pregnancy can lead to partner abandonment and isolation from their families (Drew et al., 2016; Mselle et al., 2011). This stigma and isolation often lead to loss of social support, worsening poverty and malnutrition, as well as suffering, illness, and premature death (Arrowsmith et al., 1996).

Because the physical, economic, and social consequences of obstetric fistula add difficulty and stress to the lives of these women, obstetric fistula can negatively affect psychiatric health (Weston et al., 2011). The pooled estimated prevalence of depression among women with obstetric fistula in African countries is greater than 50% (Duko et al., 2020), and high rates of suicidal ideation have been reported (Weston et al., 2011). These statistics are particularly concerning since access to mental health care is limited in areas where obstetric fistula is common. Therefore, when implementing holistic approaches to fistula management, programs should provide mental health care and family support to address the psychiatric dimensions of fistula patients' well-being (Weston et al., 2011). Without appropriate care, women with obstetric fistula will continue to suffer physically, psychologically, socially, and economically. Therefore, the health and human rights of women who have endured obstetric fistula must be prioritized as we move toward eradicating obstetric fistula by 2030.

2.4   Progress Toward Obstetric Fistula Eradication

2.4.1   Expanding Data Collection: Challenges in Knowing the True Burden of Obstetric Fistula

In locations where most births occur outside of healthcare facilities and facilities may have poor record-keeping on births, accurate and nationally representative data on the incidence and prevalence of maternal mortalities and morbidities are scant (Johnson & Peterman, 2008). Additionally, hospital records are not nationally representative and they only capture women with obstetric fistula who reach a facility, which underestimates the true burden of this childbirth injury. Hospital records on births from facilities are also prone to selection bias, since these data are not representative of women who give birth outside facilities. Determining the burden of obstetric fistula worldwide is further complicated because many of these women are marginalized and isolated from society with little economic, social, or political power (Baker et al., 2017); therefore, they often do not know that repair is possible or available. These challenges contribute to the paucity of reliable data on the incidence and prevalence of obstetric fistula, particularly at the national level.

The most common data sources on obstetric fistula are medical records, which are not nationally representative and remain dependent upon women with obstetric fistula reaching a healthcare facility, and self-reported surveys (Saifuddin Ahmed & Tunçalp, 2015), including Demographic and Health Surveys (DHS), which gather incontinence data as a proxy measure of obstetric fistula on nationally representative household surveys (Johnson & Peterman, 2008). The true prevalence of obstetric fistula is unknown as this number could only be calculated if all women with obstetric fistula were diagnosed upon clinical examination. Additionally, hospital-based studies fail to elucidate the magnitude and geographic distribution of obstetric fistula (Stanton et al., 2007). Therefore, the DHS attempted to establish baseline national-level prevalence estimates by including questions on symptoms, etiology of the problem, care-seeking behavior, and treatment outcomes in their household surveys (Johnson & Peterman, 2008). These efforts are applauded as they provide baseline prevalence estimates that are nationally representative and can be used to assess the impact of programmatic and policy interventions on obstetric fistula over time (Johnson & Peterman, 2008).

Compared to other maternal morbidities, the symptom of fistula, i.e., unrelenting incontinence after labor, is unlikely to be subject to recall bias; it is easy for women to accurately report compared to other symptoms that may be less apparent and/or associated with multiple maternal morbidities (Johnson & Peterman, 2008), which makes household surveys a useful method to capture this information. However, the DHS questions do have limitations. Notably, respondents, including women who have received obstetric fistula repair, may deny ever experiencing incontinence after labor due to shame (Johnson & Peterman, 2008), which would lead to underreporting. Additionally, overreporting could occur because a woman's incontinence may actually be due to urinary tract infections, stress incontinence, and in some cases, perineal tears (Johnson & Peterman, 2008). Therefore, the proxy measurement of incontinence symptoms for obstetric fistula in DHS may contribute to some inaccuracy in national-level obstetric fistula estimates. Additionally, misestimation may occur because DHS is a household-based survey; therefore, women who are either at fistula repair facilities or have been shunned and are subsequently homeless are not captured by DHS's survey administration methods (Johnson & Peterman, 2008).

Although there may be some inaccuracy in the estimations, the data from DHS do provide meaningful and informative lifetime obstetric fistula prevalence estimates that may be fairly accurate. For example, the lifetime prevalence of fistula in Malawi in 2006 and Uganda in 2004 was estimated to be 4.7% and 2.6%, respectively (Johnson & Peterman, 2008). This aligns with Malawi's maternal mortality ratio also being double that in Uganda (984 and 435 per 100,000 live births, respectively) and supports previous observations that obstetric fistula prevalence is correlated with national maternal mortality ratios (Danso et al., 1996; Johnson & Peterman, 2008). Nevertheless, in settings without national health information systems and where the majority of women give birth outside of facilities, DHS remains the primary method to capture representative information on maternal morbidities, including obstetric fistula, and to ensure comparable data are collected across national settings (Johnson & Peterman, 2008).

Estimating the global prevalence of obstetric fistula has been challenging, and the estimates have varied greatly. A literature review on population-based estimates of obstetric fistula found the original estimates were quoted from studies, background sources, and introductions (Stanton et al., 2007); however, these were secondary and tertiary citations, and in some cases, the original reference was personal communication (Bangser et al., 2002; United Nations Population Fund & EngenderHealth, 2003; Wall, 2002). Other population-based estimates were based upon surgeons' estimations and studies that described estimation methods with varying degrees of transparency (Stanton et al., 2007). Previously, the most commonly cited estimates of global obstetric fistula prevalence varied between two and three million cases with 50,000–100,000 incident cases per year (Bangser et al., 2002; Browning, 2004; Cook et al., 2004; Danso et al., 1996; Donnay & Weil, 2004; Hilton, 2003; United Nations Population Fund, 2012; United Nations Population Fund & EngenderHealth, 2003; Wall, 1998, 2006). Additionally, the review by Stanton et al. found global fistula prevalence estimates are sometimes incorrectly used to describe the prevalence of obstetric fistula in Africa and Asia (Kelly, 2004; World Health Organization, 2021a), which has added more inconsistencies to prevalence estimates across publications.

Although most publications have previously stated there are two to three million estimated cases of obstetric fistula across the globe, recent research suggests this number overestimates the true burden. A recent meta-analysis and systematic review found a pooled prevalence of 0.29 obstetric fistula per 1000 women of reproductive age in all regions, and in sub-Saharan Africa the prevalence was 1.60 obstetric fistula per 1000 women of reproductive age (Adler et al., 2013). Given there were approximately 1.865 billion women of reproductive age across the globe in 2015 (World Health Organization, 2021b), the global prevalence of obstetric fistula among women of reproductive age at that time would have been closer to 540,000 using the pooled prevalence estimate from Adler et al. The most recent estimate is closer to this number and suggests 500,000 women and girls are currently suffering from obstetric fistula (Ahmed, 2020; United Nations General Assembly, 2020). This remarkable reduction from two to three million to 500,000 estimated prevalent cases suggests significant progress has been made in the eradication of obstetric fistula, including increasing access to obstetric fistula repairs (United Nations General Assembly, 2020). However, new, preventable cases will continue to develop each year without significant improvements in access, quality, and affordability of maternal health services, including emergency obstetric care, which may lag behind incident cases of obstetric fistula (Wall, 2006). As we move forward in our efforts to eradicate obstetric fistula, epidemiologic data and population-based estimates on the incidence and prevalence of obstetric fistula continue to be needed (Stanton et al., 2007). This data is the only way we can accurately measure the impact of our efforts toward achieving obstetric fistula eradication.

2.4.2   Preventing Obstetric Fistula

The medical and social impacts of obstetric fistula on women's lives elucidate the urgent need to reduce fistula incidence as a matter of human rights and women's dignity (Bangser, 2007). Therefore, we must prevent incident cases of obstetric fistula through targeted interventions that promote safe motherhood and increase access to skilled attendance at birth (Fig. 2.2). The WHO classifies fistula prevention strategies into the following categories: 1) prevention strategies that focus on contraception and family planning; 2) secondary prevention strategies to ensure women have access to skilled care during delivery; and 3) tertiary prevention strategies, which focus on early fistula screening among women at increased risk (de Bernis, 2007). Collectively, these prevention strategies recognize obstetric fistula persists solely because structural factors, including gender inequality and inequity in healthcare access and quality, allow this preventable childbirth injury to continue. Therefore, any efforts that focus on obstetric fistula prevention must prioritize the SRHR of women and girls.

Successful strategies to prevent obstetric fistula include educating communities about the cultural, social, and physiologic factors that increase risk of obstetric fistula (Miller et al., 2005). Because cephalopelvic disproportion increases risk of obstructed labor and obstetric fistula development, delaying childbearing for several years after menarche can prevent the sequelae of prolonged, obstructed labor (Miller et al., 2005). Therefore, while being sensitive to social and cultural factors,

Fig. 2.2 Aberdeen Women's Centre outside Freetown, Sierra Leone. The facility provides comprehensive maternal health care, including family planning, skilled attendance during delivery, and obstetric fistula repair. (Photograph credit: Laura Briggs Drew)

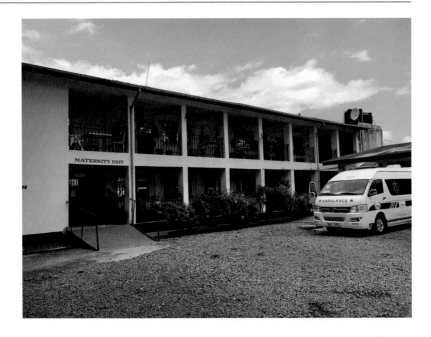

prevention efforts should focus on working with communities to emphasize the need to delay marriage and childbearing at a young age. Additionally, the special nutritional needs of girls should be emphasized to prevent chronic malnutrition and improve the physical maturity of young mothers (Miller et al., 2005).

Efforts to prevent obstetric fistula must also focus on ensuring women who are in need of modern contraception have access to these methods. In 2019, 1.9 billion women were of reproductive age (15–49 years), of which 1.1 billion had a need for family planning, yet 270 million women who wanted family planning methods did not have access to modern contraceptive methods (Kantorová et al., 2020). Ensuring access to and use of preferred contraceptive methods advances the human right of people to determine the number and spacing of their children (World Health Organization, 2020). For adolescent girls in particular, contraception use can prevent pregnancy-related health risks, including obstructed labor and obstetric fistula, and it offers a range of potential non-health benefits, including education opportunities which can advance women's empowerment and gender equality (World Health Organization, 2020).

In rural areas, midwives have a critical role in obstetric fistula prevention efforts as they can promote preventative health practices within communities. Additionally, midwives' training and skills allow for early detection of cephalopelvic disproportion, malpresentation, and prolonged, obstructed labor (Miller et al., 2005), which can encourage a family's decision to transport a mother to a maternity waiting home prior to delivery or a healthcare facility when complications arise during labor. In areas where obstetric fistula is common, increasing access to skilled attendance at birth is critical, and curriculums on obstetric fistula prevention have been developed for nurses and midwives in these settings (East, Central, and Southern African Health Community (ECSA-HC) and Fistula Care/ EngenderHealth, 2012).

The absence of skilled attendants during delivery and the lack of accessible high-quality emergency obstetric care perpetuate obstetric fistula development in resource-limited settings. For many countries within the "fistula belt," less than half of live births occur with the assistance of skilled birth attendants (World Health Organization, 2021c). The World Health Organization has prioritized the need to expand skilled attendance at delivery, particularly in countries where coverage of skilled attendance at birth is below 85% (World Health Organization, 2004). For many women, TBAs—non-formally trained and community-based providers of care during pregnancy, childbirth, and the post-natal period who are independent of the health system—are often the only available source of care during pregnancy (World Health Organization, 2004), and their assistance may be preferred for cultural, traditional, and financial reasons. Because skilled attendance at birth can threaten the livelihood of TBAs and since they work outside of the healthcare system, TBAs may have tense relationships with government healthcare systems and vice versa (World Health Organization, 2004). Therefore, it has been difficult to successfully incorporate their involvement in safe motherhood strategies (World Health Organization, 2004). Additionally, training TBAs has not been effective in reducing maternal mortality (World Health Organization, 2004).

Although it may be challenging to incorporate TBAs into safe motherhood strategies, they have a longstanding role and cultural importance in their communities, and TBAs can serve as partners to increase the number of births that occur in the presence of a skilled birth attendant (World Health Organization, 2004). The WHO points to Malaysia as an example of how to successfully incorporate TBAs into safe motherhood strategies; TBAs were registered in a separate section of the Midwives' Register, trained in avoidance of harmful practices, and given delivery allowances and hygienic childbirth kits, and they contributed valuable services, such as postnatal massages, while government midwives oversaw the delivery process (Pathmanathan et al., 2003). Additionally, TBAs reported cases to the government midwife and had their supplies renewed, and under this strategy, home deliveries shifted from being TBA-assisted to being under the supervision of government-trained midwives (Pathmanathan et al., 2003). Therefore, when trying to ensure safe motherhood, it is important to recognize that TBAs, although not formally trained, can be incorporated into such strategies. Indeed, creative and holistic solutions are needed if we are to achieve sustainable impact in reducing global maternal mortality and morbidity, including eradicating obstetric fistula by 2030.

2.4.3 Increasing Access to Obstetric Fistula Repair

When discussing the progress that has been made toward the eradication of obstetric fistula, it would be remiss to fail to highlight the work of Dr. Catherine Hamlin and her husband, Dr. Reg Hamlin, who were pioneers and devoted their lives to providing obstetric fistula repair surgery in Ethiopia. In 1974, they cofounded the Addis Ababa Fistula Hospital, which is a global center of expertise and training on obstetric fistula repair (Hamlin & Fleck, 2013). Through their work, they dramatically remodeled the maternal healthcare landscape for women in Ethiopia; more than 60,000 women with obstetric fistula received skilled surgical repair and had their lives transformed (Catherine Hamlin Fistula Foundation, 2018). Similar models have been replicated in other settings where fistula is common, which have provided life-changing surgeries for women who have suffered from obstetric fistula. More recently, the Hamlin College of Midwives was founded to ensure more women in Ethiopia have skilled attendance during their deliveries. This program recruits high school graduates from the provinces to receive midwifery training so they can return to the provinces and work with the regional fistula centers (Hamlin Fistula Ethiopia, 2014). Their pioneering work has propelled positive action to address obstetric fistula, and without their dedicated efforts, obstetric fistula would not be internationally recognized as a neglected public health and human rights issue.

As obstetric fistula has gained more prominence as a public health issue, the surgical community has also shown increased attention to improving access to obstetric fistula treatment, and these services are almost always at no cost to the patient. When women and girls have access to skilled fistula surgeons, obstetric fistula repair is successful in more than 90% of cases (Barone et al., 2015; Nardos et al., 2009, 2012; Sori et al., 2016). Therefore, the International Federation of Gynecology and

Obstetrics (FIGO) established a standardized global fistula training program to ensure surgeons can be trained in the latest techniques (Browning & Syed, 2020). This education and training program will improve women's access to high-quality fistula repair surgery and make strides toward bridging the obstetric fistula treatment gap. FIGO's effort is promising, since although the exact prevalence of obstetric fistula is unknown, there is general agreement that it considerably outweighs the number of local, skilled fistula surgeons who can repair this childbirth injury (Slinger & Trautvetter, 2020). However, in addition to these efforts, resources must be mobilized and countries should be empowered to develop their own sustainable fistula eradication plans, including access to safe delivery and emergency obstetric care (Slinger & Trautvetter, 2020).

As we expand training for the next generation of fistula surgeons, we must also continue to evaluate novel surgical techniques and ways to improve continence and sexual health after repair (Browning & Syed, 2020). Currently, there is a research gap in obstetric fistula repair techniques, and in settings where obstetric fistula is more common, there are unique challenges that may preclude the feasibility of such research studies (Pope & Beddow, 2020). Additionally, iatrogenic fistula is on the rise in settings where obstetric fistula is common, which indicates a need for additional research on the prevention and treatment of these injuries (Pope & Beddow, 2020). As international efforts are employed to gather evidence on successful surgical techniques while training local fistula surgeons to bridge the fistula treatment gap, the number of women who suffer lifelong consequences of obstetric fistula will shrink, and we will be one step closer toward eradicating this preventable and treatable childbirth injury.

However, availability of skilled fistula surgeons does not equate to accessibility; women who need fistula repair may be unable to reach these services due to barriers such as poverty, distance, and social isolation. For many women, the absence or cost of transportation is a significant barrier to reaching and receiving obstetric fistula repair services (United Nations General Assembly, 2020). Additionally, they may not know that their condition is treatable or they may be unfamiliar with healthcare services and reluctant to seek treatment. Sociocultural factors, including use of cultural and traditional practices to treat fistula, have also been identified as reasons that can contribute to delays in seeking obstetric fistula repair (Lyimo & Mosha, 2019). In some settings, decision making may be predominantly made by men, and this can lead to unequal opportunities in women's health education as well as women's lack of decision-making authority on where they can seek healthcare services (Lyimo & Mosha, 2019). To reduce these barriers to fistula repair, a number of programs have been implemented, including hospital outreach programs, mobile surgical outreach programs, community-based screening for obstetric fistula, fistula ambassador programs to identify women in need of repair, and programs to reduce financial transportation barriers (Fiander et al., 2013; Freedom from Fistula Foundation, 2016; Maroyi et al., 2020; Tunçalp et al., 2014; Umoiyoho et al., 2012; United Nations Population Fund, 2019). As similar programs are implemented in additional settings, their feasibility and impact should be evaluated, so we can achieve progress in identifying women who are in need of obstetric fistula repair and ensure that they are able to reach these life-changing services.

2.4.4 Strengthening Reintegration: Providing Continuing Support and Prioritizing SRHR After Obstetric Fistula Repair

In recent years, access to obstetric fistula repair has improved in sub-Saharan Africa and many women report improvements in physical and mental health after repair (Drew et al., 2016; El Ayadi et al., 2020). However, because of the stigmatizing nature of obstetric fistula, which a woman may have endured for many years before surgery, reintegration may be more challenging for some women than others as they adjust to new circumstances and attempt to resume their prior roles. Depending on the severity of their fistula and surgical outcomes, some women may experience ongoing physical and psychological challenges when they reintegrate into their communities, and they may need additional medical care and continuing follow-up (El Ayadi et al., 2020). For a woman who has an unsuccessful fistula repair and continues to suffer from incontinence, stigma and discrimination may worsen because her fistula is considered irreparable, and this may lead to ongoing social, economic, and psychological suffering. For women who have a successful repair but continue to suffer from incontinence (stress, urge, or low capacity), they may require further follow-up to determine and address the cause of their incontinence (Drew et al., 2016). Therefore, in addition to capacity building and strengthening health systems to prevent and treat obstetric fistula, fistula care should be comprehensive and holistic to facilitate the reintegration process and restore women's dignity (Bomboka et al., 2019). Such efforts should be based on individualized assessments of women's social reintegration needs (Emasu et al., 2019), including economic security, social support, health education, relationship desires, and family planning. A number of programs incorporate education, training in income-generating skills, and group therapy as part of obstetric fistula treatment (El Ayadi et al., 2020); however, it is imperative that women's SRHR also be prioritized as they reintegrate into their communities after obstetric fistula repair.

Interviews with women in sub-Saharan Africa have revealed that resuming their social roles as wives and mothers is a predominant positive experience during reintegration after fistula repair (Lombard et al., 2015). However, many factors may influence how quickly and successfully these roles can be resumed, particularly sexual activity, pregnancy, and childbirth. A challenging part of the discharge process is encouraging women to abstain from sexual activities for up to 6 months to allow the vaginal tissues to heal; however, this extended period of abstinence may unintendedly discourage some women from seeking obstetric fistula repair (Drew et al., 2016). Additionally, because women are encouraged to abstain from sexual activity during this prolonged period, they may be less likely to seek and use family planning methods, which could lead to unintended pregnancies and increased risk of future labor complications among women who have undergone obstetric fistula repair (Drew et al., 2016). Although many women may be able to re-establish intimate relationships after repair, the surgery can reduce vaginal caliber and women commonly report sexual dysfunction, including painful intercourse, after repair (Anzaku et al., 2017; Drew et al., 2016; Pope et al., 2018). Sexual activity can be a stigmatized health care topic; however, obstetric fistula repair centers can be used as safe spaces to discuss such issues (Mernoff et al., 2020), and these discussions may be helpful for women as they attempt to resume their intimate relationships after obstetric fistula repair. Therefore, comprehensive discharge processes that include family planning and discussions on sexual activity are encouraged. Counseling and treatment to address sexual dysfunction after obstetric fistula repair are also warranted.

In many contexts, motherhood is a critical component of a woman's identity; it defines her position in her kinship group and community (Mselle et al., 2011). Therefore, it is not surprising that a recent review on women's reintegration experiences after obstetric fistula repair found most women were concerned over their fertility (Lombard et al., 2015). However, contrary to reintegration recommendations expressed by healthcare providers (Mselle et al., 2012), women did not recommend for services that address fertility to be part of the discharge and reintegration process after obstetric fistula repair (Lombard et al., 2015). This dichotomy suggests that although healthcare providers may be able to address this need, women from low-income backgrounds may not be informed about clinical options to address their fertility concerns (Lombard et al., 2015). Indeed, most family planning services in settings with high fertility, like sub-Saharan Africa, focus on contraceptive access and promoting women's agency and decision-making for delaying and/or preventing future pregnancies, while little resources are allocated toward addressing infertility. This finding further reflects institutional failures to address the totality of issues pertaining to the SRHR of women and girls, including their fertility desires.

As we gain progress toward eradicating obstetric fistula, additional research is needed to better understand women's needs during reintegration and long-term outcomes after obstetric fistula repair, including their sexual and reproductive health. To inform the development and implementation of effective reintegration programs, such research should include patients' perspectives and recommendations rather than solely focusing on institutional perspectives (Lombard et al., 2015). Researchers and service providers should additionally implement more robust evaluations of their programs, and standardization of objectives and patient outcomes would enable evaluations of reintegration programs to be compared with one another (El Ayadi et al., 2020).

2.5 Increasing Public Awareness, Advocacy, and Action on Obstetric Fistula Through a Human Rights Approach

Although great progress was achieved in the United Nations' Millennium Development Goals, which sought to significantly decrease global maternal mortality and morbidity by 2015, disparities continue to persist across the globe, particularly in resource-limited settings. Therefore, more work needs to be done in order to achieve the United Nations' Sustainable Development Goals that pertain to advancing the health of women and girls by 2030. These targets include improving maternal health, achieving universal healthcare coverage, the eradication of child and early marriage, and ensuring universal access to sexual and reproductive healthcare services, including family planning, education, and integrating reproductive health into national strategies and programs (United Nations, 2015). In addition to these targets, the United Nations Secretary-General has put forward the goal to eradicate obstetric fistula by 2030 (United Nations General Assembly, 2020). While this goal is ambitious, it is also achievable if we prioritize the SRHR of women and girls.

If we fail to propel positive action toward preventing severe birth injuries, like obstetric fistula, women will continue to suffer from lifelong disabilities and poor quality of life. In addition to the United Nations, many partners, including EngenderHealth, FIGO, Freedom from Fistula Foundation, the Fistula Foundation, the Hamlin Hospital, Mercy Ships, Médecins Sans Frontières, and others have called for increased action to improvements in maternal health, including addressing obstetric fistula (United Nations General Assembly, 2020). In order to successfully eradicate obstetric fistula by 2030, global strategies must be developed to strengthen health systems to provide cost-effective fistula surgery, and the many risk factors that lead to prolonged, obstructed labor in low- and lower-middle income countries must be addressed (Epiu et al., 2018), including issues of human rights and social justice.

The upsetting and troubling reality is most maternal mortalities, and morbidities, including obstetric fistula, are often entirely preventable (United Nations Population Fund, 2020), but factors at the individual, interpersonal, and societal levels perpetuate the problem. For these reasons, it is imperative that there are collaborative efforts to recognize the importance of ensuring safe motherhood across the globe and prioritize women's health issues as issues of human rights. Additionally, accelerating progress in SRHR is recognized as being essential to people's health and survival, to global economic development and to the overall well-being of humanity (Starrs et al., 2018). However, despite the evidence of these benefits, progress in prioritizing SRHR has historically been stalled due to weak political commitment, inadequate resources, gender inequality, discrimination against women and girls, and hesitation to address issues that pertain to women's sexuality (Starrs et al., 2018). Given many of the United Nations' Sustainable Development Goals are targeted toward advancing the health of women and girls by 2030, it is imperative that governments and institutions collaborate to prioritize the SRHR of women and girls.

Furthermore, given that a woman's health is inextricably linked to that of her family, advancements in women's health will not only improve health and well-being for women, but they will also extend to their families. Specifically, maternal morbidities often affect more than the mother's health, as her morbidities can impact the health and development of the next generation, as well as the well-being of the family, including its social and economic standing (Koblinsky et al., 2012). This relationship is particularly evident in cases of obstetric fistula, as women who suffer from this childbirth injury are often stigmatized, abandoned, and unable to work because of their chronic incontinence. Therefore, the consequences of obstetric fistula can also affect the social and economic well-being of her family. For too long, reducing maternal morbidities has been a neglected agenda in maternal health (Koblinsky et al., 2012). However, if we prioritize and protect the SRHR of women and girls, we can achieve discernible impact and progress (Liljestrand, 2006), including making strides toward the eradication of obstetric fistula. These efforts will lead to improvements in women's health as well as the health of their families.

2.6   Conclusion

In order to successfully eradicate obstetric fistula by 2030, the human rights of women and girls must be protected, and the social determinants of health that lead to regional disparities in maternal mortality and morbidity should be addressed. As a first step, governments must make concerted efforts to prioritize the SRHR of women and girls. Governments, agencies, and organizations must also address the myriad of direct and indirect factors that negatively impact women's health. In addition to inadequate healthcare access, quality, and affordability, these factors include social and economic inequities, gender inequality, low education attainment, poverty, child marriage, and pregnancy at a young age (Anastasi et al., 2020). Obstetric fistula eradication also depends upon building and strengthening programs that target prevention and treatment (Capes et al., 2011), and research is needed to evaluate the impact and effectiveness of these programs. As we move toward eradicating obstetric fistula by expanding data collection to monitor progress, implementing strategies to prevent obstetric fistula development, and strengthening systems to ensure women's reintegration needs are met, fistula treatment must be accessible, affordable, and evidence-based. Unfortunately, there remains a backlog of women who need obstetric fistula repair, and more evidence-based practices are needed to provide high-quality, accessible, and comprehensive care (Pope, 2018).

At the core of these efforts, it must be recognized that obstetric fistula is a problem of gross inequity; it persists only because systems have failed to prioritize and protect the human rights of women and girls. Therefore, programs and policies must address the underlying determinants of obstetric fistula, including gender inequality, poverty, and disempowerment of women in these settings (Lombard et al., 2015). Moreover, if the SRHR of women and girls are not protected and prioritized, preventable maternal mortality and morbidity will continue across the globe. Obstetric fistula eradication can be achieved by 2030, but meeting this goal will only be possible if collaborations and political will recognize human rights violations perpetuate global disparities in maternal health outcomes, including obstetric fistula.

References

Adler, A. J., Ronsmans, C., Calvert, C., & Filippi, V. (2013). Estimating the prevalence of obstetric fistula: A systematic review and meta-analysis. *BMC Pregnancy and Childbirth, 13*, 246. https://doi.org/10.1186/1471-2393-13-246

Ahmed, S. (2020). Personal communication regarding forthcoming publication on global, regional, and national estimates of obstetric fistula, as cited in UN General Assembly.

Ahmed, S., & Holtz, S. A. (2007). Social and economic consequences of obstetric fistula: Life changed forever? *International Journal of Gynaecology and Obstetrics, 99*(Suppl 1), S10–S15. https://doi.org/10.1016/j.ijgo.2007.06.011

Ahmed, S., & Tunçalp, Ö. (2015). Burden of obstetric fistula: From measurement to action. *The Lancet Global Health, 3*(5), e243–e244. https://doi.org/10.1016/S2214-109X(15)70105-1

Ahmed, S., Anastasi, E., & Laski, L. (2016). Double burden of tragedy: Stillbirth and obstetric fistula. *The Lancet Global Health, 4*(2), e80–e82. https://doi.org/10.1016/S2214-109X(15)00290-9

American College of Obstetricians and Gynecologists. (2016). *Severe maternal morbidity: Screening and review.* Author. Retrieved January 10, 2021, from https://www.acog.org/clinical/clinical-guidance/obstetric-care-consensus/articles/2016/09/severe-maternal-morbidity-screening-and-review

Ampofo, E. K., Omotara, B. A., Otu, T., & Uchebo, G. (1990). Risk factors of vesico-vaginal fistulae in Maiduguri, Nigeria: A case-control study. *Tropical Doctor, 20*(3), 138–139. https://doi.org/10.1177/004947559002000320

Anastasi, E., Asiamah, B., & Lal, G. (2020). Leaving no one behind: Is the achievement of the Sustainable Development Goals possible without securing the dignity, rights, and well-being of those who are "invisible"? *International Journal of Gynaecology and Obstetrics, 148*(Suppl 1), 3–5. https://doi.org/10.1002/ijgo.13031

Anzaku, S. A., Lengmang, S. J., Mikah, S., Shephard, S. N., & Edem, B. E. (2017). Sexual activity among Nigerian women following successful obstetric fistula repair. *International Journal of Gynecology & Obstetrics, 137*(1), 67–71. https://doi.org/10.1002/ijgo.12083

Arrowsmith, S., Hamlin, E. C., & Wall, L. L. (1996). Obstructed labor injury complex: Obstetric fistula formation and the multifaceted morbidity of maternal birth trauma in the developing world. *Obstetrical & Gynecological Survey, 51*(9), 568–574.

Babiker, E. E. (2017). Gender inequality and nutritional status in patriarchal societies: The case of primary school students in Riyadh City, Saudi Arabia. *Advances in Obesity, Weight Management & Control, 6*(4), 135. https://doi.org/10.15406/aowmc.2017.06.00165

Baker, Z., Bellows, B., Bach, R., & Warren, C. (2017). Barriers to obstetric fistula treatment in low-income countries: A systematic review. *Tropical Medicine & International Health, 22*(8), 938–959. https://doi.org/10.1111/tmi.12893

Bangser, M. (2007). Strengthening public health priority-setting through research on fistula, maternal health, and health inequities. *International Journal of Gynecology & Obstetrics, 99*(S1), S16–S20. https://doi.org/10.1016/j.ijgo.2007.06.016

Bangser, M., Women's Dignity Project, Tanzania, & Wizara ya Afya. (2002). *Tanzania fistula survey 2001.* Women's Dignity Project & Ministry of Health.

Barnes-Josiah, D., Myntti, C., & Augustin, A. (1998). The "three delays" as a framework for examining maternal mortality in Haiti. *Social Science & Medicine, 46*(8), 981–993. https://doi.org/10.1016/s0277-9536(97)10018-1

Barone, M. A., Widmer, M., Arrowsmith, S., Ruminjo, J., Seuc, A., Landry, E., Barry, T. H., Danladi, D., Djangnikpo, L., Gbawuru-Mansaray, T., Harou, I., Lewis, A., Muleta, M., Nembunzu, D., Olupot, R., Sunday-Adeoye, I., Wakasiaka, W. K., Landoulsi, S., Delamou, A., … Gülmezoglu, A. M. (2015). Breakdown of simple female genital fistula repair after 7 day versus 14 day postoperative bladder catheterisation: A randomised, controlled, open-label, non-inferiority trial. *Lancet, 386*(9988), 56–62. https://doi.org/10.1016/S0140-6736(14)62337-0

de Bernis, L. (2007). Obstetric fistula: Guiding principles for clinical management and programme development, a new WHO guideline. *International Journal of Gynecology & Obstetrics, 99*(S1), S117–S121. https://doi.org/10.1016/j.ijgo.2007.06.032

Bomboka, J. B., N-Mboowa, M. G., & Nakilembe, J. (2019). Post-effects of obstetric fistula in Uganda; a case study of fistula survivors in KITOVU mission hospital (MASAKA), Uganda. *BMC Public Health, 19*(1), 696. https://doi.org/10.1186/s12889-019-7023-7

Browning, A. (2004). Obstetric fistula in Ilorin, Nigeria. *PLoS Medicine, 1*(1), e2. https://doi.org/10.1371/journal.pmed.0010002

Browning, A., & Syed, S. (2020). Where we currently stand on obstetric fistula treatment and prevention. *International Journal of Gynaecology and Obstetrics, 148*(S1), 1–2. https://doi.org/10.1002/ijgo.13030

Capes, T., Ascher-Walsh, C., Abdoulaye, I., & Brodman, M. (2011). Obstetric fistula in low and middle income countries. *Mount Sinai Journal of Medicine, 78*(3), 352–361. https://doi.org/10.1002/msj.20265

Catherine Hamlin Fistula Foundation. (2018). Retrieved March 4, 2021, from https://hamlin.org.au/catherine-hamlin/

Cook, R. J., Dickens, B. M., & Syed, S. (2004). Obstetric fistula: The challenge to human rights. *International Journal of Gynaecology and Obstetrics, 87*(1), 72–77. https://doi.org/10.1016/j.ijgo.2004.07.005

Danso, K. A., Martey, J. O., Wall, L. L., & Elkins, T. E. (1996). The epidemiology of genitourinary fistulae in Kumasi, Ghana, 1977-1992. *International Urogynecology Journal and Pelvic Floor Dysfunction, 7*(3), 117–120. https://doi.org/10.1007/BF01894198

Dolea, C., & AbouZahr, C. (2000). Global burden of obstructed labour in the year 2000. *Global Burden of Disease*, 17. Retrieved from https://www.who.int/healthinfo/statistics/bod_obstructedlabour.pdf

Donnay, F., & Weil, L. (2004). Obstetric fistula: The international response. *Lancet, 363*(9402), 71–72. https://doi.org/10.1016/S0140-6736(03)15177-X

Drew, L. B., Wilkinson, J. P., Nundwe, W., Moyo, M., Mataya, R., Mwale, M., & Tang, J. H. (2016). Long-term outcomes for women after obstetric fistula repair in Lilongwe, Malawi: A qualitative study. *BMC Pregnancy and Childbirth, 16*, 2. https://doi.org/10.1186/s12884-015-0755-1

Duko, B., Wolka, S., Seyoum, M., & Tantu, T. (2020). Prevalence of depression among women with obstetric fistula in low-income African countries: A systematic review and meta-analysis. *Archives of Women's Mental Health, 24*(1), 1–9. https://doi.org/10.1007/s00737-020-01028-w

East, Central, and Southern African Health Community (ECSA-HC) and Fistula Care/EngenderHealth. (2012). *The prevention and management of obstetric fistula a curriculum for nurses and midwives*. EngenderHealth/Fistula Care.

El Ayadi, A. M., Painter, C. E., Delamou, A., Barr-Walker, J., Korn, A., Obore, S., Byamugisha, J., & Barageine, J. K. (2020). Rehabilitation and reintegration programming adjunct to female genital fistula surgery: A systematic scoping review. *International Journal of Gynaecology and Obstetrics, 148*(S1), 42–58. https://doi.org/10.1002/ijgo.13039

Emasu, A., Ruder, B., Wall, L. L., Matovu, A., Alia, G., & Barageine, J. K. (2019). Reintegration needs of young women following genitourinary fistula surgery in Uganda. *International Urogynecology Journal, 30*(7), 1101–1110. https://doi.org/10.1007/s00192-019-03896-y

EngenderHealth. (2015). *End the inequity: The journey to eradicate obstetric fistula*. Author. Retrieved December 10, 2020, from https://www.engenderhealth.org/2015/05/22/05-21-end-inequality-fistula/

Epiu, I., Alia, G., Mukisa, J., Tavrow, P., Lamorde, M., & Kuznik, A. (2018). Estimating the cost and cost-effectiveness for obstetric fistula repair in hospitals in Uganda: A low income country. *Health Policy and Planning, 33*(9), 999–1008. https://doi.org/10.1093/heapol/czy078

Fiander, A., Ndahani, C., Mmuya, K., & Vanneste, T. (2013). Results from 2011 for the transportMYpatient program for overcoming transport costs among women seeking treatment for obstetric fistula in Tanzania. *International Journal of Gynecology & Obstetrics, 120*(3), 292–295. https://doi.org/10.1016/j.ijgo.2012.09.026

Firoz, T., Chou, D., von Dadelszen, P., Agrawal, P., Vanderkruik, R., Tunçalp, O., Magee, L. A., van Den Broek, N., & Say, L. (2013). Measuring maternal health: Focus on maternal morbidity. *Bulletin of the World Health Organization, 91*(10), 794–796. https://doi.org/10.2471/BLT.13.117564

Freedom from Fistula Foundation. (2016). *Fistula ambassadors*. Author. Retrieved February 20, 2021, from https://www.freedomfromfistula.org/programs/fistula-ambassadors

Geller, S. E., Koch, A. R., Garland, C. E., MacDonald, E. J., Storey, F., & Lawton, B. (2018). A global view of severe maternal morbidity: Moving beyond maternal mortality. *Reproductive Health, 15*(1), 98. https://doi.org/10.1186/s12978-018-0527-2

Hamlin Fistula Ethiopia. (2014). *About Us*. Author. Retrieved February 20, 2021, from https://hamlinfistula.org/about-us/

Hamlin, C., & Fleck, F. (2013). Giving hope to rural women with obstetric fistula in Ethiopia. *Bulletin of the World Health Organization, 91*(10), 724–725. https://doi.org/10.2471/BLT.13.031013

Hilton, P. (2003). Vesico-vaginal fistulas in developing countries. *International Journal of Gynaecology and Obstetrics, 82*(3), 285–295. https://doi.org/10.1016/s0020-7292(03)00222-4

Johnson, K., & Peterman, A. (2008). *Incontinence data from the Demographic and Health Surveys: Comparative analysis of a proxy measurement of vaginal fistula and recommendations for future population-based data collection*. DHS analytical studies no. 17. Macro International Inc.. Retrieved January 3, 2021, from https://dhsprogram.com/pubs/pdf/AS17/AS17.pdf

Kantorová, V., Wheldon, M. C., Ueffing, P., & Dasgupta, A. N. Z. (2020). Estimating progress towards meeting women's contraceptive needs in 185 countries: A Bayesian hierarchical modelling study. *PLoS Medicine, 17*(2), e1003026. https://doi.org/10.1371/journal.pmed.1003026

Kelly, J. (2004). Outreach programmes for obstetric fistulae. *Journal of Obstetrics and Gynaecology, 24*(2), 117–118. https://doi.org/10.1080/01443610410001645352

Khan, K. S., Wojdyla, D., Say, L., Gülmezoglu, A. M., & Van Look, P. F. (2006). WHO analysis of causes of maternal death: A systematic review. *The Lancet, 367*(9516), 1066–1074. https://doi.org/10.1016/S0140-6736(06)68397-9

Koblinsky, M., Chowdhury, M. E., Moran, A., & Ronsmans, C. (2012). Maternal morbidity and disability and their consequences: Neglected agenda in maternal health. *Journal of Health, Population, and Nutrition, 30*(2), 124–130.

Liljestrand, J. (2006). Trends in maternal health/healthcare in low-income countries and the implications on neonatal health. *Seminars in Fetal & Neonatal Medicine, 11*(1), 3–6. https://doi.org/10.1016/j.siny.2005.10.001

Lombard, L., de St Jorre, J., Geddes, R., El Ayadi, A. M., & Grant, L. (2015). Rehabilitation experiences after obstetric fistula repair: Systematic review of qualitative studies. *Tropical Medicine & International Health, 20*(5), 554–568. https://doi.org/10.1111/tmi.12469

Lyimo, M. A., & Mosha, I. H. (2019). Reasons for delay in seeking treatment among women with obstetric fistula in Tanzania: A qualitative study. *BMC Women's Health, 19*(1), 1–8. https://doi.org/10.1186/s12905-019-0799-x

Maroyi, R., Keyser, L., Hosterman, L., Notia, A., & Mukwege, D. (2020). The mobile surgical outreach program for management of patients with genital fistula in the Democratic Republic of Congo. *International Journal of Gynecology & Obstetrics, 148*(S1), 27–32. https://doi.org/10.1002/ijgo.13036

Mernoff, R., Chigwale, S., & Pope, R. (2020). Obstetric fistula and safe spaces: Discussions of stigmatised healthcare topics at a fistula centre. *Culture, Health & Sexuality, 22*(12), 1429–1438. https://doi.org/10.1080/13691058.2019.1682196

Miller, S., Lester, F., Webster, M., & Cowan, B. (2005). Obstetric fistula: A preventable tragedy. *Journal of Midwifery & Women's Health, 50*(4), 286–294. https://doi.org/10.1016/j.jmwh.2005.03.009

Moerman, M. L. (1982). Growth of the birth canal in adolescent girls. *American Journal of Obstetrics and Gynecology, 143*(5), 528–532. https://doi.org/10.1016/0002-9378(82)90542-7

Mselle, L. T., Moland, K. M., Evjen-Olsen, B., Mvungi, A., & Kohi, T. W. (2011). "I am nothing": Experiences of loss among women suffering from severe birth injuries in Tanzania. *BMC Women's Health, 11*, 49. https://doi.org/10.1186/1472-6874-11-49

Mselle, L., Evjen-Olsen, B., Moland, K. M., Mvungi, A., & Kohi, T. W. (2012). "Hoping for a normal life again": Reintegration after fistula repair in rural Tanzania. *Journal of Obstetrics and Gynaecology Canada, 34*(10), 927–938. https://doi.org/10.1016/S1701-2163(16)35406-8

Nardos, R., Browning, A., & Chen, C. C. G. (2009). Risk factors that predict failure after vaginal repair of obstetric vesicovaginal fistulae. *American Journal of Obstetrics and Gynecology, 200*(5), 578.e1–578.e4. https://doi.org/10.1016/j.ajog.2008.12.008

Nardos, R., Menber, B., & Browning, A. (2012). Outcome of obstetric fistula repair after 10-day versus 14-day Foley catheterization. *International Journal of Gynecology & Obstetrics, 118*(1), 21–23. https://doi.org/10.1016/j.ijgo.2012.01.024

Pacagnella, R. C., Cecatti, J. G., Osis, M. J., & Souza, J. P. (2012). The role of delays in severe maternal morbidity and mortality: Expanding the conceptual framework. *Reproductive Health Matters, 20*(39), 155–163. https://doi.org/10.1016/S0968-8080(12)39601-8

Pathmanathan, I., Liljestrand, J., Martins, J., Rajapaksa, L., Lissner, C., de Silva, A., Selvaraju, S., & Singh, P. (2003). *Investing in maternal health: Learning from Malaysia and Sri Lanka.* The World Bank. Retrieved March 1, 2021, from http://documents1.worldbank.org/curated/en/367761468760748311/pdf/259010REPLACEM10082135362401PUBLIC1.pdf

Pope, R. (2018). Research in obstetric fistula: Addressing gaps and unmet needs. *Obstetrics and Gynecology, 131*(5), 863–870. https://doi.org/10.1097/AOG.0000000000002578

Pope, R., & Beddow, M. (2020). A review of surgical procedures to repair obstetric fistula. *International Journal of Gynaecology and Obstetrics, 148*(S1), 22–26. https://doi.org/10.1002/ijgo.13035

Pope, R., Ganesh, P., Chalamanda, C., Nundwe, W., & Wilkinson, J. (2018). Sexual function before and after vesicovaginal fistula repair. *The Journal of Sexual Medicine, 15*(8), 1125–1132. https://doi.org/10.1016/j.jsxm.2018.06.006

Slinger, G., & Trautvetter, L. (2020). Addressing the fistula treatment gap and rising to the 2030 challenge. *International Journal of Gynecology & Obstetrics, 148*(S1), 9–15. https://doi.org/10.1002/ijgo.13033

Sori, D. A., Azale, A. W., & Gemeda, D. H. (2016). Characteristics and repair outcome of patients with vesicovaginal fistula managed in Jimma University teaching Hospital, Ethiopia. *BMC Urology, 16*(1), 41. https://doi.org/10.1186/s12894-016-0152-8

Stanton, C., Holtz, S. A., & Ahmed, S. (2007). Challenges in measuring obstetric fistula. *International Journal of Gynecology & Obstetrics, 99*(S1), S4–S9. https://doi.org/10.1016/j.ijgo.2007.06.010

Starrs, A. M., Ezeh, A. C., Barker, G., Basu, A., Bertrand, J. T., Blum, R., Coll-Seck, A. M., Grover, A., Laski, L., Roa, M., Sathar, Z. A., Say, L., Serour, G. I., Singh, S., Stenberg, K., Temmerman, M., Biddlecom, A., Popinchalk, A., Summers, C., & Ashford, L. S. (2018). Accelerate progress-sexual and reproductive health and rights for all: Report of the Guttmacher-Lancet Commission. *Lancet, 391*(10140), 2642–2692. https://doi.org/10.1016/S0140-6736(18)30293-9

Tebeu, P. M., Fomulu, J. N., Khaddaj, S., de Bernis, L., Delvaux, T., & Rochat, C. H. (2012). Risk factors for obstetric fistula: A clinical review. *International Urogynecology Journal, 23*(4), 387–394. https://doi.org/10.1007/s00192-011-1622-x

Tunçalp, Ö., Isah, A., Landry, E., & Stanton, C. K. (2014). Community-based screening for obstetric fistula in Nigeria: A novel approach. *BMC Pregnancy and Childbirth, 14*, 44. https://doi.org/10.1186/1471-2393-14-44

Umoiyoho, A. J., Inyang-Etoh, E. C., & Etukumana, E. A. (2012). Obstetric fistula repair: Experience with hospital-based outreach approach in Nigeria. *Global Journal of Health Science, 4*(5), 40–45. https://doi.org/10.5539/gjhs.v4n5p40

UNICEF. (2019). *Early childbearing. Monitoring the situation of children and women.* Author. Retrieved March 5, 2021, from https://data.unicef.org/topic/child-health/adolescent-health/

United Nations. (2015). Transforming our world: The 2030 agenda for sustainable development. In *A new era in global health.* Author. Retrieved December 10, 2020, from https://sdgs.un.org/sites/default/files/publications/21252030%20Agenda%20for%20Sustainable%20Development%20web.pdf

United Nations General Assembly. (2020). *Intensifying efforts to end obstetric fistula within a decade: Report of the Secretary-General.* United Nations. Retrieved December 10, 2020, from http://www.endfistula.org/sites/default/files/pub-pdf/Intensifying%20efforts%20to%20end%20obstetric%20fistula%20within%20a%20decade.pdf

United Nations Population Fund. (2012). *When childbirth harms: Obstetric fistula*. Author. Retrieved December 10, 2020, from https://www.unfpa.org/sites/default/files/resource-pdf/EN-SRH%20fact%20sheet-Fistula.pdf

United Nations Population Fund. (2019). *Ending obstetric fistula: Devastating and preventable childbirth injury continues to haunt women*. Author. Retrieved December 10, 2020, from https://www.unfpa.org/news/ending-obstetric-fistula-devastating-and-preventable-childbirth-injury-continues-haunt-women

United Nations Population Fund. (2020). *Maternal health*. Author. Retrieved December 10, 2020, from https://www.unfpa.org/maternal-health

United Nations Population Fund, & EngenderHealth. (2003). *Obstetric fistula needs assessment report: Findings from nine African countries*. United Nations Population Fund. Retrieved December 10, 2020, from https://www.unfpa.org/sites/default/files/pub-pdf/fistula-needs-assessment.pdf

United Nations Population Fund, World Health Organization, UNICEF, World Bank Group, & United Nations Population Division. (2019). *Trends in maternal mortality: 2000 to 2017*. World Health Organization. Retrieved December 10, 2020, from https://www.unfpa.org/sites/default/files/pub-pdf/Maternal_mortality_report.pdf

Velez, A., Ramsey, K., & Tell, K. (2007). The campaign to end fistula: What have we learned? Findings of facility and community needs assessments. *International Journal of Gynaecology and Obstetrics, 99*(S1), S143–S150. https://doi.org/10.1016/j.ijgo.2007.06.036

Wall, L. L. (1998). Dead mothers and injured wives: The social context of maternal morbidity and mortality among the Hausa of northern Nigeria. *Studies in Family Planning, 29*(4), 341–359.

Wall, L. L. (2002). Fitsari 'dan Duniya. An African (Hausa) praise song about vesicovaginal fistulas. *Obstetrics and Gynecology, 100*(6), 1328–1332. https://doi.org/10.1016/s0029-7844(02)02498-5

Wall, L. L. (2006). Obstetric vesicovaginal fistula as an international public-health problem. *Lancet, 368*(9542), 1201–1209. https://doi.org/10.1016/S0140-6736(06)69476-2

Wall, L. L., Karshima, J. A., Kirschner, C., & Arrowsmith, S. D. (2004). The obstetric vesicovaginal fistula: Characteristics of 899 patients from Jos, Nigeria. *American Journal of Obstetrics and Gynecology, 190*(4), 1011–1019. https://doi.org/10.1016/j.ajog.2004.02.007

Weston, K., Mutiso, S., Mwangi, J., Qureshi, Z., Beard, J., & Venkat, P. (2011). Depression among women with obstetric fistula in Kenya. *International Journal of Gynaecology and Obstetrics, 115*(1), 31–33. https://doi.org/10.1016/j.ijgo.2011.04.015

World Health Organization. (2004). *Making pregnancy safer: The critical role of the skilled attendant: A joint statement by WHO, ICM and FIGO*. Author. Retrieved March 6, 2021, from https://apps.who.int/iris/bitstream/handle/10665/42955/9241591692.pdf;jsessionid=9E3DA8EC37B669936637A04B39697B69?sequence=1

World Health Organization. (2019). *Maternal mortality*. Author. Retrieved December 10, 2020, from https://www.who.int/news-room/fact-sheets/detail/maternal-mortality

World Health Organization. (2020). *Family planning/contraception methods*. Author. Retrieved March 1, 2021, from https://www.who.int/news-room/fact-sheets/detail/family-planning-contraception

World Health Organization. (2021a). *Improving access to high quality care for obstetric fistula*. Author. Retrieved January 14, 2021, from http://www.who.int/reproductivehealth/topics/maternal_perinatal/fistula-study/en/

World Health Organization. (2021b). *Women of reproductive age (15-49 years) population (thousands)*. Author. Retrieved March 6, 2021, from https://www.who.int/data/maternal-newborn-child-adolescent-ageing/indicator-explorer-new/mca/women-of-reproductive-age-(15-49-years)-population-(thousands)

World Health Organization. (2021c). *Global health observatory data: Skilled attendants at birth*. Author. Retrieved March 6, 2021, from http://www.who.int/gho/maternal_health/skilled_care/skilled_birth_attendance/en/

World Health Organization, & Human Reproduction Programme. (2015). *WHO statement on caesarean section rates*. World Health Organization. Retrieved March 6, 2021, from http://www.who.int/reproductivehealth/publications/maternal_perinatal_health/cs-statement/en/

Zabin, L. S., & Kiragu, K. (1998). The health consequences of adolescent sexual and fertility behavior in sub-Saharan Africa. *Studies in Family Planning, 29*(2), 210–232.

Archeological Basis for Obstetrical Fistula: A Condition That Is as Ancient as Human Themselves

David A. Schwartz

3.1 Evolutionary Origins of Obstructed Delivery

Obstructed labor occurs more frequently in humans than in any other animals. The development of bipedalism in human evolution resulted in skeletal changes together with enlargement of the human brain that together are responsible for this birth complication. Even compared with other primates, childbirth in humans is slow and particularly difficult as a result of the small size of the maternal pelvis and the large size of the fetal head. Bipedal locomotion together with encephalization has resulted in increased demands placed on the human female pelvis. This process of decreased size of the human birth canal resulting from maintaining an upright bipedal mechanism of locomotion and the progressively larger human cranial capacity throughout evolution has been termed the "obstetric dilemma" by Sherwood Washburn (Washburn, 1960; Wittman & Wall, 2007). The resulting "tight fit" between the dimensions of the fetal head and the maternal birth canal is the result of millions of years of human evolution, but has led to rates of cephalopelvic disproportion and consequently obstructed labor in from 1% to 8% of all childbirths in different regions of the world (Dolea & AbouZahr, 2003; Wittman & Wall, 2007). If obstructed labor is not relieved, maternal exhaustion, dehydration, infection, and ketosis can develop. Obstructed labor is a major cause of maternal death in resource-poor nations of the world, in which cases the immediate causes of death include sepsis, uterine rupture, hemorrhage, and shock. Fetal death is also a common occurrence, and if the fetus and placenta are left in situ, maternal complications and death can also ensue (Pavličev et al., 2020; Schwartz, 2015). In those mothers who survive an obstructed delivery, a frequent complication is the development of an obstetric fistula.

3.2 Archeology of Obstetric Fistula and Obstructed Birth

The archeological record provides evidence for a number of diseases in antiquity that includes both infectious and noninfectious conditions. Paleopathology, the study of ancient diseases, utilizes a number of tools to identify these conditions. They include examination of human remains to identify

D. A. Schwartz (✉)
Perinatal Pathology Consulting, Atlanta, GA, USA
e-mail: davidalanschwartz@gmail.com

© Springer Nature Switzerland AG 2022
L. B. Drew et al. (eds.), *A Multidisciplinary Approach to Obstetric Fistula in Africa*, Global Maternal and Child Health, https://doi.org/10.1007/978-3-031-06314-5_3

osteological disease, analysis of preserved soft tissues, chemical analysis, pathology and histological examination, radiological methods, and, most recently, molecular biology techniques.

For the overwhelming majority of human history, pregnancy and childbirth have been dangerous, and even life-threatening, conditions for girls and women (Schwartz, 2018). Although fetal and newborn skeletal remains are not as well preserved as are adult osteological materials, there still exist physical anthropology and archeology evidence of obstetrical death as a result of childbirth in many parts of the ancient world (Wells, 1975; Wells et al., 2012). Examples include the occurrence of a third-trimester fetus associated with the body of the famed "rich Athenian lady" who was cremated c.a. 850 BCE in Greece (Liston & Papadopoulos, 2004); death of a young mother and her unborn full-term breech fetus at the Neolithic site of An Son in Vietnam c.a. 2100–1050 BCE (Willis & Oxenham, 2013); three maternal deaths in medieval Stockholm (Högberg et al., 1987); two maternal deaths from ancient Egypt in which each woman had a deformed pelvis and a fetal head present within the pelvic cavity (Elliot-Smith & Wood Jones, 1910); a woman having a "coffin birth" in medieval Aebelholt, Denmark (Moller-Christensen, 1958; Wells, 1975); and an obstetric death from Kings Worthy, Great Britain, in which a Saxon woman was interred with an infant that appeared to lie half in and half out of her vagina (Hawkes & Wells, 1975; Wells, 1975).

It should not be surprising that one of the leading causes of pregnancy-related death both in ancient and contemporary times is obstructed delivery. As a result, in ancient times the mortality rate of pregnant women with obstructed deliveries was extremely high, and if the dead fetus was not quickly removed (often by decapitation and withdrawal of the remains piece by piece), there would be a high likelihood of maternal sepsis, coagulopathy, hemorrhage, shock, and death. Those who survived the immediate period of childbirth would frequently develop obstetric fistula. In more recent times, still prior to the advent of cesarean section and anesthesia in the nineteenth century, the sole potential treatment for an obstructed delivery was by use of the obstetrical forceps, a tool that had been invented in the seventeenth century and used in secrecy by members of the Chamberlen family of surgeons (Dunn, 1999).

Mummies can be especially rewarding to study in documenting the spectrum and patterns of disease in antiquity, including disorders of pregnancy. This is because in many cases the body, especially the soft tissues including organs, has been preserved due to mortuary rituals or, in some cases, climatological factors. An analysis of female mummies representing seven pre-Columbian Andean populations of Arica, Chile, ranging in age from the Early Formative Period in the Azapa Valley (1300 BCE) up to the Gentilar period (1400 CE), revealed that 18 (14% of the total) had died from childbirth-complicated death. The majority of these women appear to have died during the puerperium, including three without completing delivery (Arriaza et al., 1988).

The best evidence for obstetrical fistula in the archeological record comes from ancient Egypt—a time and place where mummification reached its zenith as a method for preserving human remains. The well-preserved mummy of Queen Henhenit from 4000 years ago demonstrates the type of obstetrical fistula that still occurs today, and the condition is likely discussed in the Ebers Papyrus. Avicenna, a Persian polymath and physician and the Father of Early Modern Medicine, also described the association between obstructed birth and vesicovaginal fistulas in the eleventh century.

3.3   Queen Henhenit

The mummy of Queen Henhenit (also Henhenet) is the oldest physical evidence of obstetric fistula. She lived during the Eleventh Dynasty, around 2025 BCE, the start of ancient Egypt's Middle Kingdom period (2040–1710 BCE) and immediately following the First Intermediate Period (2081–2040 BCE). As a young woman, Henhenit was a priestess of the goddess Hathor. This deity was a loving mother figure, a protectress, goddess of childbirth and fertility, and the patroness of music, dance, and wine (Wall, 2018). She became the wife of Pharaoh Nebhepetre Mentuhotep (Mentuhotep II), also known by his prenomen Nephepetre, who ruled Egypt for 51 years as the first pharaoh of the Middle Kingdom. He had many wives who were interred with him or near his mortuary temple located in the Theban necropolis at Deir el-Bahri. Henhenit, in addition to Sadeh, Ashayet, and Kemsit, was a secondary wife of the pharaoh, and all were priestesses of Hathor. They were titled *Hmt-nswt mryt.f*, meaning "King's wife, his beloved" and *khkrt-nswt-w3tit*, "Unique embellishment of the King."

Beginning in 1893, excavations began at Deir-al-Bahri by Henri Édouard Naville and his team of archaeologists and workmen on behalf of the Egypt Exploration Fund (Fig. 3.1). After working for 10 years, they discovered the funerary temple of the Pharaoh Mentuhotep II. Further work identified the "pit tomb number 11" located beneath a column in a colonnaded court on the Western aspect of the temple. The sarcophagus and mummy of Henhenit were discovered in this tomb, termed DBXI.11 (Figs. 3.2 and 3.3) (Winlock, 1942; Wall, 2018; Zacharin, 1988; Naville et al., 1907). Five other women, probably priestesses of Hathor, were entombed nearby. A wooden coffin was present within Queen Henhenit's sarcophagus and in this was her mummy that had apparently been robbed in antiquity. Naville stated,

> The lid had been broken into three pieces, which lay on the rubbish accumulation at the bottom of the chamber. Fragments of a large square wooden coffin were found in the shaft, with a line of hieroglyphs painted in green on a white ground; this, like the sarcophagus, bore the name of Henhenit, priestess of Hathor, and only royal favorite.
>
> Within the sarcophagus was the mummy of a woman, no doubt Henhenit, lying on the cloth wrappings. Her hands and feet are small and delicately formed, her hair short and straight. It is a very interesting mummy. It and the sarcophagus have been assigned to the Metropolitan Museum of New York.

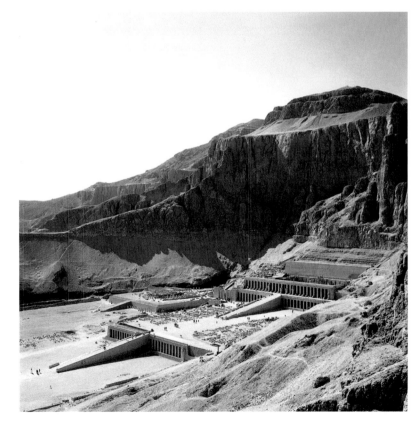

Fig. 3.1 The tomb of Henhenit (DBXI.11) and a small decorated chapel were found in the mortuary temple of King Mentuhotep II and Queen Hatshepsut (reigned 1498–1483 BCE, Dynasty XVIII), Deir el-Bahri, Thebes. The temple is a partly rock-cut and partly free-standing terraced structure. During the Graeco-Roman Period (332 BCE–CE 395), the temple became a center for healing and the upper terrace was consecrated to Imhotep. Numerous graffiti are evidence of the large number of invalids who visited it until the second-century CE. (Credit: Reeves, 1989. Licensed under the terms of the Creative Commons Attribution 4.0 International License, http://creativecommons.org/licenses/by/4.0/)

Fig. 3.2 Massive stone sarcophagus of Queen Henhenit on display at the Metropolitan Museum, New York. It was buried in a shaft tomb beneath the platform of King Mentuhotep II's temple at Deir el Bahri. (From the Metropolitan Museum of Art. https:// www.metmuseum.org/ art/collection/ search/100000424, licensed under the terms of the Creative Commons Zero (CC0) License, https:// creativecommons.org/ publicdomain/zero/1.0/)

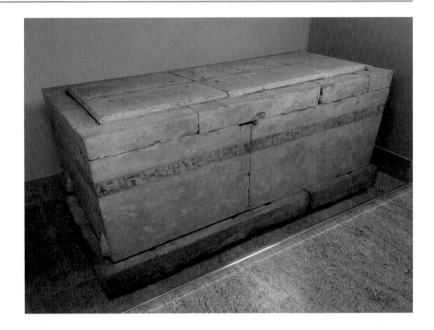

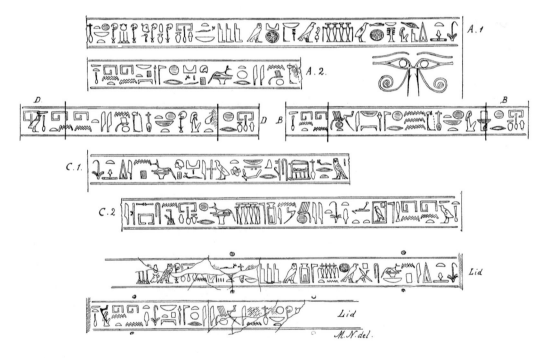

INSCRIPTIONS OF THE SARCOPHAGUS OF HENHENIT.

Fig. 3.3 Hieroglyphic inscriptions on the sarcophagus of Queen Henhenit. (From Naville et al., 1907)

In 1907, Naville sent both Queen Henhenit's mummy and her sarcophagus to the Metropolitan Museum of Art in New York in gratitude for having received financial support for his archeological work. Once at the Metropolitan Museum, the mummy was observed that a 10 cm long portion of tissue, probably intestine, was protruding through the anus. In 1923, the Metropolitan Museum Trustees had the mummy returned to Cairo for additional examination. The famed Egyptologist Herbert Winlock returned the mummy for examination to Professor D.E. Derry of the Egyptian University (Wall, 2018; Derry, 1935).

According to the Australian gynecologist and author Dr. Robert Zacharin (1988), Derry found that the Queen's body was very well-preserved, with no abdominal incision present. Mummies from this period typically failed to show that the abdomen had been entered through the customary left flank incision in order to remove the visceral organs. The body showed a widely dilated vagina and rectum. Professor Derry's examination of the interior of the mummy revealed significant anatomical abnormalities of a vesical–vaginal fistula from an unrelieved obstructed delivery (Figs. 3.4, 3.5, and 3.6) (Cron, 2003; Derry, 1935; Zacharin, 1988).

Fig. 3.4 A large vesicovaginal fistula in the mummy of Queen Henhenit. The pelvic cavity of Henhenit shows excessive anteroposterior pelvic diameter and rupture of the vagina into the bladder; (1) bladder cavity enormously dilated; (2) thickened, infected bladder mucosa; (3) large vesicovaginal fistula; and (4) right arm. (From: Derry, 1935. Figure 2a. Used with permission of John Wiley and Sons)

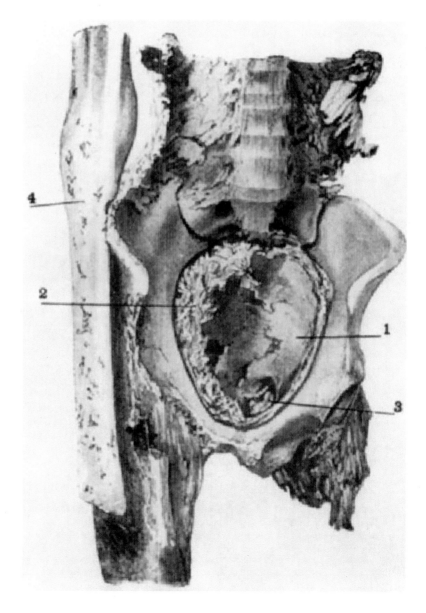

Fig. 3.5 A close-up image of the large vesicovaginal fistula in the mummy of Queen Henhenit. (From: Derry, 1935. Figure 2b. Used with permission of John Wiley and Sons)

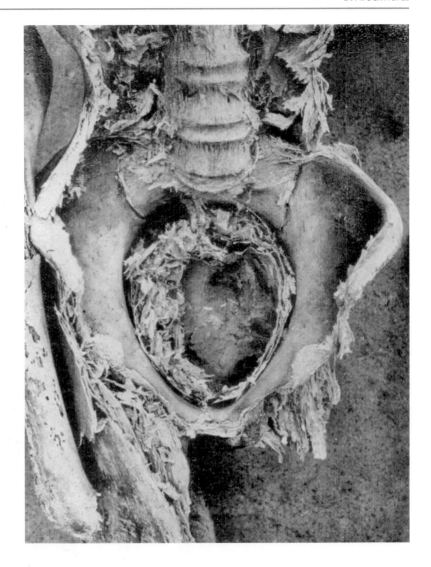

When the abdominal cavity was opened, Derry discovered a rent in the bladder communicating directly with the vagina and so the exterior, and what had appeared as dilated vagina when seen through the vulva, in reality was the bladder. In addition the pelvis was an abnormal shape with a much reduced transverse diameter and the antero- posterior, exceptionally long. The pelvic brim index approximated that of apes and the pelvis illustrated a further ape-like condition, namely a high standing sacral promontory. Also, there were only four lumbar vertebrae, and six sacral (Figs. 2 a, b and 3). Even allowing for the present dried up tissues, Derry believed it would have been difficult for a fetal head to pass, and that the severe damage discovered, probably occurred at the time of parturition resulting in Henhenit's death.

Dr. Zacharin (1988) also believed that the pelvis of Queen Henhenit was abnormally small,

The injury was considered to be a tear from the vagina into the bladder due to the abnormally narrow pelvis through which the child had to be dragged by force. The vagina was discovered crushed between the distended bladder and rectum, which itself was obliterated by descent of the lower part of the large bowel which protruded outside. The presence of this dried up intestine protruding through the anal orifice outside the body, suggested an attempt had been made to remove some of the organs at least by this route. It is likely Henhenit was Nubian, and if her pelvis had been examined in isolation, it would have been considered grossly deformed the measurements corresponding to those of a chimpanzee, but with four other mummies exhibiting similar characteristics although of lesser degree, it seemed her pelvis was only an extreme example of a racial characteristic common to all five women. Only one pelvis even approximated brim diameters common in Europe.

Fig. 3.6 Posterior surface of mummy of Queen Henhenit showing a complete perineal tear. (1) anus; (2) perineal tear; and (3) vagina. (From Derry, 1935. Fig. 3. Used with permission of John Wiley and Sons)

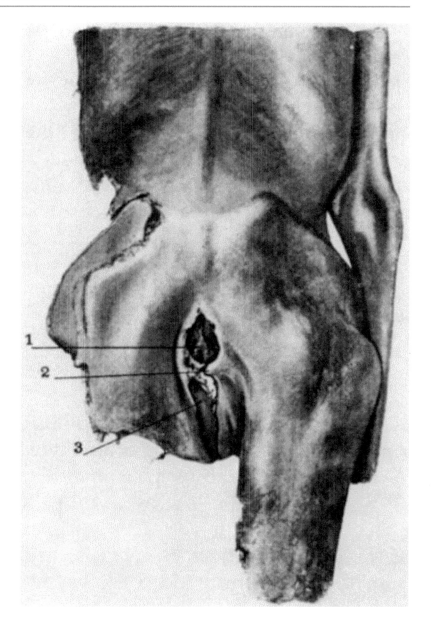

The mummy of Queen Henhenit, the most ancient women displaying anatomical findings of an obstetric fistula from childbirth, presently resides in the Egyptian Museum in Cairo, and her sarcophagus is displayed at The Metropolitan Museum of Art (n.d.) in New York City.

3.4   Ebers Papyrus

There are two ancient Egyptian papyri that contain medical references, the Kahun Papyrus and Ebers Papyrus. The Ebers Papyrus (Fig. 3.7) was written in hieratic Egyptian script sometime around 1500 BCE and contains the most extensive description of ancient Egyptian medicine known. Although the exact origin of the papyrus is unknown, it is believed to have been discovered lying between the

Fig. 3.7 A page from the Ebers Papyrus, written circa 1500 BCE (Wellcome Collection, n.d. Licensed under the terms of the Creative Commons Attribution 4.0 International License, http://creativecommons.org/licenses/by/4.0/)

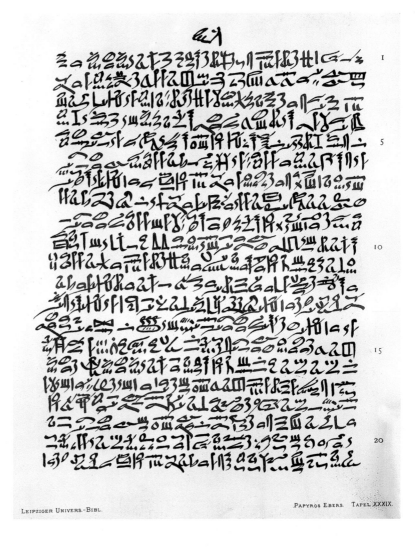

legs of a mummy in the El-Assasif District located in the Theban necropolis. Within this 18.63 m long, 200-page scroll is approximately well-preserved 700 remedies, incantations, and formulas that include references to topics on the health of women. The Ebers Papyrus was first translated by H. Joachim in 1890. On page 3, two fragmentary prescriptions occur (Zacharin, 1988). One of these can be interpreted as relating to vesicovaginal fistula, advising the physician against attempting to cure it

> *Prescription for a woman whose urine is in an irksome place: if the urine keeps coming and she distinguishes it, she will be like this forever.*

The Ebers Papyrus is kept at the University Library of Leipzig in Germany.

3.5 Kahun Gynecological Papyrus

The Kahun Gynecological Papyrus is the oldest remaining record of medicine in ancient Egypt, having been written during the Twelfth Dynasty, approximately 1800 BCE (Figs. 3.8 and 3.9). This papyrus is divided into 34 paragraphs, each discussing a specific medical problem or complaint, and

Fig. 3.8 Page 1 and part of page 2 of the Kahun Gynecological Papyrus. The papyrus was written in hieratic script. (From Francis Llewellyn. *Hieratic papyri from Kahun and Gurob (principally of the middle kingdom).* London: Quaritch. 1898)

Fig. 3.9 Page 3 of the Kahun Gynecological Papyrus. (From Francis Llewellyn. *Hieratic papyri from Kahun and Gurob (principally of the middle kingdom).* London: Quaritch. 1898)

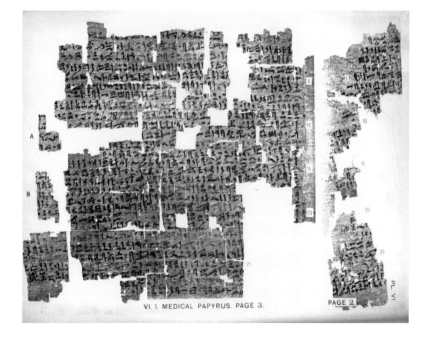

contains a large amount of materials relating to women's health, birth, and gynecology (Smith, 2011). The papyrus dates to the reign of the last ruler of the Twelfth Dynasty, pharaoh Sobekneferu (Stevens, 1975). Sobekneferu was the daughter of King Amenemhat III and was a childless woman whose interest in gynecology might have originated when her elder sister, Neferuptah, died at an early age.

According to the interpretation of Reeves (1992) and Bouwer (2012), the Kahun Gynecological Papyrus contains a prescription that is based on a vesicovaginal fistula. It reads as follows:

> *Prescription for a woman whose urine is in an irksome place: if urine keeps coming … and she distinguishes it, she will be like this forever ….*

The Kahun Gynecological Papyrus is preserved at the University College London, Great Britain.

3.6   Avicenna

Avicenna, or Ibn Sina, was a Persian physician, astronomer, and philosopher who lived from 980 to 1037 CE and is generally considered one of the founders of modern medicine. He is believed to have written over 400 books, and among his most famous was *The Canon of Medicine*, a compendium of five books completed in 1025 CE (Fig. 3.10). It was the standard medical textbook relied upon in many

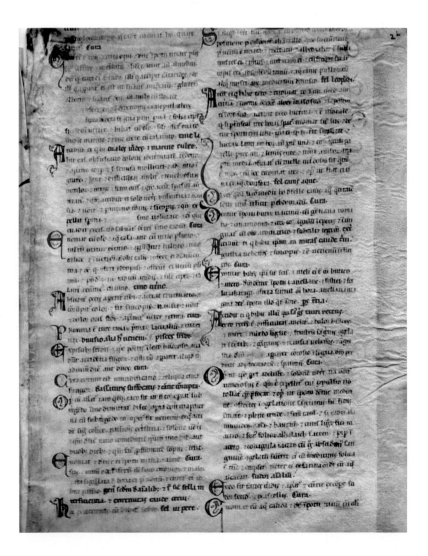

Fig. 3.10 Handwritten page from a manuscript copy of the Canon Medicine by Avicenna. This rubricated manuscript was written in Italy circa thirteenth century. (From the author's collection)

medieval universities, remaining in use in Europe as late as the eighteenth century. Avicenna provided the following advice in his chapter on pregnancy prevention (Zacharin, 1988):

> *In cases in which women are married too young, and in patients who have weak*
> *bladders, the physician should instruct the patient in the ways of prevention*
> *of pregnancy. In these patients the bulk of foetus may cause a tear in the*
> *bladder which results in incontinence of urine. The condition is incurable*
> *and remains so till death.*

This statement by Avicenna is believed to refer to the development of vesicovaginal fistulas resulting from obstructed deliveries.

3.7 Conclusions

Obstructed labor has been a topic in the medical literature for hundreds of years. In the absence of the availability of cesarean section, obstructed labor can result in not only maternal and fetal injuries but also maternal and infant mortality. Obstetric fistula is an unfortunate complication of unrelieved obstructed delivery. Evidence for obstructed delivery and obstetrical fistula has also been demonstrated in the physical anthropology and archeology records, as well as from written documents, from many parts of the ancient world. The oldest evidence of obstructed labor can be found in the remains of Queen Henhenit, the wife of Egypt's ruler around the time of 2050 BCE. It has been hypothesized that severe damage to Queen Henhenit's bladder and vagina occurred at the time of parturition, likely resulting in her death. As was stated by Cron (2003), "to Queen Henhenit belongs the dubious honor of having suffered the most antique vesicovaginal fistula documented."

References

Arriaza, B., Allison, M., & Gerszten, E. (1988). Maternal mortality in pre-Columbian Indians of Arica, Chile. *American Journal of Physical Anthropology, 77*(1), 35–41. https://doi.org/10.1002/ajpa.1330770107

Bouwer, D.S. (2012). *Ancient Egyptian health related to women: Obstetrics and gynaecology*. Masters thesis. University of South Africa. Retrieved September 15, 2020, from http://uir.unisa.ac.za/bitstream/handle/10500/8786/dissertation_bouwer_ds.pdf?isAllowed=y&sequence=1

Cron, J. (2003). Lessons from the developing world: Obstructed labor and the vesico-vaginal fistula. *Medscape General Medicine, 5*(3), 24.

Derry, D. E. (1935). Note on five pelves of women of the Eleventh Dynasty in Egypt. *BJOG: An International Journal of Obstetrics & Gynaecology, 42*, 490–495. https://doi.org/10.1111/j.1471-0528.1935.tb12160.x

Dolea, C., & AbouZahr, C. (2003). *Global burden of obstructed labor in the year 2000*. World Health Organization. Retrieved September 18, 2020, from https://www.who.int/healthinfo/statistics/bod_obstructedlabour.pdf

Dunn, P. M. (1999). The Chamberlen family (1560-1728) and obstetric forceps. *Archives of Disease in Childhood. Fetal and Neonatal Edition, 81*(3), F232–F234. https://doi.org/10.1136/fn.81.3.f232

Elliot-Smith, G. B., & Wood Jones, F. (1910). *The archaeological survey of Nubia report for 1907-1908, volume II: Report on human remains*. National Printing Department.

Griffith, F. L. (1898). *Hieratic papyri from Kahun and Gurob (principally of the middle kingdom)*. [Photograph]. Quaritch. Retrieved from https://archive.org/details/hieraticpapyrifr00grifuoft/page/n31/mode/2up

Hawkes, S. C., & Wells, C. (1975). An Anglo-Saxon obstetric calamity from Kingsworthy, Hampshire. *Medical & Biological Illustration, 25*, 47–51.

Högberg, U., Iregren, E., Siven, C. H., & Diener, L. (1987). Maternal deaths in medieval Sweden: An osteological and life table analysis. *Journal of Biosocial Science, 19*(4), 495–503. https://doi.org/10.1017/s0021932000017120

Liston, M. A., & Papadopoulos, J. K. (2004). The 'Rich Athenian Lady' was pregnant: The anthropology of a geometric tomb reconsidered. *Hesperia: The Journal of the American School of Classical Studies at Athens, 73*(1), 7–38.

Moller-Christensen, V. (1958). *Bogen om Aebelholt kloster*. Dansk Videnskabs Forlag.

Naville, E., Hall, H. R., & Ayrton, E. R. (1907). *The XI Dynasty Temple at Deir el-Bahari. Part I*. Offices of the Egypt Exploration Fund.

Pavličev, M., Romero, R., & Mitteroecker, P. (2020). Evolution of the human pelvis and obstructed labor: New explanations of an old obstetrical dilemma. *American Journal of Obstetrics and Gynecology, 222*(1), 3–16. https://doi.org/10.1016/j.ajog.2019.06.043

Reeves, C. (1989). *Mortuary temple of Queen Hatshepsut (reigned 1498-1483 BCE, dynasty XVIII), Deir el-Bahri, Thebes.* [Photograph]. Wellcome Collection. Retrieved from https://wellcomecollection.org/works/bgz9ja34

Reeves, C. (1992). *Egyptian medicine.* Shire Publications Ltd.

Schwartz, D. A. (2015). *Maternal mortality: Risk factors, anthropological perspectives, prevalence in developing countries and preventive strategies for pregnancy-related death.* Nova Science Publishers.

Schwartz, D. A. (2018). Aztec pregnancy – Archaeological & cultural foundations for motherhood & childbearing in ancient Mesoamerica. In D. A. Schwartz (Ed.), *Maternal death and pregnancy-related morbidity among indigenous women of Mexico and Central America: An anthropological, epidemiological and biomedical approach.* Springer. Retrieved from https://link.springer.com/chapter/10.1007/978-3-319-71538-4_2

Smith, L. (2011). The Kahun Gynaecological Papyrus: Ancient Egyptian medicine. *The Journal of Family Planning and Reproductive Health Care, 37*(1), 54–55. https://doi.org/10.1136/jfprhc.2010.0019

Stevens, J. M. (1975). Gynaecology from ancient Egypt: The papyrus Kahun: A translation of the oldest treatise on gynaecology that has survived from the ancient world. *Medical Journal of Australia, 2*(25–26), 949–952.

The Metropolitan Museum of Art. (n.d.). *Sarcophagus of the Hathor Priestess Henhenet, ca. 2051–2030 B.C.* [Photograph]. Author. Retrieved from https://www.metmuseum.org/art/collection/search/100000424

Wall, L. L. W. (2018). *Tears for my sisters. The tragedy of obstetric fistula.* Johns Hopkins University Press. ISBN-10:1421424177.

Washburn, S. L. (1960). Tools and human evolution. *Scientific American, 203*, 3–15.

Wellcome Collection. (n.d.). *A page from the Ebers Papyrus, written c. 1500 B.C.* Author. Retrieved from https://wellcomecollection.org/works/yzg97evz

Wells, C. (1975). Ancient obstetric hazards and female mortality. *Bulletin of the New York Academy of Medicine, 51*(11), 1235–1249. Retrieved September 15, 2020, from https://www.ncbi.nlm.nih.gov/pmc/articles/PMC1749741/pdf/bullnyacadmed00167-0035.pdf

Wells, J. C., DeSilva, J. M., & Stock, J. T. (2012). The obstetric dilemma: An ancient game of Russian roulette, or a variable dilemma sensitive to ecology? *American Journal of Physical Anthropology, 149*(Suppl 55), 40–71. https://doi.org/10.1002/ajpa.22160. Retrieved September 15, 2020, from https://onlinelibrary.wiley.com/doi/full/10.1002/ajpa.22160

Willis, A., Oxenham, M.F. (2013). A case of maternal and perinatal death in neolithic Southern Vietnam, c. 2100–1050 BCE. *International Journal of Osteoarchaeology, 23*(6), 676–684. https://doi.org/10.1002/oa.1296

Winlock, H. E. (1942). *Excavations at Deir el Bahri 1911-1931.* MacMillan.

Wittman, A. B., & Wall, L. L. (2007). The evolutionary origins of obstructed labor: Bipedalism, encephalization, and the human obstetric dilemma. *Obstetrical & Gynecological Survey, 62*(11), 739–748. https://doi.org/10.1097/01.ogx.0000286584.04310.5c

Zacharin, R. F. (1988). *Obstetric fistula.* Springer. ISBN 978-3-7091-8921-4.

Obstetric Fistula in Context

4

L. Lewis Wall

4.1 Defining the Problem

A fistula is an abnormal communication between two epithelialized body cavities that normally are not connected. Fistulas are named with reference to the structures that have become connected with one another: e.g., a vesicovaginal fistula is an abnormal opening between the bladder and the vagina. Fistulas sometimes arise as the result of errors in embryological development (e.g., congenital urethrovaginal fistula) (Martinez Escoriza et al., 2014; Ohno et al., 2015); more commonly, however, they are caused by trauma (Wall, 2006, 2018). In females, the most common (and most troubling) fistulas are genitourinary fistulas (vesicovaginal fistula, urethrovaginal fistula, ureterovaginal fistula, etc.) and genito-enteric fistulas (especially rectovaginal fistula). An obstetric fistula is a genitourinary or genito-enteric fistula that develops as the result of complications of the pregnant state (pregnancy, labor, delivery, and the puerperium) or from interventions, omissions, incorrect treatment, or a chain of events resulting from any of the above. Some authors use the terms "obstetric fistula" and "genitourinary fistula" interchangeably. This is incorrect. Using these terms as synonyms obscures important differences between them, which are important for their treatment and subsequent prognosis.

4.2 Pathophysiology in Context

In wealthy countries with well-developed healthcare systems, vesicovaginal fistulas are rare. Fistulas arising in these countries occur most commonly as a complication of pelvic surgery, usually hysterectomy (Hilton & Crowell, 2012; Brown et al., 2012; Hillary et al., 2016). For example, in 2016 a national referral center in Norway reported a series of 280 genital fistulas (98 genitourinary fistulas and 182 genito-enteric fistulas) seen between 1995 and 2014 (Trovik et al., 2016). Only 16% of these fistulas (42 cases) were of obstetric origin (and of these, two women had delivered outside Norway). Of the 40 obstetric fistula cases remaining, 36 were genito-enteric fistulas and only four were genitourinary fistulas. The vast majority of these injuries were rectovaginal (24) or recto-perineal lacerations

L. L. Wall (✉)
Departments of Anthropology and Obstetrics &
Gynecology, Washington University in St. Louis,
St. Louis, MO, USA
e-mail: walll@wustl.edu

© Springer Nature Switzerland AG 2022
L. B. Drew et al. (eds.), *A Multidisciplinary Approach to Obstetric Fistula in Africa*, Global
Maternal and Child Health, https://doi.org/10.1007/978-3-031-06314-5_4

(12) that failed to heal properly after delivery, with subsequent formation of a fistula. The four geni-tourinary fistulas occurred as complications of cesarean section (2), cervical cerclage (1), and uterine rupture (1). None of the genitourinary fistulas were crush injuries resulting from prolonged obstructed labor. In contrast to their rarity in wealthy Norway, genitourinary fistulas are common in low-resource countries, where thousands of women suffer avoidable obstetric trauma (Vangeenderhuysen et al., 2001; Wall, 2006; Adler et al., 2013; Cowgill et al., 2015). In Malawi, for example, the prevalence of obstetric fistula is estimated to be as high as 1.6 cases per 1000 women (Kalilani-Phiri et al., 2010).

The injury process (pathophysiology) by which a fistula is created is extremely important; it relates directly to how much difficulty is encountered during fistula repair, and this affects the prognosis for healing. The different etiologies of obstetric fistula formation are also related to different underlying socioeconomic realities in the societies where these injuries occur. In high-resource countries, fistulas occur infrequently and are complications of acute lacerations at delivery (generally rectovaginal fistu-las), whereas in the impoverished countries of Africa and Asia where obstetric fistulas are common, they often result from a prolonged crush injury of the affected tissues, rather than from an acute lac-eration. These differences in nature of the injuries explain the serious comorbidities that often accom-pany obstructed labor.

A vesicovaginal fistula occurring as a surgical complication (e.g., a post-hysterectomy fistula) is a discrete injury to otherwise healthy tissues. The fistula develops because urinary leakage from the injured bladder interferes with normal tissue healing at the surgical incision in the vaginal cuff. Incomplete healing of the incision allows a fistula to form between the bladder and vagina. In per-forming a hysterectomy, the surgeon must mobilize the bladder away from the underlying uterus and cervix before severing their attachments to the vagina. In most cases of post-hysterectomy fistula, an unrecognized injury occurs to the bladder at the time of the operation. Urine escaping from the injured bladder pools over the vaginal cuff. The continued leakage of urine through the unrecognized hole in the bladder prevents normal healing of the incision at the top of the vagina where the cervix was removed. Eventually, the urine drains into the vagina through the non-healing surgical incision, the bladder and vagina form a communication, and a fistula forms. Post-hysterectomy fistulas are gener-ally small (2–3 mm in size) but still permit large volumes of urine to escape; the tissues surrounding the fistula are uninjured, however, and this improves the prognosis for surgical repair.

Obstructed labor produces vesicovaginal fistulas through an entirely different mechanism (Wall, 2018). The fistula from obstructed labor is far more serious, is much more likely to be complicated, and has a much worse prognosis for repair than does the post-hysterectomy fistula. This distinction is critical for understanding the contextual complexities in which obstetric fistulas develop in poor countries.

Unlike the post-hysterectomy fistula from an unrecognized bladder laceration, the fistula that develops after obstructed labor is a crush injury. Whereas the post-hysterectomy fistula is a discrete injury to otherwise normal tissues, the obstetric fistula from obstructed labor is a *field injury*, which affects broad swaths of pelvic tissue and often produces a much larger, much more extensive injury.

Labor is obstructed when the fetus cannot progress through the birth canal during labor despite adequate uterine contractions (Neilson et al., 2003). This occurs in roughly 5% of labors. Obstructed labor results from a mismatch between the size of the fetus (usually the fetal head) and the space through which it must pass in the maternal pelvis (Fig. 4.1).

This condition is called "fetopelvic disproportion" or "cephalopelvic disproportion." Humans are uniquely predisposed to this problem because of two competing influences in human evolution: bipedal locomotion and encephalization (Wittman & Wall, 2007). Humans walk upright on two legs. In evolving to this mode of locomotion, the human pelvis underwent numerous architectural changes, altering the size, shape, and alignment of the pelvic inlet, the mid-pelvis, and the pelvic outlet through which a fetus must pass during labor. These changes—which were needed to maintain balance and

Fig. 4.1 Illustration of
obstructed labor in
which there is an
absolute disproportion
between the fetal head
and the available space
in the pelvis. (Smellie,
1754, public domain)

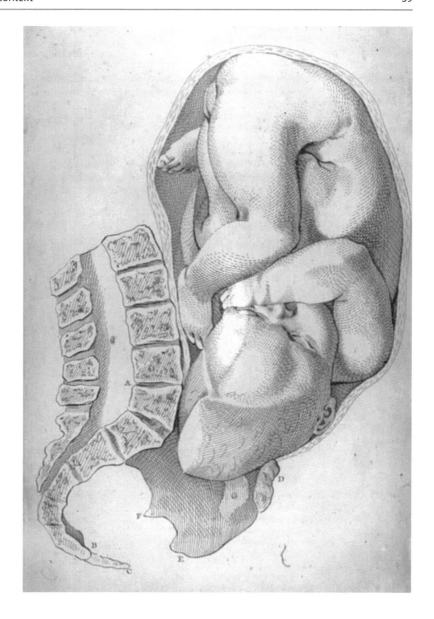

locomotive efficiency in the upright posture—also reduced the space available for fetal transit during delivery. Human evolution was also characterized by a progressive increase in brain size ("encephalization") that led to the increases in the size of the fetal head. These competing forces created what anthropologist Sherwood Washburn called the "human obstetrical dilemma:" how to get an increasingly large fetus through a diminishing pelvic space (Washburn, 1960).

The evolutionary response to this dilemma was the development of a complicated rotational mechanism during the process of delivery. Human parturition involves a seven-step process in which the fetus constantly readjusts its position as it moves through the three misaligned planes of the pelvis during labor: engagement, descent, flexion, internal rotation, extension, external rotation, and, finally, expulsion from the pelvis (Wall, 2018). If the fetus cannot successfully execute these maneuvers, labor is obstructed. The presenting fetal part (usually, but not always, the fetal head) comes to rest against the bones of the maternal pelvis. Once labor begins, labor is programmed to continue until it is completed. When labor is obstructed, the uterus continues to contract in an attempt to force the fetus past the point of obstruction. The fetal head becomes wedged deeper and more tightly into the pelvis, gradually compressing the maternal soft tissues between the pelvic bones and the fetal head (Fig. 4.2).

Eventually, enough force is exerted to cut off the blood supply to the impacted tissues. If the process is not relieved, the compressed tissues will die and slough away, producing catastrophic injuries such as a vesicovaginal fistula.

In parts of the world where maternal healthcare systems are poor and access to emergency obstetric care is limited, obstructed labor may last for several days. In the vast majority of these cases, the fetus dies from asphyxiation during labor. If the pregnant woman does not herself die from exhaustion, infection, hemorrhage, or uterine rupture (and many do), the fetus dies in her birth canal, starts to decompose, and is gradually expelled when it has softened sufficiently to slide past the point of obstruction. The injured vaginal tissues separate a few days later and slough away, producing the fistula (Fig. 4.3).

This process of pelvic crush injury may also produce a broad range of associated injuries known as the "obstructed labor injury complex" (Arrowsmith et al., 1996; Wall, 2018). The extent and severity of the resulting injuries can be breathtaking (Table 4.1): The entire bladder base may be destroyed, the raw surfaces of the pubic bones may be exposed within the vagina, the vaginal lumen may be reduced by scarring to only a pin hole, the nerves to the lower extremities may be compressed so severely that the woman can no longer walk or even stand, etc. The fetus rarely survives, and in addition to the loss of her child, the woman herself may be injured so terribly that she becomes a social outcast (Wall, 1998, 2018; Barageine et al., 2015; Mselle et al., 2011; Weston et al., 2011).

Fig. 4.2 Pathophysiology of fistula formation in obstructed labor. The bladder is wedged between the descending fetal head and the boney pelvis. Over time, the pressure exerted shuts off the blood supply to the entrapped tissues, resulting in the formation of a fistula. (Copyright © Worldwide Fistula Fund, used by permission)

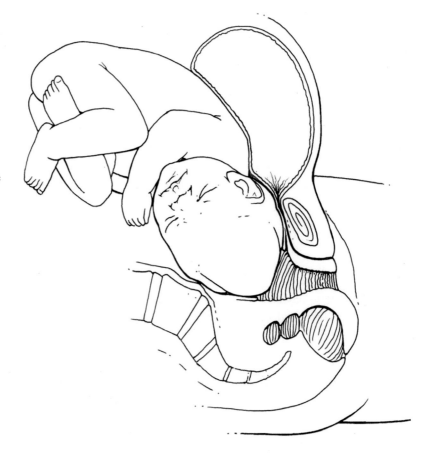

Fig. 4.3 A vesicovaginal fistula from prolonged obstructed labor. (Photograph by Andrew Browning (Wall, 2012d). Reprinted from Wall, L.L. (2012). Obstetric Fistula Is a "Neglected Tropical Disease". *PLoS Negl Trop Dis.* 6(8):e1769, Figure 1. https://doi.org/10.1371/journal.pntd.0001769. g001, licensed under the terms of the Creative Commons Attribution 4.0 International License, http://creativecommons.org/licenses/by/4.0/)

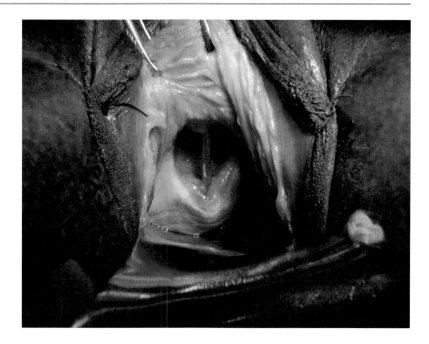

4.3 Risk Factors in Context

Since obstructed labor is caused by fetopelvic or cephalopelvic disproportion, the risk that obstruction will occur is affected by anything that increases the amount of disproportion. This can be due either to an increase in the size of the fetus or a decrease in maternal pelvic capacity. The point at which fetal descent becomes obstructed during labor and the nature and extent of the injuries that may occur depend on factors unique to each delivery.

The factors influencing disproportion may occur by biological chance alone; at other times, modifiable social or cultural factors may be present (Wall et al., 2005, 2017; Onolemhemhen & Ekwempu, 1999; Melah et al., 2007; Wright et al., 2016; Browning et al., 2014; Barageine et al., 2014; Tebu et al., 2009; Ampofo et. al. 1990; Hamed et. al. 2017). For example, male fetuses are usually larger and heavier than female fetuses. If conception results in a male fetus (determined by paternal gametes), a woman with a small pelvis has an increased risk of obstructed labor compared to the risk she has in the presence of a female fetus (but obstructed labor could still develop in either case, depending on other factors). An occiput-posterior presentation or a transverse fetal lie in labor (compared to the normal occiput-anterior presentation of the fetus) also increases the chance of obstruction. Uncontrolled diabetes results in larger fetuses, with a greater risk of obstruction during labor. Poor nutrition in childhood (perhaps worsened by cultural patterns of nutritional discrimination in which males are fed preferentially over females) may result in reduced growth and a smaller pelvic capacity, with a relative increase in the risk of obstructed labor. Adult pelvic capacity in girls is not reached until late adolescence, but menarche (with the potential for pregnancy) usually occurs much earlier than this (Moerman, 1982). Thus, girls who become pregnant in early adolescence are at relatively higher risk of obstructed labor than those who become pregnant after pelvic growth is complete (Wall et al., 2004; Akpan, 2003). Societies in which cultural tradition mandates marriage soon after menarche will therefore likely see an increase in cases of obstructed labor compared to societies in which marriage is deferred to a later age, especially if maternal healthcare systems are poorly developed. It is nonetheless true that *every* woman is potentially at risk of developing obstructed labor due to the nature of the "human

Table 4.1 Spectrum of injuries in the "obstructed labor injury complex"

Acute obstetric injury
Hemorrhage, especially post-partum hemorrhage from uterine atony
Intrauterine infection and/or systemic sepsis
Deep venous thrombosis
Massive vulvar edema
Pathological uterine retraction ring (Bandl's ring)
Uterine rupture
Urologic injury
Genitourinary fistulas (vesicovaginal fistula and complex combinations of injuries)
Urethral damage, including complete loss of the urethra
Bladder stone formation
Urinary stress incontinence
Acute and chronic ureteral injury (hydroureteronephrosis)
Acute and chronic urinary tract infection (chronic pyelonephritis)
Kidney failure
Gynecologic injury
Cessation of menstruation (amenorrhea)
Vagina scarring and narrowing, leading to loss of sexual capability
Damage to the cervix, including complete loss of the cervix
Pelvic inflammatory disease
Infertility and childlessness
Gastrointestinal injury
Rectovaginal fistula
Scarring and narrowing of the rectum
Anal sphincter injury and anal incontinence
Musculoskeletal injury
Inflammation and injury of the pubic bone
Diffuse trauma to the pelvic floor
Neurological injury
Foot drop
Neuropathic bladder dysfunction
Dermatological injury
Chronic excoriation of the skin from maceration by urine and feces
Fetal/neonatal injury
Over 90% stillbirth rate with a high death rate among living newborns
Neonatal asphyxiation, infection, and birth injuries (such as scalp damage, nerve palsies, and bleeding in the brain)
Psycho-social injury
Social isolation
Separation and divorce
Worsening poverty
Malnutrition
Post-traumatic stress disorder
Depression, sometimes leading to suicide

obstetrical dilemma" (Wittman & Wall, 2007). Many cases of obstructed labor occur in older women who have previously delivered successfully. Since fetal weight tends to increase with subsequent deliveries and since other health and life-course issues may also affect the pelvis, grand multiparous women may develop a fistula even after successfully delivering 10 or 12 children. The final factor in fistula formation in these cases is whether or not obstructed labor is recognized as soon as it occurs and whether or not it is treated effectively and in a timely fashion (Wall, 2018).

Certain harmful traditional medical practices, including the use of herbal medicines (Adaji et al., 2013), salt packing of the vagina (Underhill, 1964), and various forms of genital cutting may produce fistulas by direct trauma in pregnancy, labor, the puerperium, or completely apart from pregnancy (Tukur et al., 2006; Ouedraogo et al., 2018a, b). Female genital cutting is also strongly associated with a low status of women in societies where these practices are prevalent and, more than a specific risk factor for obstructed labor, cutting practices appear to be associated with lack of access to emergency obstetric care, low socioeconomic status, early marriage, and diminished female autonomy, all of which increase the risk of obstetric fistula (Browning et al., 2010).

4.4   The Context of Delay

Obstetric fistulas in resource-poor countries result primarily from obstructed labor that lasts long enough for necrosis of the compressed tissues to develop (Figs. 4.1 and 4.2). There is no absolute time limit beyond which this happens; rather, fistula formation depends upon how numerous variables intersect in any individual case (Fig. 4.4). The formation of an obstetric fistula can almost always be prevented if the diagnosis of obstructed labor is made early and if intervention (usually cesarean delivery) occurs promptly. It is delay in the relief of the obstruction that leads to formation of a fistula. Why do these delays occur?

In an influential article on the social context of maternal mortality, Sereen Thaddeus and Deborah Maine described three phases of delay that lead to maternal death by hindering timely, appropriate treatment of obstetrical complications (Thaddeus & Maine, 1994). The same framework applies to obstetric fistula formation, a non-fatal obstetric morbidity (Wall, 2012a, b, 2018). Obstetric fistulas develop when women in obstructed labor do not receive effective care in a timely manner.

The first delay is delay in deciding to seek care (Thaddeus & Maine, 1994; Wall, 2012c, 2018). This delay occurs when obstructed labor is not recognized as a problem that needs special help. Delays in deciding to seek care are impacted by numerous cultural factors including beliefs concerning what is normal during labor and how long labor should last. Even when labor is recognized as having lasted too long, cultural perceptions of why this is occurring and what should be done about it

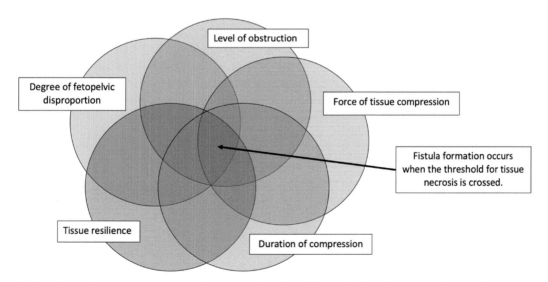

Fig. 4.4 Determinants of obstetric fistula formation. (Copyright © Worldwide Fistula Fund, used by permission)

influence decision-making. In many parts of the world, prolonged labor is attributed to misbehavior on the part of the laboring woman, rather than to mechanical obstruction (Wall, 2018). If spiritual forces are believed to be causing delayed delivery, the patient may be taken to a church, a mosque, or other centers of spiritual care for prayer or ritual intervention, rather than to a clinical facility (Udoma et al., 1999). Who makes the decision to seek care, and why? The laboring woman may lack the personal agency to seek help, the decision residing with her husband or other family members, or she may be unable to travel. The family may recognize a problem, but not know where to go, or decide that the perceived benefit of going to a nearby health facility is not worth the trouble it would take to get there. The economic costs of seeking obstetrical care (including opportunity costs) may preclude the attempt to seek care.

Once the decision to seek care has been made, the second delay is the delay in arriving at an appropriate obstetric care facility (Thaddeus & Maine, 1994; Wilson et al., 2013; Wall, 2018). Ensuring that patients know where to go when a serious problem arises is probably the most important contribution made by prenatal care programs in poor countries. In rural Africa and Asia, transportation to a clinical center may be unpredictable, unreliable, and expensive. Roads are often hazardous, particularly at night and during the rainy season. Even assuming that patients know where to go, the prospect of getting there can be daunting—and expensive. In one famous West African case study, for example, researchers in the northern town of Farafenni in the Gambia (where maternal mortality was high and obstetrical care was provided only at a dispensary manned by a dresser and one midwife) it was discovered that a woman requiring advanced obstetric care had to be transferred to the capital city of Banjul, 200 km away—a trip that took hours and required crossing the River Gambia by ferry (Greenwood et al., 1987).

The third delay is delay in receiving appropriate care after arrival at a healthcare facility (Thaddeus & Maine, 1994; Wall, 2018). This is the most tragic delay because a patient in desperate need has finally arrived at the threshold, only to find that she cannot or does not get the care she needs. There are many reasons this happens, including lack of basic resources (no electricity, water, drugs, surgical instruments, suture, intravenous fluids, blood, etc.), lack of technical capacity (no one is trained to perform a cesarean section, etc.), lack of adequate staff (lack of trained nurses, absent doctors, midwives, anesthetists, and so on), corruption (requests for bribes before care is provided), indifference, disrespect, ethnic or racial hostility, religious discrimination—the potential list of obstructive factors is long (Wall, 2018). Administrative incompetence, overwork, poor staff morale, lack of clearly delineated protocols for emergency care, and lack of funding all contribute to woefully inadequate healthcare facilities in many parts of the world (Sundari, 1992; Knight et al., 2013; Wall, 2018).

Women who survive prolonged obstructed labor only to develop a fistula often experience the so-called fourth delay—delay in receiving competent care for their injuries (Ruder et al., 2018). The experiences of women seeking care for an obstetric fistula mirror the delays experienced by women seeking help in obstructed labor. As result, many women with fistulas live with their condition for decades without gaining any relief, turning into what Reginald Hamlin called "fistula pilgrims" engaged in an endless round of travel from city to city, clinic to clinic, and hospital to hospital seeking relief (Maulet et al., 2013; Wall, 2018).

4.5   Fistula Treatment in Context

Women with an obstetric fistula face considerable challenges. Their daily lives are dominated by the need to manage the constant leakage of urine. The constant maceration of the skin may lead to painful sores and ulcers. If the urine cannot be contained or washed away regularly, it starts to smell. The afflicted woman may be burdened by additional disabilities, unable to walk or to care for her daily needs. The worst cases of childbirth injury are heart-wrenching. Johannes Dieffenbach, a nineteenth-century plastic surgery pioneer, described the spectrum of injury in a dozen patients he had collected for treatment, writing: "The extent of the disease in these 12 cases is very different. In some the orifice is very small; in others, the communication between the bladder and vagina is large. The smallest admits only a very fine probe, while others give passage to the little, or even index, finger; finally, some will admit the passage of several fingers united into the abnormal opening. In one case the uterus and vagina are prolapsed, and the perineum lacerated completely back to the anus. … The most unfortunate of all the patients is a woman 30 years of age, healthy and strong. The whole anterior wall of the vagina is split up, from behind the orifice of the urethra to the os uteri, and the bladder hangs down between the thighs, and is inverted; there is also complete rupture of the perineum, and the anus, with a part of the rectum, is equally torn through. For 17 years this unfortunate woman has been compelled to sit on a seat made for the purpose, the excretions of urine and faeces passing away under her" (Dieffenbach, 1836). It is no wonder that women afflicted in this way persist in their attempts to find a cure. The treatment challenges presented by these cases are also severe. Frequently, they are beyond what the local healthcare system can provide.

It is ironic that both the prevention of the injury and its cure are surgical. Prompt access to cesarean delivery when labor is obstructed could eliminate most of these injuries, but they continue to occur because healthcare systems in poor countries do not provide timely emergency obstetric care to many women who need it. Because surgical care is not generally available in the first place, after they develop an obstetric fistula many women cannot get competent care to repair their injuries, leading to the problem of the "fourth delay" (Ruder et al., 2018).

It has been abundantly clear for over 150 years that the best chance of repairing an obstetric fistula lies with the first attempt. As the American fistula surgeon Nathan Bozeman observed when presenting his experience to the New York Medical Society in 1868, "Any surgeon who bases his hopes upon the chances of reaching the maximum limit of success by repeated operations in the same case will surely meet with sad disappointment. It is a well known fact that every unsuccessful operation lessens the chances of an ultimate cure, by diminishing the vitality of the parts, and but few patients can be found in whom faith and power of endurance will not diminish in a like ratio" (Bozeman, 1869).

There is a debate as to where fistula repair surgery should take place (Wall, 2007). In the hands of a competent, experienced surgeon, uncomplicated cases could certainly be repaired at the local level; but considering the rudimentary nature of surgical care at most district hospitals in developing nations, a better strategy is the development of specialist referral centers in countries where these injuries are highly prevalent. This approach allows better treatment for more complex cases, assures that the simpler cases are done by surgeons with extensive experience (ensuring better outcomes), and also allows for the development of needed ancillary services such as nutritional support, physical therapy, psychological counseling, job skill training, and other forms of social rehabilitation. There are several examples of such centers in developing countries, the most famous of which is the Addis Ababa Fistula Hospital founded by Drs. Catherine and Reginald Hamlin (Wall, 2018).

An alternative approach, heavily promoted by UNFPA since 2003, has been the development of so-called fistula camps in which large numbers of women with obstetric fistulas are gathered together at temporary locations for purposes of carrying out a mass surgical campaign in which scores (or even hundreds) of cases are done over a 2-week period (UNFPA, 2006). This approach is fraught with potential problems, including not only managing the daunting logistics of coordinating the care of a large number of women who descend on the designated site, but also ensuring high standards of care during high-volume surgery, maintaining individualized treatment instead of resorting to a standardized "cookbook" approach, which ignores the vastly divergent nature of fistula cases, ensuring that patients receive proper education and give truly informed consent before undergoing surgery, and most critically, arranging competent, accessible, ongoing care to deal with postoperative complications that may arise after the surgical team has left the area (Wall et al., 2006; Wall, 2011, 2018).

4.6   Treatment Outcomes in Context

In the early nineteenth century, when the repair of obstetric fistulas was regarded as an almost hopeless endeavor that was achieved only occasionally (and then usually only by serendipity), the goal of most surgeons was simply to try to close the hole in the bladder. Because relatively few surgeons achieved even this modest goal, it was assumed that if the hole was closed, all would be well. Even early on, however, it was obvious that many women with fistulas also had other serious comorbidities that were part of the obstructed labor injury complex. Two early surgical pioneers, Thomas Addis Emmet and Nathan Bozeman, emphasized the importance of the "preparatory treatment" of the patient prior to attempted fistula repair. Great importance was attached to rehabilitating injured tissues and mobilizing extensive vaginal scarring to maximize the chances of successful closure. Often, this required operations to be carried out in stages to achieve the desired surgical goals (Emmet, 1867; Bozeman, 1887). As fistula closure became more reliable, surgeons often used "closure of the defect" as their criterion for "success," even though many patients whose fistulas were closed continued to experience persistent trans-urethral urine loss. McConnachie noted as far back as 1958 that even "though a fistulous opening is successfully closed by operation, the case is not … a cure unless she also has complete urinary continence and control" (McConnachie, 1958).

This discrepancy between fistula closure and the achievement of continence has been called the "continence gap" (Wall & Arrowsmith, 2007). Persistent incontinence can have many different causes, including irreversible damage to the normal closing mechanism of the urethra and bladder neck, reduced bladder capacity and compliance due to fibrosis, detrusor muscle over-activity ("bladder spasms"), the presence of bladder stones, and combinations of such pathologies. A more honest and realistic approach to reporting surgical outcomes is to classify patients as "closed and dry," "failed closure," or "closed but wet" (Ouedraogo et al., 2018b). It is also extremely important to provide realistic assessment of the outcomes that can and cannot be achieved to women who are about to undergo fistula surgery, particularly if achieving total continence seems unlikely based on their history and the nature of their injuries.

These comments regarding "success" apply only to regaining urinary control. It is obvious that many women with an obstetric fistula also have other complications as part of the larger obstructed labor injury complex (Arrowsmith et al., 1996; Wall, 2018). These women will not consider themselves "cured" until all of their comorbidities have been resolved. In 1966, Coetzee and Lithgow advanced the stringent view that no fistula patient should be considered "cured" unless she has complete urinary continence by day and by night with an adequate bladder capacity (~170 mL); does not lose urine with coughing or straining; has a vagina that permits normal intercourse without pain; has regular menstrual periods; and can bear children if she so desires (Coetzee & Lithgow, 1966). If standards like these are used, "success" rates will plummet—and even then no mention has yet been made of the damage to self-image that a fistula inflicts, the disrupted marital and social relationships that often result, the economic hardships that many such women endure, and the ongoing need that many women have for counseling, for reassurance, for social support, and for economic assistance during the prolonged period of their recovery.

4.7   The Human Rights Context

The brutal reality is that obstetric fistula is a "neglected tropical disease" (Wall, 2012d). Like leprosy, sleeping sickness, filariasis, and the other "NTDs," obstetric fistula is also a preventable, treatable, stigmatizing condition that primarily afflicts members of the world's "bottom billion." It is a disease of poverty; only rarely does it affect the educated, the prosperous, and the socially secure. As the British fistula surgeon Lawson Tait pointedly remarked in 1889, "I have … said that operations for vaginal fistulae are rarely paid for, except in gratitude, because the patients are nearly always poor. I must have operated on 200 or 300 cases, and I have not yet been remunerated to an extent which would pay for the instruments I have bought for the purpose" (Tait, 1889).

Most pointedly, obstetric fistula is an affliction of poor *women*. Obstetric fistula is a disorder of childbearing, the health risks and burdens of which are borne exclusively by females. Women with obstetric fistulas are innocent victims of parturition gone awry, injured through no fault of their own. In many countries where obstetric fistulas are common, women have little say in when—or even if— they become pregnant. Their control over their reproductive lives—and often even their control over their sexual activity—is heavily constrained by economics, family structure, marriage practices, imbalances in gender power, and cultural expectations of proper feminine social roles. Without reproductive choice, the pregnancies they carry are often unintended and are also frequently unwanted. Obstetric fistulas and other devastating injuries occur because women are denied their right to safe motherhood by inadequate infrastructure and inattentive policy priorities. Access to cesarean delivery in poor countries is heavily skewed toward the wealthiest quintiles of society, especially in urban areas (Ronsmans et al., 2006). The capacity to provide trained attendants at all deliveries and to ensure prompt access to emergency obstetrical care for all childbearing women is economically possible in every country in the world, but the political will to do so is often absent. This is the great medical scandal of the twenty-first century (Wall, 2018).

Equally as scandalous as the fact that obstetric fistulas continue to occur on a regular basis in the poor countries of the world is the delay that these injured women experience in getting proper care. The "fourth delay" (Ruder et al., 2018) is real, and it is made worse by the abuse these women frequently receive as they search for effective treatment. Women with fistulas are often poor, uneducated, vulnerable, and sometimes marginalized. As a result, they are often ignored or treated rudely, and sometimes, they are exploited by unscrupulous members of the community, by healthcare workers, and even by governmental and nongovernmental organizations. The human rights of women with fistulas must be emphasized as we work to eliminate this persistent scourge of childbearing.

The proper care of the obstetric fistula sufferer must be guided by sound principles of human rights. These principles should include the following (Wall, 2014):

- Every woman with an obstetric fistula has the right to be treated with compassion, dignity, and respect, irrespective of her socioeconomic status.
- Every woman with an obstetric fistula has a right to privacy. She has the right to refuse to be interviewed, photographed, or displayed in any fashion without her express consent. Receiving care at any institution where patients with fistulas are treated should not be contingent upon interviews, photographs, or displays that are not relevant to a woman's immediate clinical care.
- Every woman with an obstetric fistula has the right to have the nature of her condition—its causes, prognosis, and possible treatments—explained to her fully and completely in a language she can understand. She has the right to ask questions about these subjects and to participate actively in deliberations about her care.
- Every woman with an obstetric fistula has the right to food, clothing, and shelter sufficient to sustain her basic needs while receiving care for her condition.
- Every woman with an obstetric fistula has the right to self-determination. She has the right to be free from coercion, proselytizing, or exposure to any form of undue influence when making decisions about how, when, where, or if she is to undergo treatment.

- Every woman with an obstetric fistula has the right to refuse treatment, to refuse to participate in research studies, and to leave obstetric fistula treatment centers whenever she chooses to do so without penalty or retribution.
- Every woman with an obstetric fistula has the right to receive competent care from qualified doctors, nurses, social workers, and therapists during the course of her treatment.

Women with obstetric fistulas have full human rights and deserve to be treated with compassion, respect, and justice, as equal members of the human community. Adherence to this philosophy will help reduce the overall level of human suffering as we strive toward a world in which safe motherhood is expected for every child-bearer, no matter what her social or economic status, and no matter where on this planet she lives.

References

Adaji, S. E., Bature, S. B., & Shittu, O. S. (2013). Vaginally inserted herbs causing vesico-vaginal fistula and vaginal stenosis. *International Urogynecology Journal, 14*, 1057–1058.

Adler, A. J., Ronsmans, C., Calvert, C., & Vilippi, V. (2013). Estimating the prevalence of obstetric fistula: A systematic review and meta-analysis. *BMC Pregnancy and Childbirth, 13*, 246.

Akpan, E. O. (2003). Early marriage in eastern Nigeria and the health consequences of vesicovaginal fistulae (VVF) among young mothers. *Gender and Development, 11*(2), 70–76.

Ampofo, E. K., Omotara, B. A., Out, T., & Uchebo, G. (1990). Risk factors of vesico-vaginal fistulae in Maiduguri, Nigeria: A case-control study. *Tropical Doctor, 20*, 138–139.

Arrowsmith, S., Hamlin, E. C., & Wall, L. L. (1996). "Obstructed labor injury complex:" Obstetric fistula formation and the multifaceted morbidity of maternal birth trauma in the developing world. *Obstetrical and Gynecological Survey, 51*, 568–574.

Barageine, J. K., Tumwesigye, N. M., Byamugisha, J. K., Almroth, L., & Faxelid, E. (2014). Risk factors for obstetric fistula in western Uganda: A case-control study. *PLoS One, 9*, 11.

Barageine, J. K., Beyeza-Kashesya, J., Byamugisha, J. K., Tumwesigye, N. M., Almrosh, L., & Faxelid, E. (2015). 'I am alone and isolated': A qualitative study of experiences of women living with genital fistula in Uganda. *BMC Women's Health, 15*, 73.

Bozeman, N. (1869). Vesico-vaginal fistule and its successful treatment by the button suture. In *Extracted from the Proceedings of the New York State Medical Society*. Weed, Parsons, and Company.

Bozeman, N. (1887). The gradual preparatory treatment of the complications of urinary and fecal fistule in women, including a special consideration of the treatment of pyelitis by a new method and the prevention of the evils of incontinency of the urine by a new system of drainage. In J. B. Hamilton (Ed.), *Transactions of the International Medical Congress, 9th Session, Washington, DC* (Vol. 2, pp. 514–558).

Brown, H. W., Wang, L., Bunker, C. H., & Lowder, J. L. (2012). Lower reproductive tract fistula repair in inpatient US women, 1979-2006. *International Urogynecology Journal, 23*, 403–410.

Browning, A., Allwsorth, J. E., & Wall, L. L. (2010). The relationship between female genital cutting and obstetric fistulae. *Obstetrics & Gynecology, 115*, 578.

Browning, A., Lewis, A., & Whiteside, S. (2014). Predicting women at risk for developing obstetric fistula: A fistula index? An observational study comparison of two cohorts. *BJOG, 121*, 604–609.

Coetzee, T., & Lithgow, D. M. (1966). Obstetric fistulae of the urinary tract. *The Journal of Obstetrics and Gynaecology of the British Commonwealth, 73*, 837–844.

Cowgill, K. D., Bishop, J., Norgaard, A. K., Rubens, C. E., & Gravett, M. G. (2015). Obstetric fistula in low-resource countries: An under-valued and under-studied problem—Systematic review of its incidence, prevalence, and association with stillbirth. *BMC Pregnancy and Childbirth, 15*, 193.

Dieffenbach, J. (1836). On the cure of vesico-vaginal fistula, and laceration of the bladder and vagina. *Lancet, 26*(678), 754–758.

Emmet, T. A. (1867). Vesico-vaginal fistula: The preparatory treatment and mode of operation. *American Journal of the Medical Sciences, 54*(108), 313–321.

Greenwood, A. M., Greenwood, B. M., Bradley, A. K., Williams, K., Shenton, F. C., Tulloch, S., Byass, P., & Oldfield, F. S. J. (1987). A prospective survey of the outcome of pregnancy in a rural area of the Gambia. *Bulletin of the World Health Organization, 65*, 635–643.

Hamed, S., Ahlberg, B. M., & Trenholm, J. (2017). Powerlessness, normalization, and resistance: A Foucauldian discourse analysis of women's narratives of obstetric fistula in eastern Sudan. *Qualitative Health Research, 27*(12), 1828–1841.

Hillary, C. J., Osman, N. I., Hilton, P., & Chapple, C. R. (2016). The aetiology, treatment, and outcome of urogenital fistulae managed in well- and low-resourced countries: A systematic review. *European Urology, 70*, 478–492.

Hilton, P., & Crowell, A. D. (2012). The risk of vesicovaginal and urethrovaginal fistula after hysterectomy performed in the English National Health Service—A retrospective cohort study examining patterns of care between 2000 and 2008. *BJOG, 119*, 1447–1454.

Kalilani-Phiri, A. V., Umar, E., Lazaro, D., Lunguzi, J., & Bhilungo, A. (2010). Prevalence of obstetric fistula in Malawi. *International Journal of Gynecology & Obstetrics, 109*, 204–208.

Knight, H. E., Self, A., & Kennedy, S. H. (2013). Why are women dying when they reach the hospital on time? A systematic review of the 'third delay'. *PLoS One, 8*(5), E63846.

Martinez Escoriza, J. C., Palacios Marques, A. M., Lopez Fernandez, J. A., Feliu Rey, E., Martin Medina, P., Herraiz Romero, I., et al. (2014). Congenital vesicovaginal fistula with or without menouria: A literature review. *European Journal of Obstetrics & Gynecology and Reproductive Biology, 175*, 38–48.

Maulet, N., Keita, M., & Macq, J. (2013). Medico-social pathways of obstetric fistula patients in Mali and Niger: An 18-month cohort follow-up. *Tropical Medicine and International Health, 18*(5), 524–533.

McConnachie, E. L. F. (1958). Fistulae of the urinary tract in the female. *South African Medical Journal, 32*, 524–527.

Melah, G. S., Massa, A. A., Yahaya, U. R., Bukar, M., Kizaya, D., & El-Nafaty, A. U. (2007). Risk factors for obstetric fistulae in north-eastern Nigeria. *Journal of Obstetrics and Gynaecology, 27*(8), 819–823.

Moerman, M. L. (1982). Growth of the birth canal in adolescent girls. *American Journal of Obstetrics and Gynecology, 143*, 528–532.

Mselle, L. Z. T., Moland, K. M., Evjen-Olsen, B., Mvungi, A., & Kohi, T. W. (2011). 'I am nothing:' experiences of loss among women suffering from severe birth injuries in Tanzania. *BMC Women's Health, 11*, 49.

Neilson, J. P., Lavender, T., Quenby, S., & Wray, S. (2003). Obstructed labour. *British Medical Bulletin, 67*, 191–2004.

Ohno, K., Nakaoka, T., Takama, Y., Higashio, A., Santo, K., & Yoneda, A. (2015). Congenital urethrovaginal fistula associated with imperforate hymen causing fetal urinary ascites and abdominal cystic lesions: A case report and literature review. *Journal of Pediatric Surgery Case Reports, 3*, 48–52.

Onolemhemhen, D. O., & Ekwempu, C. C. (1999). An investigation of sociomedical risk factors associated with vaginal fistula in northern Nigeria. *Women & Health, 23*(3), 103–116.

Ouedraogo, I., McConley, R., Payne, C., Heller, A., & Wall, L. L. (2018a). Gurya cutting and female genital fistulas in Niger: Ten cases. *International Urogynecology Journal, 29*, 363–368.

Ouedraogo, I., Payne, C., Nardos, R., Adelman, A. J., & Wall, L. L. (2018b). Obstetric fistula in Niger: Six-month post-operative follow-up on 384 patients from the Danja Fistula Center. *International Urogynecology Journal, 29*, 345–351.

Ronsmans, C., Holtz, S., & Stanton, C. (2006). Socioeconomic differentials in caesarean rates in developing countries: A retrospective analysis. *Lancet, 368*, 1516–1523.

Ruder, B., Cheyney, M., & Emasu, A. A. (2018). Too long to wait: Obstetric fistula and the sociopolitical dynamics of the fourth delay in Soroti, Uganda. *Qualitative Health Research, 28*(5), 721–732.

Smellie, W. (1754). *A set of anatomical tables with explanations and an abridgment of the practice of midwifery.* Author.

Sundari, T. K. (1992). The untold story: How the health care system in developing countries contribute to maternal mortality. *International Journal of Health Services, 22*(3), 513–528.

Tait, L. (1889). *Diseases of women and abdominal surgery* (Vol. I, p. 91). Lea Brothers and Company.

Tebu, R. M., de Bernis, L., Doh, A. S., Rochat, C. H., & Delvaux, T. (2009). Risk factors for obstetric fistula in the Far North Province of Cameroon. *International Journal of Gynecology & Obstetrics, 107*, 12–15.

Thaddeus, S., & Maine, D. (1994). Too far to walk: Maternal mortality in context. *Social Science and Medicine, 38*(8), 1091–1110.

Trovik, J., Thornhill, H. F., & Kiserud, T. (2016). Incidence of obstetric fistula in Norway: A population-based prospective cohort study. *Acta Obstetricia et Gynecologica, 95*, 405–410.

Tukur, J., Jido, T. A., & Uzoho, C. C. (2006). The contribution of gishiri cut to vesicovaginal fistula in Birnin Kudu, northern Nigeria. *African Journal of Urology, 12*(3), 121–125.

Udoma, E. J., Asuquo, E. E. J., & Ekott, M. I. (1999). Maternal mortality from obstructed labor in south-eastern Nigeria: The role of spiritual churches. *International Journal of Gynecology & Obstetrics, 67*, 103–105.

Underhill, B. M. L. (1964). Salt-induced vaginal stenosis of Arabia. *The Journal of Obstetrics and Gynaecology of the British Commonwealth, 71*, 293–298.

United Nations Population Fund (UNFPA). (2006). *The fistula fortnight: Healing wounds, renewing hope (21 February – 6 March 2005) Kano, Katsina, Kebbi and Sokoto States, Nigeria.* Author.

Vangeenderhuysen, C., Prual, A., & Ould el Joud, D. (2001). Obstetric fistulae: incidence estimates for sub-Saharan Africa. *International Journal of Gynecology & Obstetrics, 73*, 65–66.

Wall, L. L. (1998). Dead mothers and injured wives: The social context of maternal morbidity and mortality among the Hausa of northern Nigeria. *Studies in Family Planning, 29*(4), 341–359.

Wall, L. L. (2006). Obstetric vesicovaginal fistula as an international public health problem. *Lancet, 368*(9542), 1201–1209.

Wall, L. L. (2007). Where should obstetric fistulas be repaired: At the district general hospital or a specialized fistula center? *International Journal of Gynecology & Obstetrics, 99*(Suppl.1), S28–S31.

Wall, L. L. (2011). Ethical concerns regarding surgical operations on vulnerable patient populations: The case of obstetric fistula. *HEC Forum, 23*(2), 115–127.

Wall, L. L. (2012a). Preventing obstetric fistulas in low-resource countries: Insights from a Haddon Matrix. *Obstetrical and Gynecological Survey, 67*, 111–121.

Wall, L. L. (2012b). A framework for analyzing the determinants of obstetric fistula formation. *Studies in Family Planning, 43*(4), 255–272.

Wall, L. L. (2012c). Overcoming Phase I delays: The critical component in obstetric fistula prevention programs in low-resource countries. *BMC Pregnancy and Childbirth, 12*, 68.

Wall, L. L. (2012d). Obstetric fistula is a 'neglected tropical disease'. *PLoS Neglected Tropical Diseases, 6*(8), E1769.

Wall, L. L. (2014). A bill of rights for patients with obstetric fistula. *International Journal of Gynecology & Obstetrics, 127*, 301–304.

Wall, L. L. (2018). *Tears for my sisters: The tragedy of obstetric fistula*. Johns Hopkins University Press.

Wall, L. L., & Arrowsmith, S. D. (2007). The "Continence Gap:" A critical concept in obstetric fistula repair. *International Urogynecology Journal, 8*(8), 843–844.

Wall, L. L., Karshima, J. A., Kirschner, C., & Arrowsmith, S. D. (2004). The obstetrical vesicovaginal fistula: Characteristics of 899 patients from Jos, Nigeria. *American Journal of Obstetrics and Gynecology, 190*, 1011–1019.

Wall, L. L., Arrowsmith, S. D., Briggs, N. D., Browning, A., & Lassey, A. T. (2005). The obstetric vesicovaginal fistula in the developing world. *Obstetrical and Gynecology Survey, 60*(Suppl 1), S1–S55.

Wall, L. L., Arrowsmith, S. D., Lassey, A. T., & Danso, K. A. (2006). Humanitarian ventures or 'fistula tourism'? The ethical perils of pelvic surgery in the developing world. *International Urogynecology Journal, 17*(6), 559–562.

Wall, L. L., Belay, S., Hargeot, T., Dukes, J., Berhan, E., & Abreha, M. (2017). A case-control study of the risk factors for obstetric fistula in Tigray, Ethiopia. *International Urogynecology Journal, 28*, 1817–1824.

Washburn, S. (1960). Tools and human evolution. *Scientific American, 203*, 3–15.

Weston, K., Muytiso, S., Mwangi, J. W., Qureshi, Z., Beard, J., & Venkat, P. (2011). Depression among women with obstetric fistula in Kenya. *International Journal of Gynecology & Obstetrics, 115*, 31–33.

Wilson, A., Hillman, S., Rosato, M., Skelton, J., Costello, A., Jussein, J., MacArthur, C., & Coomarasamy, A. (2013). A systematic review and thematic synthesis of qualitative studies on maternal emergency transport in low- and middle-income countries. *International Journal of Gynecology & Obstetrics, 122*, 192–201.

Wittman, A. B., & Wall, L. L. (2007). The evolutionary origins of obstructed labor: Bipedalism, encephalization, and the human obstetric dilemma. *Obstetrical and Gynecological Survey, 62*(11), 739–748.

Wright, J., Ayenachew, F., & Ballard, K. D. (2016). The changing face of obstetric fistula surgery in Ethiopia. *International Journal of Women's Health, 8*, 243–248.

Co-occurrence of Obstetric Fistula and Stillbirth in Sub-Saharan Africa

5

Karen D. Cowgill

Abbreviations

DHS	Demographic and Health Survey
EmOC	Emergency Obstetric Care
EmONC	Emergency Obstetric and Neonatal Care
GBD	Global Burden of Disease
HDI	Human Development Index
OF	Obstetric fistula
SB	Stillbirth
VF	Vaginal fistula

5.1 Background

Prolonged obstructed labor can lead to a host of physical and psychosocial injuries to the laboring woman, collectively known as "obstructed labor injury complex" (Wall, 2012d), when emergency obstetric care (EmOC) is unavailable or inaccessible. One potentially life-altering birth injury to the mother that follows from prolonged obstructed labor is obstetric fistula (OF). A potential consequence of obstructed labor to the fetus is stillbirth (SB). Both of these events are often surrounded by stigma or shame and not disclosed or discussed at either the personal or community level (Changole et al., 2017; Desalliers et al., 2017; Heller, 2018). Consequently, they have been both underappreciated and undercounted in the realms of health policy and research.

In this chapter, I make the case that because SB so often occurs with the development of OF, these two events should routinely be considered together. A holistic view that encompasses the woman and her fetus should be embraced in the context of prevention efforts, measurement of years lived with

K. D. Cowgill (✉)
University of Washington Tacoma, Tacoma, WA, USA

University of Washington, Seattle, WA, USA
e-mail: kdc8@uw.edu

© Springer Nature Switzerland AG 2022
L. B. Drew et al. (eds.), *A Multidisciplinary Approach to Obstetric Fistula in Africa*, Global Maternal and Child Health, https://doi.org/10.1007/978-3-031-06314-5_5

disability and years of life lost, and in the care extended to women who have developed OF. This chapter starts by defining OF and describing its risk factors and repercussions and then reviews estimates of its prevalence and incidence in sub-Saharan Africa. This is followed by a brief definition of SB and its risk factors and a review of global and regional estimates of its incidence. Finally, the chapter reviews reports from sub-Saharan Africa of SB in conjunction with OF, arguing for improved surveillance and prevention of these two events.

5.2   Obstetric Fistula in Sub-Saharan Africa

Obstetric fistula (OF) is caused when the presenting fetal part continually compresses the birth canal tissues, bladder base, urethra or rectum causing ischemia (loss of circulation) and necrosis (cell death) of the tissues, resulting in a fistula—an abnormal opening, or passageway. In most cases, the fistula occurs between the vagina and bladder (i.e., vesicovaginal), but it may also occur between the vagina and rectum (i.e., rectovaginal) (Wall et al., 2005). As a result of the fistula, women leak urine and/or feces out of the vagina continually without control and can experience medical complications, including infection (Ramphal & Moodley, 2006).

In countries where EmOC is available and accessible, OF has been virtually eliminated; when it does occur, it is often iatrogenic in origin and relatively minor, due to errant cuts during cesarean sections rather than to prolonged obstructed labor, and it is promptly repaired (Ismail, 2015; Naidoo et al., 2018; Osman et al., 2018; Reisenauer, 2016; Trovik et al., 2016). However, severe OF continues to be prevalent and problematic in many less-developed regions of the world despite the fact that it is preventable and treatable (Wall, 2006). Surgical repair can be successful, but success depends on the extent of the damage, the skill of the surgeon, management of the urinary catheter in the vulnerable post-operative period, and resistance of the repair to the stress of sexual intercourse or the exertions associated with physical labor or subsequent childbirth (Delamou et al., 2015). For example, Ouedraogo et al. (2018) reported that only 57% of the most difficult cases as compared to 92% of the simplest cases were repaired at their fistula center in Niger. Quality of life may improve substantially for women following surgery, but remain poor for some women who remain incontinent (Drew et al., 2016; Mafo Degge et al., 2017; Wilson et al., 2016). Surgery to repair OF can be difficult for women to access or afford (Miller et al., 2005), especially since fistula repair facilities or campaigns are relatively few and far between, women may not be aware of them or of the services they provide, quality of care may be poor, and there are substantial opportunity costs involved in the long waits for and recuperation from surgery (Baker et al., 2017; Keya et al., 2018; Khisa et al., 2017; Mselle & Kohi, 2015).

From a biological perspective, OF results from prolonged obstructed labor, which is most often due to cephalopelvic disproportion, meaning the head of the fetus is too large to pass through the woman's pelvis, or else to a malpresentation of the fetus, in which it is bottom- or leg-first instead of head-first (Miller et al., 2005). Underdeveloped pelvic bony structure in pregnant women is therefore a risk factor for obstructed labor and OF. In regions where young girls become pregnant, or where malnutrition that leads to stunting is prevalent, obstructed labor and OF are more common (Tsui et al., 2007; Wall, 2012d).

Seen from a biosocial perspective, OF results from inadequate EmOC due to the three delays that contribute to maternal death, described by Thaddeus and Maine in a seminal 1994 paper (Thaddeus & Maine, 1994) and discussed by Wall in the context of OF (Wall, 2012a). OF has been associated with a range of social factors and conditions that are associated with poor health outcomes for women and their children: women's lack of autonomy (Kaplan et al., 2017; Mselle & Kohi, 2016), lack of education or knowledge, and gender-based violence (Mallick & Tripathi, 2018). Women with OF often

suffer significant psychosocial repercussions, including isolation, divorce, loss of income, stigmatization, shame, diminished self-esteem, and loss of social roles, including the role of mother, for those
whose infants are stillborn (Roush, 2009).

While there is work underway on the part of governments and non-governmental organizations to
find, treat, and prevent OF in low-resource countries, reliable population-based estimates of its incidence and prevalence are lacking (Stanton et al., 2007; Tunçalp et al., 2015; Wall et al., 2005). These
data are needed to inform policy and to make visible the costs in human suffering and potential lives
lost from lack of effective EmOC. Improvements in access to and quality of obstetric surgical care can
reduce the incidence of OF, as demonstrated by disease burden modeling (Higashi et al., 2015), provider training initiatives (Elneil & Browning, 2009), and prompt referral of women with prolonged
labor (Ballard et al., 2016; Seim et al., 2014).

This chapter updates an earlier systematic review (Cowgill et al., 2015) in which we identified and
screened 1541 records and included 19 with OF incidence or prevalence data worldwide. For this
chapter, the author updated earlier searches in PubMed and CAB Global (see search terms in Box 5.1)
and limited results to those published after January 1, 1995, and indexed by December 31, 2018,
reporting data from sub-Saharan Africa and included an additional five articles with OF incidence or
prevalence data; see Table 5.1 for information from the 16 included references.

We reviewed titles and/or abstracts of all search results and selected articles addressing obstetric
fistula incidence or prevalence in sub-Saharan African countries for full-text review. An ancestry
search of references in reviewed articles yielded additional resources.

Published or grey literature articles obtained through ancestry searches or in response to email
requests were included if they were published after January 1, 1995, and met the following inclusion
criteria: (1) They provided original population-based OF incidence and/or prevalence data, (2) data
were from sub-Saharan Africa, and (3) the resource was in English, Spanish, French, Chinese,
Portuguese, Polish, or German.

We extracted data on OF and standardized fistula incidence or prevalence estimates to be expressed
per 1000 to facilitate comparisons. For primary data from non-weighted samples, we obtained exact
95% confidence intervals using OpenEpi.com, a free open-access tool that permits simple epidemiologic calculations. We assessed risk of bias in individual OF studies by taking into account the study
design, clarity of the documentation of methods, the definition of and the precision of the estimated
size of the reference population, whether samples were selected randomly, the case definition of OF
applied, whether cases were determined based on self-report alone or on physical examination, and
peer-review status. We did not conduct a meta-analysis due to the clinical heterogeneity of the data
(Pai et al., 2004).

Box 5.1 Search Terms for Articles on Obstetric Fistula Indexed in PubMed and CAB Global
((vaginal OR vesicovaginal OR rectovaginal OR obstetric OR ureterovaginal OR urethrovaginal
OR genitourinary OR urogenital) AND (fistula OR fistulas OR fistulae)) NOT (iatrogenic OR
penis OR testicular OR testicle OR scrotal OR scrotum OR hypospadias OR congenital OR
cancer OR radiation OR renal OR kidney OR dialysis OR crohn's OR diverticular OR diverticu-
losis OR diverticulitis OR esophageal OR behcet's OR cholelithiasis).

Table 5.1 Obstetric fistula incidence/prevalence estimates by country, sub-Saharan Africa 1995–2018

Author, year	Country	Sample	Data source	Obstetric fistula incidence estimates	Obstetric fistula prevalence estimates	Risk of bias—potential source of bias
Low risk of bias						
Prual et al. (2000), Vangeenderhuysen et al. (2001)	West Africa: Abidjan (Côte d'Ivoire), Bamako (Mali), Niamey (Niger), Nouakchott (Mauritania), Ouagadougou (Burkina Faso), Saint-Louis (Senegal), and rural Kaolack (Senegal)	19,342 post-partum women of 21,557 pregnant women identified in door-to-door census	Multicenter, prospective, population-based surveys and gynecologic examination	Overall: **0.103** (95% CI 0–0.37) per 1000 deliveries Urban: **0** (95% CI 0–0.18) per 1000 deliveries Rural: **1.24** (95% CI 0.15–4.46) per 1000 deliveries		*Low*
Walraven et al. (2001)	Farafenni, The Gambia	1056 (56.0%) of 1871 women aged 15–54 years living in one of 20 semi-randomly sampled villages in a demographic surveillance area	Survey and gynecologic examination		**0.95** per 1000 women aged 15–54 years (95% CI 0.03–5.27) 1/1056	*Low*
Muleta et al. (2007)	Seven of 11 administrative regions of Ethiopia	Random multistage sampling of regions 22,826 women aged 15–49 years	House-to-house survey to identify women with any problem of bowel or bladder control followed by physical examination		Any OF every **2.45** per 1000 women 15–49 years (95% CI 1.87–3.17) 56/22,826 Estimated number of fistula patients in rural Ethiopia is approximately 26,819	*Low*

Adler et al. (2013a, b)	South Sudan (Western Bahr el Ghazal State)	8865 women of childbearing age estimate based on 20% of population	Key informants identified probable cases which were confirmed by physical examination	**0.34** per 1000 women aged 15–49 years 3/8865 (95% CI 0.07–1.0)	*Low*
Ballard et al. (2016)	Three rural zones of Ethiopia	Cross-sectional population-based study of maternal health experiences in eight health centers supported by Hamlin Fistula Ethiopia and 18 control health centers Women aged 15–49 years	DHS fistula screening question asked if women ever experienced a condition in which she continuously leaked urine and/or feces following childbirth followed by clinical examination with methylene blue dye test	**0.56** per 1000 (95% CI 0.31–0.94) 13 of 23,023 women screened were confirmed on examination to have VVF	*Low*
Mocumbi et al. (2017)	Maputo and Gaza provinces in Mozambique	Cross-sectional population-based study nested in a prospective cohort Women 12–49 years old who had delivered in previous 12 months	Structured interview to determine self-reported urinary incontinence with fistula confirmed on clinical examination	**1.1** per 1000 (95% CI 0.4–2.5) five fistulas among 4358 women interviewed	*Low*
Moderate risk of bias					
Mabeya (2004)	West Pokot, Kenya	Recruitment of cases via community outreach	Hospital Medical Records 1999–2003 Estimated district population WRA 150,000	**0.44** per 1000 WRA[a] (95% CI 0.34–0.56) 66 OF repairs/150,000 WRA	*Moderate* – grey literature conference proceeding – estimated reference population – relied on medical record review

(continued)

Table 5.1 (continued)

Author, year	Country	Sample	Data source	Obstetric fistula incidence estimates	Obstetric fistula prevalence estimates	Risk of bias—potential source of bias
High risk of bias						
NSO and ORC Macro (2005)	Malawi	DHS[b] systematic sample of households within clusters	Probable fistula determined by asking if women who gave birth in past 5 years had leakage of urine or stool from vagina following most recent birth		**16.1** per 1000 (95% CI 13.4–19.2) 117/7272 women	*High* – self-report of OF status – proxy measure of OF
Uganda Bureau of Statistics (UBOS) and Macro International Inc (2006)	Uganda	DHS systematic sample of households within clusters	Probable fistula determined by asking if parous women had leakage of urine or stool from vagina following delivery		**26.4** per 1000 women aged 15–49 years reported ever experiencing uncontrollable leakage of urine or stool from vagina (95% CI 23.1–30.0) likely overestimate 225/8531 women	*High* – self-report of OF status – proxy measure of OF
Johnson (2007)	Malawi	DHS systematic sample of households within clusters	DHS interview Probable fistula determined by asking if women who gave birth in past 5 years had leakage of urine or stool from vagina following most recent birth		**15.6** per 1000 live births (95% CI 13.5–18.1) 183 OF/11,699 live births Lifetime prevalence of vaginal fistula symptoms in women aged 15–49 years 4.7% (assuming all fistulas were obstetric in origin)	*High* – self-report of OF status – proxy measure of OF
Tsui et al. (2007)	Nigeria	DHS systematic sample of households within clusters	Models based on 1999 DHS prolonged labor data, UN population data, and probability of obstructed labor given prolonged labor + probability of OF given obstructed labor	Projected OF incidence: **2.11** per 1000 deliveries in women 12–49 years; **4.09** per 1000 deliveries in women <20 years		*High* – estimated conditional probabilities

Kalilani-Phiri et al. (2010)	Nine districts in Malawi	Cross-sectional population-based study with multistage random sampling, respondents reported their own or others' OF + hospital records were reviewed Denominator estimated as 60% of female population in 2008 Malawi census	Community survey asking if women who gave birth in past 5 years had leakage of urine or stool from vagina following a delivery or if their sisters had; also hospital record review	**81.0**/1000 survey respondents (95% CI 72.1–90.8) 266/3282 respondents and **22.9**/1000 siblings (95% CI 18.2–28.4) 75/3279 siblings reported fistula symptoms Combined estimate from all sources: lifetime prevalence **1.6** per 1000 women, excluding repaired OF	*High* – excluded women with repaired OF – estimated denominator of women 12–45 years old
Biadgilign et al. (2013)	Ethiopia	DHS systematic sample of households within clusters	DHS survey 2005 Probable fistula determined by asking if parous women had leakage of urine or stool from vagina following delivery	**10.6**/1000 (95% CI 8.7–12.8) parturient women aged 15–49 years ever experienced uncontrollable leakage of urine or stool from vagina 103/9713	*High* – self-report of OF status – proxy measure of OF
Maheu-Giroux et al. (2015b)	Ethiopia Mali Democratic Republic of the Congo Nigeria Kenya Burkina Faso Senegal Chad Togo Malawi Tanzania Republic of Congo Cameroon Benin Uganda Niger Guinea Comoros Sierra Leone	MICS in Chad and Togo, DHS in all others systematic sample of households within clusters	Household surveys 2005–2013 Probable fistula determined by asking if women ever experienced fistula symptoms (questions varied by survey)	*Lifetime OF prevalence* corrected for imperfect sensitivity and specificity Ethiopia **7.1** per 1000 Mali **0.7** per 1000 Democratic Republic of the Congo **1.8** per 1000 Nigeria **3.2** per 1000 Kenya **9.1** per 1000 Burkina Faso **0.4** per 1000 Senegal **0.5** per 1000 Chad **1.9** per 1000 Togo **2.3** per 1000 Malawi **5.1** per 1000 Tanzania **5.4** per 1000 Republic of Congo **1.7** per 1000 Cameroon **3.2** per 1000 Benin **6.5** per 1000 Uganda **19.2** per 1000 Niger **0.8** per 1000 Guinea **5.5** per 1000 Comoros **14.1** per 1000 Sierra Leone **6.0** per 1000	*High* – self-report of OF status – proxy measure of OF – insufficient correction for specificity

Table 5.1 (continued)

Author, year	Country	Sample	Data source	Obstetric fistula incidence estimates	Obstetric fistula prevalence estimates	Risk of bias—potential source of bias
Mallick and Tripathi (2018)	Cameroon Comoros Ethiopia Kenya Malawi Mali Nigeria Sierra Leone Tanzania Togo Uganda Zambia	DHS systematic sample of households within clusters	DHS surveys 2008–2016 DHS interview Probable fistula determined by asking if women ever experienced a constant leakage of urine or stool from their vagina during the day and night		*Fistula due to any cause* Cameroon **3** per 1000 Comoros **15** per 1000 Ethiopia **5** per 1000 Kenya **10** per 1000 Malawi **4** per 1000 Mali **7** per 1000 Nigeria **4** per 1000 Sierra Leone **9** per 1000 Tanzania **5** per 1000 Togo **10** per 1000 Uganda **18** per 1000 Zambia **6** per 1000	*High* – self-report of gynecologic fistula status – proxy measure of gynecologic fistula – proportion due to delivery between 50% and 90%

[a]*WRA* women of reproductive age
[b]*DHS* Demographic and Health Surveys

5.3   Obstetric Fistula Incidence/Prevalence

Obstetric fistula incidence and/or prevalence data were available for 25 countries in Africa. Estimates varied widely, ranging from less than 1 to more than 80 cases of OF per 1000 deliveries. The reference populations for estimates differed, with most based on women of reproductive age, defined as 15–44, 49, or 54 years, and some limited to women who had ever married or ever been pregnant. Table 5.1 describes the included obstetric fistula incidence/prevalence studies and groups them by risk of bias. Studies in which estimates were based on interview alone were classified as having high risk of bias, because interviews may misclassify other conditions that cause incontinence as fistula unless they are confirmed by physical examination. All studies in which initial report of fistula symptoms was followed by a confirmatory physical examination were classified as having low risk of bias.

Only two of the 15 included studies reported OF incidence. In one of these, a research group in West Africa reported 0.1 OF cases per 1000 deliveries based on physical examinations of post-partum women (Prual et al., 2000; Vangeenderhuysen et al., 2001), with a higher incidence in rural than urban residents (1.2 (95% confidence interval (CI) 0.15–4.46) vs. 0 (95% CI 0–0.18) cases per 1000 among post-partum women). The other study reporting incidence used a model based on Demographic and Health Survey (DHS) data from Nigeria. It projected 4.09 OF cases per 1000 deliveries in women under 20 years of age, and 2.11 per 1000 deliveries in women aged 12–49 years (Tsui et al., 2007). This model extrapolated OF incidence by using data about the frequency of prolonged labor and applying a probability of obstruction given prolonged labor and then a probability of fistula given obstruction.

Of the 13 articles reporting period or lifetime OF prevalence estimates, seven were based on data obtained from DHS surveys. Estimates based on surveys alone tended to be much higher. One study (Ballard et al., 2016) was conducted independently using the question developed for the DHS survey; in this case, the authors identified 35 cases of suspected fistula, of which 13 were confirmed on physical examination, for an estimated incidence of 0.56 cases per 1000 women aged 15–49 years.

A note that we did not include two studies by Filippi and colleagues (Filippi et al., 2007, 2010) that were included in Adler et al.'s 2013 review of OF prevalence (Adler et al., 2013b) because the participants in those studies were selected based on having severe obstetric complications and thus did not represent prevalence in the general population. Similarly, we excluded a hospital-based study from Nigeria (Ijaiya & Aboyeji, 2004) out of concern that the numerator and denominator estimates were not clearly based on the same source populations.

5.4   Stillbirth

Another potential consequence of prolonged obstructed labor is stillbirth (SB), defined by the World Health Organization (WHO) as fetal death at 1000 g or greater body weight, 28 or more weeks of completed gestation, or 35 cm or longer body length (World Health Organization, 2016). However, WHO and other authors acknowledge that the line between a miscarriage in which the fetus would not be considered viable and a SB varies from one setting to another depending on medical care (Blencowe et al., 2016).

Groups have approached the question of how best to count SB from various angles. Some have used existing data to model SB rates and project numbers worldwide. For example, WHO estimated 2.6 million stillbirths worldwide in 2009; Cousens et al. (2011) similarly estimated the number in that same year to be between 2.14 and 3.82 million SB, three-quarters of which were in south Asia and sub-Saharan Africa (Cousens et al., 2011). The same group (Blencowe et al., 2016) estimated 2.4–3 million SB in 2015, with a rate in sub-Saharan Africa at 28.7 per 1000, for a total of 1.06 million SB in sub-Saharan Africa alone that year. They estimate that the rate of SB has been falling, but as the world's population is increasing, the absolute number has remained about the same. The Global Burden of Disease (GBD) models estimate a 68% decline in SB rates between 1970 and 2016; their estimate of the number of SB worldwide in 2016 is one-third lower than that of Blencowe et al. (2016) at 1.7 million (GBD 2016 Mortality Collaborators, 2017).

Models such as these which are based on existing data have limitations because data on SBs are often incomplete or of poor quality. Another approach is illustrated by research groups who have prospectively followed all pregnancies at sites in several countries to produce population-based estimates; these studies avoid the data quality pitfall but have the disadvantage of being more limited in scope. The Global Network's Maternal Newborn Health Registry (McClure et al., 2015) prospectively followed women who were pregnant over 4 years at ten sites in six LMICs in South Asia, sub-Saharan Africa, and Latin America where civil registration and vital statistics are lacking. They used a modified WHO definition of SB in which fetuses of 20 weeks' gestation or greater or 500 g or more were counted and classified as fresh or macerated (maceration indicates fetal death at least 6 h before delivery, World Health Organization, 2016). They found increased risk of SB in deliveries not attended by a healthcare professional. Operative delivery reduced the risk of SB, but still 7.6% of the SB they counted were delivered by cesarean section, most commonly because of obstructed labor. They found the highest rates of SB at their South Asian study sites, as did another multi-country prospective cohort study of stillbirths (AMANHI, 2018). Of note, the results from these prospective studies conflict with the model-based estimates from the 2017 Global Burden of Disease (GBD) study (GBD 2016 Mortality Collaborators, 2017), which projected the highest rates in central sub-Saharan Africa.

Regardless of the approach used, all authors agree that SB is an important and overlooked issue and that most SBs—98%, by some estimates (McClure et al., 2015)—now occur in low- and middle-income countries (LMICs). Between one-third (Lawn et al., 2010) and one-half (Blencowe et al., 2016) of these occur in the intrapartum period, indicating that the fetus might have survived if adequate obstetric care had been received. Indeed, fetal death during labor is as much as 50 times greater in developing than developed countries (McClure et al., 2006). Antepartum SBs, in which the fetus dies before the start of labor, are associated with conditions such as chronic or acute disease or nutritional deficiencies in the mother or with placental malfunction or fetal anomalies; interventions that improve the pre-pregnancy health of girls and women and antenatal care that addresses the health of the woman and her fetus during pregnancy may reduce the occurrence of antepartum SB (Haws et al., 2009). However, in many cases of intrapartum SB, the fetus is viable, but complications during delivery and lack of EmOC and/or emergency neonatal care (EmNC) cause it to die. These SB are preventable with appropriate EmONC, and it is these intrapartum SBs that make up a larger proportion of SB in LMICs (Blencowe et al., 2016). An editorial in *The Lancet* puts it this way: "*The truly horrific figure is 1.3 million intrapartum stillbirths. The idea of a child being alive at the beginning of labour and dying for entirely preventable reasons during the next few hours should be a health scandal of international proportions*" (Horton & Samarasekera, 2016).

SB rates are underreported and undervalued (Lawn et al., 2014; Phillips & Millum, 2014), but are known to be closely associated with maternal mortality rates (Lawn et al., 2010). Little has been reported about the association of SB with maternal *morbidity* rates, which may be ten to hundreds of times higher than maternal mortality rates (Prual et al., 1998; Wall et al., 2005). The treatment most likely to improve both maternal and fetal outcomes in obstructed labor is cesarean section, so increasing access to EmOC is a cornerstone of preventing both OF and SB (Dolea & Abouzahr, 2003; Wall, 2012c).

5.5   Stillbirth with Obstetric Fistula

Intrapartum SB associated with prolonged obstructed labor often occurs with OF, and many women who experience OF must also grieve a stillborn baby (Roush, 2009). Some take it as a given that without intervention, a fetus will almost certainly die during prolonged obstructed labor—that in fact, what often resolves the obstruction is the death and decomposition of the fetus that allows its head to compress enough to pass through the vaginal canal (Wall, 2018). Indeed, many case series of women with OF report that 100% of fetuses in the delivery that caused the OF were stillborn. However, others report that some infants were born living and survived.

We reviewed titles and/or abstracts of all search results (see Box 5.2 for search terms) and selected articles addressing obstetric fistula incidence, prevalence, or the correlation between obstetric fistula and stillbirth in sub-Saharan African countries for full-text review. An ancestry search of references in reviewed articles yielded additional resources. Published or grey literature articles obtained through database, manual, and ancestry searches were included if they were published after January 1, 1995, and provided frequency of SB associated with OF from countries in sub-Saharan Africa. Twelve articles published since our earlier review met the inclusion criteria.

For studies reporting the proportion of SB among deliveries that led to OF, we did not perform an explicit assessment of bias, as these estimates were generally not part of the studies' main objectives. Instead, we commented on factors that might decrease the validity of estimates, recognizing that small sample size, while it may decrease precision of estimates, is not in itself a source of bias. We did not conduct a meta-analysis due to the clinical heterogeneity of the data.

Table 5.2 describes data from 53 studies that reported SB and OF data from sub-Saharan Africa; one study (Barone et al., 2012) included information about both Africa and Bangladesh. The reported proportion of infants stillborn to women who developed OF at the same delivery ranged from 64% to 100%. Three articles did not report if SB was the outcome of the OF-inducing delivery or a previous one (Holme et al., 2007; Kirby et al., 2012; Savan et al., 2010). Two articles reported a large percentage of unknown fetal outcomes; one of these (Hawkins et al., 2013) reported a SB proportion of 55%, with an additional 38% of unknown outcomes, while the other (Roenneburg et al., 2006) reported 46% stillborn with fistula and 45% with unknown fetal outcome; it is likely that many deliveries with unknown outcomes also resulted in stillbirths. Another article (Husain et al., 2005) did not report fetal outcome, but noted that in 21 women (56% of cases), "the mode of delivery associated with fistula was 'destructive delivery' (evacuation of a stillborn fetus)." Fetal outcome of the remaining 44% of cases was not reported.

In one study that reported SB statistics for both cesarean section deliveries and spontaneous vaginal deliveries (Onsrud et al., 2011), SB proportions were higher in the vaginal delivery groups (96.4%) than the cesarean group (87.2%), consistent with the idea that cesarean can reduce fetal mortality. In another study of nearly 15,000 women with OF, more than half of infants were male (635 cases, 70.6%), and SB rates were higher for boy (91.9%) than girl (78.9%) fetuses (Muleta et al., 2010), consistent with male fetuses being larger.

It would be ideal to have population-based data linking OF and SB, but only two (Ballard et al., 2016; Mocumbi et al., 2017) of the articles included here are population-based. The rest are facility-based estimates of SB in births that caused OF. It is hard to judge how accurately these reflect the true

---

Box 5.2 Search Terms to Identify Articles on Stillbirth and Obstetric Fistula in Africa

(stillbirth OR perinatal mortality OR fetal death) AND (fistula OR fistulae OR fistulas OR obstructed labor) AND Africa.

Table 5.2 Articles reporting on co-occurrence of obstetric fistula and stillbirth, sub-Saharan Africa, 1995–2018

Article	Country	Fistula cases, obstetric etiology	% of fistula cases with stillbirth or perinatal death	Comments
Barone et al. (2012)	(Bangladesh)	1243	88%	Includes 46 early neonatal deaths
	Guinea			
	Nigeria			
	Niger			
	Uganda			
Nathan et al. (2009)	Benin	37	95%	
Tebeu et al. (2009)	Cameroon	42	83%	
Tebeu et al. (2012)	Cameroon	38	74%	
Benfield et al. (2011)	Democratic Republic of the Congo	57	88%	
Onsrud et al. (2011)	Democratic Republic of the Congo	440	92%	Stillbirth occurred in 95% of vaginal and 87% of cesarean deliveries
Benfield et al. (2019)	Democratic Republic of the Congo	171	74%	Fistula repair patients at a single hospital, 2009–2012
				44% delivered by cesarean section, 19% with assistance
				18/40 live births were by spontaneous vaginal delivery
Loposso et al. (2015)	Democratic Republic of the Congo	117	100%	Fistula repair patients at a single hospital, 2006–2011
				>63% were delivered by cesarean section after mean duration of 31 h (range 8–61 h)
Bulanda Nsambi et al. (2018)	Democratic Republic of the Congo	242	93.4%	Fistula repair campaign attendees
				229 fistulas resulted from vaginal and 13 from cesarean deliveries
				No information on the proportion of stillbirths occurring for each type of delivery
Turan et al. (2007)	Eritrea	26	100%	
Browning et al. (2007)	Ethiopia	51	98%	
Goh (1998)	Ethiopia	110	95.5%	
Browning (2006)	Ethiopia	481	95.2%	
Browning et al. (2010)	Ethiopia	489	94%	
Kelly (1995)	Ethiopia	300	93%	

Table 5.2 (continued)

Article	Country	Fistula cases, obstetric etiology	% of fistula cases with stillbirth or perinatal death	Comments
Muleta et al. (2010)	Ethiopia	14,822	92%	Cases accrued between 1974 and 2008. 434 cases reported baby's sex; 91.1% of males and 78.9% of females were stillborn
Gessessew and Mesfin (2003)	Ethiopia	184	88.6%	
Ballard et al. (2016)	Ethiopia	13	77%	Population-based data
				Two delivered by cesarean section
Sori et al. (2016)	Ethiopia	168	86%	
Delamou et al. (2015)	Guinea	2116	94%	65% delivered vaginally, 33% by cesarean section, 2% unknown
				Case series of fistula repair patients 2007–2013
Khisa and Nyamongo (2012)	Kenya	8	88%	
McFadden et al. (2011)	Kenya	77	87%	Includes 11 early neonatal deaths
Mabeya (2004)	Kenya	64	73%	Grey literature. Includes three early neonatal deaths
Weston et al. (2011)	Kenya	70	64%	
Hawkins et al. (2013)	Kenya	303	76%	Includes eight neonatal deaths; excludes 180 births with unknown outcome
Roka et al. (2013)	Kenya	70	78.6%	
Raassen et al. (2008)	Kenya, Tanzania and Uganda	579	88%	Includes 18 neonatal deaths in first week. Stillbirth occurred in 90% of vaginal and 87% of cesarean deliveries
Rijken and Chilopora (2007)	Malawi	379	87%	Includes 23 early neonatal deaths
Mocumbi et al. (2017)	Malawi	5	100%	Population-based data
				Includes one early neonatal death

Table 5.2 (continued)

Article	Country	Fistula cases, obstetric etiology	% of fistula cases with stillbirth or perinatal death	Comments
Savan et al. (2010)	Niger	21	92% of 24	24 fistula cases total, 21 of obstetric etiology, three traumatic. Stillbirth numbers reported as outcome of "most recent delivery" not specified if associated with birth causing fistula and included traumatic cases
Alio et al. (2011)	Niger	20	100%	Stillborn or neonatal death within 2 days of birth
Nafiou and Idrissa (2007)	Niger	111	100%	Perinatal deaths
Meyer et al. (2007)	Niger	58	97%	
Cam et al. (2010)	Niger	51	61%	
Roenneburg et al. (2006)	Niger	56	89%	
Kay et al. (2014)	Niger	345	83%	Women presenting for fistula repair at campaigns from 2003 to 2009; 28% of women reported cesarean delivery, but data do not correlate stillbirth with mode of delivery
Ouedraogo et al. (2018)	Niger	384	89%	In addition, eight early neonatal deaths; denominator excludes 20 missing/other
Wall et al. (2004)	Nigeria	899	92%	In addition, of 75 live births, 14 died within the first 4 weeks, most within 7 days
Orji et al. (2007)	Nigeria	68	90%	
Hilton (1998)	Nigeria	2202	90%	Stillbirth occurred in 97% of spontaneous vaginal, 89% of assisted vaginal, and 77% of cesarean deliveries
Ezegwui and Nwogu-Ikojo (2005)	Nigeria	68	84%	Includes four early neonatal deaths

(continued)

Table 5.2 (continued)

Article	Country	Fistula cases, obstetric etiology	% of fistula cases with stillbirth or perinatal death	Comments
Kirby et al. (2012)	Nigeria	83	66%	55 of the 83 participants had a history of a stillborn child, but it was not specified if it was experienced with the same birth that caused the fistula
Tunçalp et al. (2014)	Nigeria	50 and 29	84% and 74%	80% and 56% of OF cases were delivered by cesarean section
Lawani et al. (2015)	Nigeria	188	99%	Women with successful fistula repairs between 2011 and 2013
Washington et al. (2015)	Rwanda	59	73%	Data available for 59 of 65 women undergoing fistula repair
Kamara (2012)	Sierra Leone/Aberdeen Women's Centre	641	95.2%	Unpublished dissertation
Ramphal et al. (2008), Ramphal et al. (2007)	South Africa	41	87%	
Mohamed et al. (2009)	Sudan	47	89%	
Pope et al. (2011)	Tanzania	25	88%	
Browning et al. (2017)	Tanzania	270	89%	Outcome of delivery that caused OF; however, many of these women were delivered by cesarean section (no information re: survival by mode of delivery)
Kayondo et al. (2011)	Uganda	77	90%	
Bangser et al. (2011)	Uganda and Tanzania	124	90%	
Holme et al. (2007)	Zambia	237	78%	Stillbirth numbers were reported as outcome of most recent delivery not reported if it was the same birth associated with fistula

co-occurrence of these conditions. The key piece of information that is missing from many of these reports is whether there was an intervention that relieved the obstruction, since cesarean section, if performed early enough, can save the fetus' life.

An article from the Maternal and Newborn Health Registry—the same prospective population-based study described above (McClure et al., 2015)—reported on fetal outcomes in selected rural and semi-urban communities. In the two African countries included, Kenya and Zambia, the authors observed that 340/4860 (7%) of infants were stillborn in cases where labor was obstructed, prolonged, or failed to progress, as compared with 909/57,615 (1.6%) in other cases (Harrison et al., 2015). In a hospital-based prospective study in Uganda, 230 fetuses and newborns died due to complications of obstructed labor: 64 were stillborn, 46 died in the early neonatal period, and 120 died of birth asphyxia related to obstructed labor; no information on whether the mother developed fistula was reported (Nakimuli et al., 2015).

5.6   Discussion

Both OF and SB occur at much higher rates in countries that lack resources or political will to extend EmOC to all women; these are also settings in which documentation, surveillance, and reporting of these conditions are likely to be incomplete. Thus, it is difficult to reliably estimate the frequency with which these events occur.

In recent years, several initiatives, such as the Campaign to End Fistula (Campaign to End Fistula, n.d.) and the Every Newborn Action Plan (Lawn et al., 2014), have aimed to increase the visibility and reporting of both OF and SB, but there is still relatively little information about their co-occurrence. This has implications for the quantification of the burden of years of life lived with disability due to OF or lost due to SB and the consequent allocation of resources to promote respectful, high-quality EmOC (White Ribbon Alliance, 2011), as well as for the provision of services, including mental health services (such as that provided by Watt et al., 2015), to women and families who have experienced prolonged obstructed labor that resulted in either or both an OF and SB.

Reported rates of OF vary widely; some of the variations represent true differences in incidence, while others are artifacts of study design. Most available research is facility-based, accounting only for women who can access health care. Many women who might have developed OF had they survived a difficult childbirth instead die, so are not included in estimates (Bacon, 2003). Women living in rural areas are at higher risk for labor complications (Johnson, 2007), so OF occurs more often in rural areas (Vangeenderhuysen et al., 2001). OF may be hidden from view, as those afflicted often experience shame and isolation from their communities (Weston et al., 2011) and/or hide the condition from others (Heller, 2018).

Where health systems are weak and vital registration systems spotty or nonexistent, policymakers and health service providers do not have surveillance data to track vital events and measure population size (Ye et al., 2012). Reliable population-based estimates of OF and associated SB are needed to guide and evaluate prevention and treatment programs, but population-based studies are difficult to conduct. Studies of OF prevalence are more prone to bias than studies of incidence; studies of incidence may be based on cohorts of pregnant or post-partum women that can be reliably followed over a defined period, while studies of prevalence require surveying or examining all parous women in a population. Both are complicated by the relative rarity of OF (Tunçalp et al., 2015); although the absolute number of women with OF is large, the incidence rate may be only a few per 1000. The few population-based OF incidence and prevalence estimates that are available have used different definitions of fistula as well as different methods of sampling and case ascertainment. Questions about the prevalence of symptoms associated with OF were added to the Demographic and Health Survey in the mid-to-late 2000s and have begun to provide data, but these questions alone cannot confirm OF—clinical examination is required for that. For example, several of the estimates we report here are based on DHS interviews, which, as a proxy measure of OF, asked parous women whether they had experienced uncontrollable leakage of urine or stool from the vagina (Johnson, 2007). The DHS estimates are much higher than estimates based on other definitions of OF, and in fact, in studies where women were both asked if they had symptoms of OF and also examined, the frequency of OF on examination was lower than by self-report (Bhatia et al., 1997; Fronczak et al., 2005; Jokhio et al., 2014), in one case by two-thirds (Ballard et al., 2016). Thus, physical examination is required to reliably establish OF and to rule out stress incontinence, pelvic organ prolapse, vaginal discharge (Ballard et al., 2016), or other conditions like unrepaired third- and fourth-degree perineal tears (Lozo et al., 2016; Pinder et al., 2017) that might lead women to respond affirmatively to the DHS survey question. Tunçalp et al. (2014) reported a positive predictive value of the 2008 Nigeria DHS questions of only 47%, and this in a subsample of women who presented for fistula screening; the predictive value would be much lower in the general population, where the prevalence of OF would doubtless be lower than among those who participated in a screening program.

In the absence of reliable data, an interesting approach some authors have taken is to estimate OF incidence using data about prolonged labor. They estimate the probability of obstructed labor, given prolonged labor, and of OF, given obstructed labor, to estimate OF incidence (Tsui et al., 2007; Wall et al., 2005).

However, even the best estimates cannot replace hard data. As noted above, in response to the paucity of reliable data, in 2007 Stanton et al. (2007) proposed a series of questions to be added to the DHS that would be more specific for OF incidence and prevalence and that would also capture cases in deceased siblings of survey respondents, thus generating comparable population-based estimates and avoiding the survival bias resulting from collecting data only on living subjects. But even these questions produce false positives, since the surveys are not followed by gold-standard gynecological examinations. If these surveys were followed with physical examinations where feasible, as in the case of Adler et al. (2013a, b) and Ballard et al. (2016) in their studies using a similar approach, it would provide a measure of survey validity and improve data quality even further.

We included results of a meta-analysis of DHS and Multiple Indicators Cluster Surveys (MICS) data on vaginal fistula (VF) collected between 2005 and 2013 from nineteen sub-Saharan African countries (Maheu-Giroux et al., 2015b), but these results should be interpreted with caution, despite our earlier endorsement (Cowgill et al., 2015). In their paper, Maheu-Giroux et al. (2015b) report that their best estimates of lifetime and point VF prevalence per 1000 women aged 15–49 years in these countries was 3.0 cases (95% credible interval (CrI) 1.3–5.5) and 1.0 case (95% CrI 0.3–2.4), respectively. However, others challenged these estimates because, as noted above, the DHS questions only poorly approximate the case definition for OF (Ballard et al., 2015). The authors of the meta-analysis acknowledge this and other limitations of the data (Maheu-Giroux et al., 2015a) and state that they compensated for imperfect sensitivity and specificity of the fistula screening questions in their calculations. However, it is not clear that they compensated enough for the poor specificity of the questions or that they assessed the clinical heterogeneity of their data.

We did not conduct a meta-analysis of OF data; OF is not an outcome that occurs at a consistent rate around the world, within regions, or even at national and subnational levels in a single country. Instead, it is an indicator of weak emergency obstetric care systems (Wall, 2012b). We concur with Stanton et al. (2007), Wall et al. (2005), and Zheng and Anderson (2009) that current published estimates of OF incidence and prevalence are unreliable and do not support the conduct of a meta-analysis given the poor quality of the data. We found risk of bias was moderate or high in most studies, especially those in grey literature. Different researchers used different definitions of fistula, and some fistulas may not have been obstetric in origin. Study populations were variably defined as women who had ever borne children, or recently borne children, or who were of childbearing age—excluding older women who might no longer be fertile but could still suffer from an earlier OF, as noted in a community-based screening in Nigeria (Sunday-Adeoye & Landry, 2012). One study inexplicably excluded women with repaired fistula from its estimate of lifetime OF prevalence (Kalilani-Phiri et al., 2010). Fetal and neonatal deaths that occur at home are often not reported (McClure et al., 2006). Stillbirth may be more common with male babies, perhaps because male fetuses are larger on average (Wall et al., 2004). There was incomplete reporting of birth outcomes in some studies that mentioned SB. Many studies did not differentiate between SB and early neonatal mortality.

Aside from the risk of bias inherent in the studies themselves, an important limitation of this review is that the search strategy we used may not have been sensitive enough to capture studies of reproductive morbidity in which fistula was neither explicitly sought nor found, but where it would have been reported had it been found. As Adler et al. (2013a, b) point out, excluding studies with negative findings when attempting to generate an overall estimate of OF rates constitute search bias (Felson, 1992). We did not attempt to generate an overall estimate of OF rates, so we do not feel that the possible omission of studies with negative findings substantially weakens our review. A strength of our review is that we calculated 95% confidence intervals around all OF estimates to illustrate their inherent variability, and as a reminder that observing zero cases does not always mean the true incidence is zero: with small sample sizes, an event that occurs on the order of <5 times per 1000 births could easily be missed.

SB rates are high in women who develop OF but estimates of the proportion of cases in which the two co-occur are variable and imprecise. While we cannot say for sure exactly how often OF and associated stillbirth co-occur, we do know, to a large extent, why they do. The reasons are systemic: Prenatal care is difficult to obtain because of cost, availability, and/or accessibility (Pope et al., 2011); longstanding traditions or cultural expectations to give birth at home without assistance, or with an unskilled birth attendant, may carry more weight than programs to promote facility-based births and/ or skilled birth attendance (Hawkins et al., 2013; Johnson, 2007; Wall et al., 2004); emergency obstetric facilities and care, when they exist, are often inadequate and of poor quality; and impediments to treatment, such as waiting for permission to seek care, lack of transportation, desire to try traditional treatments, unawareness of available services, or distance from healthcare facilities, may limit the use of EmOC (Hawkins et al., 2013).

5.7 Conclusions

In summary, OF remains a significant obstetric problem in low-resource countries. It is strongly associated with stillbirth, as both are related to obstructed labor in the absence of emergency obstetric care. Reliable data on OF and associated SB in low-resource countries are lacking, underscoring the relative invisibility of these issues; sound numbers are needed to guide policy and fund responses to these neglected conditions of poverty.

Acknowledgments For contributions to the article this chapter was based on, the author thanks Jennifer Bishop, Amanda K. Norgaard, Craig E. Rubens, and Michael G. Gravett. Thanks, too, to Hao Bao for Chinese translation and to Danuta Wojnar for Polish translation.

Competing Interests The authors declare no competing interests.

References

Adler, A. J., Fox, S., Campbell, O. M. R., & Kuper, H. (2013a). Obstetric fistula in Southern Sudan: Situational analysis and Key Informant Method to estimate prevalence. *BMC Pregnancy and Childbirth, 13*(1), 64. https://doi.org/10.1186/1471-2393-13-64

Adler, A., Ronsmans, C., Calvert, C., & Filippi, V. (2013b). Estimating the prevalence of obstetric fistula: A systematic review and meta-analysis. *BMC Pregnancy and Childbirth, 13*(1), 246. https://doi.org/10.1186/1471-2393-13-246. Retrieved August 23, 2019, from https://www.ncbi.nlm.nih.gov/pmc/articles/PMC3937166/

Alio, A. P., Merrell, L., Roxburgh, K., Clayton, H. B., Marty, P. J., Bomboka, L., et al. (2011). The psychosocial impact of vesico-vaginal fistula in Niger. *Archives of Gynecology and Obstetrics, 284*(2), 371–378. https://doi.org/10.1007/s00404-010-1652-5

AMANHI. (2018). Population-based rates, timing, and causes of maternal deaths, stillbirths, and neonatal deaths in south Asia and sub-Saharan Africa: A multi-country prospective cohort study. *The Lancet Global Health, 6*, 1297–1308. https://doi.org/10.1016/S2214-109X(18)30385-1

Bacon, C. (Ed.). (2003). *Obstetric fistula: Needs assessment report: Findings from nine African countries.* UNFPA and EngenderHealth. Retrieved August 28, 2019, from http://www.unfpa.org/fistula/docs/fistula-needs-assessment.pdf

Baker, Z., Bellows, B., Bach, R., & Warren, C. (2017). Barriers to obstetric fistula treatment in low-income countries: A systematic review. *Tropical Medicine and International Health, 22*(8), 938–959.

Ballard, K., Ayenachew, F., Wright, J., Atnafu, H., & Andrews, M. (2015). Correspondence fistula in sub-Saharan. *The Lancet Global Health, 3*(8), e441. https://doi.org/10.1016/S2214-109X(15)00028-5

Ballard, K., Ayenachew, F., Wright, J., & Atnafu, H. (2016). Prevalence of obstetric fistula and symptomatic pelvic organ prolapse in rural Ethiopia. *International Urogynecology Journal, 27*, 1063–1067. https://doi.org/10.1007/s00192-015-2933-0

Bangser, M., Mehta, M., Singer, J., Daly, C., Kamugumya, C., & Mwangomale, A. (2011). Childbirth experiences of women with obstetric fistula in Tanzania and Uganda and their implications for fistula program development. *International Urogynecology Journal, 22*(1), 91–98. https://doi.org/10.1007/s00192-010-1236-8

Barone, M. A., Frajzyngier, V., Ruminjo, J., Asiimwe, F., Barry, T. H., Bello, A., et al. (2012). Determinants of postoperative outcomes of female genital fistula repair surgery. *Obstetrics and Gynecology, 120*(3), 524–531. https://doi.org/10.1097/AOG.0b013e31826579e8

Benfield, N., Kinsindja, R. M., Kimona, C., Masoda, M., Ndume, J., & Steinauer, J. (2011). Fertility desires and the feasibility of contraception counseling among genital fistula patients in eastern Democratic Republic of the Congo. *International Journal of Gynaecology and Obstetrics, 114*(3), 265–267. https://doi.org/10.1016/j.ijgo.2011.02.024

Benfield, N., Young-Lin, N., Kimona, C., Kalisya, L. M., & Kisindja, R. M. (2019). Fistula after attended delivery and the challenge of obstetric care capacity in the eastern Democratic Republic of Congo. *International Journal of Gynaecology and Obstetrics, 130*(2015), 157–160. https://doi.org/10.1016/j.ijgo.2015.02.032

Bhatia, J. C., Bhagavan, L., & Rao, N. S. N. (1997). Levels and determinants of gynecological in a district morbidity of South India. *Studies in Family Planning, 28*(2), 95–103.

Biadgilign, S., Lakew, Y., Reda, A. A., & Deribe, K. (2013). A population based survey in Ethiopia using questionnaire as proxy to estimate obstetric fistula prevalence: Results from demographic and health survey. *Reproductive Health, 10*(1), 14. https://doi.org/10.1186/1742-4755-10-14

Blencowe, H., Cousens, S., Jassir, F. B., Say, L., Chou, D., Mathers, C., et al. (2016). National, regional, and worldwide estimates of stillbirth rates in 2015, with trends from 2000: A systematic analysis. *The Lancet Global Health, 4*(2), e98–e108. https://doi.org/10.1016/S2214-109X(15)00275-2

Browning, A. (2006). Risk factors for developing residual urinary incontinence after obstetric fistula repair. *BJOG : An International Journal of Obstetrics and Gynaecology, 113*(4), 482–485. https://doi.org/10.1111/j.1471-0528.2006.00875.x

Browning, A., Fentahun, W., & Goh, J. (2007). The impact of surgical treatment on the mental health of women with obstetric fistula. *BJOG : An International Journal of Obstetrics and Gynaecology, 114*, 1439–1441. https://doi.org/10.1111/j.1471-0528.2007.01419.x

Browning, A., Allsworth, J. E., & Wall, L. L. (2010). The relationship between female genital cutting and obstetric fistulae. *Obstetrics & Gynecology, 115*(3), 578–583.

Browning, A., Mbise, F., & Foden, P. (2017). The effect of early pregnancy on the formation of obstetric fistula. *International Journal of Gynaecology and Obstetrics, 138*, 288–292. https://doi.org/10.1002/ijgo.12228

Bulanda Nsambi, J., Mukuku, O., Foma Yunga, J.-D., Kinenkinda, X., Kakudji, P., Kizonde, J., et al. (2018). Fistules obstetricales dans la province du Haut-Katanga, Republique Democratique du Congo: A propos de 242 cas. *The Pan African Medical Journal, 29*, 34. https://doi.org/10.11604/pamj.2018.29.34.14576. Retrieved August 29, 2019, from https://www.ncbi.nlm.nih.gov/pmc/articles/PMC5987152/

Cam, C., Karateke, A., Ozdemir, A., Gunes, C., Celik, C., Guney, B., et al. (2010). Fistula campaigns--Are they of any benefit? *Taiwanese Journal of Obstetrics & Gynecology, 49*(3), 291–296. https://doi.org/10.1016/S1028-4559(10)60063-0

Campaign to End Fistula. (n.d.). Retrieved April 19, 2019, from www.endfistula.org

Changole, J., Thorsen, V., & Kafulafula, U. (2017). "I am a person but I am not a person": Experiences of women living with obstetric fistula in the central region of Malawi. *BMC Pregnancy and Childbirth, 17*(1), 433. https://doi.org/10.1186/s12884-017-1604-1. Retrieved August 29, 2019, from https://www.ncbi.nlm.nih.gov/pmc/articles/PMC5740704/

Cousens, S., Blencowe, H., Stanton, C., Chou, D., Ahmed, S., Steinhardt, L., et al. (2011). National, regional, and worldwide estimates of stillbirth rates in 2009 with trends since 1995: A systematic analysis. *Lancet, 377*(9774), 1319–1330. https://doi.org/10.1016/S0140-6736(10)62310-0

Cowgill, K. D., Bishop, J., Norgaard, A. K., Rubens, C. E., & Gravett, M. G. (2015). Obstetric fistula in low-resource countries: An under-valued and under-studied problem - Systematic review of its incidence, prevalence, and association with stillbirth. *BMC Pregnancy and Childbirth, 15*(1), 193. https://doi.org/10.1186/s12884-015-0592-2. Retrieved August 28, 2019, from https://www.ncbi.nlm.nih.gov/pmc/articles/PMC4550077/

Delamou, A., Diallo, M., Beavogui, A. H., Delvaux, T., Millimono, S., Kourouma, M., et al. (2015). Good clinical outcomes from a 7-year holistic programme of fistula repair in Guinea. *Tropical Medicine and International Health, 20*(6), 813–819. https://doi.org/10.1111/tmi.12489

Desalliers, J., Pare, M., Kouraogo, S., & Corcos, J. (2017). Impact of surgery on quality of life of women with obstetrical fistula: A qualitative study in Burkina Faso. *International Urogynecology Journal, 28*(7), 1091–1100. https://doi.org/10.1007/s00192-016-3235-x

Dolea, C., & Abouzahr, C. (2003). *Global burden of obstructed labour in the year 2000*. World Health Organization. Retrieved from http://www.who.int/healthinfo/statistics/bod_obstructedlabour.pdf

Drew, L., Wilkinson, J., Nundwe, W., Moyo, M., Mataya, R., Mwale, M., et al. (2016). Long-term outcomes for women after obstetric fistula repair in Lilongwe, Malawi: A qualitative study. *BMC Pregnancy and Childbirth, 16*, 2. https://doi.org/10.1186/s12884-015-0755-1. Retrieved September 3, 2019, from https://bmcpregnancychildbirth.biomedcentral.com/articles/10.1186/s12884-015-0755-1

Elneil, S., & Browning, A. (2009). Obstetric fistula--A new way forward. *BJOG : An International Journal of Obstetrics and Gynaecology, 116*(Suppl), 30–32. https://doi.org/10.1111/j.1471-0528.2009.02309.x

Ezegwui, H. U., & Nwogu-Ikojo, E. E. (2005). Vesico-vaginal fistula in Eastern Nigeria. *Journal of Obstetrics and Gynaecology, 25*(6), 589–591. https://doi.org/10.1080/01443610500239479

Felson, D. T. (1992). Bias in meta-analytic research. *Journal of Clinical Epidemiology, 45*(8), 885–892.

Filippi, V., Ganaba, R., Baggaley, R. F., Marshall, T., Storeng, K. T., Sombié, I., et al. (2007). Health of women after severe obstetric complications in Burkina Faso: A longitudinal study. *Lancet, 370*(9595), 1329–1337. https://doi.org/10.1016/S0140-6736(07)61574-8

Filippi, V., Goufodji, S., Sismanidis, C., Kanhonou, L., Fottrell, E., Ronsmans, C., et al. (2010). Effects of severe obstetric complications on women's health and infant mortality in Benin. *Tropical Medicine & International Health, 15*(6), 733–742. https://doi.org/10.1111/j.1365-3156.2010.02534.x

Fronczak, N., Antelman, G., Moran, A. C., Caulfield, L. E., & Baqui, A. H. (2005). Delivery-related complications and early postpartum morbidity in Dhaka, Bangladesh. *International Journal of Gynaecology and Obstetrics, 91*(3), 271–278. https://doi.org/10.1016/j.ijgo.2005.09.006

GBD 2016 Mortality Collaborators. (2017). Global, regional, and national under-5 mortality, adult mortality, age-specific mortality, and life expectancy, 1970 – 2016: A systematic analysis for the Global Burden of Disease Study 2016. *Lancet, 390*, 1084–1150. https://doi.org/10.1016/S0140-6736(17)31833-0. Retrieved September 3, 2019, from https://www.thelancet.com/journals/lancet/article/PIIS0140-6736(17)31833-0/fulltext

Gessessew, A., & Mesfin, M. (2003). Genitourinary and rectovaginal fistulae in Adigrat Zonal Hospital, Tigray, North Ethiopia. *Ethiopian Medical Journal, 41*(2), 123–130.

Goh, J. T. W. (1998). Genital tract fistula repair on 116 women. *Australian and New Zealand Journal of Obstetrics and Gynaecology, 38*(2), 158–161. https://doi.org/10.1111/j.1479-828x.1998.tb02991.x

Harrison, M. S., Ali, S., Pasha, O., Saleem, S., Althabe, F., Berrueta, M., et al. (2015). A prospective population-based study of maternal, fetal, and neonatal outcomes in the setting of prolonged labor, obstructed labor and failure to progress in low- and middle-income countries. *Reproductive Health, 12*(Suppl 2), S9. https://doi.org/10.1186/1742-4755-12-S2-S9. Retrieved September 3, 2019, from https://www.ncbi.nlm.nih.gov/pmc/articles/PMC4464213/

Hawkins, L., Spitzer, R. F., Christoffersen-Deb, A., Leah, J., & Mabeya, H. (2013). Characteristics and surgical success of patients presenting for repair of obstetric fistula in western Kenya. *International Journal of Gynaecology and Obstetrics, 120*(2), 178–182. https://doi.org/10.1016/j.ijgo.2012.08.014

Haws, R. A., Yakoob, M. Y., Soomro, T., Menezes, E. V., Darmstadt, G. L., & Bhutta, Z. A. (2009). Reducing stillbirths: Screening and monitoring during pregnancy and labour. *BMC Pregnancy and Childbirth, 48*, 1–48. https://doi.org/10.1186/1471-2393-9-S1-S5. Retrieved August 5, 2019, from https://bmcpregnancychildbirth.biomedcentral.com/articles/10.1186/1471-2393-9-S1-S

Heller, A. (2018). Transforming obstetric fistula through concealment in Niger. *Human Organization, 77*(3), 239–248. https://doi.org/10.17730/0018-7259.77.3.239

Higashi, H., Barendregt, J. J., Kassebaum, N. J., Weiser, T. G., Bickler, S. W., & Vos, T. (2015). Surgically avertable burden of obstetric conditions in low- and middle-income regions: A modelled analysis. *BJOG: An International Journal of Obstetrics & Gynaecology, 122*, 228–237. https://doi.org/10.1111/1471-0528.13198

Hilton, P. (1998). Urodynamic findings in patients with urogenital fistulae. *British Journal of Urology, 81*, 539–542.

Holme, A., Breen, M., & MacArthur, C. (2007). Obstetric fistulae: A study of women managed at the Monze Mission Hospital, Zambia. *BJOG : An International Journal of Obstetrics and Gynaecology, 114*(8), 1010–1017. https://doi.org/10.1111/j.1471-0528.2007.01353.x

Horton, R., & Samarasekera, U. (2016). Stillbirths: Ending an epidemic of grief. *The Lancet, 387*, 515–516. https://doi.org/10.1016/S0140-6736(15)01276-3

Husain, A., Johnson, K., Glowacki, C. A., Osias, J., Wheeless, C. R., Asrat, K., et al. (2005). Surgical management of complex obstetric fistula in Eritrea. *Journal of Women's Health, 14*(9), 839–845. https://doi.org/10.1089/jwh.2005.14.839

Ijaiya, M. A., & Aboyeji, P. A. (2004). Obstetric urogenital fistula: The Ilorin experience, Nigeria. *West African Journal of Medicine, 23*(1), 7–9.

Ismail, S. I. M. F. (2015). The increasing number of surgical procedures for female genital fistula in England: Analysis of hospital episode statistics (HES) data. *Journal of Obstetrics and Gynaecology, 35*, 57–59. https://doi.org/10.3109/01443615.2014.935714

Johnson, K. (2007). Incontinence in Malawi: Analysis of a proxy measure of vaginal fistula in a national survey. *International Journal of Gynaecology and Obstetrics, 99*(Suppl 1), S122–S129. https://doi.org/10.1016/j.ijgo.2007.06.033

Jokhio, A., Rizvi, R. M., Rizvi, J., & MacArthur, C. (2014). Prevalence of obstetric fistula: A population-based study in rural Pakistan. *BJOG : An International Journal of Obstetrics and Gynaecology, 121*(8), 1039–1046. https://doi.org/10.1111/1471-0528.12739

Kalilani-Phiri, L. V., Umar, E., Lazaro, D., Lunguzi, J., & Chilungo, A. (2010). Prevalence of obstetric fistula in Malawi. *International Journal of Gynecology & Obstetrics, 109*(3), 204–208. https://doi.org/10.1016/j.ijgo.2009.12.019

Kamara, M. M. (2012). *A study on obstetric fistulae at the Aberdeen Women's Centre and Bo Government Hospital from 1st January, 2010 to 31st December, 2011*. University of Sierra Leone.

Kaplan, J. A., Kandodo, J., Sclafani, J., Raine, S., Blumenthal-Barby, J., Norris, A., et al. (2017). An investigation of the relationship between autonomy, childbirth practices, and obstetric fistula among women in rural Lilongwe District, Malawi. *BMC International Health and Human Rights, 17*(1), 1–10. https://doi.org/10.1186/s12914-017-0125-3. Retrieved August 18, 2019, from https://www.ncbi.nlm.nih.gov/pmc/articles/PMC5477240/

Kay, A., Idrissa, A., & Hampton, B. S. (2014). Epidemiologic profile of women presenting to the National Hospital of Niamey, Niger for vaginal fistula repair. *International Journal of Gynecology & Obstetrics, 126*(2), 136–139. https://doi.org/10.1016/j.ijgo.2014.03.022

Kayondo, M., Wasswa, S., Kabakyenga, J., Mukiibi, N., Senkungu, J., Stenson, A., et al. (2011). Predictors and outcome of surgical repair of obstetric fistula at a regional referral hospital, Mbarara, western Uganda. *BMC Urology, 11*(1), 23. https://doi.org/10.1186/1471-2490-11-23. Retrieved August 11, 2019, from https://www.ncbi.nlm.nih.gov/pmc/articles/PMC3252285/

Kelly, J. (1995). Ethiopia an epidemiological study of vesicovaginal fistula in Addis Ababa. *World Health Statistics Quarterly, 48*(1), 15–17.

Keya, K. T., Sripad, P., Nwala, E., & Warren, C. E. (2018). "Poverty is the big thing": Exploring financial, transportation, and opportunity costs associated with fistula management and repair in Nigeria and Uganda. *International Journal for Equity in Health, 17*(1), 70. https://doi.org/10.1186/s12939-018-0777-1

Khisa, A. M., & Nyamongo, I. K. (2012). Still living with fistula: An exploratory study of the experience of women with obstetric fistula following corrective surgery in West Pokot, Kenya. *Reproductive Health Matters, 20*(40), 59–66. https://doi.org/10.1016/S0968-8080(12)40661-9

Khisa, W., Wakasiaka, S., McGowan, L., Campbell, M., & Lavender, T. (2017). Understanding the lived experience of women before and after fistula repair: A qualitative study in Kenya. *BJOG: An International Journal of Obstetrics & Gynaecology, 124*(3), 503–510. Retrieved August 24, 2019, from https://obgyn.onlinelibrary.wiley.com/doi/full/10.1111/1471-0528.13902

Kirby, A. C. A., Gleason, J. J. L., Greer, W. J., Norman, A. J., Lengmang, S., & Richter, H. E. (2012). Characterization of colorectal symptoms in women with vesicovaginal fistulas. *International Journal of Gynaecology and Obstetrics, 116*(1), 64–66. https://doi.org/10.1016/j.ijgo.2011.08.005.Characterization

Lawani, L. O., Iyoke, C. A., & Ezeonu, P. O. (2015). Contraceptive practice after surgical repair of obstetric fistula in southeast Nigeria. *International Journal of Gynecology & Obstetrics, 129*(3), 256–259. https://doi.org/10.1016/j.ijgo.2014.11.028

Lawn, J. E., Gravett, M. G., Nunes, T. M., Rubens, C. E., Stanton, C., & Group, R. (2010). Global report on preterm birth and stillbirth (1 of 7): Definitions, description of the burden and opportunities to improve data. *BMC Pregnancy and Childbirth, 10*(Suppl 1), S1. https://doi.org/10.1186/1471-2393-S1-S1. Retrieved August 27, 2019, from https://www.ncbi.nlm.nih.gov/pmc/articles/PMC2841772/

Lawn, J. E., Blencowe, H., Oza, S., You, D., Lee, A. C. C., Waiswa, P., et al. (2014). Every newborn: Progress, priorities, and potential beyond survival. *Lancet, 384*(9938), 189–205. https://doi.org/10.1016/S0140-6736(14)60496-7

Loposso, M. N., Ndundu, J., De Win, G., Ost, D., Punga, A. M., & De Ridder, D. (2015). Obstetric fistula in a district hospital in DR Congo: Fistula still occur despite access to caesarean section. *Neurourology and Urodynamics, 34*, 434–437. https://doi.org/10.1002/nau

Lozo, S., Eckardt, M. J., Altawil, Z., Nelson, B. D., Ahn, R., Weston, K., et al. (2016). Prevalence of unrepariied third- and fourth-degree tears among women taken to the operating room for repair of presumed obstetric fistula during two fistula camps in Kenya. *International Urogynecology Journal, 27*, 463–466. https://doi.org/10.1007/s00192-015-2850-2

Mabeya, H. (2004). Characteristics of women admitted with obstetric fistula. In *Postgraduate training course in reproductive health 2004*. Retrieved from http://www.gfmer.ch/Medical_education_En/PGC_RH_2004/Obstetric_fistula_Kenya.htm

Mafo Degge, H., Hayter, M., & Laurenson, M. (2017). An integrative review on women living with obstetric fistula and after treatment experiences. *Journal of Clinical Nursing, 26*, 11–12. https://doi.org/10.1111/jocn.13590

Maheu-Giroux, M., Filippi, V., Samadoulougou, S., Castro, M. C., Maulet, N., Meda, N., et al. (2015a). Fistula in sub-Saharan Africa – Authors' reply. *The Lancet Global Health, 3*(8), e442. https://doi.org/10.1016/S2214-109X(15)00030-3

Maheu-Giroux, M., Filippi, V., Samadoulougou, S., Castro, M. C., Maulet, N., Meda, N., et al. (2015b). Prevalence of symptoms of vaginal fistula in 19 sub-Saharan Africa countries: A meta-analysis of national household. *The Lancet Global Health, 3*(5), e271–e278. https://doi.org/10.1016/S2214-109X(14)70348-1

Mallick, L., & Tripathi, V. (2018). The association between female genital fistula symptoms and gender-based violence: A multicountry secondary analysis of household survey data. *Tropical Medicine and International Health, 23*(1), 106–119. https://doi.org/10.1111/tmi.13008

McClure, E. M., Nalubamba-Phiri, M., & Goldenberg, R. L. (2006). Stillbirth in developing countries. *International Journal of Gynaecology and Obstetrics, 94*(2), 82–90. https://doi.org/10.1016/j.ijgo.2006.03.023

McClure, E. M., Saleem, S., Goudar, S. S., Moore, J. L., Garces, A., Esamai, F., et al. (2015). Stillbirth rates in low-middle income countries 2010 - 2013: A population-based, multi-country study from the Global Network. *Reproductive Health, 12*(Suppl 2), S7. Retrieved September 3, 2019, from https://reproductive-health-journal.biomedcentral.com/articles/10.1186/1742-4755-12-S2-S7

McFadden, E., Taleski, S. S. J., Bocking, A., Spitzer, R. F., & Mabeya, H. (2011). Retrospective review of predisposing factors and surgical outcomes in obstetric fistula patients at a single teaching hospital in Western Kenya. *Journal of Obstetrics and Gynaecology Canada, 33*(1), 30–35. https://doi.org/10.1016/S1701-2163(16)34769-7

Meyer, L., Ascher-Walsh, C. J., Norman, R., Idrissa, A., Herbert, H., Kimso, O., et al. (2007). Commonalities among women who experienced vesicovaginal fistulae as a result of obstetric trauma in Niger: Results from a survey given at the National Hospital Fistula Center, Niamey, Niger. *American Journal of Obstetrics and Gynecology, 197*(1), 90.e1–90.e4. https://doi.org/10.1016/j.ajog.2007.03.071

Miller, S., Lester, F., Webster, M., & Cowan, B. (2005). Obstetric fistula: A preventable tragedy. *Journal of Midwifery & Women's Health, 50*(4), 286–294. https://doi.org/10.1016/j.jmwh.2005.03.009

Mocumbi, S., Hanson, C., Högberg, U., Boene, H., von Dadelszen, P., Bergström, A., et al. (2017). Obstetric fistulae in southern Mozambique: Incidence, obstetric characteristics and treatment. *Reproductive Health, 14*, 147. https://doi.org/10.1186/s12978-017-0408-0. Retrieved August 21, 2019, from https://www.ncbi.nlm.nih.gov/pmc/articles/PMC5681779/

Mohamed, E. Y., Boctor, M. F. A., Ahmed, H. A., Seedahmed, H., Abdelgadir, M. A., & Abdalla, S. M. (2009). Contributing factors of vesico-vaginal fistula (VVF) among fistula patients in Dr. Abbo's National Fistula & Urogynecology Centre - Khartoum 2008. *Sudanese Journal of Public Health, 4*(2), 259–264.

Mselle, L. T., & Kohi, T. W. (2015). Perceived health system causes of obstetric fistula from accounts of affected women in rural Tanzania: A qualitative study. *African Journal of Reproductive Health, 19*(1), 124–132. Retrieved September 3, 2019, from http://www.bioline.org.br/pdf?rh15013

Mselle, L. T., & Kohi, T. W. (2016). Healthcare access and quality of birth care: Narratives of women living with obstetric fistula in rural Tanzania. *Reproductive Health, 13*, 1–9. https://doi.org/10.1186/s12978-016-0189-x

Muleta, M., Fantahun, M., Tafesse, B., Hamlin, E., & Kennedy, R. (2007). Obstetric fistula in rural Ethiopia. *East African Medical Journal, 84*(11), 525–533.

Muleta, M., Rasmussen, S., & Kiserud, T. (2010). Obstetric fistula in 14,928 Ethiopian women. *Acta Obstetricia et Gynecologica Scandinavica, 89*(7), 945–951. https://doi.org/10.3109/00016341003801698

Nafiou, I., & Idrissa, A. (2007). Obstetric vesico-vaginal fistulas at the National Hospital of Niamey, Niger. *International Journal of Gynecology & Obstetrics, 99*(Suppl 1), S71–S74. https://doi.org/10.1016/j.ijgo.2007.06.012

Naidoo, T., Moodley, J., & Naidoo, S. (2018). Genital tract fistula: A case series from a tertiary centre in South Africa. *International Urogynecology Journal, 29*(3), 383–389. https://doi.org/10.1007/s00192-017-3396-2

Nakimuli, A., Mbalinda, S. N., Nabirye, R. C., Kakaire, O., Nakubulwa, S., Osinde, M. O., et al. (2015). Still births, neonatal deaths and neonatal near miss cases attributable to severe obstetric complications: A prospective cohort study in two referral hospitals in Uganda. *BMC Pediatrics, 15*, 44. https://doi.org/10.1186/s12887-015-0362-3. Retrieved August 15, 2019, from https://bmcpediatr.biomedcentral.com/articles/10.1186/s12887-015-0362-3

Nathan, L. M. L., Rochat, C. H., Grigorescu, B., & Banks, E. (2009). Obstetric fistulae in West Africa: Patient perspectives. *American Journal of Obstetrics and Gynecology, 200*(5), e40–e42. https://doi.org/10.1016/j.ajog.2008.10.014

NSO, & ORC Macro. (2005). *Malawi Demographic and Health Survey 2004*. DHS. Retrieved from http://dhsprogram.com/pubs/pdf/FR175/FR-175-MW04.pdf

Onsrud, M., Sjøveian, S., & Mukwege, D. (2011). Cesarean delivery-related fistulae in the Democratic Republic of Congo. *International Journal of Gynaecology and Obstetrics, 114*(1), 10–14. https://doi.org/10.1016/j.ijgo.2011.01.018

Orji, E., Aduloju, O., & Orji, V. (2007). Correlation and impact of obstetric fistula on motherhood. *Journal of Chinese Clinical Medicine, 2*(8), 448–454.

Osman, S., Al-Badr, A., Malabarey, O., Dawood, A., AlMosaieed, B., & Rizk, D. (2018). Causes and management of urogenital fistulas. A retrospective cohort study from a tertiary referral center in Saudi Arabia. *Saudi Medical Journal, 39*(4), 373–378. https://doi.org/10.15537/smj.2018.4.21515

Ouedraogo, I., Payne, C., Nardos, R., & Adelman, A. J. (2018). Obstetric fistula in Niger: 6-month postoperative follow-up of 384 patients from the Danja Fistula Center. *International Urogynecology Journal, 29*, 345–351. https://doi.org/10.1007/s00192-017-3375-7

Pai, M., Mcculloch, M., Gorman, J. D., Pai, N., Enanoria, W., Kennedy, G., et al. (2004). Systematic reviews and meta-analyses: An illustrated, step-by-step guide. *The National Medical Journal of India, 17*(2), 86–95.

Phillips, J., & Millum, J. (2014). Valuing stillbirths. *Bioethics, 29*(6), 413–423. https://doi.org/10.1111/bioe.12120

Pinder, L. F., Natsuhara, K. H., Burke, T. F., Lozo, S., Oguttu, M., Miller, L., et al. (2017). Nurse-midwives' ability to diagnose acute third- and fourth-degree obstetric lacerations in western Kenya. *BMC Pregnancy and Childbirth, 17*, 308. https://doi.org/10.1186/s12884-017-1484-4. Retrieved August 2, 2019, from https://www.ncbi.nlm.nih.gov/pmc/articles/PMC5604156/

Pope, R., Bangser, M., & Requejo, J. H. (2011). Restoring dignity: Social reintegration after obstetric fistula repair in Ukerewe, Tanzania. *Global Public Health, 6*(8), 859–873. https://doi.org/10.1080/17441692.2010.551519

Prual, A., Huguet, D., Garbin, O., & Rabe, G. (1998). Severe obstetric morbidity of the third trimester, delivery and early puerperium in Niamey (Niger). *African Journal of Reproductive Health, 2*(1), 10–19.

Prual, A., De Bernis, L., Bre, G., Bouvier-Colle, M. H., de Bernis, L., & Bréart, G. (2000). Severe maternal morbidity from direct obstetric causes in West Africa: Incidence and case fatality rates. *Bulletin of the World Health Organization, 78*(5), 593–602. Retrieved August 3, 2019, from https://www.who.int/bulletin/archives/78(5)593.pdf

Raassen, T. J. I. P., Verdaasdonk, E. G. G., & Vierhout, M. E. (2008). Prospective results after first-time surgery for obstetric fistulas in East African women. *International Urogynecology Journal and Pelvic Floor Dysfunction, 19*(1), 73–79. https://doi.org/10.1007/s00192-007-0389-6

Ramphal, S., & Moodley, J. (2006). Vesicovaginal fistula: Obstetric causes. *Current Opinion in Obstetrics & Gynecology, 18*(2), 147–151. https://doi.org/10.1097/01.gco.0000192980.92223.2d

Ramphal, S., Kalane, G., Fourie, T., & Moodley, J. (2007). Obstetric urinary fistulas in KwaZulu-Natal - What is the extent of this tragedy? *South African Journal of Obstetrics and Gynaecology, 13*(3), 92–94.

Ramphal, S. R., Kalane, G., Fourie, T., & Moodley, J. (2008). An audit of obstetric fistulae in a teaching hospital in South Africa. *Tropical Doctor, 38*(3), 162–163. https://doi.org/10.1258/td.2007.070087

Reisenauer, C. (2016). Presentation and management of rectovaginal fistulas after delivery. *International Urogynecology Journal, 27*(6), 859–864. https://doi.org/10.1007/s00192-015-2860-0

Rijken, Y., & Chilopora, G. (2007). Urogenital and recto-vaginal fistulas in southern Malawi: A report on 407 patients. *International Journal of Gynecology & Obstetrics, 99*(1), 85–89. https://doi.org/10.1016/j.ijgo.2007.06.015

Roenneburg, M. L., Genadry, R., & Wheeless, C. R. (2006). Repair of obstetric vesicovaginal fistulas in Africa. *American Journal of Obstetrics and Gynecology, 195*(6), 1748–1752. https://doi.org/10.1016/j.ajog.2006.07.031

Roka, Z. G., Akech, M., Wanzala, P., Omolo, J., Gitta, S., & Waiswa, P. (2013). Factors associated with obstetric fistulae occurrence among patients attending selected hospitals in Kenya, 2010: A case control study. *BMC Pregnancy and Childbirth, 13*(1), 56. https://doi.org/10.1186/1471-2393-13-56. Retrieved August 10, 2019, from https://bmcpregnancychildbirth.biomedcentral.com/articles/10.1186/1471-2393-13-56

Roush, K. M. (2009). Social implications of obstetric fistula: An integrative review. *Journal of Midwifery & Women's Health, 54*(2), e21–e33. https://doi.org/10.1016/j.jmwh.2008.09.005

Savan, K., Ekin, M., Kupelioglu, L., Oral, S., & Yasar, L. (2010). Surgical repair of genitourinary fistulae: Comparison of our experience at Turkey and Niger. *Archives of Gynecology and Obstetrics, 282*(6), 649–653. https://doi.org/10.1007/s00404-009-1311-x

Seim, A. R., Alassoum, Z., Bronzan, R. N., Alou, A., Jacobsen, J. L., & Asma, Y. (2014). Pilot community-mobilization program reduces maternal and perinatal mortality and prevents obstetric fistula in Niger. *International Journal of Gynecology & Obstetrics, 127*, 269–274. https://doi.org/10.1016/j.ijgo.2014.06.016

Sori, D. A., Azale, A. W., & Gemeda, D. H. (2016). Characteristics and repair outcome of patients with Vesicovaginal fistula managed in Jimma University teaching. *BMC Urology, 16*(1), 1–6. https://doi.org/10.1186/s12894-016-0152-8. Retrieved August 25, 2019, from https://www.ncbi.nlm.nih.gov/pmc/articles/PMC4942998/

Stanton, C., Holtz, S., & Ahmed, S. (2007). Challenges in measuring obstetric fistula. *International Journal of Gynaecology and Obstetrics, 99*(Suppl 1), S4–S9. https://doi.org/10.1016/j.ijgo.2007.06.010

Sunday-Adeoye, I., & Landry, E. (2012). *Community-based screening for obstetric fistula in Ebonyi State, Nigeria.* USAID Fistula Care. Retrieved August 27, 2019, from https://fistulacare.org/wp-fcp/wp-content/uploads/pdf/technical-briefs/ebonyi_community_screening4.5.2012.pdf

Tebeu, P. M., de Bernis, L., Doh, A. S., Rochat, C. H., & Delvaux, T. (2009). Risk factors for obstetric fistula in the Far North Province of Cameroon. *International Journal of Gynaecology and Obstetrics, 107*(1), 12–15. https://doi.org/10.1016/j.ijgo.2009.05.019

Tebeu, P. M., Maninzou, S. D., Kengne Fosso, G., Jemea, B., Fomulu, J. N., & Rochat, C. H. (2012). Risk factors for obstetric vesicovaginal fistula at University Teaching Hospital, Yaoundé, Cameroon. *International Journal of Gynaecology and Obstetrics, 118*(3), 256–258. https://doi.org/10.1016/j.ijgo.2012.04.011

Thaddeus, S., & Maine, D. (1994). Too far to walk: Maternal mortality in context. *Social Science & Medicine (1982), 38*(8), 1091–1110.

Trovik, J., Thornhill, H., & Kiserud, T. (2016). Incidence of obstetric fistula in Norway: A population-based prospective cohort study. *Acta Obstetrica et Gynecologica Scandinavia, 95*(4), 405–410. https://doi.org/10.1111/aogs.12845

Tsui, A., Creanga, A., & Ahmed, S. (2007). The role of delayed childbearing in the prevention of obstetric fistulas. *International Journal of Gynaecology and Obstetrics, 99*(Suppl 1), S98–S107. https://doi.org/10.1016/j.ijgo.2007.06.024

Tunçalp, Ö., Isah, A., Landry, E., & Stanton, C. K. (2014). Community-based screening for obstetric fistula in Nigeria: A novel approach. *BMC Pregnancy and Childbirth, 14*, 44. https://doi.org/10.1186/1471-2393-14-44. Retrieved August 1, 2019, from https://bmcpregnancychildbirth.biomedcentral.com/articles/10.1186/1471-2393-14-44

Tunçalp, Ö., Tripathi, V., Landry, E., Stanton, K., & Ahmed, S. (2015). Measuring the incidence and prevalence of obstetric fistula: Approaches, needs and recommendations. *Bulletin of the World Health Organization, 93*, 60–62. Retrieved August 1, 2019, from https://www.who.int/bulletin/volumes/93/1/14-141473/en/

Turan, J. M., Johnson, K., & Polan, M. L. (2007). Experiences of women seeking medical care for obstetric fistula in Eritrea: Implications for prevention, treatment, and social reintegration. *Global Public Health, 2*(1), 64–77. https://doi.org/10.1080/17441690600648728

Uganda Bureau of Statistics (UBOS), & Macro International Inc. (2006). *Uganda Demographic and Health Survey 2006.* DHS.

Vangeenderhuysen, C., Prual, A., & Ould, D. (2001). Obstetric fistulae: Incidence estimates for sub-Saharan Africa. *International Journal of Gynaecology and Obstetrics, 73*, 65–66. https://doi.org/10.1016/s0020-7292(00)00374-x

Wall, L. L. (2006). Obstetric vesicovaginal fistula as an international public-health problem. *Lancet, 368*, 1201–1209. https://doi.org/10.1016/S0140-6736(06)69476-2

Wall, L. L. (2012a). A framework for analyzing the determinants of obstetric fistula formation. *Studies in Family Planning, 43*(4), 255–272. https://doi.org/10.1111/j.1728-4465.2012.00325.x

Wall, L. L. (2012b). Obstetric fistula is a "neglected tropical disease". *PLoS Neglected Tropical Diseases, 6*(8), e1769. https://doi.org/10.1371/journal.pntd.0001769. Retrieved August 5, 2019, from https://journals.plos.org/plosntds/article?id=10.1371/journal.pntd.0001769

Wall, L. L. (2012c). Overcoming phase 1 delays: The critical component of obstetric fistula prevention programs in resource-poor countries. *BMC Pregnancy and Childbirth, 12*(1), 68. https://doi.org/10.1186/1471-2393-12-68. Retrieved July 30, 2019, from https://bmcpregnancychildbirth.biomedcentral.com/articles/10.1186/1471-2393-12-68

Wall, L. L. (2012d). Preventing obstetric fistulas in low-resource countries: Insights from a Haddon matrix. *Obstetrical & Gynecological Survey, 67*(2), 111–121. https://doi.org/10.1097/OGX.0b013e3182438788

Wall, L. L. (2018). *Tears for my sisters: The tragedy of obstetric fistula.* Johns Hopkins University Press.

Wall, L. L., Karshima, J. A., Kirschner, C., & Arrowsmith, S. D. (2004). The obstetric vesicovaginal fistula: Characteristics of 899 patients from Jos, Nigeria. *American Journal of Obstetrics and Gynecology, 190*(4), 1011–1019. https://doi.org/10.1016/j.ajog.2004.02.007

Wall, L. L., Arrowsmith, S. D., Briggs, N., Browning, A., & Lassey, A. (2005). The obstetric vesicovaginal fistula in the developing world. In P. Abrams, L. Cardozo, S. Khoury, & A. Wein (Eds.), *Incontinence, vol. 2, Management: Report on the 3rd International Consultation on Incontinence* (pp. 1403–1454). Health Publications Ltd.. Retrieved from http://www.ics.org/Publications/ICI_3/v2.pdf/chap22.pdf

Walraven, G., Scherf, C., West, B., Ekpo, G., Paine, K., Coleman, R., et al. (2001). The burden of reproductive-organ disease in rural women in The Gambia, West Africa. *Lancet, 357*(9263), 1161–1167. https://doi.org/10.1016/S0140-6736(00)04333-6

Washington, B. B., Raker, C. A., Kabeja, G. A., Kay, A., & Hampton, B. S. (2015). Demographic and delivery characteristics associated with obstetric fistula in Kigali, Rwanda. *International Journal of Gynecology & Obstetrics, 129*, 34–37. https://doi.org/10.1016/j.ijgo.2014.09.033

Watt, M. H., Wilson, S. M., Sikkema, K. J., Velloza, J., Mosha, M. V., Masenga, G. G., Bangser, M., Browning, A., & Nyindo, P. M. (2015). Development of an intervention to improve mental health for obstetric fistula patients in Tanzania. *Evaluation and Program Planning, 50*, 1–9. https://doi.org/10.1016/j.evalprogplan.2015.01.007

Weston, K., Mutiso, S., Mwangi, J. W., Qureshi, Z., Beard, J., & Venkat, P. (2011). Depression among women with obstetric fistula in Kenya. *International Journal of Gynecology & Obstetrics, 115*(1), 31–33. https://doi.org/10.1016/j.ijgo.2011.04.015

White Ribbon Alliance. (2011). *Respectful maternity care: The universal rights of childbearing women*. Author. Retrieved August 27, 2019, from https://www.whiteribbonalliance.org/wp-content/uploads/2017/11/Final_RMC_Charter.pdf

Wilson, S., Sikkema, K., Watt, M., Masenga, G., & Mosha, M. (2016). Psychological symptoms and social functioning following repair of obstetric fistula in a low-income setting. *Maternal and Child Health Journal, 20*(5), 941–945. https://doi.org/10.1007/s10995-016-1950-z

World Health Organization. (2016). *Making every baby count: Audit and review of stillbirths and neonatal deaths*. Author. Retrieved August 29, 2019, from https://apps.who.int/iris/bitstream/handle/10665/249523/9789241511223-eng.pdf;jsessionid=5A1A96A9462737020273D6B395F1A2D2?sequence=1

Ye, Y., Wamukoya, M., Ezeh, A., Emina, J. B. O., & Sankoh, O. (2012). Health and demographic surveillance systems: A step towards full civil registration and vital statistics system in sub-Sahara Africa? *BMC Public Health, 12*, 741. https://doi.org/10.1186/1471-2458-12-741. Retrieved July 30, 2019, from https://www.ncbi.nlm.nih.gov/pmc/articles/PMC3509035/

Zheng, A. X., & Anderson, F. W. J. (2009). Obstetric fistula in low-income countries. *International Journal of Gynaecology and Obstetrics, 104*(2), 85–89. https://doi.org/10.1016/j.ijgo.2008.09.011

A Multidisciplinary Approach to Obstetric Fistula in Africa: Public Health, Sociological, and Medical Perspectives

6

Tina Lavender, Sabina Wakasiaka, and Weston Khisa

6.1   Introduction

After her fistula healed, a woman once said, "*I wouldn't wish a fistula even on my worst enemy; this thing is devastating and negates a woman's very existence.*" This is the twenty-first century, yet women continue to suffer the pain and stigma that accompanies this debilitating condition.

A fistula is described as a hole between two epithelial tissues. The abnormal communication can occur anywhere between the reproductive system of a woman and urinary system or rectum. The most common cause of fistula in low-income countries is childbirth, especially when prolonged and obstructed labor is not relieved on time (Orach, 2000). During obstructed labor, the fetus fails to progress along the birth canal, leading to compression of the mother's pelvic tissues between her bony pelvis and the fetal head (Wall, 1998). The subsequent obstruction of blood flow, or perfusion, to the soft tissues of the maternal bladder, rectum, and vagina leads to lack of oxygen (ischemia), tissue necrosis, and the development of a fistula through which faces or urine continually stream from the vagina (World Health Organization, 2006; Ali & Adam, 2010). The uncontrollable flow of waste leaves women with an offensive odor; causes dermatitis of her vulva and thighs; and can lead to early mortality from infection or kidney failure (Arrowsmith et al., 1996; UNFPA, 2018). The obstructed labor may also result in foot drop (as a result of sciatic nerve injury) in one or both legs, severely restricting a woman's mobility (Waaldijk & Elkins, 1994).

Other emerging causes of fistula include pelvic surgeries and gynecologic cancers or radiation-related factors (Velez et al., 2007). Although cancer or radiation-related fistulas still occur in developed countries, the care is usually prompt and women are not exposed to psychosocial trauma associated with living with fistula.

T. Lavender (✉)
Department of International Public Health, Liverpool School of Tropical Medicine, Liverpool, Great Britain
e-mail: Tina.lavender@lstmed.ac.uk

S. Wakasiaka
College of Health Sciences, University of Nairobi, Nairobi, Kenya

W. Khisa
Reproductive Health Department, Kenyatta National Hospital, Nairobi, Kenya

© Springer Nature Switzerland AG 2022
L. B. Drew et al. (eds.), *A Multidisciplinary Approach to Obstetric Fistula in Africa*, Global Maternal and Child Health, https://doi.org/10.1007/978-3-031-06314-5_6

Women with a fistula are easily identified because of the classical urine leakage, stool leakage, or both. Indeed, it could be argued that getting to know a woman with fistula is challenging because of their neglected appearance and strong odor. In Khisa et al. (2017) research, women were referred to as "mongoose" by community members, who compared them to an animal with a foul stench who is often left isolated. These unfortunate events unfold each day, especially in Africa, yet prevention options are cheap and easily accessible. Fistula development is not determined by health workers alone, it is surrounded by multiple factors which need long-term multi-faceted approaches. Unfortunately, many health workers do not know about the basic approach to fistula care (Omari et al., 2015). Trainers and curriculum developers for health workers are also silent on this issue. The lack of information among health workers may lead to women being discharged home without a clear plan of care amid poor health infrastructure. Partly, this contributes to the prolonged periods that women live with fistula in highly stigmatizing communities (Khisa et al., 2017).

Regardless of the cause, fistulas are classified according to size and location whereby Type 1 refers to small fistulas (Fig. 6.1), Type 2—medium size fistulas (Fig. 6.2), and Type 3—large fistulas (Fig. 6.3). The diagnosis and care of fistula are not complicated as long as patients are under skilled hands.

6.2   Prevalence of Obstetric Fistula

The prevalence of obstetric fistula is very difficult to accurately determine due to poor or absent documentation and lack of effective surveillance and case-reporting. This factor contributes to the poor services offered to affected women, as resource allocation and capacity development are reliant on evidence, which is currently very weak in this case. Thus, the prevalence and incidence of obstetric fistula vary significantly owing to challenges in data collection procedures and methods that vary from country to country and study to study. A review of 19 studies, aimed at assessing the global prevalence and incidence of obstetric fistula, failed due to the lack of studies that used a nationally representative sample (Adler et al., 2013). However, estimates show that over two million women live with fistula around the world, out of which, over one million are located in sub-Saharan Africa and South Asia

Fig. 6.1 Appearance of a small recto-vaginal fistula. (Courtesy of Dr. Weston Khisa)

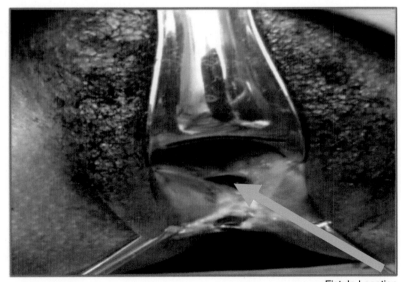

Fistula Location

Fig. 6.2 A medium-sized Type IIAb obstetric fistula with circumferential defect. (Courtesy of Dr. Weston Khisa)

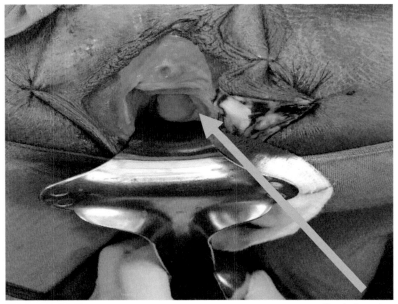

Fistula Location

Fig. 6.3 Appearance of a large Type III uretero-obstetric fistula illustrating a dilated ureter. (Courtesy of Dr. Weston Khisa)

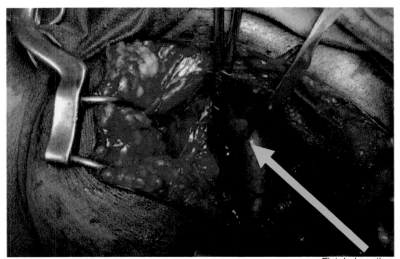

Fistula Location

(World Health Organization, 2018). It is suggested that a further 50,000–100,000 new cases of fistula develop each year (World Health Organization, 2018), although, as stated, the methodology has inherent challenges. This is equivalent to approximately 2 per 1000 women of reproductive age in sub-Saharan Africa and South Asia who are at risk of developing a fistula in any given year.

However, similar to so many conditions affecting pregnant women in this part of the world, the true prevalence of obstetric fistula is likely to be even greater than that reported. The prevalence relies on self-reporting from women or from surgeons who, in most cases, only collect data at the facility level (Tunçalp et al., 2014). Furthermore, the lack of a standardized data collection system at national, regional, and international platforms makes room for uncoordinated, unstandardized approaches to fistula surveillance. Such haphazard processes make accurate data reporting very difficult. This is because in most cases only women presenting for fistula care services at the hospitals are identified. With such a stigmatized condition (Khisa et al., 2017), many women live in silence; thus, the true prevalence of fistula remains unknown.

The unavailability of accurate data is compounded by the inaccessibility and remoteness of the many regions in Africa and Asia where girls and women are at highest risk. Poverty and low literacy levels are common in most rural settings, leaving women with limited employment opportunities. Without an income and access to modern technologies, women continue their plight, not knowing there is a solution; one of the authors of this chapter (WK) has conducted surgery on women who have experienced fistula for more than 30 years. In part, such a scenario explains why research reports conclude that fistula is a condition for the poor, rural woman (Keya et al., 2018). In our experience, women often only learn about fistula through awareness-raising programs, and not through core health services.

6.3   Social Aspects of Obstetric Fistula

The plight of fistula sufferers is compounded by the studious silence that families and communities maintain toward a woman experiencing fistula (Lavender et al., 2016). Neither women, their partners, nor healthcare providers openly talk about fistula; thus, the stigmatization is reinforced. This is evident in a quote from a partner of a woman who had a fistula, in a previous study (Lavender et al., 2016):

> You know I understand her very well ... she is mine ... So, this fistula problem that she has is not something to go announcing out there ... it is my problem ... it is our secret the two of us. I understand my wife and love her the way she is and I can't start telling people about her issue what for? I consider this VVF issue my private agenda. (p. 57)

In this grounded theory study (Lavender et al., 2016), the core theme was revealed as "secrecy hinders support." This theme describes how the stigmatization stops people talking about fistula, which in turn acts as a barrier to women being made aware that they can access help, thus compounding the problem.

The social environment is pivotal to women accessing, receiving, and recovering from obstetric treatments. The poorest women are the most vulnerable (Keya et al., 2018) but also have less decision-making power (Roush et al., 2012), resulting in less access to essential services including emergency obstetric care. A typical example of how fistula is related to the social environment in general and poverty in particular can be seen in Box 6.1.

Box 6.1 An Exemplar of the Social Impact on Women

Karen (pseudonym), from Kenya, was married off to a polygamous man aged 68; at the time, she was aged 15 years and in primary school. Her father was given 30 cows as a dowry, which is in keeping with the tradition of the region. The family needed the cows to help educate her younger brother (who was seen as a priority for education) and take care of her father's medical bills. Karen was never involved in the marriage arrangement nor did she know the man until the day they came for her. When she arrived at his home, she was shocked to find he had three other wives and many children. A year later she became a mother. Unfortunately, she was a mother without a baby. Her baby died at birth and an obstetric fistula developed. Her husband did not accept this predicament since all his wives had babies normally and were not leaking urine. As a consequence, Karen found herself alone; she was rejected by the people around her but also had no baby to hold and console her. A year after the fistula developed, her husband married another young wife and his life went on unperturbed.

Karen had no source of income or a skill to help her survive. The stress of her lifestyle, particularly her isolation, was too much and on many occasions she contemplated taking her own life. One day, the village health workers organized a health talk which she attended. Karen learnt that her condition was curable and that she did not have to pay for the service. Again, explaining and convincing her husband that she needed to travel to the city for treatment were a real challenge. However, finally he agreed. Karen arrived at the fistula center where she received fistula surgery, which healed without complications. At this point, Karen had lived with the fistula for 14 years.

Although Karen was delighted to now be continent, her relationship with her husband had already broken down and could not be regained. Because she had no education and no family support, her life did not change much since the stigma still persisted even after she healed. In many instances, she felt hopeless and wanted to die and escape the pain of rejection even after fistula healed.

Karen's story highlights the complexities around fistula and how women's experiences are embedded in a cultural context which fails to empower or support women.

Women with obstetric fistula are often neglected and rejected by the very society where they were born and grew up. In our qualitative work (Khisa et al., 2017), women having fistula would find it difficult to use public transport or attend community gatherings; some were even banned by the church. Many of the women we have studied were abandoned by their husbands or were made to sleep in animal dwellings.

The question one has to ask is whether the world would still be silent if fistula affected men in the same way it affects women today. What would be different and why? Furthermore, how long can women wait for a global voice to end fistula? It is an unfortunate fact that gender inequalities exist across all societal strata's in many low-income settings, including the health system (Murunga, 2017). However, there is some optimism, particularly if the fifth Sustainable Development Goal (SDG) (United Nations, 2015), which focuses on achieving gender equality and empowerment of all women and girls, can be operationalized.

6.4   Impact of Women's Position in Society

Poverty and the poor status of women in some traditional cultures underpin a combination of economic, biological and social risk factors that ensure developing countries bear the global burden of obstetric fistula (Wall, 2006). Factors that put women at risk of developing obstetric fistula include early age of marriage, malnutrition, and underdeveloped pelvis (Miller et al., 2005); lack of skilled birth attendants (Wall, 2012); and women's reliance on gaining familial permission to access those healthcare services that do exist (Roush et al., 2012). Female genital mutilation and traditional intrapartum vulvar cutting have also been linked by some investigators to development of obstetric fistula (Berg & Underland, 2013; World Health Organisation, 2019), although others disputed this association, as obstetric fistula tends to occur at the pelvic brim or cavity and not at the pelvic outlet, where such cutting predominantly takes place (Wall et al., 2005). It may be, however, that the association is more related to the demographics of women receiving female genital mutilation as opposed to a clinical rationale; i.e., poor women in rural settings are more likely to have female genital mutilation and are more likely to give birth without a skilled birth attendant, resulting in fistula.

Seen as both physically and spiritually unclean, women with obstetric fistula are highly stigmatized by their communities. They are excluded from religious and social life (Gebresilase, 2015; Lavender et al., 2016; Khisa et al., 2017) and may be forced to live in total isolation (Khisa et al., 2017). As women with obstetric fistula are physically incapable of carrying out agrarian work, they become economically dependent (Khisa et al., 2017) or fend for themselves through begging and prostitution (Fenta, 2010). Not only will many women with obstetric fistula have lost their babies due to asphyxia during obstructed labor (estimated to be as much as 90% by Ahmed et al., 2016), but their condition can render them infertile (Kopp et al., 2017) and make them more at risk of sexual dysfunction (Pope et al., 2018). This failure to meet gender expectations leads to domestic abuse and/or high rates of divorce (Khisa et al., 2017), increasing a woman's social and economic isolation. These physical, economic, and sociocultural burdens have a tremendous impact on women's psychological well-being and greatly increase their risk of depression and suicidal ideation (Khisa et al., 2011; Wilson et al., 2015).

6.5   Impact of Fistula on Children

A neglected area of investigation related to fistula is the impact it has on the children of suffering women; there is a dearth of information in the published literature. We have found that fistula has a huge impact on the children of affected mothers, who often take on the burden of being home keeper, particularly when the husband has abandoned the family. In Khisa's work (Khisa et al., 2017), there were many examples of the impact on children; one example is in Box 6.2.

Box 6.2 An Exemplar of the Impact of Fistula on Children

One mother described how other women humiliated her son, who was 11 years old, when he went to collect water from the well. While at the well, a female neighbor asked him his age, and when he told her, she said:

At age 11 and you are still fetching water for your mother to go wash her urine hahahaha ... she laughed.

The boy's education suffered as he had to spend his time supporting his mother by constantly washing her bedding and clothing. On the rare occasion that he invited school friends home, they would tease him saying:

Eh! your mother leaks urine may be the urine drops in the drinking water since ... Do you really expect us to eat and drink urine the way you do? Tell us, tell us, they ask, laughing all the way to or from school.

The son was clearly very upset by this behavior, and his mother told him just to ignore these people. However, the mother also expressed the hurt she felt for her son and she expressed hope that one day her healing would bring some joy to her son's life.

The story related in Box 6.2 is typical of the experiences of children of women who have an obstetric fistula. They often take on the parental role and sacrifice their own existence to care for their mother. These children are often forgotten about in such scenarios, and there are no national programs to support them.

6.6   Fistula Prevention

Prevention of fistula is reliant on a number of social, financial, clinical, and political factors. It is well known, for example, that enabling the girl child to attend school and to delay marriage is a very important step in fistula prevention (Shefren, 2009). The ability to read and write enables the girl to understand and make health-promoting choices in her life; these include family planning choices. In fact, health literacy is regarded as one of the key contributors to fistula prevention (Banke-Thomas et al., 2013). A good education optimizes chances of economic stability, increasing autonomy when health decisions are to be made. For instance, ambassadors to end fistula advocate for women's empowerment, such that when labor starts they are able to travel to the nearest facility, access skilled care, and avert fistula formation (Velez et al., 2007).

At the national and facility level, strengthened health delivery systems, including highly skilled workforces, are required to prevent fistulas. When a woman overcomes individual and community level barriers such as permission to attend the facility, long traveling distances, and travel costs, her care on arrival needs to be prompt and skilled. This is an important aspect of quality maternal health services because unskilled hands are attributed to iatrogenic fistulas (Wall, 2012).

Prolonged and obstructed labors are the main contributors to fistula development, with reports suggesting a mean duration of labor, among fistula patients, of between 2.5 and 4 days (Tebeu et al., 2012; Egziabher et al., 2015). Recognition of prolonged labor is thus imperative; but inadequate resources, in terms of facilities and trained personnel, mean that a downward trend is not imminent. It disappointing to note, however, that the majority of fistulas could be prevented with timely, evidence-based intrapartum care.

A further issue is the lack of feedback to health providers. Women in many low-income settings do not receive any postnatal care. This means that midwives and obstetricians are not always aware of the impact of the care that they have provided in the intrapartum period. This was evident in a workshop that the authors conducted, in which prolonged labor and fistula were discussed. The midwifery participants failed to link the two conditions stating that "fistula does not concern us." It was not that the midwives did not care about the plight of these women, but as they were not seeing the problem they had not considered the direct association. Such disconnect between services needs further attention. Clearly training is required for all health providers who support women of reproductive age. Some classroom training sessions are available for health providers to also gain some experiential learning by working in the fistula clinics, observing the fistula surgery and talking to women who have experienced a fistula.

6.7   Medical Management

The management of obstetric fistula has one principal goal to help girls and women regain full continence without undue delays so that they can resume their activities from their pre-fistula life. Such activities include regaining employment to earn an income to help support herself/family, resuming education, and reintegration into societal structures, among others. In many cases, women living with fistula are courageous enough to tell their story. This is essential, as storytelling enables informative discourse, enabling the woman to learn more about the causes and treatment of fistula. Those that remain in silence may never get treatment and, sadly, may live with the fistula for the remainder of their lives.

All women with obstetric fistula must be accorded the highest standards of care through a sensitive team approach to case management which includes counseling and social rehabilitation. The basic team comprises of fistula surgeons, nurses, midwives, nutritionists, counselors, physiotherapists, social workers and the family, and all play their part in a woman's recovery.

The management of a woman presenting with a fistula problem starts from the admission desk where a comprehensive history is taken by the admitting staff. To provide a conducive environment and accurate data entry, the staff should be sensitized and utilize a standardized checklist which guides data collection at this point. The checklist documents the woman's social and medical background including a detailed obstetric history. This history includes events that took place before, during and after fistula formation; the duration of labor and management; mode of birth, with or without episiotomy, symphysiotomy or destructive surgery; and whether the baby died or lived. The latter is particularly important for care planning as these women often have a "double tragedy" (Ahmed et al., 2016) of losing their baby and their dignity during the same birth. In fact, it has been suggested that the risk of stillbirth is 99 times higher when women develop fistula than if they have a normal birth (Ahmed et al., 2016). These events are rarely brought to the limelight owing to either culture, lack of interest by health workers, or other unknown reasons. The place and characteristics of the birth attendant are also collected to help understand the background of those present at the time fistula occurred and to assess what may have gone wrong before the woman arrived at the health facility.

Thereafter, a comprehensive characterization of the fistula is done to determine whether the woman has experienced a vesico-vaginal fistula or recto-vaginal fistula. Women with vesico-vaginal fistula often present with continuous urine leakage that may have an offensive odor, while recto-vaginal fistula presents with stool leakage with a foul smell. In rare circumstances, a woman may have a coexisting vesico-vaginal and recto-vaginal fistula; she will give a history of leaking both stool and urine.

Once a comprehensive history is completed, the woman is settled into a comfortable bed and prepared for a pelvic examination. Willing and consenting fistula patients are then placed in the exaggerated lithotomy position. This position allows the surgeon to fully examine the woman to ascertain key fistula characteristics, i.e., type, size, location, whether anal sphincter is involved or rectal stricture or circumferential defect is observed. The presence of scarring tissue is noted. After the pelvic examination, a dye test is necessary to help locate the fistula. Once a fistula diagnosis is made, basic laboratory tests are done which include urinalysis, renal function, a hemoglobin (Hb) count, blood typing, and cross-matching. In instances of a fresh fistula, a conservative approach is preferred. This refers to gently inserting an indwelling Foley catheter that is left in place for 4–6 weeks and advising the woman to maintain her perineal hygiene and take plenty of fluids. Adequate fluid intake is important to help flush out bacteria, keep the woman hydrated, and promote tissue healing.

6.8   Conservative Management

Not all fistula patients require surgery to close their fistula. Conservative management refers to a noninvasive approach to fistula management whereby the patient does not receive surgery; instead, simple catheterization is performed. Such management applies in instances where the fistula is small and there is a chance that the fistula may heal spontaneously. The primary objective of conservative management is to spare the woman from the knife and prevent stigma and complications such infections and excoriations that occur due to constant urine leakage. However, this mode of treatment is used only where the fistula is fresh and small in size. Fresh fistulas refer to those that present within 3 months of formation. The period (0–3 months) is also referred to as the physiologic healing period because tissue oxygenation is still good and necrosis has not occurred. Those tissues that were damaged during labor and childbirth may heal spontaneously. The catheter is left in place for 4–6 weeks, which allows continuous urine flow. During the time the patient is catheterized, weekly evaluation and debridement are advised and, as soon as the fistula edges become clean, adaptation of the fistula is performed to promote healing with or without anesthesia.

In other instances, the patient develops stress or overflow incontinence as a result of obstructed and prolonged labor. Overflow incontinence is commonly caused by atonic bladder due to overstretching of the bladder muscle, especially when the woman labors for a long time with a full bladder. Left unattended, women's lives suddenly take a sharp spin downhill. The bladder muscle is left atonic, and the woman is unable to contract her bladder for normal expulsion of urine. Ordinarily, such cases present as a suprapubic tender mass (usually representing a full bladder) and continuous urine leakage through the urethral opening. To confirm that the woman has regained continence, a dye test is done prior to catheter insertion.

It is important to note that routine antibiotics are not administered during the 4–6-week period because fistula is caused by pressure necrosis and tissue ischemic injury and not local or systemic infection. Studies show that 30% of small and fresh fistulas heal spontaneously by catheterization and plenty of fluids intake alone (Waaldijk, 2004). The patients are advised on the need to have hematinics to boost their hemoglobin which helps promote healing. In addition, mobilization is encouraged as soon as possible to prevent permanent foot drop, a common complication among women who experience obstructed labor. Regular vaginal hygiene and debridement of the sloughing tissues are done— these actions promote wound healing. These practices tend to promote spontaneous healing of the bladder especially where the fistula is small, saving the woman from the stigma, rejection, and surgeon's knife.

6.9   Surgical Management

If the conservative approach fails, the woman is informed of the need for a surgical procedure to close the fistula. The surgery is done once the fistula edges are clean.

In theater, surgical principals (Blaivas et al., 1995) guide the surgeon in closing the fistula. The practice is that the fistula is repaired as soon as the woman presents to the hospital to yield better outcomes. This is because early repairs tend to heal better, protecting the woman from stigma and rejection that follows fistula formation.

Women that present with mature fistulas should be prepared for a less conservative approach that involves surgery, while knowing that the first attempt at fistula repair has better outcomes than subsequent repairs. Once surgery has been carried out, the women will be returned to the ward for postoperative care. During this period, women are advised to maintain perineal hygiene, have a high fluid intake, and conduct pelvic exercises. They should also maintain a continuous flow of urine through the catheter. After 2 weeks post-operatively, a dye test is performed to confirm that the fistula has healed. If healed, the catheter is removed, and if not, the catheter can be kept for an extra 2 weeks.

Before discharge, women should be counseled about family planning options and the need to abstain from sexual intercourse for at least 6 months to allow complete healing. For women of reproductive age, the importance of spacing childbirth is emphasized as it allows for proper fistula healing and allows the woman adequate time to rest and recuperate. In addition, the woman is advised on the great need for antenatal care in all future pregnancies; this way, women at risk can be identified earlier and birth plans drawn in response to individual needs. Similar information is given to partners and the family because a supportive system is central to the full recovery and social reintegration of these women.

6.10   Social Reintegration Following Fistula Repair

Following successful fistula repair, women's immediate reaction is one of elation, as they realize that they are continent. However, recently healthcare providers have begun to realize that surgery alone is insufficient to restore women's dignity. Khisa et al. (2017), in his phenomenological study, described "miracle" and "post-miracle" phases, based on qualitative interviews with women. The "miracle" phase represents how women feel prior discharge, knowing that they can resume activities of daily living without the leakage of urine and faces. However, the post-miracle phase comes into play when the woman returns home; the reality is that women find it difficult to re-enter a community that abandoned them in their time of need. It is at this point that women realize that, although they are physically healed, emotionally they remain scarred.

Others (Khisa et al., 2019), in their grounded theory study, have suggested four potential outcomes following surgery: (1) reintegration fully into their previous community, (2) reintegration partially back into their previous communities, (3) no integration at all, and (4) integration into a new community. Given the different scenarios, any programs to support these women need to be tailored to individual needs and circumstances. Women's expectations need to be managed appropriately before surgery, so that they know what to expect after surgery. Social and psychological support should be offered to women both pre- and post-surgery, and this should include developing an individualized short- and long-term post-operative action plan.

6.11   Fistula and Politics

A recent literature review describes nine direct types of barriers to accessing fistula repair: psychosocial, social, political, financial, along with awareness, transportation, facility, and care quality (Baker et al., 2017). The political barriers have probably received the least attention, yet are fundamental to positive changes.

At the surface level, a fistula can be viewed as a medical problem that can be easily fixed for a moderate cost. However, when we hear of women living with fistula for several decades, then one has to question why? At the international level, fistula provides a strong example of global inequity, particularly as we know that it has been totally eradicated in the Global North (Adler et al., 2013). While greater communication systems and increased international travel, as a result of globalization, have raised awareness of the problem, fistula care is still not a priority focus for programmatic interventions, international aid or research prioritization.

Exploring fistula from a reproductive health lens, one can see why fistula prevention and repair have received little investment. Imbedded in large resource-poor facilities, women's health is uncompetitive for two reasons. Firstly, women have a lower status in the countries where fistula is prevalent; thus, their views are rarely sought or valued. Dismissed as "women's business," facility personnel often fail to understand the impact on the woman and the family as a whole. Secondly, cash-strapped facilities usually prioritize funding in areas where disease can be "cured" and where it affects a cross-section of individuals. Treatment of cancer, for example, which affects people, regardless of gender, economic status, or place of residence, receives greater funding than fistula care which affects poor, rural, and women.

Although international communities have begun publicizing the unacceptability of fistula, fistula surgery is still not seen as a desirable career. Fistula surgeons are often applauded for their commitment to women's health, but they will never get rich. There is no money in fistula surgery, and although young medics are often trained in conducting repairs, our personal experience is that the majority do not continue. Most women who have a fistula are poor and therefore cannot pay for health care. In countries where private practice is flourishing, women who have a fistula have nothing to offer.

6.12   Clinician's Perspectives

In his own words, a fistula surgeon said *"training specialized fistula teams helps reduce the burden of fistula in many countries where the condition is prevalent."* However, most of these countries lack structural frameworks that guide fistula care and prevention. This is best exemplified in the lack of fistula training curricula and clinical guidelines. In these settings, it is common to find trained fistula surgeons and midwives working in non-fistula related fields where their specialized knowledge and skills are not applied. Over time, the skills and motivation to do fistula work wanes; meanwhile, women continue to live with the fistula in silence for many years (Khisa et al., 2019).

Lack of a coordinated mechanism, compounded by unavailability of accurate fistula data, makes it difficult to know the fistula prevalence in a given area or those who have been attended to at each healthcare facility or country.

Establishing the quality of fistula services presents as an uphill task because of paucity of well-designed local research on actual number of successful or repeat surgeries. The disconnect between healthcare delivery systems and communities can be seen when women with fistula have undergone surgery and healed and still face rejection by their communities. The rejection is partially attributed to ignorance in fistula knowledge.

6.13   Conclusion

It is unacceptable in this century for women to suffer a condition that is largely preventable and usually treatable. Obstetric fistula provides a heart-breaking example of women's value in some low-income settings. As tweeted by the past First Lady of the United States, Michelle Obama, on October 13, 2016, "The measure of any society is how it treats women and girls."

Education of the girl child has been linked to delayed age of marriage and better employment opportunities. These factors also influence access to emergency obstetric care and fistula services. Equal access to community and family resources for all persons regardless of gender and age is thus vital (Lavender et al., 2016).

Politics aside, fistula remains a major public health issues despite treatment being surgically feasible. A holistic approach including mental health is critical in restoration of women's dignity and for the benefits of the whole family.

Health system strengthening, health professional training, and community engagement are the first steps toward eradication of this debilitating condition. A multidisciplinary approach is pivotal to women receiving the care they deserve. The most affected countries should strive to formulate policy frameworks that guide targeted activities for fistula care and prevention. We should strive for eradication of fistula, but until we have achieved this, women should be provided with, sensitive, evidenced based care. Psychological and social support is also warranted, and this should include support for family members.

References

Adler, A. J., Ronsmans, C., Calvert, C., & Filippi, V. (2013). Estimating the prevalence of obstetric fistula: A systematic review and meta-analysis. *BMC Pregnancy and Childbirth, 13*, 246. https://doi.org/10.1186/1471-2393-13-246. Retrieved June 20, 2019, from https://www.ncbi.nlm.nih.gov/pmc/articles/PMC3937166/

Ahmed, S., Anastasi, E., & Laski, L. (2016). Double burden of tragedy: stillbirth and obstetric fistula. *The Lancet Global Health, 4*(2), e80–e82.

Ali, A., & Adam, I. (2010). Maternal and perinatal outcomes of obstructed labour in Kassala hospital, Sudan. *Journal of Obstetrics and Gynaecology, 30*(4), 376–377. https://doi.org/10.3109/01443611003672096

Arrowsmith, S., Hamlin, E. C., & Wall, L. L. (1996). Obstructed labor injury complex: Obstetric fistula formation and the multifaceted morbidity of maternal birth trauma in the developing world. *Obstetrical & Gynecological Survey, 51*(9), 568–574.

Baker, Z., Bellows, B., Bach, R., & Warren, C. (2017). Barriers to obstetric fistula treatment in low-income countries: A systematic review. *Tropical Medicine & International Health, 22*(8), 938–959. Retrieved June 18, 2019, from https://onlinelibrary.wiley.com/doi/10.1111/tmi.12893

Banke-Thomas, A. O., Kouraogo, S. F., Siribie, A., Taddese, H. B., & Mueller, J. E. (2013). Knowledge of obstetric fistula prevention amongst young women in urban and rural Burkina Faso: A cross-sectional study. *PLoS One, 8*(12), e85921. https://doi.org/10.1371/journal.pone.0085921. Retrieved June 5, 2019, from https://journals.plos.org/plosone/article?id=10.1371/journal.pone.0085921

Berg, R. C., & Underland, V. (2013). *Obstetric consequences of female genital mutilation/cutting (FGM/C).* Report from Norwegian Knowledge Centre for the Health Services (NOKC) No. 06-2013. NOKC. Retrieved August 30, 2019, from https://www.fhi.no/globalassets/dokumenterfiler/rapporter/2013/rapport_2013_06_obstetric_consequences_fgm_v6.pdf

Blaivas, J. G., Heritz, D. M., & Romanzi, L. J. (1995). Early versus late repair of vesicovaginal fistulas: Vaginal and abdominal approaches. *Journal of Urology, 153*(4), 1110–1112.

Egziabher, T. G., Eugene, N., Ben, K., & Fredrick, K. (2015). Obstetric fistula management and predictors of successful closure among women attending a public tertiary hospital in Rwanda: A retrospective review of records. *BMC Research Notes, 8*, 744. https://doi.org/10.1186/s13104-015-1771-y. Retrieved May 20, 2019, from https://www.ncbi.nlm.nih.gov/pmc/articles/PMC4676892/

Fenta, T. A. (2010). From trauma to rehabilitation and reintegration: Experiences of women facing the challenge of obstetric fistula in Addis Ababa, Ethiopia. *International Institute of Social Studies*, 1–62. Retrieved March 10, 2019, from https://thesis.eur.nl/pub/8768

Gebresilase, Y. T. (2015). A qualitative study of the experience of obstetric fistula survivors in Addis Ababa, Ethiopia. *International Journal of Women's Health, 6*, 1033–1043. Retrieved June 30, 2019, from https://www.ncbi.nlm.nih.gov/pmc/articles/PMC4266262/

Keya, K. T., Sripad, P., Nwala, E., & Warren, C. E. (2018). "Poverty is the big thing": Exploring financial, transportation, and opportunity costs associated with fistula management and repair in Nigeria and Uganda. *International Journal for Equity in Health, 17*(1), 70. https://doi.org/10.1186/s12939-018-0777-1. Retrieved June 15, 2019, from https://www.ncbi.nlm.nih.gov/pmc/articles/PMC5984775/

Khisa, W., Mutiso, S., Mwangi, J., Qureshi, Z., Beard, J., & Venkat, P. (2011). Depression among women with obstetric fistula in Kenya. *International Journal of Gynaecology and Obstetrics, 115*(1), 31–33. https://doi.org/10.1016/j.ijgo.2011.04.015

Khisa, W., Wakasiaka, S., McGowan, L., Campbell, M., & Lavender, T. (2017). Understanding the lived experience of women before and after fistula repair: A qualitative study in Kenya. *British Journal of Obstetrics and Gynaecology, 124*(3), 503–510. Retrieved May 10, 2019, from https://obgyn.onlinelibrary.wiley.com/doi/full/10.1111/1471-0528.13902

Khisa, A. M., Nyamongo, I. K., Omoni, G. M., & Spitzer, R. F. (2019). A grounded theory of regaining normalcy and reintegration of women with obstetric fistula in Kenya. *Reproductive Health, 16*(1), 29. Retrieved May 25, 2019, from https://reproductive-health-journal.biomedcentral.com/articles/10.1186/s12978-019-0692-y

Kopp, D. M., Wilkinson, J., Bengtson, A., Chipungu, E., Pope, R. J., Moyo, M., et al. (2017). Fertility outcomes following obstetric fistula repair: A prospective cohort study. *Reproductive Health, 14*(1), 159. https://doi.org/10.1186/s12978-017-0415-1. Retrieved June 28, 2019, from https://www.ncbi.nlm.nih.gov/pmc/articles/PMC5704560/

Lavender, T., Wakasiaka, S., McGowan, L., Moraa, M., Omari, J., & Khisa, W. (2016). Secrecy inhibits support: A grounded theory of community perspectives of women suffering from obstetric fistula, in Kenya. *Midwifery, 42*, 54–60. https://doi.org/10.1016/j.midw.2016.10.001

Miller, S., Lester, F., Webster, M., & Cowan, B. (2005). Obstetric fistula: A preventable tragedy. *Journal of Midwifery and Women's Health, 50*(4), 286–294.

Murunga, V. (2017). *Africa's progress on gender equality and women's empowerment is notable but gender inequality persists.* Africa Up Close. Retrieved June 30, 2019, from https://africaupclose.wilsoncenter.org/africas-progress-on-gender-equality-and-womens-empowerment-is-notable-but-gender-inequality-persists/

Omari, J., Wakasiaka, S., Khisa, W., Omoni, G., & Lavender, T. (2015). Women and men's awareness of obstetric fistula in facilities in Kisii and Nyamira Counties, Kenya. *African Journal of Midwifery and Women's Health, 9*, 12–16.

Orach, C. G. (2000). Maternal mortality estimated using the Sisterhood method in Gulu district Uganda. *Tropical Doctor, 30*(2), 72–74. https://doi.org/10.1177/004947550003000205

Pope, R., Ganesh, P., Chalamanda, C., Nundwe, W., & Wilkinson, J. (2018). Sexual function before and after vesicovaginal fistula repair. *The Journal of Sexual Medicine, 15*(8), 1125–1132. https://doi.org/10.1016/j.jsxm.2018.06.006

Roush, K., Kurth, A., Hutchinson, M. K., & Van Devanter, N. (2012). Obstetric fistula: What about gender power? *Health Care for Women International, 33*(9), 787–798.

Shefren, J. M. (2009). The tragedy of obstetric fistula and strategies for prevention. *American Journal of Obstetrics and Gynecology, 200*(6), 668–671. https://doi.org/10.1016/j.ajog.2009.03.008

Tunçalp, O., Tripathi, V., Landry, E., Stanton, C. K., & Ahmed, S. (2014). Measuring the incidence and prevalence of obstetric fistula: Approaches, needs and recommendations. *Bulletin of the World Health Organization, 93*(1), 60–62. https://doi.org/10.2471/BLT.14.141473. Retrieved March 10, 2019, from https://www.who.int/bulletin/volumes/93/1/14-141473/en/

Tebeu, P. M., Fomulu, J. N., Khaddaj, S., de Bernis, L., Delvaux, T., & Rochat, C. H. (2012). Risk factors for obstetric fistula: a clinical review. *International urogynecology journal, 23*(4), 387–394.

UNFPA. (2018). *Obstetric fistula.* Author. Retrieved February 1, 2019, from https://www.unfpa.org/obstetric-fistula

United Nations. (2015). *Sustainable development goals.* Author. Retrieved June 26, 2019, from https://sustainabledevelopment.un.org/?menu=1300

Velez, V. A., Ramsey, K., & Tell, K. (2007). The Campaign to End Fistula: What have we learned? Findings of facility and community needs assessments. *International Journal of Gynaecology and Obstetrics, 99*(Suppl 1), S143–S150. https://doi.org/10.1016/j.ijgo.2007.06.036

Waaldijk, K. (2004). The immediate management of fresh obstetric fistulas. *American Journal of Obstetrics and Gynaecology, 191*(3), 795–799.

Waaldijk, K., & Elkins, T. E. (1994). The obstetric fistula and peroneal nerve injury: An analysis of 947 consecutive patients. *International Urogynecology Journal, 5*(1), 12–14.

Wall, L. L. (1998). Dead mothers and injured wives: The social context of maternal morbidity and mortality among the Hausa of northern Nigeria. *Studies in Family Planning, 29*(4), 341–359.

Wall L. L, Arrowsmith S. D, Briggs N. D, Browning A, Lassey A. T. (2005) The obstetric vesicovaginal fistula in the developing world. *Obstet Gynecol Survey, 60*(suppl 1), S1–51

Wall, W. L. (2006). Obstetric vesico-vaginal fistula as an international public-health problem. *The Lancet, 368*(9542), 1201–1209. https://doi.org/10.1016/S0140-6736(06)69476-2

Wall, L. L. (2012). Preventing obstetric fistulas in low-resource countries: Insights from a Haddon matrix. *Obstetrical & Gynecological Survey, 67*(2), 111–121. https://doi.org/10.1097/OGX.0b013e3182438788

Wilson, S. M., Sikkema, K. J., Watt, M. H., & Masenga, G. G. (2015). Psychological symptoms among obstetric fistula patients compared to gynecology outpatients in Tanzania. *International Journal of Behavioral Medicine, 22*(5), 605–613. https://doi.org/10.1007/s12529-015-9466-2. Retrieved May 2, 2019, from https://www.ncbi.nlm.nih.gov/pmc/articles/PMC4779591/

World Health Organisation. (2019). *Health risks of female genital mutilation (FGM).* Author. Retrieved June 30, 2019, from http://www.who.int/reproductivehealth/topics/fgm/health_consequences_fgm/en/

World Health Organization. (2006). *Obstetric fistula: Guiding principles for clinical management and program development.* Author. ISBN 9241593679. Retrieved January 9, 2019, from http://whqlibdoc.who.int/publications/2006/9241593679_eng.pdf

World Health Organization. (2018). *10 Facts on obstetric fistula.* Author. Retrieved March 10, 2019, from http://www.who.int/features/factfiles/obstetric_fistula/en/

Women Who Lose Their Lives While Giving Life: Exploring Obstetric Fistula as a Public Health Issue in Kenya

7

Kathomi Gatwiri

7.1 Introduction

Obstetric fistula is referred to in many euphemisms. The United Nations Population Fund and the World Health Organisation call it the "hidden disease" (UNFPA, 2001; World Health Organization, 2006), Graham (1998) calls pregnancy-related deaths and injuries such as fistulas the "scandal of the century", and Wall (2012) calls it the most "neglected problem" in the world. About 10 years ago, the World Health Organization estimated (although not through concrete data) that globally, more than two million women were living with an obstetric-related fistula (OF), with the vast majority of those located in developing countries in Asia and Africa (DeBernis, 2007). Although a systematic review and meta-analysis conducted by (Adler et al., 2013) suggests that the prevalence of fistula could be lower than what is often reported, their study does not consider the overwhelming majority of women who never report their fistulas in medical facilities. I have also argued elsewhere in (Gatwiri, 2018) that the magnitude of the problem, and particularly in sub-Saharan Africa where data records are quite unsophisticated and where majority of cases go unreported, could be much greater. Despite this staggering number, the obstetric fistula condition remains hidden and neglected, with profound consequences for sufferers as well as their families and communities. Velez et al. (2007) cited the concerns of the World Health Organization (WHO), arguing that for *"For each of the half million women who die in pregnancy and childbirth each year, approximately 20–50 experience morbidities which, if left untreated, can cause lifelong [injuries]"*. Life during the most healthy and productive years of the fistula-affected women becomes wasted in a constant and non-ending negotiation with the intricacies and the complexities of the shame that living with an incontinent body fosters.

Perhaps the biggest tragedy about the obstetric fistula "scandal" is that it is completely preventable and treatable but due to inadequate and/or absent maternal health care for women in most African countries during childbirth, the devastating and widespread outcomes continue to impacts millions of women's lives. As Wall et al. (2005) argue, *"the fistula problem in third world countries will not be solved until those nations also develop effective systems of maternal health care"*. As of 2005, when Lewis Wall and colleagues wrote the seminal text, *"Obstetric Vesico-Vaginal Fistula in the Developing World"*, only 13 countries accounted for the 70% of all global maternal deaths. These were, "*India,*

77

777

7777

K. Gatwiri (✉)
Faculty of Health, Centre for Children & Young People, Southern Cross University,
Gold Coast, Australia
e-mail: Kathomi.Gatwiri@scu.edu.au

© Springer Nature Switzerland AG 2022
L. B. Drew et al. (eds.), *A Multidisciplinary Approach to Obstetric Fistula in Africa*, Global Maternal and Child Health, https://doi.org/10.1007/978-3-031-06314-5_7

Nigeria, Pakistan, DRC, Ethiopia, Tanzania, Afghanistan, Bangladesh, Angola, China, Kenya, Indonesia and Uganda … [however] when ranked according to [the obstetric risk present], the most dangerous countries for pregnant women are all in sub-Saharan Africa" (Wall et al., 2005). These include Sierra Leone, Malawi, Zimbabwe, Chad, Central African Republic, Guinea Bissau, Kenya, Mozambique, Burkina Faso and Burundi. That these data and statistics did not inform drastic policy changes in the sub-Sahara begs us to question the commitment and the goodwill channelled at ending suffering for millions of women. In 2019, no woman should literally or figuratively lose their lives while trying to give one.

7.2   Defining and Contextualising Fistulas in Kenya

As established in literature, obstetric fistulas are mostly caused by prolonged obstructed labour (Cowgill et al., 2015; Kelly, 1992; Cichowitz et al., 2018; Wall, 2006, 2018; Gatwiri & Fraser, 2017; Gatwiri & McLaren, 2017). When labour is obstructed, there is often enormous and persistent pressure from the baby's head against the pelvic tissues of the mother. Wall (2006) states that this occurs due to cephalopelvic disproportion, a situation in which the baby's head becomes trapped in the mother's pelvis *because of a discrepancy between the size of the foetus and the space available in her pelvis*". Sometimes, obstructed labour occurs from the manner in which the baby is positioned during labour or a combination of the two. When labour is obstructed, a woman is unable to push the baby through her birth canal, leading to compression of blood vessels, decreased blood flow, and causing prolonged tissue ischemia and consequent irreversible cell death (necrosis) that leads to tissue breakdown and the formation of a vesico- or recto-vaginal fistula. However, Khisa (2009, cited in Human Rights Watch, 2010) argues that although "*medically fistula is caused by obstructed labour … there is [also] obstructed transport, obstructed family planning, obstructed emergency care, obstructed rights*".

A vesico-vaginal fistula and a recto-vaginal fistula are often formed through a tearing between the woman's vagina and her bladder and/or rectum, resulting in the incontinence of urine or faeces or at times both (Bashah et al., 2018; Beattle, 2005). In his book "*Tears for my Sisters*", Wall (2018) states that obstetric fistulas need to also be understood in the context of the "*human obstetrical dilemma*". He makes the argument that as "*we need to deliver larger babies with bigger brains through a narrower, constricted pelvis … the consequences of these biological constraints are amplified*" for women during childbirth. For African women, the stakes are higher because as Wall (2006) posits, African women are more predisposed to dystocia due to their relatively narrower construction of their pelvises as compared to women of European descent.

Compounding these possible evolutionary consequences, obstetric fistulas often demonstrate a range of various socioeconomic and structural complexities and dynamics within the contexts where they are most prevalent. The prevalence of obstetric fistulas problematises the ranking and marginalisation of women's sexual and reproductive health needs, which are often pushed to the periphery to function as a "by the way" by legislators and makers of health policies. The gendered framing of obstetric fistulas complicates the preventative and curative efforts as legislators (who are almost always men) tend to view them solely as a "women's issue" and not as a "public health" issue. I have argued elsewhere in (Gatwiri & Fraser, 2017) that if obstetric fistulas were a condition that exclusively affected men in their millions, ruined their families, halted their sexual lives, led to their diminished productivity in the social and economic sphere and attached shame to their masculine identities, then elaborate measures would have already been employed to eradicate the condition at least in the African context.

Amidst the policy marginalisation in the most affected countries such as Kenya, the medical and social consequences of obstetric fistula remain dire, with women in several studies reporting experiences of depression, suicidal ideation and attempts, hopelessness, powerlessness, and an overall diminished quality of life in terms of their health and well-being (Khisa & Nyamongo, 2012; Khisa et al., 2017; Weston et al., 2011; Mselle & Kohi, 2015a; Gatwiri, 2018; Mwanri & Gatwiri, 2017). The impact of living with an obstetric fistula and the experience of living with a *leaking* and incontinent body generate extensive feelings of loss of control and uncleanliness. Often, though, the consequences of obstetric fistulas are social. These may include broken or fractured marriages, relationships and friendships, unemployment, exclusion from community gatherings and a further lowering of women's social status in community. However, the personalised nature of reporting and theorising the impacts of fistulas, though necessary, takes the focus away from where it needs to be. That is, how structural systems fail these women and condemning them to a life of shame and stigmatisation that lacks dignity.

When the Kenya Ministry of Health and the United Nations Population Fund (UNFPA) conducted a needs assessment of women with obstetric fistula in 2004, they reported that approximately 3000 women and girls developed fistula annually (in Kenya this constitutes 1 out of every 500 live births) and that there were an estimated 300,000 cases of untreated fistulas in the ever-increasing backlog. In 2018, 15 years after this study, Kenya is still described as one of the most dangerous countries in the world to be a woman and pregnant. Citing a World Bank report, Burbano-Herrera (2017) noted that in Kenya "*only 44% of births are delivered under the supervision of a skilled birth attendant*", with the remainder being attended to by traditional birth attendants as well as by female relatives and friends from community. To put this in an even more direr context, "*In Kenya in [the year] 2015 alone, 8000 expectant mothers died from pregnancy related complications*", and many more developed lifelong obstetric injuries such as fistulas. "*This means that each single day in Kenya 22 women die from preventable causes related to pregnancy and childbirth*" (Burbano-Herrera, 2017). In a country with more than 3000 new cases of fistulas each year, only one-third of those are treated due to lack of fistula specialist clinics and doctors. The national newspaper in Kenya reported recently that the country has only eight fistula surgeons, against the backlog of almost 300,000 women already living with fistulas and an additional 3000 new cases annually (Bii, 2017). Clearly, this is more than a "women's issue". The data tell us that it is a public health crisis.

In continuing to demystify the myth that obstetric fistulas are a women's issue rather than a public health one, I must also address the commonly asked question; who are the typical fistula patients? Hawkins et al. (2013) found that in Kenya it was mostly poor, young girls with minimal formal education, living in geographically remote areas who were most predisposed to developing fistulas. This suggests that in contexts where women and girls have limited access to formal education, they are more likely to marry young and have less sexual and reproductive health knowledge to inform their bodily autonomy and decision-making. The other structural issue includes the inadequacies in the healthcare system which are often unavailable to provide emergency care when girls/women report with critical obstetric needs. The study by Hawkins et al. (2013) suggested that it is structural issues that underpin the problem, trends and dimensions of obstetric fistulas. They reported that, "*Poverty, long distances to maternity facilities, inaccurate obstetric knowledge, and Kenya's rugged landscape were identified as major barriers to prevention of obstetric fistula*". Women living with fistula represent the significant absence of maternal health care that exists in the Kenyan context. As McFadden et al. (2011) state, obstetric fistulas as a health care phenomenon and the suffering many women endure during childbirth are directly related to the limited availability of obstetrical care.

In 2010, Human Rights Watch (2010) released the *I Am Not Dead, But I Am Not Living: Barriers to Fistula Prevention and Treatment in Kenya* report which highlighted the multiple ways that the Kenyan state, despite being a signatory of various reproductive health charters, violates and infringes on the rights of fistula sufferers. This occurs through "*denying them their internationally-guaranteed access to the highest attainable standard of health, to health information critical to women's and girls' wellbeing, to their reproductive and maternal health, and to a remedy for the injustices and denial of service that they face*" (Human Rights Watch, 2010). The Kenyan government has a responsibility to the national and international law to abide by its commitment to protect the human rights of women and girls by providing them with adequate sexual and reproductive health care. Women living with fistula are an acute example of how the Kenyan government has contributed, through its lack of action and political goodwill, to the rise and prevalence of obstetric fistulas in this country.

7.3   Barriers to Accessing Emergency Obstetric Care in Kenya

To be a pregnant woman in Africa is to have one foot in the grave – An African Proverb

7.3.1   Kagandu's Story

I met Kagandu[1] in the December of 2014 when I was in Kenya collecting data for my doctoral project[2] which sought to investigate how Kenyan women with vaginal fistulas negotiated their fistula diagnosis. Kagandu was waiting for her turn to receive a restorative fistula surgery at the Kenyatta National Hospital in Nairobi. She was a 39-year-old woman living in rural Meru County (location changed for anonymity) and had been married for close to two decades and had five children. Kagandu reported that her last child was significantly "bigger" which caused her to experience labour that lasted for more than 2 days. She mentioned that she had been trying to give birth at home with the help of a Traditional Birth Attendant (TBA) but because the labour was "*not progressing*", the TBA decided that Kagandu should be taken to the nearest hospital.

Kagandu's experience of seeking obstetric care was thwarted when she arrived at the hospital in a critical condition after a complicated, obstructed, and prolonged labour nearing 3 days. She was informed that the doctor on call was "very tired" and that if she *really* needed a doctor, he would be called. She was made aware at the hospital reception that it had been a "very busy day at the hospital and that there were others in the waiting room in more critical conditions". As the pain progressed, and with no one to help her, Kagandu's situation got worse. It is not until she fainted on the floor from the pain that the nurses rushed to call the doctor. The next thing she recalls was waking up in the theatre. She had not only lost her baby-but as she would also discover later, she had developed a vesico-vaginal fistula which she would live with for the next several years. I use this story as a backdrop to theorise these challenges in more detail next.

7.3.2   The Barriers and Their Causes

Different complications can arise during childbirth leading to devastating lifelong injuries or even death to the mother, infant or both. Access to quality Emergency Obstetric Care (EmOC) when these complications arise can be a matter of life and death (World Health Organization, 2006). Citing the UNFPA handbook which monitors emergency obstetric care in different countries, Geleto et al. (2018) state that there are two different but complementary emergency obstetric services. One is the Basic

---

[1] Pseudonyms have been used to protect the anonymity of the study participants.

[2] The research was approved by Flinders University as well as Kenya's research ethics boards.

Emergency Obstetric Service (BEmOS) and the other is a Comprehensive Emergency Obstetric Service (CEmOC). A BEmOC facility provides six critical obstetric services which are also referred to as the "signal functions". They include administration of parenteral antibiotics, parenteral anticonvulsants, parenteral uterotonics, removal of retained products, manual removal of placenta and assisted vaginal delivery. CEmOC comprehensive emergency care facilities on the other hand deliver caesarean sections as well as blood transfusion services in addition to the signal functions of BEmOC. If every pregnancy is a risk, as Graham (1998) posits, then it is necessary that women are able to access the above-listed emergency obstetric services if and when it becomes necessary. Unfortunately, in most sub-Saharan countries including Kenya, access to both BEmOS and CEmOC is limited or unavailable.

As established earlier, a woman's locality (urban or rural), level of education, socioeconomic status, tribal affiliation and religion and cultural attitudes on childbirth greatly determine where they deliver their babies (Kitui et al., 2013). These factors may prevent many women in Kenya from accessing quality maternal health care. Physically and geographically, many women in rural and remote areas live far away from healthcare facilities. It may take such women several hours if not days to arrive at the nearest hospital. In some places where roads and bridges may be impassable (due to rain or terrain), access to transportation can be impossible. For some, the time taken to negotiate access to a hospital or clinic may be too late to save themselves and/or their baby. Educationally and culturally, there is also a vast number of women who lack basic knowledge on obstetric complexities and birthing preparedness (Kabakyenga et al., 2011; Udofia et al., 2013). Some women may have cultural or social traditional beliefs that may exacerbate complications during birth (Maimbolwa et al., 2003). For example, traditional beliefs that associate prolonged or obstructed labour with infidelity (Hadley & Tuba, 2011) or spiritual practices such as offering prayers instead of medical assistance (Aziato & Cephas, 2018) may have devastating obstetric consequences that can lead to the formation of fistulas.

In addition, numerous other structural and systemic barriers from also accessing dignified maternal health care exist. Studies show that some women deliberately avoid healthcare facilities because of the alarming cases of abuse, disrespect, maltreatment and malpractice during childbirth (McMahon et al., 2014; Bohren et al., 2015; Abuya et al., 2015; Warren et al., 2013). For some, the fear of being victimised, disrespected and abused by medical staff functions is a key barrier to seeking help in health facilities. As an example, Moyer et al. (2014) showed that many women in labour were treated "*like they [were] not human beings*". This study found that women suffered obstetric violence in the form of physical abuse, verbal abuse, neglect and other various forms of overt and covert discrimination.

In *Please Understand When I Cry Out In Pain* (D'Ambruoso et al., 2005) details harrowing accounts of women's experiences in maternity services during labour. While also exploring the different trends of disrespect and abuse during childbirth, Bowser and Hill (2010) showed that abuse and disrespect can take various forms and manifestations. These may include physical or verbal abuse (e.g. slapping, spitting, making derogatory comments about one's body or sex life); non-consented care (e.g. being handled or touched intimately without any priori communication); non-confidential care (e.g. one's private and intimate details being disclosed in front of others); non-dignified care (e.g. exposure of one's nudity in front of others, sharing hospital beds, no clean sheets or privacy); discrimination (due to socioeconomic class, religion or tribe); abandonment of care (e.g. being left without support); and detention in facilities (e.g. being held indefinitely in a hospital due outstanding maternity bills).

Studies have indicated that this trend persists where there is a lack of patient-centred treatment approaches, absence of professional accountability and deficient maternal policies to protect women who have experienced abuse while giving birth (Ishola et al., 2017; Asefa & Bekele, 2015; Sethi et al., 2017; Rosen et al., 2015). Without development of a compassionate system of maternal care, a kind of care that centres on women and their needs during childbirth (sometimes referred to as femifocal care), a majority of women will continue giving birth at home where they feel more respected and supported-regardless of the risks involved. Economically, women may also "choose" to give birth at home because they may not have enough money to finance the hospital bills. Montagu et al. (2011) showed that most poor women in developing countries give birth at home because of the costs associated with delivery. In fact, Izugbara et al. (2008) found that one of the key reasons why 60% of Kenyan women still use traditional birth attendants is because "*hospital-based obstetric care [was] out of the economic reach of [many] women*" (p. 41).

7.3.3   The 3D Model to Understanding Barriers of Obstetric Care

In *Too Long to Walk*, Thaddeus and Maine (1994) proposed the seminal 3D model that underscores the major barriers to seeking obstetric health care. In this model, they argue that three things determine the delays in seeking health care: (1) delay in making a decision to seek care in a health facility, (2) delay in reaching the hospital, and (3) delay in receiving adequate care at the hospitals once there. The 3Ds function both *before* and *after* the development of obstetric injuries such as fistulas. In my doctoral research, for example, I interviewed women who were *still* living with obstetric fistulas but were currently seeking restorative surgeries in hospitals. They gave heartbreaking stories that involved their experiences with the three Ds. As with the findings from other studies, my research found that some of the factors that influence the first delay in making a decision to seek care are distance, cost, family and cultural attitudes, and scepticism in the quality of care—particularly due to corruption.

The factors influencing the second delay include shortage and inaccessibility of healthcare facilities, the latter due to remoteness of geographical terrain, long distance to be travelled and the lack of transportation. Often in rural areas in developing countries, there are few public transport vehicles, and when they are available, they are often overcrowded and have little ventilation. The third delay suggests that women can sometimes reach the hospital on time but still die there or develop serious injuries due to delayed or denial of proper care. This is due to underequipped and understaffed facilities (refer to Kagandu's story above for context). Izugbara et al. (2008) noted, "*Kenya's public health sector is [grossly] under-financed and characterized by [severe] shortages of [the] most basic [medical] essentials*". The shortage of medical staff and essential equipment affects the waiting period a woman has to endure before seeing a doctor (Mselle et al., 2011). At times too, the "doctor" is not really a fully trained doctor but a clinical officer or a student intern who may lack competence on how to address complex labour obstructions. At other times, even when the doctors are present and know what to do, they may lack essential tools and equipment to perform a safe operation or caesarean section (Schwartz, 2015). As Schwartz states,

> *... a pregnant woman's life may hang by a thread, even when they are able to reach a health facility, a haemorrhaging woman dies because the blood bank staff are on their break and have taken their keys with them; a caesarean section for an adolescent with an obstructed labour is postponed because the washing machine has broken and the operating room could not be prepared, resulting in her death; a pregnant woman with eclampsia and foetal distress cannot get oxygen because the hospital assistant is absent and the staff do not know how to connect the oxygen cylinder; a woman with a severe infection cannot have her fever measured because the thermometer is broken; a young woman with preeclampsia cannot have her blood pressure monitored because the blood pressure cuff is missing; there are no needles remaining for the life-saving blood test ... the list of breakdowns in the human sequence of maternal care goes on and on.*

This structural failure in the healthcare infrastructure can result in life and death situations for women needing emergency obstetric care. To summarise how the three delays function (Thaddeus &

Maine, 1994), reflect on a letter that they received from a colleague articulating how the three domains intersect and interact across the aforementioned barriers,

> *By the time they have found a vehicle to go to hospital, by the time they [have] struggled to get her an admission card. By the time she [is] admitted, by the time her file [is] made up, by the time the midwife [is] called, by the time the midwife finishes eating, by the time the midwife comes, by the time the husband goes and brings some gloves, by the time the gloves are brought to the hospital … by the time the midwife examines the woman, by the time the bleeding starts, by the time the doctor is called, by the time the doctor can be found, by the time the ambulance goes to [get] the doctor, by the time the doctor comes … by the time the t's had been properly crossed and all the i's dotted and the husband signs the consent form, the woman has died* (p. 1102).

This shows that obstetric fistulas are not accidental—they are a predictable outcome of poor structural failures and reinforce the African proverb that commenced this section. That is; to be "pregnant in Africa, is to have one foot in the grave".

7.4 Moving from the Personal to the Political: Rethinking the Cultural Discourse of Obstetric Fistulas

The popularised "single story" image of a typical fistula sufferer is problematic. As I established earlier, the "typical fistula sufferer" implies a personal and individualised discourse of fistula. My suggestion is to rethink this narrative and position fistulas in a structural and political paradigm. In the following statement, Heller and Hannig (2017) reflect on how a "typical fistula sufferer" is mostly presented in discourse and in media.

> *The narrative zeroes in on a particular type of fistula sufferer: she is young, innocent, and physically underdeveloped. Those with fistula are rarely portrayed as women, but widely referred to as "girls". The fistula narrative routinely focuses on "child" marriage as a principal cause of obstructed labour, resulting in pregnancies among girls whose pelvises are too small and "immature" to birth a fully developed child. Invoking images of abused, despoiled, or tainted youth, fistula is then framed as the physical evidence of corrupted "cultural" practices–of children who are no longer allowed to be children, as they are drafted into marriage and its onerous duties. The narrative's emphasis on first pregnancies means that the young girl is left without living children, leaving her alone and without value in cultures portrayed as aggressively pronatalist* (pp. 84–85).

The public discourse on obstetric fistulas is often dominated by the above narrative and is preoccupied with synonymising culture and fistulas. The rhetoric of fistulas today focuses much on issues of early marriage, child marriages, early childbirth and female genital mutilation, with these "cultural" nuances being summoned often as the "causes" of fistula (Heller & Hannig, 2017). Fistulas are commonly theorised through the lens of harmful traditional practices and "backward cultures" that place women at the bottom of the social hierarchy. These "backward practices" are often cited as the reason why the incidence of fistulas is so prevalent in *those* countries with "bad culture".

Positioning "bad culture" as the cause of fistulas is an inadequate way of exploring the phenomenon of obstetric fistulas in all its complex nuances. This is because, it allows theorisation of fistulas to mostly fall back on old and tired stereotypes about Africa and African women. By pathologising African traditions and culture, the continent is essentialised and its women are positioned as backward, helpless and passive victims of "primitive" cultural practices. This framing postions African women as more susceptible to developing and suffering from conditions "that do not affect Westerners". The theorisation here, locates culture as an immovable, permanent and irreversible obstacle that enters the lives of African women right from when they are children and *ruins* their lives. This argument assumes that culture ensures that girls/women are denied education, married young to older men and become pregnant early—and with their lives now "ruined"—they spend the rest of their lives in servitude to the "bad" men who married them to elevate their social status. This "bad culture" follows the woman, robbing her of all agency, and is summoned again during labour where the child/girl/woman is pressured to give birth at home (like a real woman) where she is attended to by traditional birth attendants with no medical skills. When a fistula develops, culture follows her, where she is abandoned and shunned by her community due to not meeting her "womanly and wifely" roles and falling short of her "cultural expectations". Her success as a human being is weighed and measured through cultural lenses where notions of purity and corporeality are constantly evoked and summoned. All through, the structures surrounding her—the political and systemic barriers, which continually fail her on a daily basis—are erased from the narrative.

A focus on culture as the "cause" of fistulas overrides and overshadows a more pertinent focus on the economic, political and environmental conditions under which African women live and work. As Heller and Hannig (2017) note, the *"focus on pathological "culture" has fashioned a reality in which the structural dimensions of how women sustain obstetric fistula and how they navigate their injury have become obscured. As a result, the solution to the problem of fistula seems to lie in reforming cultural habits, such as "child" marriage, rather than instituting complex health access reforms"*. In part, the popularised accounts of fistula in Western media and in most published research on the topic unwittingly reproduce a historicised and colonised representation of Africa—once again portraying Africans as being obsessed and submerged in traditions and cultures that are dysfunctional. The dominant cultural narrative of obstetric fistulas has been overtaken by Western media constructing an incomplete picture that over-exaggerated the "cultural cruelty" that leads to the development of fistulas.

Women with fistula are also mostly painted as being "voiceless, modern-day lepers" who embody the perfect imagery of the modern-day social pariah (Hannig, 2012). This is not in any way to say that fistula sufferers do not experience anguish, pain, humiliation, shame and stigma—but rather, to unsettle the dominant fistula narrative and to disrupt the oversensationalised discourse that is mostly packaged for the consumption of the Western audiences at the expense of the dignity of the African women living with the fistula. Indeed, African women suffering from fistulas are mostly positioned as objects of pity and cultural curiosity. In McLaren and Gatwiri (2016), we argued that even through internet imagery, *"[African] with vaginal fistulas become represented in Internet images … as deviant, diseased, abnormal or as curiosities"*. Through this perception, *"visual imageries of [their] abject bodies are created, contained and exploited through hegemonic politics that reinforce stereotypes of race, gender and disability"*. We further argued that through the undignified and dehumanised manner in which African *"women's bodies with fistulas are portrayed in media, the complexity of the social, cultural, economic and political circumstances surrounding the fistula is therefore silenced and disregarded"*.

Let us consider this, before the institutionalisation of birthing, obstetric fistulas were just as prevalent in Western countries as they are in Africa and in parts of Asia now. The numerous attempts by Doctor J. Marion Sims[3] to close obstetric fistulas, mostly in black women in the USA, show that the problem dates back to the last few centuries. Interestingly, culture is never mentioned as a "cause" of fistulas while describing the prevalence of fistulas in Western countries in the previous centuries. The Western prevalence of fistula is always theorised through the lens of "lack of proper maternal health care". In addition, the "immature" and "pudendal" pelvic muscles of adolescent and young girls are often seen as the reason why obstructed deliveries occur in this age group. However, fistulas still occur in adult women (such as Kagandu). The only difference is that in Western countries, women have bet-

---

[3] J. J. Marion Sims, MD (1813–1883) was an American physician known as the "father of modern gynaecology". Sims practiced and perfected his surgical techniques on enslaved black women without the use of anaesthesia which had just recently been developed. Between seeing his first patient with vesico-vaginal fistula in 1845 until 1849, Sims conducted experimental surgery on 12 enslaved women with fistulas in his backyard hospital in Alabama. His "experimentation" on Black women's bodies has now been criticised by Black scholars as racist.

ter and more comprehensive access to emergency obstetric care. Western women who develop obstetric fistulas during childbirth are "fixed" straight away before being discharged to go home.

Put simply, while at first glance it might seem that the main variables for developing obstetric fistulas are poverty, age, marital status, low levels of education, geographical location and residence, age of first pregnancy, and early marriage (Sagna et al., 2011), obstetric fistulas are solely caused by obstructed labour—which if not addressed in a timely way through accessible emergency obstetric care leads to tears and tissue necrosis that creates the fistula. This can happen to women of any age, race, socioeconomic group, educational background, physical stature, nationality, ethnicity, and religion. Numerous studies continue to indicate that it is the inaccessibility to quality obstetric care when experiencing complicated and obstructed labour that leads to the development of fistulas (Mselle & Kohi, 2015b; Mselle et al., 2011; Human Rights Watch, 2010; Pope, 2018). Despite these structural shortfalls, giving birth at home is still discussed as a "personal choice" or a "cultural preference" rather than as a structural failure by the health situations in the most affected countries like Kenya.

The problem of fistula therefore needs to be discussed as a structural issue, one that is perpetuated by broken health infrastructures and as a consequence of the geo-political and economic systems. As Heller and Hannig (2017) advice, the complexity of the problem *"extends well beyond the specificity of fistula and applies to other global health initiatives whose focus on cultural inadequacies and individual behaviours obscures vast structural inequalities"*. The cultural fixation and the pathological obsession with putting African cultures under scrutiny while discussing fistulas, often with the minimisation of the structural factors, poses more risk to the theorisation of conditions like fistulas because it "misses the mark", whereas there is more to gain from long-term, contextual and systemic analysis *"that takes seriously the complex structural obstacles faced by those who experience illness and injury, while also understanding that their lives do not cave under the force of these constraint"* (Heller & Hannig, 2017).

Summoning an individualised lens that blames women, their families and their communities for their "choices", or accusing them of refusing to embrace "modern medicine and technology" surrounding childbirth practice, serves to minimise the difficulties surrounding their access to such facilities and services. The medical facilities which are stated to be the "ultimate solution" to the fistula problem are often understaffed, underequipped and inaccessible. Qualified obstetric and gynaecological specialists are still largely unavailable, the antibiotics are still late in arrival, the blood banks are still empty, and surgical equipment and "stuff" are still in shortage. Additionally, the abuse and mistreatment of women during childbirth still linger in Kenyan hospitals.

7.5 Reimagining Kenya Without the Burden of Obstetric Fistulas: Framing the Conclusion and the Way Forward

Seen as one the most dangerous places for a pregnant woman, it is almost hard to imagine Kenya as a country free of obstetric fistulas and as a space and place that is safe for birthing women. Kenya has one of the highest maternal mortality rates in the world—with a significant number of the women who survive a complicated and traumatising childbirth acquiring debilitating, life-altering injuries such as fistulas (Neilson et al., 2003; AbouZahr, 2003). These statistics of women dying and developing fistulas through complicated births in Kenya indicate a lagging commitment by the government to address this reality. The government of Kenya has a duty and a responsibility to remedy this situation. The interaction between the political and the health system and women's rights demonstrates that Kenya is not "responsive to women's needs [before or] during fistula illness" (Khisa et al., 2017). As a signatory to international charters and treaties that protect the rights of women to give birth safely, and according to the national and international guidelines, the Kenyan government is currently participating in the violation of women's rights by choosing inaction. The government has a solemn duty to correct and undo these maternal injustices perpetrated towards women—through developing a system of accountability and correcting systemic failures that lead to the development of preventable obstetric complications conditions such as fistulas.

It has been long said that women rights are human rights but without accountability and access to these rights, they remain no more than lip service and decorative speech. Ahmed and Tunçalp (2015) state *"That [obstetric fistulas are] still a public health problem in some countries shows the enormous gap in maternal health care between high-income and low-income nations and is a result of the egregious failure of health systems in these regions to provide safe maternity care"*. The good news is that all cases of obstetric fistula can be prevented with timely intervention and access to emergency obstetric care. This has been true of all industrialised countries, where virtually all fistulas have been eliminated because of advanced medical technology, expertise and availability of obstetric care for women.

To bring this to a close, the key message remains this; to understand the full picture of the obstetric crisis in Kenya, one has to look at the structural face of health care and the gendered way in which it stratifies and marginalises women. The general theorising of obstetric fistulas from a structural rather than a cultural perspective enables us to gain some insight about the overall plight of women living with this condition. I have argued in this chapter that largely due to the unresponsiveness of the healthcare system in Kenya, women are forced to seek alternative forms of care such as prayer, home remedies, unsupervised home births, with less than desired outcomes—sometimes fatal. Unfortunately, as established, the deaths of women who die from these "women issues" are not always taken seriously. But as Walley (as cited in Moulton, 2001) reminds us, *"death is death whether it occurs on the end of a bullet or giving birth"*.

References

Abouzahr, C. (2003). Global burden of maternal death and disability. *British Medical Bulletin, 67*(1), 1–11. Retrieved January 26, 2019, from https://academic.oup.com/bmb/article/67/1/1/330397

Abuya, T., Warren, C. E., Miller, N., Njuki, R., Ndwiga, C., Maranga, A., et al. (2015). Exploring the prevalence of disrespect and abuse during childbirth in Kenya. *PLoS One, 10*(4), E0123606. https://doi.org/10.1371/Fjournal.pone.0123606

Adler, A. J., Ronsmans, C., Calvert, C., & Filippi, V. (2013). Estimating the prevalence of obstetric fistula: A systematic review and meta-analysis. *BMC Pregnancy and Childbirth, 13*, 246. https://doi.org/10.1186/1471-2393-13-246

Ahmed, S., & Tunçalp, Ö. (2015). Burden of obstetric fistula: From measurement to action. *The Lancet Global Health, 3*(5), e243–e244. Retrieved February 4, 2019, from https://www.thelancet.com/journals/langlo/article/PIIS2214-109X%2815%2970105-1/fulltext

Asefa, A., & Bekele, D. (2015). Status of respectful and non-abusive care during facility-based childbirth in a hospital and health centers in Addis Ababa, Ethiopia. *BMC Reproductive Health, 12*, 33. https://doi.org/10.1186/s12978-015-0024-9

Aziato, L., & Cephas, N. (2018). Initiation of traditional birth attendants and their traditional and spiritual practices during pregnancy and childbirth in Ghana. *BMC Pregnancy and Childbirth, 18*, 64. https://doi.org/10.1186/s12884-018-1691-7

Bashah, D. T., Worku, A. G., & Mengistu, M. Y. (2018). Consequences of obstetric fistula in sub Sahara African countries, from patients' perspective: A systematic review of qualitative studies. *BMC Women's Health, 18*, 106. Retrieved February 3, 2019, from https://bmcwomenshealth.biomedcentral.com/articles/10.1186/s12905-018-0605-1#Sec1

Beattle, J. B. (2005). Life shattering but preventable: Obstetric fistula. *UN Chronicle, 42*, 60–62. Retrieved January 31, 2019, from https://www.questia.com/magazine/1G1-141814475/obstetric-fistula-life-shattering-but-preventable

Bii, B. (2017). Lack of specialists hinders treatment of fistula cases. *Daily Nation*. Retrieved January 27, 2019, from https://www.nation.co.ke/health/Lack-of-specialists-hinders-treatment-of-fistula-cases/3476990-3956802-2sl2v7/index.html

Bohren, M. A., Vogel, J. P., Hunter, E. C., Lutsiv, O., Makh, S. K., Souza, J. P., et al. (2015). The mistreatment of women during childbirth in health facilities globally: A mixed-methods systematic review. *PLoS Medicine, 12*(6), E1001847. https://doi.org/10.1371/journal.pmed.1001847

Bowser, D., & Hill, K. (2010). *Exploring evidence for disrespect and abuse in facility-based childbirth: report of a landscape analysis*. USAID-TRAction Project. USAID. Retrieved January 24, 2019, from https://cdn2.sph.harvard.edu/wp-content/uploads/sites/32/2014/05/Exploring-Evidence-RMC_Bowser_rep_2010.pdf

Burbano-Herrera, C. (2017). Examining high rates of preventable maternal mortality in Kenya: Could provisional measures be an effective tool to Guarantee safe pregnancy?'. *Journal of African Law, 61*(2), 197. https://doi.org/10.1017/S002185531700016X

Cichowitz, C., Watt, M. H., Mchome, B., & Masenga, G. G. (2018). Delays contributing to the development and repair of obstetric fistula in northern Tanzania. *International Urogynecology Journal, 29*(3), 397–405. https://doi.org/10.1007/s00192-017-3416-2

Cowgill, K. D., Bishop, J., Norgaard, A. K., Rubens, C. E., & Gravett, M. G. (2015). Obstetric fistula in low-resource countries: An under-valued and under-studied problem: Systematic review of its incidence, prevalence, and association with stillbirth. *BMC Pregnancy and Childbirth, 15*(193), 1–7. https://doi.org/10.1186/s12884-015-0592-2

D'ambruoso, L., Abbey, M., & Hussein, J. (2005). Please understand when I cry out in pain: Women's accounts of maternity services during labour and delivery in Ghana. *BMC Public Health, 5*, 140. https://doi.org/10.1186/1471-2458-5-140

DeBernis, L. (2007). Obstetric fistula: Guiding principles for clinical management and programme development, a new WHO guideline. *International Journal of Gynecology & Obstetrics, 99*, S117–S121. https://doi.org/10.1016/j.ijgo.2007.06.032

Gatwiri, K. (2018). *African womanhood and incontinent bodies: Kenyan women with vaginal fistulas*. Springer.

Gatwiri, G., & Fraser, H. (2017). Putting vaginal fistulas on the international social work map: A critical perspective. *International Social Work, 60*, 1039–1050. https://doi.org/10.1177/0020872815594865

Gatwiri, G., & Mclaren, H. J. (2017). Better off dead' – Sasha's story of living with vaginal fistula. *Journal of International Women's Studies, 18*(2), 247–259.

Geleto, A., Chojenta, C., Mussa, A., & Loxton, D. (2018). Barriers to access and utilization of emergency obstetric care at health facilities in sub-Saharan Africa - A systematic review protocol. *Systematic Reviews, 7*(1), 183. https://doi.org/10.1186/s13643-018-0720-y

Graham, W. (1998). The scandal of the century. *British Journal of Obstetrics and Gynaecology, 105*, 375–376. https://doi.org/10.1111/j.1471-0528.1998.tb10116.x

Hadley, M. B., & Tuba, M. J. (2011). Local problems; local solutions: An innovative approach to investigating and addressing causes of maternal deaths in Zambia's Copperbelt. *BMC Reproductive Health, 8*, 17. https://doi.org/10.1186/1742-4755-8-17

Hannig, A. (2012). *The gift of cure: Childbirth injuries, clinical structures, and religious subjects in Ethiopia*. University of Chicago.

Hawkins, L., Spitzer, R. F., Christoffersen-Deb, A., Leah, J., & Mabeya, H. (2013). Characteristics and surgical success of patients presenting for repair of obstetric fistula in western Kenya. *International Journal of Gynecology & Obstetrics, 120*(2), 178–182. https://doi.org/10.1016/j.ijgo.2012.08.014

Heller, A., & Hannig, A. (2017). Unsettling the fistula narrative: Cultural pathology, biomedical redemption, and inequities of health access in Niger and Ethiopia. *Anthropology & Medicine, 24*(1), 81–95. https://doi.org/10.1080/13648470.2016.1249252

Human Rights Watch. (2010). *I am not dead, but I am not living: Barriers to fistula prevention and treatment in Kenya*. Author. Retrieved January 4, 2019, from https://www.hrw.org/report/2010/07/15/i-am-not-dead-i-am-not-living/barriers-fistula-prevention-and-treatment-kenya

Ishola, F., Owolabi, O., & Filippi, V. (2017). Disrespect and abuse of women during childbirth in Nigeria: A systematic review. *PLoS One, 12*(3), e0174084. https://doi.org/10.1371/journal.pone.0174084

Izugbara, C., Ezeh, A., & Fotso, J. C. (2008). The persistence and challenges of homebirths: Perspectives of traditional birth attendants in urban Kenya. *Health Policy and Planning, 24*(1), 36–45. https://doi.org/10.1093/heapol/czn042

Kabakyenga, J. K., Östergren, P. O., Turyakira, E., & Pettersson, K. O. (2011). Knowledge of obstetric danger signs and birth preparedness practices among women in rural Uganda. *BMC Reproductive Health, 8*, 33. https://doi.org/10.1186/1742-4755-8-33

Kelly, J. (1992). Vesico-vaginal and recto-vaginal fistulae. *Journal of the Royal Society of Medicine, 85*(5), 257–258.

Khisa, A. M., & Nyamongo, I. K. (2012). Still living with fistula: An exploratory study of the experience of women with obstetric fistula following corrective surgery in West Pokot, Kenya. *Reproductive Health Matters, 20*(40), 59–66. https://doi.org/10.1016/S0968-8080(12)40661-9

Khisa, A. M., Omoni, G. M., Nyamongo, I. K., & Spitzer, R. F. (2017). 'I stayed with my illness': A grounded theory study of health seeking behaviour and treatment pathways of patients with obstetric fistula in Kenya. *BMC Women's Health, 17*(92), 1–14. https://doi.org/10.1186/s12905-017-0451-6

Kitui, J., Lewis, S., & Davey, G. (2013). Factors influencing place of delivery for women in Kenya: An analysis of the Kenya demographic and health survey, 2008/2009. *BMC Pregnancy and Childbirth, 13*, 40. Retrieved February 5, 2019, from https://www.ncbi.nlm.nih.gov/pmc/articles/PMC5622500/

Maimbolwa, M. C., Yamba, B., Diwan, V., & Ransjö-Arvidson, A. B. (2003). Cultural childbirth practices and beliefs in Zambia. *Journal of Advanced Nursing, 43*(3), 263–274.

Mcfadden, E., Taleski, S. J., Bocking, A., Spitzer, R. F., & Mabeya, H. (2011). Retrospective review of predisposing factors and surgical outcomes in obstetric fistula patients at a single teaching hospital in western Kenya. *Journal of Obstetrics and Gynaecology Canada, 33*(1), 30–35. https://doi.org/10.1016/S1701-2163(16)34769-7

Mclaren, H. J., & Gatwiri, G. (2016). Black women with vaginal fistula: The power to silence via internet imagery. *Social Alternatives, 35*(1), 47–52.

Mcmahon, S. A., George, A. S., Chebet, J. J., Mosha, I. H., Mpembeni, R. N., & Winch, P. J. (2014). Experiences of and responses to disrespectful maternity care and abuse during childbirth; a qualitative study with women and men in Morogoro Region, Tanzania. *BMC Pregnancy and Childbirth, 14*, 268. https://doi.org/10.1186/1471-2393-14-268

Montagu, D., Yamey, G., Visconti, A., Harding, A., & Yoong, J. J. (2011). Where do poor women in developing countries give birth? A multi-country analysis of demographic and health survey data. *PLoS One, 6*(2), e17155. https://doi.org/10.1371/journal.pone.0017155

Moulton, D. (2001). Death is death whether it occurs on the end of a bullet or giving birth. *Canadian Medical Association Journal, 165*(3), 384.

Moyer, C. A., Adongo, P. B., Aborigo, R. A., Hodgson, A., & Engmann, C. M. (2014). They treat you like you are not a human being: Maltreatment during labour and delivery in rural northern Ghana. *Midwifery, 30*(2), 262–268. https://doi.org/10.1016/j.midw.2013.05.006

Mselle, L. T., & Kohi, T. W. (2015a). Living with constant leaking of urine and odour: Thematic analysis of socio-cultural experiences of women affected by obstetric fistula in rural Tanzania. *BMC Women's Health, 15*, 107. https://doi.org/10.1186/s12905-015-0267-1

Mselle, L. T., & Kohi, T. W. (2015b). Perceived Health System Causes of Obstetric Fistula from Accounts of Affected Women in Rural Tanzania: A qualitative study. *African Journal of Reproductive Health, 19*(1), 124–132.

Mselle, L. T., Kohi, T. W., Mvungi, A., Evjen-Olsen, B., & Moland, K. M. (2011). Waiting for attention and care: Birthing accounts of women in rural Tanzania who developed obstetric fistula as an outcome of labour. *BMC Pregnancy and Childbirth, 11*, 75. https://doi.org/10.1186/1471-2393-11-75

Mwanri, L., & Gatwiri, G. J. (2017). Injured bodies, damaged lives: Experiences and narratives of Kenyan women with obstetric fistula and Female Genital Mutilation/Cutting. *BMC Reproductive Health, 14*, 38. https://doi.org/10.1186/s12978-017-0300-y

Neilson, J., Lavender, T., Quenby, S., & Wray, S. J. (2003). Obstructed labour: Reducing maternal death and disability during pregnancy. *British Medical Bulletin, 67*(1), 191–204. https://doi.org/10.1093/bmb/ldg018

Pope, R. (2018). Research in obstetric fistula: Addressing gaps and unmet needs. *Journal of Obstetrics and Gynecology, 131*(5), 863–870.

Rosen, H. E., Lynam, P. F., Carr, C., Reis, V., Ricca, J., Bazant, E. S., & Bartlett, L. A. (2015). Direct observation of respectful maternity care in five countries: A cross-sectional study of health facilities in East and Southern Africa. *BMC Pregnancy and Childbirth, 15*, 306. https://doi.org/10.1186/s12884-015-0728-4

Sagna, M. L., Hoque, N., & Sunil, T. (2011). Are some women more at risk of obstetric fistula in Uganda? Evidence from the Uganda demographic and health survey. *Journal of Public Health in Africa, 2*(2), 108–111.

Schwartz, D. A. (2015). Interface of epidemiology, anthropology and health care in maternal death prevention in resource-poor nations. In D. A. Schwartz (Ed.), *Maternal mortality: Risk factors, anthropological perspectives, prevalence in developing countries and preventive strategies for pregnancy-related death* (pp. ix–xiv). Nova Science Publishers.

Sethi, R., Gupta, S., Oseni, L., Mtimuni, A., Rashidi, T., & Kachale, F. (2017). The prevalence of disrespect and abuse during facility-based maternity care in Malawi: Evidence from direct observations of labor and delivery. *Reproductive Health, 14*, 111. https://doi.org/10.1186/s12978-017-0370-x

Thaddeus, S., & Maine, D. (1994). Too far to walk: Maternal mortality in context. *Social Science & Medicine, 38*(8), 1091–1110.

Udofia, E. A., Obed, S. A., Calys-Tagoe, B. N., & Nimo, K. P. (2013). Birth and emergency planning: A cross sectional survey of postnatal women at Korle Bu Teaching Hospital, Accra, Ghana. *African Journal of Reproductive Health, 17*(1), 27–40.

UNFPA. (2001). *Obstetric fistula: United Nations and International Obstetricians Meet to Combat Hidden Disease.* Author. Retrieved January 24, 2019, from https://www.unfpa.org/press/obstetric-fistula-united-nations-and-international-obstetricians-meet-combat-hidden-disease

Velez, A., Ramsey, K., & Tell, K. (2007). The campaign to end fistula: What have we learned? Findings of facility and community needs assessments. *International Journal of Gynaecology and Obstetrics, 99*(1), S143–S150.

Wall, L. (2006). Obstetric vesicovaginal fistula as an international public-health problem. *Lancet, 368*(9542), 1201–1209.

Wall, L. (2012). Obstetric fistula is a "neglected tropical disease". *PLoS One, 6*(8), e1769. https://doi.org/10.1371/journal.pntd.0001769

Wall, L. (2018). *Tears for my sister: The tragedy of obstetric fistulas.* John Hopkins University Press.

Wall, L., Arrowsmith, S. D., Briggs, N. D., Browning, A., & Lassey, A. (2005). The obstetric vesicovaginal fistula in the developing world. *Obstetrical and Gynecological Survey, 60*(1), s3–s51.

Warren, C., Njuki, R., Abuya, T., Ndwiga, C., Maingi, G., Serwanga, J., et al. (2013). Study protocol for promoting respectful maternity care initiative to assess, measure and design interventions to reduce disrespect and abuse during childbirth in Kenya'. *BMC Pregnancy and Childbirth, 13*, 21. https://doi.org/10.1186/1471-2393-13-21

Weston, K., Mutiso, S., Mwangi, J. W., Qureshi, Z., Beard, J., & Venkat, P. (2011). 'Depression among women with obstetric fistula in Kenya. *International Journal of Gynecology & Obstetrics, 115*(1), 31–33. https://doi.org/10.1016/j.ijgo.2011.04.015

World Health Organization. (2006). *Obstetric fistula: Guiding principles for clinical management and programme development.* Author. Retrieved January 24, 2019, from https://apps.who.int/iris/bitstream/handle/10665/43343/9241593679_eng.pdf?sequence=1&isAllowed=y

Kathomi Gatwiri   is the author of "*African Womanhood and Incontinent Bodies*" (Springer ISBN 978-981-13-0564-1) and an award-winning researcher, currently residing in Australia. Dr. Gatwiri is a social worker and psychotherapist who holds a Bachelor of Social Work from the Catholic University of Eastern Africa, a Master's in Counselling and Psychotherapy from the Cairnmillar Institute in Melbourne and a PhD from Flinders University in South Australia. In 2017, Gatwiri was named Young Kenyan of the Year by the Kenya Association of South Australia for her achievements and service in the African community in Australia.

Part II

Perspectives and Experiences from Women and Girls with Obstetric Fistula

Obstetric Fistula: A Case of Miscommunication—Social Experiences of Women with Obstetric Fistula

8

Marielle E. Meurice, Saifuddin Ahmed, and René Génadry

8.1 Introduction

Obstetric fistula (OF) is an abnormal communication between the vaginal canal and the bladder and/or rectum most commonly caused by an obstructed labor or a traumatic delivery. This preventable condition has been eliminated in high-income countries from obstetric causes but remains prevalent where emergency obstetric care (EmOC) services are unavailable, inaccessible, unaffordable, inadequate, and/or untimely. Delays in recognition of prolonged or obstructed labor in seeking care and obtaining proper management are the three main risk factors facilitating the development of an OF. This chapter looks at miscommunication at the core of the development of an abnormal communication between the various pelvic organs resulting in the flow of their contents (urine, feces) outside their natural pathway into the vagina. Such miscommunication also applies to individual, community, and national levels, where the outflow of this critical information on prevention and treatment to who it should be disseminated and acted upon is deficient or defective. This has allowed obstetric fistula to persist and thus creates challenges in eradicating this disastrous condition.

M. E. Meurice (✉)
Department of Obstetrics & Gynecology, University of California, Irvine, CA, USA
e-mail: mmeurice@uci.edu

S. Ahmed
Department of Population, Family, and Reproductive Health, Johns Hopkins University Bloomberg School of Public Health, Baltimore, Maryland, USA

R. Génadry
Department of Obstetrics & Gynecology, University of Iowa, Iowa City, IA, USA

© Springer Nature Switzerland AG 2022
L. B. Drew et al. (eds.), *A Multidisciplinary Approach to Obstetric Fistula in Africa*, Global Maternal and Child Health, https://doi.org/10.1007/978-3-031-06314-5_8

8.2   Anatomical Miscommunication

8.2.1   Mechanisms of Development

Obstructed labor can occur secondary to cephalopelvic disproportion (CPD), malpresentation or in a protracted or prolonged labor course. Also, women that experience malnutrition or under-nutrition and younger women with immature anatomy can have smaller pelvic sizes that create a situation where operative delivery including cesarean section becomes necessary, but in resource-poor areas it is often not available and particularly not in a timely manner (Konje & Ladipo, 2000). With ongoing obstruction that sometimes lasts several days, the head of the fetus exerts a force on the pelvic bones and ultimately causes the intervening tissue to undergo necrosis due to ischemia. This damaged area eventually sloughs off, allowing the breakdown of a critical barrier between the involved organs and leaving behind a fistula wherever the pressure was exerted (bladder, urethra, rectum, etc.) (Creanga & Genadry, 2007). This pathologic process often results in dense scarring of the surrounding tissues, and nervous structures can also be affected (Wall, 2006). Most women with obstetric fistulas suffer injuries involving multiple organ systems: The syndrome of *obstetric labor injury complex* has been coined to encompass all morbidities associated with OF and can involve the urologic, gynecologic, gastrointestinal, neurologic, and musculoskeletal systems (Arrowsmith et al., 1996; Tennfjord et al., 2014).

8.2.2   Factors Influencing Successful Repair

Surgical treatment is the mainstay of therapy to correct an OF unless it is small and discovered early to allow conservative means of management (with urinary catheter) to have a chance of success. There are several factors that can make surgical repair difficult and the outcome less predictable. These include extensive tissue loss and development of scar tissue, irritation of urination/fecal matter, and the involvement of the urethra (Loposso et al., 2016). Patients requiring more than one procedure to close the defect add to the backlog of patients whose fistulas continue to be created daily in the developing world. The initial surgery has the best prognostic outcome.

Because it is difficult to estimate the number of actual cases, determining the best approach to addressing the back log of surgical cases has been challenging. Unfortunately, many of these countries where obstetric fistula is most prevalent are those in which access to repair will likely be at least as difficult as is access to medical care. Even a common language to facilitate communication has been difficult to agree upon. Indeed, classifying and standardizing the severity of obstetric fistula have proven challenging with more than 25 classification systems (see chapter in this book by Goh & Krause). Many academic reports utilize the Waaldijk classification system that uses three types based on the anatomic and functional structure violated with modifiers based on extent of injury (Waaldijk, 1995). An alternative classification with objective measurements has been suggested and is gaining acceptance, but properly conducted studies remain lacking. This makes comparative studies difficult and hampers progress in the proper care of the patient with OF (Goh, 2004).

Many articles discuss obstetric fistula as having a simple surgical remedy, but this is not always the case and often requires highly trained surgical teams for successful repair and extensive services for women who have been stigmatized and are suffering socially and mentally as well. One example of a comprehensive effort is described in rural Burundi, which was funded by Médecins Sans Frontières (MSF). This center has undertaken efforts to advertise its services as a dedicated center for the care of women both pre- and post-operatively, with a staff of expert surgeons who are able to help train local doctors, as well as pelvic floor physical therapy and follow-up with medical personnel and social workers (Tayler-Smith et al., 2013).

Even after a successful surgical repair, a number of morbidities—including residual incontinence—can persist in the medical and social realms and have profound effects on women, making the definition of surgical success elusive.

8.3   Individual-Level Miscommunication

Communication at the level of the individual is an essential aspect to understanding how OF develops and consequently what can be done to prevent it from occurring. Miscommunications regarding what to expect during labor can lead to delay. Once a labor complication has developed, miscommunications between the patient and their family, healthcare workers, and community members can also contribute to delays in seeking and receiving timely care. Lack of knowledge due to miscommunication regarding prolonged labor, the cause of OF, and availability of cesarean section may lead to difficulty in prevention efforts and timely treatment.

8.3.1   Barriers to Recognition of Labor Abnormality and Evaluation

Delay is often thought to be the cause of obstetric fistula with reference to the three types of delay first described by Thaddeus and Maine: (1) delay in deciding to seek treatment, (2) delay in actually arriving at health facility, and (3) delay in receiving adequate care (Fig. 8.1) (Thaddeus & Maine, 1994).

All women from a fistula study in Malawi had experienced delay arising in one of these areas. These authors cited lack of resources, lack of health literacy, poor access to health care, and lack of male involvement in the birthing process as contributing factors to delay in seeking care. One woman's experience included being treated by a traditional birth attendant (TBA) who did not realize she was pregnant with twins until she noted the arm of the second twin presenting and was unable to proceed with delivery. After 3 h of waiting, they called an ambulance. The trip to the hospital then took 10 h. This description provides a glimpse into some of the horrors that women experience in developing a fistula. Improving education at the level of the individual during pregnancy, together with warning signs of prolonged or obstructed labor, are suggested as methods to help prevent delay at the level of the individual. However, in actual practice, this proves more challenging than in theory (Changole et al., 2018).

When labor becomes obstructed, the duration of time in which the intervening body tissues are compressed from onset of obstruction to delivery is of critical importance, further emphasizing how miscommunication allows this obstetric fistula to develop. The degree of ischemic damage to the compressed tissues is dependent upon rapid and accurate diagnosis, mobilization of resources to obtain transportation, and identifying and reaching a healthcare provider capable of relieving the

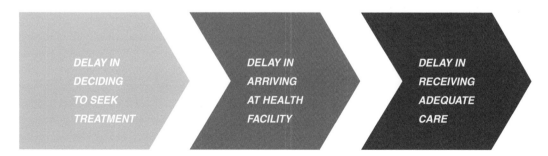

Fig. 8.1 Three delays leading to obstetric fistula

obstruction competently. The first level of delay may be from confusion as what to do next for treatment, gender inequalities in deciding to seek care, fear of hospitals and misinformation on treatments available, and cost (Wall, 2012). In many settings, women are not empowered to seek treatment without the consent of their husband or mother-in-law. Additionally, defining prolonged labor can be difficult, as it takes many variables into account including phase of labor, parity, frequency of contractions, membrane status, and many other factors. This further complicates educating others on what defines a normal labor course; nonetheless, partograms and labor curves can be used to help diagnose a labor dystocia. However, this requires skills and training.

In a study from Tanzania, a 20-year-old woman recounted her story of developing OF (Mselle et al., 2011). She had attended antenatal care, and when she started having contractions, a TBA was called. She labored all night without progress and was sent to the village dispensary. There she was told to push without an examination or assessment of her progress. She pushed without success, so others were called from the village.

"Some put cloths into my mouth; others tightened my legs, while others pinched me, as they were telling me I must push. In the end, I was exhausted, and foam started coming out of my mouth. There was no progress; the baby was stuck in the pelvis, when I raised my legs the baby could easily be seen. It was stuck between my legs. After many hours my legs became numb and I could not walk."

It was not until the third day that she was seen by her physician to be told of fetal demise and the need to be referred to the hospital with further delay and to proceed to secure funds for transportation. Following a forceps delivery, she started leaking urine and fecal material (Mselle et al., 2011). This story illustrates how many delays and miscommunications occurred leading to loss of her child, developing a fistula, and the consequent suffering of this young woman.

Understanding the cause of OF is critical for the prevention at the individual level, but miscommunication persists as well as lack of women's control over delivery location and resources. In a study in Niger, the average labor lasted 3 days and 92% had a stillborn infant. The majority of patients were illiterate and from rural areas. Although antenatal care clinic attendance was high, the information regarding labor and risk of fistula was not shared (Meurice et al., 2016).

From the individual patient's perspective, trauma from operative delivery and lack of financial resources are more commonly cited as causing an OF and few patients seem to relate the development of fistula to prolonged and obstructed labor (Nathan et al., 2009). Likewise in southern Tanzania, operative trauma was implicated in the development of fistula. Such perception of OF resulting from trauma due to surgery or mishandling of patients by hospital personnel has a strong negative impact on encouraging people to promptly seeking obstetric care and accessibility to emergency services. This points to the importance of maternal health education, not only to women but also to men, family members, and the society (Kazaura et al., 2011). Another study in Uganda corroborates, this lack of understanding of how fistula was acquired, with many thinking that the baby "kicked the bladder"; however, others were able identify that having large baby and a long/painful labor may have been the cause. In discussing further, many believed that healthcare providers were directly the cause of the fistula, which again could thwart efforts in preventing OF (Meurice et al., 2017).

There are known risk factors at the level of the individual that could be theoretically used to help communicate risk to patients and consequently prevent the incidence of OF. Recognizing those women with immature pelvic anatomy, severe female genital cutting, malnutrition, and primiparity could help to identify those at risk during the antenatal period. During labor, the identification of mothers with suspected fetal macrosomia, prolonged labor courses, and need for cesarean section could also help in identifying women at risk for developing OF. In a case–control study in Western Uganda, cesarean section, prolonged labor, macrosomic infants, short stature, and lack of education were all significant risk factors for development of OF. The authors concluded that women with short stature and suspected fetal macrosomia needed birth plans that could be implemented in time as well as monitoring labor curves (Barageine et al., 2014). However, this assumes adequate resources, training, and supplies for such warning signs to be recognized, and availability of and access to adequate emergency services to manage complications. Attempts have been made to identify those patients most likely to sustain labor obstruction including short stature, contracted pelvis, large babies, and identification of a "fistula index" or the use of an intrapartum partograph; unfortunately, these have not been effectively implemented and supported by proper and predictable preventive measures to render them effective (Browning et al., 2014). By definition, labor abnormalities occur during labor and most remain outside the realm of predictability (Abraham & Berhan, 2014; Browning et al., 2014). The education of both patients and healthcare providers has been as lacking as that of the development of the needed infrastructures to render the health system responsive and functional. The identification of waiting maternity homes has been advocated for those at risk, and the initial results have been encouraging (Gaym et al., 2012).

Moreover, successfully recovered patients with OF have been engaged as ambassadors to help sensitize pregnant women in their communities. Nonetheless, there remains a lack of proper education that allows circumstances to obviate all measures taken with the best of intentions. This should include proper maternal health education including husbands and other decision makers at households such as mothers-in-law; it should also extend to family and community to minimize the issues related to misconceptions about the causes and consequences of OF (Barageine et al., 2016).

8.3.2   Barriers to Treatment

Miscommunication and misunderstanding at the level of the individual frequently hinder treatment for obstetric fistula. A study in Niger looked specifically at women with OF and the barriers that were encountered in seeking treatment. Miscommunication is at the core of much of what caused delay, morbidity, and social consequences for these women. After initially beginning to experience postpartum leaking, few were told about their condition or made an immediate referral. Many reported long stories of going to multiple different facilities, with trips back to their homes in between, prior to finding the national referral center that actually performs the surgery (Meurice et al., 2016). Conversely, a study in Uganda found that knowing someone else with OF influenced women to seek treatment (Meurice et al., 2017). In this study, more than one-half of the patients developed OF following their first delivery despite almost everyone receiving antenatal care. Nearly every patient's social participation changed in at least one setting. In another study from Uganda, most women reported improvements in physical and psychosocial health following surgical correction of their OF (El Ayadi et al., 2019).

There were a number of barriers to getting information regarding treatment of fistula and to receiving treatment. The majority of women were delivered with physician assistance, a reflection of the significant role of delay in getting to a center where obstruction could be relieved, and delivery completed. The following barriers were noted from this study in Niger in regards to obtaining treatment: lack of information, use of traditional healers, inability to access care, delay for recovery from childbirth, permission needed to seek treatment, cost, treatment unavailable, and lack of social support. Barriers to information regarding OF included rural dwelling, lack of education, lack of understanding of cause of OF, no access to specific information where treatment could be sought, and lack of information dissemination (Meurice et al., 2016).

8.3.3 Psychosocial Experiences

Women suffering from OF face challenges in communicating within their social networks and navigating social functions and relationships. The constant leakage and resulting persistent offensive odor often displace the woman within her family and circle of friends. Their quality of life and social positions are influenced by the reaction of people around them as well as their perception of the cause of OF and the social stigma associated with it. Often the main goal of OF sufferers remains to keep clean and neat, preserve their marriage, maintain their social standing, and earn an income. If these goals cannot be easily achieved given the condition and its circumstances, more often than not, these women resort to self-imposed ostracism and withdrawal from regular activities, family and spousal relationships, and social connections. This leads to more symptoms of depression, post-traumatic stress disorder (PTSD), somatic complaints, and maladaptive coping. Compared to patients attending an outpatient gynecology clinic, they also report significantly reduced social support. Wilson et al. (2015) suggested that if healthcare workers were trained in integrating mental health into the treatment, this may help with their overall care. In Tanzania, a mental health nurse effectively delivered a psychological intervention acceptable to women who were receiving surgical for an OF. The intervention was based on theories of cognitive behavioral therapy and coping models and consisted of six individual sessions including: (1) recounting the fistula story; (2) creating a new story about the fistula; (3) loss, grief, and shame; (4) specific strategies for coping; (5) social relationships; and (6) planning for the future. Resuming mobility, increasing social interaction, improved self-esteem, reduction of internalized stigma, returning to work, meeting their own needs and the needs of dependents, reassuming other expected and desired roles, and negotiating larger life issues were themes central to women's experiences following surgery (Watt et al., 2015).

Many of these women, especially after failed surgeries, need social reintegration and support for their subsistence and bare survival. Besides, they often need to adapt their sexual and reproductive behavior to prevent the recurrence of OF. A reintegration instrument was validated in Uganda as a first step toward improving measurement of post-surgical reintegration. The reintegration score correlated significantly with quality of life, depression, self-esteem, stigma, and social support. This provides ample suggestions for national programs to assist with patients' reintegration following surgical care of OF (El Ayadi et al., 2017). In attempting to identify patient's priorities following repair, it was learned that most women were happy and relieved; but some continued to experience anguish, physical problems, and stigma despite a successful procedure. Fear of developing another fistula led some to avoid intercourse and childbearing with ensuing marital conflict, economic vulnerability, and isolation. The authors recommended OF programs to integrate post-repair counseling about fistula and risk factors for recurrence, community-based follow-up care, linkages to income-generating opportunities, engagement of women affected by fistula for community outreach, and metrics for evaluating rehabilitation and social reintegration efforts to ensure women regain healthy, productive lives—especially as most remain interested in participation in marriage, community life, and childbearing (Donnelly et al., 2015). Furthermore, adjunctive coping strategies have included group therapy and religious coping. In a comparative pre- and post-intervention design, group therapy was found to significantly reduce the proportion of those women with severe mental health status problems following fistula surgery including depression, low self-esteem, and suicidal ideation (Ojengbede et al., 2014). Religion can be an integral part of dealing with stress, distress, and reintegration of women back to their communities following surgery. Indeed, religious coping was universal in an in-depth study in Tanzania with positive coping more often reported and negative coping correlating with depression, stigma, and low social support (Watt et al., 2014).

Looking at social experiences of women with OF seeking treatment in Kampala, Uganda, a woman described her participation in social functions as "worried and unhappy" and that she would "sit until others go away and then she can move." The majority reported being "treated differently" in one or more social setting. Embarrassing events were commonly reported including wet and soiled clothes at weddings or funerals. Relationships with their husbands tended to be variable from strained to supportive. The affected women were at time blamed for their condition as resulting from "a curse" or "refusing to push it out." In any event, feelings of shame colored all descriptions of social interactions. Most women intended to return home to their families and have future pregnancies (Meurice et al., 2017).

As fertility and motherhood remains important in many societies where OF is prevalent, women with fistula may be left with a stillborn and prospects for future fertility low. In Malawi, women with OF identified fertility and continued childbearing as central concerns. Although a high rate of divorces and stigma were found, they reported a high level of support from persons close to them (Yeakey et al., 2009).

Patients referred to as "incurable" include those women who have elected to forgo a diversion procedure and live with the fistula. Major challenges remain secondary to constant leaking. From a study in rural Tanzania that explored these issues, important themes included keeping "clean and neat", income generation, maintaining relationship in marriage and associations. These women felt isolated through self-ostracism or as a result of the constant odor and were prevented from fulfilling their role as wives, mothers, and partners (Mselle & Kohi, 2015). Gainful employment was curtailed, and their social interactions were limited. Indeed, a study in Niger found that prevention of gainful activity was 4.8 times higher following the onset of OF (Ndiaye et al., 2009).

8.4   Community-Level Miscommunication

8.4.1   Culture and Traditions

The community plays a critical role in the life of people particularly in matters of religion, culture, and traditions. The latter usually regulate the life of individuals and families. While the role of husband, mother-in-law, and elders in the community all interact to determine the place of delivery, it is through them that the community can alter its conduct for the benefit of a safe delivery in encouraging delayed pregnancy and antenatal care during pregnancy and in providing a communal means of transportation. Additionally, local healthcare workers and traditional birthing attendants are an important consideration at the community level. Indeed miscommunication and misinformation at that level continue to be repeated and reinforced; it should be corrected as it often dictates the course of reproductive health and health care.

The local community and local health system may have a promising avenue for areas that need to be improved in order to help prevent and treat this condition. These include early interventions focused on the individual, a potential future patient, and her community (family, elders, local healthcare workers) through education with the aim of correcting misconceptions about the cause of OF, having a plan and a choice of health facility for safe delivery. These actions could address some of the main issues contributing to the development of OF and would also help remove the stigma associated with OF by raising awareness. Education has been shown to be critical in eliminating stigma (Changole et al., 2017).

8.4.2 Education and Training

Training and education of traditional birthing attendants are critical to manage labor and identify abnormalities occurring during this period (Keri et al., 2010). Monitoring of quality care remains critical to ensure proper compliance (Qureshi et al., 2010). Local-level contributions to eradicating obstetric fistula include infrastructure development, access to medical facilities, standardized care provided at medical facilities, family planning availability, and general education (Tayler-Smith et al., 2013). Attempting to address these systems issues may have widespread effects in helping to prevent obstetric fistula from developing (Roka et al., 2013). In Niger, a community mobilization program was piloted in which volunteers from a poor-resource village were trained to help identify and evacuate women with protracted labor. This reduced maternal mortality by 73% from year 1 to 3 of the study and decreased perinatal mortality by 61%. No OFs were reported during the final 2 years of the program (Seim et al., 2014). In Ethiopia, an attempt was made to overcome the human resources shortage to manage emergency obstetric care. The Amhara Regional Health Bureau requested help from volunteer teams of obstetricians and midwives in rural hospitals. Their role was to provide obstetrical services and also train local staff members in EmOC. This initiative resulted in a reduction of maternal mortality and morbidity while increasing the number of women delivering in the hospital over the 3-year intervention period. The number of obstetric fistulas presenting to the hospital was also reduced from 48 to 12 during the observation period. The program also resulted in a number of collateral benefits to the staff and the hospital (Browning & Menber, 2015).

Too often, rural facilities lack the communication mechanisms for consultation and referral. With the availability of mobile phone technology, this should theoretically be easily managed with proper support. A central consultation and referral phone number available 24 h/day would facilitate the process. As ambulance services are usually not available at first-level facilities, families have to secure and pay for their own transportation (Cham et al., 2005). Ideally, this function could be a community undertaking to secure timely transportation to a healthcare facility. Programs can be established at the community and national levels to allow proper access to timely care. Such is the experience in Tanzania, where mobile phone transfer of money was used to help women with OF pay for transport to treatment facility (Fiander et al., 2013). These technological advantages could be extended to EmOC and prevent consequences of obstructed labor.

8.4.3 Autonomy and Respect

The limited autonomy of the women in general and the pregnant married woman in particular is another factor in the development of OF. Decision making regarding reproduction, healthcare utilization, freedom of movement, and income disposition remain curtailed for women in many communities where OF is prevalent. A number of women report being pressured by their husband and families (mainly mothers-in-law) as well as their community at large to get pregnant as soon as possible. However, it is not uncommon for them to require their husband's permission before leaving home, and frequently older women in the community contribute to discouraging and even preventing women from delivering in a hospital (Kaplan et al., 2017).

Women report varying level of support from family and community. While initial reports based upon data from hospitalized patients have stressed the total lack of support of the patient living with OF, more recent reports have evaluated such support within the local environment (Dennis et al., 2016; Yeakey et al., 2009). Many women were found to benefit from a high level of support from family members and partners. Nonetheless, it remains critical to include additional resources to allow identification of those in need and additional supportive services for the complete care of these patients. This is a commonly recurring theme in the reported literature.

8.4.4 National-Level Miscommunication

Despite progress being made in every country dealing with the problem of OF, a great deal remains to be done in order to eradicate this scourge. In that respect, the role of international organisms to establish priorities and goals for eradication of OF helps motivate and shape policies at the national level. National policies have to rely on reliable data to establish eradication plans (Tuncalp et al., 2015). Unfortunately, the estimation of the burden of obstetric fistula in low- and middle- countries still remains a major challenge. The Demographic and Health Surveys collect self-reported symptoms of fistula in selected countries, but the accuracy of such data was never validated. The most commonly quoted estimate of obstetric fistula globally is two million prevalent cases (Cottingham et al., 1991). Other estimates range from 1 to 3 million cases globally and 352,000 cases in 19 sub-Saharan African countries (Adler et al., 2013; Maheu-Giroux et al., 2015; Wall, 2006). In the absence of reliable data on incidence or prevalence of obstetric fistula, it is difficult for the United Nations agencies, donors, NGOs, and government organizations to develop country-specific intervention programs for the treatment and prevention of obstetric fistula.

Effective and practical national strategies and plans for the prevention and treatment of obstetric fistula must be multidimensional, addressing the issues of miscommunication at every level including education, child marriage, genital mutilation, healthcare infrastructures and systems as well as monitoring and supplies of properly trained healthcare workers and the quality of care delivered. In a population-based survey of an area with large numbers of facility births, a high incidence of OF was found: There were few level 1 (deciding to seek care) and 2 (accessing healthcare facility) delays identified, but a large number of level 3 (receiving care at healthcare facility) delays, raising concerns over the quality of care (Mocumbi et al., 2017). Improving the capacity and quality of the health system is critical in caring for the women in labor and should be a national priority in the effort to eradicate the problem of OF.

8.5 Priority and Economic Development

Level 1, 2, and 3 barriers should be directly addressed, and economical barriers overcome through all means of government (Baker et al., 2017). As discussed in individual- and community-level miscommunication, patients should be closely monitored during labor by attendants well-versed in the early recognition and diagnosis of obstructed labor and have access to timely and quality obstetrical care when needed. Then, and only then, will there be a chance of eradicating OF after each country's backlog has been properly identified and managed, but the burden has to be at the national level to ensure resources are dedicated to this important cause (Tuncalp et al., 2014). In that respect, programs should be implemented to assist those patients deemed incurable and offered the means and support to be managed with urinary or GI diversion.

8.5.1 Creative and Holistic Solutions

In the meantime, a number of solutions have been piloted and offer hope including those occurring in Niger and Ethiopia mentioned above. By learning from health-seeking behaviors, Khisa et al. (2017) attempted to answer the question "what patterns of health seeking do women with obstetric fistula display in their quest for healing?". They analyzed data from narratives of women following fistula surgery in three hospitals in Kenya and identified seven key actions in that trajectory: staying home, trying home remedies, consulting with private healthcare providers, non-governmental organizations, prayer, traditional medicine and formal hospitals and clinics. The "unresponsiveness" of the hospitals at the first encounter seemed to justify the delay in further health-seeking behavior. They concluded that the current health system does not cater to the need of the patient with fistula and recommended the creation of a robust health system provided with expertise and facilities in order to treat obstetric fistula to shorten women's treatment pathways (Khisa et al., 2017).

For patients who have been managing their fistula, a holistic approach requires a variety of interventions as seen in the following example. In Ethiopia, some patients must travel over 250 miles to reach a care service area, and thus, it was recommended that maternity waiting homes be created and care standardized to improve access to comprehensive emergency obstetrical care for mother from rural areas. Indirect evidences suggested that the service improved maternal health outcome (Gaym et al., 2012).

8.5.2 Prevention, Prevention, and Prevention

In addition to improving antepartum and intrapartum care, reproductive health counseling and planning both before and after pregnancy are critical to prevent fistula from developing. Contraception is an important intervention for the avoidance of too early, too many, and too late births—all of which increase the risk of OF. Among 188 patients 1 year following OF surgery in a study in Nigeria by Lawani et al., 2015, 95% were aware of contraception but only 37% were able to use it. While fear of adverse effects and partner disapproval were commonly cited, socioeconomic reasons, religious and cultural beliefs, and myths were also operative. Contraceptive knowledge was also low in a study in Malawi by Kopp et al. (2017) with less than one-half of women intending to use it following surgical repair of their OF. In rural Malawi, fertility and pregnancy outcomes in women living with OF and following surgical repair remain poor. These studies indicate that counseling regarding family planning and delaying pregnancy following repair of an OF as well as the management of future pregnancies is critically needed in national health programs (Wilson et al., 2011).

8.6 Conclusions

Miscommunication is a core theme not only in understanding the pathologic development of obstetric fistula, but also the complexities of this condition at the individual, community, and national levels of this preventable public health problem. More can be done regarding education of individuals, family, and community to prevent and treat OF. At the level of the community, besides education and raising awareness, there is a significant need to address stigmatization of fistula sufferers and to pool resources to prevent and treat this disease. Nationally, more must be done to educate the workforce and provide resources as well as funding and overseeing more comprehensive approaches. Because OF is a global public health problem associated with low-income countries where poverty is prevalent and there is lack of access to quality health care, efforts to ameliorate this situation via the allocation of resources and aid with the backlog of patients should continue to be supported by organizations such as the World Health Organization, the United National Population Fund, and other international aid agencies. Unfortunately, communications between these global agencies and the national, local, and individual levels are often complex, involving local politics, and limited by the resources available and where OF stands in terms of other medical priorities.

Communication in the developing world paradoxically relies heavily on cellular networks to overcome the physical distances between urban centers and the rural, remote, and often isolated areas of the country. Unfortunately, this reliance can make it difficult for poor, uneducated women living in remote areas where infrastructure is deficient to have the necessary communications to access care. The result of this "electronic" isolation makes verbal communication easier, but unfortunately has not translated itself in the flow of information that should make it a tool for education and referral. This paradox of theoretically easy communication and inaccessible care helps to at least partly explain the unacceptable persistence of OF. The combination of lack of education, knowledge, empowerment, and resources determines the fate of the pregnant woman in the developing world. What needs to be implemented is well-defined, but it takes more than knowledge to put it in effect. Empowerment, education, and adequate resources are all equally critical ingredients for the eradication of obstetric fistula if the millennial goal of eliminating this preventable obstetrical complication is to be reached.

References

Abraham, W., & Berhan, Y. (2014). Predictors of labor abnormalities in university hospital: Unmatched case control study. *BMC Pregnancy and Childbirth, 14*, 256. https://doi.org/10.1186/1471-2393-14-256. Available from: https://www.ncbi.nlm.nih.gov/pmc/articles/PMC4129102/. Accessed 1 October 2019

Adler, A. J., Ronsmans, C., Calvert, C., & Filippi, V. (2013). Estimating the prevalence of obstetric fistula: A systematic review and meta-analysis. *BMC Pregnancy and Childbirth, 13*, 246. https://doi.org/10.1186/1471-2393-13-246. Available from: https://www.ncbi.nlm.nih.gov/pmc/articles/PMC3937166/. Accessed 12 October 2019

Arrowsmith, S., Hamlin, E. C., & Wall, L. L. (1996). Obstructed labor injury complex: Obstetric fistula formation and the multifaceted morbidity of maternal birth trauma in the developing world. *Obstetrical & Gynecological Survey, 51*(9), 568–574.

Baker, Z., Bellows, B., Bach, R., & Warren, C. (2017). Barriers to obstetric fistula treatment in low-income countries: A systematic review. *Tropical Medicine & International Health, 22*(8), 938–959. https://doi.org/10.1111/tmi.12893

Barageine, J. K., Faxelid, E., Byamugisha, J. K., & Rubenson, B. (2016). As a man I felt small': A qualitative study of Ugandan men's experiences of living with a wife suffering from obstetric fistula. *Culture, Health & Sexuality, 18*(4), 481–494. https://doi.org/10.1080/13691058.2015.1089325

Barageine, J. K., Tumwesigye, N. M., Byamugisha, J. K., Almroth, L., & Faxelid, E. (2014). Risk factors for obstetric fistula in Western Uganda: A case control study. *PLoS One, 9*(11), e112299. https://doi.org/10.1371/journal.pone.0112299. Available from: https://www.ncbi.nlm.nih.gov/pmc/articles/PMC4234404/. Accessed 30 September 2019

Browning, A., Lewis, A., & Whiteside, S. (2014). Predicting women at risk for developing obstetric fistula: A fistula index? An observational study comparison of two cohorts. *BJOG, 121*(5), 604–609. https://doi.org/10.1111/1471-0528.12527

Browning, A., & Menber, B. (2015). Reducing maternal morbidity and mortality in the developing world: A simple, cost-effective example. *International Journal of Women's Health, 7*, 155–159. https://doi.org/10.2147/IJWH.S75097

Cham, M., Sundby, J., & Vangen, S. (2005). Maternal mortality in the rural Gambia, a qualitative study on access to emergency obstetric care. *Reprod Health, 2*(1), 3. https://doi.org/10.1186/1742-4755-2-3. Available from: https://reproductive-health-journal.biomedcentral.com/articles/10.1186/1742-4755-2-3. Accessed 19 October 2019

Changole, J., Thorsen, V. C., & Kafulafula, U. (2018). A road to obstetric fistula in Malawi: Capturing women's perspectives through a framework of three delays. *International Journal of Women's Health, 10*, 699–713. https://doi.org/10.2147/IJWH.S171610

Changole, J., Thorsen, V. C., & Kafulafula, U. (2017). "I am a person but I am not a person": Experiences of women living with obstetric fistula in the central region of Malawi. *BMC Pregnancy Childbirth, 17*(1), 433. https://doi.org/10.1186/s12884-017-1604-1. Available from: https://www.ncbi.nlm.nih.gov/pmc/articles/PMC5740704/ Accessed 10 October 2019

Cottingham J, Royston Erica, and World Health Organization. (1991). Obstetric fistulae: A review of available information. Available from: http://www.who.int/iris/handle/10665/59781. Accessed 5 October 2019.

Creanga, A. A., & Genadry, R. R. (2007). Obstetric fistulas: a clinical review. *International Journal of Gynaecology and Obstetrics, 99*(Suppl 1), S40–S46. https://doi.org/10.1016/j.ijgo.2007.06.021

Dennis, A. C., Wilson, S. M., Mosha, M. V., Masenga, G. G., Sikkema, K. J., Terroso, K. E., & Watt, M. H. (2016). Experiences of social support among women presenting for obstetric fistula repair surgery in Tanzania. *International Journal of Women's Health, 8*, 429–439. https://doi.org/10.2147/IJWH.S110202. Available from: https://www.ncbi.nlm.nih.gov/pmc/articles/PMC5019876/. Accessed 19 October 2019

Donnelly, K., Oliveras, E., Tilahun, Y., Belachew, M., & Asnake, M. (2015). Quality of life of Ethiopian women after fistula repair: Implications on rehabilitation and social reintegration policy and programming. *Culture, Health & Sexuality, 17*(2), 150–164. https://doi.org/10.1080/13691058.2014.964320

El Ayadi, A. M., Barageine, J., Korn, A., Kakaire, O., Turan, J., Obore, S., et al. (2019). Trajectories of women's physical and psychosocial health following obstetric fistula repair in Uganda: a longitudinal study. *Trop Med Int Health, 24*(1), 53–64. https://doi.org/10.1111/tmi.13178. Available from: https://www.ncbi.nlm.nih.gov/pmc/articles/PMC6324987/. Accessed 16 October 2019

El Ayadi, A., Nalubwama, H., Barageine, J., Neilands, T. B., Obore, S., Byamugisha, J., et al. (2017). Development and preliminary validation of a post-fistula repair reintegration instrument among Ugandan women. *Reprod Health, 14*(1), 109. https://doi.org/10.1186/s12978-017-0372-8. Available from: https://reproductive-health-journal.biomedcentral.com/articles/10.1186/s12978-017-0372-8 Accessed 12 October 2019

Fiander, A., Ndahani, C., Mmuya, K., & Vanneste, T. (2013). Results from 2011 for the transportMYpatient program for overcoming transport costs among women seeking treatment for obstetric fistula in Tanzania. *International Journal of Gynaecology and Obstetrics, 120*(3), 292–295. https://doi.org/10.1016/j.ijgo.2012.09.026

Gaym, A., Pearson, L., & Soe, K. W. (2012). Maternity waiting homes in Ethiopia--three decades experience. *Ethiopian Medical Journal, 50*(3), 209–219.

Goh, J. T. (2004). A new classification for female genital tract fistula. *The Australian & New Zealand Journal of Obstetrics & Gynaecology, 44*(6), 502–504. https://doi.org/10.1111/j.1479-828X.2004.00315.x

Kaplan, J. A., Kandodo, J., Sclafani, J., Raine, S., Blumenthal-Barby, J., Norris, A., et al. (2017). An investigation of the relationship between autonomy, childbirth practices, and obstetric fistula among women in rural Lilongwe District, Malawi. *BMC Int Health Hum Rights, 17*(1), 17. https://doi.org/10.1186/s12914-017-0125-3. Available from: https://www.ncbi.nlm.nih.gov/pmc/articles/PMC5477240/ Accessed 28 September 2019

Kazaura, M. R., Kamazima, R. S., & Mangi, E. J. (2011). Perceived causes of obstetric fistulae from rural southern Tanzania. *African Health Sciences, 11*(3), 377–382.

Keri, L., Kaye, D., & Sibylle, K. (2010). Referral practices and perceived barriers to timely obstetric care among Ugandan traditional birth attendants (TBA). *African Health Sciences, 10*(1), 75–81.

Khisa, A. M., Omoni, G. M., Nyamongo, I. K., & Spitzer, R. F. (2017). "I stayed with my illness": a grounded theory study of health seeking behaviour and treatment pathways of patients with obstetric fistula in Kenya. *BMC Women's Health, 17*(1), 92. https://doi.org/10.1186/s12905-017-0451-6. Available from: https://www.ncbi.nlm.nih.gov/pmc/articles/PMC5622500/ Accessed 18 October 2019

Konje, J. C., & Ladipo, O. A. (2000). Nutrition and obstructed labor. *American Journal of Clinical Nutrition, 72*(1 Suppl), 291S–297S. https://doi.org/10.1093/ajcn/72.1.291S

Kopp, D. M., Bengtson, A., Wilkinson, J., Chipungu, E., Moyo, M., & Tang, J. H. (2017). Contraceptive knowledge, use and intentions of Malawian women undergoing obstetric fistula repair. *The European Journal of Contraception & Reproductive Health Care, 22*(5), 375–380. https://doi.org/10.1080/13625187.2017.1397111

Lawani, L. O., Iyoke, C. A., & Ezeonu, P. O. (2015). Contraceptive practice after surgical repair of obstetric fistula in Southeast Nigeria. *International Journal of Gynaecology and Obstetrics, 129*(3), 256–259. https://doi.org/10.1016/j.ijgo.2014.11.028

Loposso, M., Hakim, L., Ndundu, J., Lufuma, S., Punga, A., & De Ridder, D. (2016). Predictors of recurrence and successful treatment following obstetric fistula surgery. *Urology, 97*, 80–85. https://doi.org/10.1016/j.urology.2016.03.079

Maheu-Giroux, M., Filippi, V., Samadoulougou, S., Castro, M. C., Maulet, N., Meda, N., & Kirakoya-Samadoulougou, F. (2015). Prevalence of symptoms of vaginal fistula in 19 sub-Saharan Africa countries: A meta-analysis of national household survey data. *The Lancet Global Health, 3*(5), e271–e278. https://doi.org/10.1016/S2214-109X(14)70348-1. Available from: https://www.thelancet.com/action/showPdf?pii=S2214-109X%2814%2970348-1 Accessed 17 October 2–19.

Meurice, M. E., Genadry, R. R., Bradly, C. S., Majors, B., & Gand, S. O. (2016). Identifying barriers to accessing information and treatment for obstetric fistula in Niamey, Niger. *Proceedings in Obstetrics and Gynecology, 6, 13*(2). https://doi.org/10.17077/2154-4751.1304. Available from: https://pdfs.semanticscholar.org/d945/a8a8221160bd1d9b-78607c09208b101d8858.pdf?_ga=2.79668820.1964168836.1571582332–398277846.1510768166. Accessed 16 October 2019

Meurice, M., Genadry, R., Heimer, C., Ruffer, G., & Kafunjo, B. J. (2017). Social experiences of women with obstetric fistula seeking treatment in Kampala, Uganda. *Ann Glob Health, 83*(3–4), 541–549. https://doi.org/10.1016/j.aogh.2017.07.003. Available from: https://www.researchgate.net/publication/318919501_Social_Experiences_of_Women_with_Obstetric_Fistula_Seeking_Treatment_in_Kampala_Uganda Accessed 20 October 2019

Mocumbi, S., Hanson, C., Hogberg, U., Boene, H., von Dadelszen, P., Bergstrom, A., et al. (2017). Obstetric fistulae in southern Mozambique: Incidence, obstetric characteristics and treatment. *Reprod Health, 14*(1), 147. 10.1186/s12978-017-0408-0. Available from: https://www.ncbi.nlm.nih.gov/pmc/articles/PMC5681779/ Accessed 11 October 2019

Mselle, L. T., Kohi, T. W., Mvungi, A., Evjen-Olsen, B., & Moland, K. M. (2011). Waiting for attention and care: Birthing accounts of women in rural Tanzania who developed obstetric fistula as an outcome of labour. *BMC Pregnancy and Childbirth, 11*, 75. https://doi.org/10.1186/1471-2393-11-75. Available from: https://bmcpregnancychildbirth.biomedcentral.com/articles/10.1186/1471-2393-11-75 Accessed 15 October 2019.

Nathan, L. M., Rochat, C. H., Grigorescu, B., & Banks, E. (2009). Obstetric fistulae in West Africa: Patient perspectives. *American Journal of Obstetrics and Gynecology, 200*(5), e40–e42. https://doi.org/10.1016/j.ajog.2008.10.014

Mselle, L. T., & Kohi, T. W. (2015). Living with constant leaking of urine and odour: Thematic analysis of socio-cultural experiences of women affected by obstetric fistula in rural Tanzania. *BMC Womens Health, 15*, 107. https://doi.org/10.1186/s12905-015-0267-1. Available from: https://www.ncbi.nlm.nih.gov/pmc/articles/PMC4658753/. Accessed 3 October 2019

Ndiaye, P., Amoul Kini, G., Abdoulaye, I., Diagne Camara, M., & Tal-Dia, A. (2009). Epidemiology of women suffering from obstetric fistula in Niger. *Med Trop (Mars), 69*(1), 61–65.

Ojengbede, O. A., Baba, Y., Morhason-Bello, I. O., Armah, M., Dimiti, A., Buwa, D., & Kariom, M. (2014). Group psychological therapy in obstetric fistula care: A complementary recipe for the accompanying mental ill health morbidities? *African Journal of Reproductive Health, 18*(1), 155–159.

Qureshi, Z. P., Sekadde-Kigondu, C., & Mutiso, S. M. (2010). Rapid assessment of partograph utilisation in selected maternity units in Kenya. *East African Medical Journal, 87*(6), 235–241.

Roka, Z. G., Akech, M., Wanzala, P., Omolo, J., Gitta, S., & Waiswa, P. (2013). Factors associated with obstetric fistulae occurrence among patients attending selected hospitals in Kenya, 2010: A case control study. *BMC Pregnancy and Childbirth, 13*, 56. https://doi.org/10.1186/1471-2393-13-56. Available from: https://bmcpregnancychildbirth.biomedcentral.com/articles/10.1186/1471-2393-13-56. Accessed 10 October 2019

Seim, A. R., Alassoum, Z., Bronzan, R. N., Mainassara, A. A., Jacobsen, J. L., & Gali, Y. A. (2014). Pilot community-mobilization program reduces maternal and perinatal mortality and prevents obstetric fistula in Niger. *Int J Gynaecol Obstet, 127*(3), 269–274. https://doi.org/10.1016/j.ijgo.2014.06.016. Available from: https://www.researchgate.net/publication/264386036_Pilot_community-mobilization_program_reduces_maternal_and_perinatal_mortality_and_prevents_obsetric_fistula_in_Niger. Accessed 20 October 2019

Tayler-Smith, K., Zachariah, R., Manzi, M., van den Boogaard, W., Vandeborne, A., Bishinga, A., et al. (2013). Obstetric fistula in Burundi: A comprehensive approach to managing women with this neglected disease. *BMC Pregnancy and Childbirth, 13*, 164. https://doi.org/10.1186/1471-2393-13-164. Available from: https://bmcpregnancychildbirth.biomedcentral.com/articles/10.1186/1471-2393-13-164. Accessed 8 October 2019

Tennfjord, M. K., Muleta, M., & Kiserud, T. (2014). Musculoskeletal sequelae in patients with obstetric fistula - a case-control study. *BMC Womens Health, 14*, 136. https://doi.org/10.1186/s12905-014-0136-3. Available from: https://www.ncbi.nlm.nih.gov/pmc/articles/PMC4228064/. Accessed 15 August 2019

Thaddeus, S., & Maine, D. (1994). Too far to walk: Maternal mortality in context. *Social Science & Medicine, 38*(8), 1091–1110.

Tuncalp, O., Tripathi, V., Landry, E., Stanton, C. K., & Ahmed, S. (2015). Measuring the incidence and prevalence of obstetric fistula: Approaches, needs and recommendations. *Bull World Health Organ, 93*(1), 60–62. https://doi.org/10.2471/BLT.14.141473. Available from: https://www.ncbi.nlm.nih.gov/pmc/articles/PMC4271685/. Accessed 19 October 2019

Tuncalp, O., Isah, A., Landry, E., & Stanton, C. K. (2014). Community-based screening for obstetric fistula in Nigeria: A novel approach. *BMC Pregnancy and Childbirth, 14*, 44. https://doi.org/10.1186/1471-2393-14-44. Available from: https://bmcpregnancychildbirth.biomedcentral.com/articles/10.1186/1471-2393-14-44. Accessed 18 October 2019

Waaldijk, K. (1995). Surgical classification of obstetric fistulas. *International Journal of Gynaecology and Obstetrics, 49*(2), 161–163.

Wall, L. L. (2006). Obstetric vesicovaginal fistula as an international public-health problem. *Lancet, 368(9542)*, 1201–1209. https://doi.org/10.1016/S0140-6736(06)69476-2

Wall, L. L. (2012). Overcoming phase 1 delays: The critical component of obstetric fistula prevention programs in resource-poor countries. *BMC Pregnancy and Childbirth, 12*, 68. https://doi.org/10.1186/1471-2393-12-68. Available from: https://bmcpregnancychildbirth.biomedcentral.com/articles/10.1186/1471-2393-12-68 Accessed 29 September 2019.

Watt, M. H., Wilson, S. M., Sikkema, K. J., Velloza, J., Mosha, M. V., Masenga, G. G., et al. (2015). Development of an intervention to improve mental health for obstetric fistula patients in Tanzania. *Evaluation and Program Planning, 50*, 1–9. https://doi.org/10.1016/j.evalprogplan.2015.01.007

Watt, M. H., Wilson, S. M., Joseph, M., Masenga, G., MacFarlane, J. C., Oneko, O., & Sikkema, K. J. (2014). Religious coping among women with obstetric fistula in Tanzania. *Glob Public Health, 9*(5), 516–527. https://doi.org/10.1080/17441692.2014.903988. Available from: https://www.ncbi.nlm.nih.gov/pmc/articles/PMC4046104/. Accessed 18 October 2019

Wilson, S. M., Sikkema, K. J., Watt, M. H., & Masenga, G. G. (2015). Psychological symptoms among obstetric fistula patients compared to gynecology outpatients in Tanzania. *International Journal of Behavioral Medicine, 22*(5), 605–613. https://doi.org/10.1007/s12529-015-9466-2

Wilson, A. L., Chipeta, E., Kalilani-Phiri, L., Taulo, F., & Tsui, A. O. (2011). Fertility and pregnancy outcomes among women with obstetric fistula in rural Malawi. *International Journal of Gynaecology and Obstetrics, 113*(3), 196–198. https://doi.org/10.1016/j.ijgo.2011.01.006

Yeakey, M. P., Chipeta, E., Taulo, F., & Tsui, A. O. (2009). The lived experience of Malawian women with obstetric fistula. *Culture, Health & Sexuality, 11*(5), 499–513. https://doi.org/10.1080/13691050902874777

The Experience of Childbirth and Obstetric Fistula: Perspectives of Women in Northern Ghana

9

F. Beryl Pilkington, Prudence Mwini-Nyaledzigbor, and Alice Abokai Agana

9.1   Introduction

This chapter provides perspectives from women in northern Ghana to document the experiences of women living with obstetric fistula.[1] The present discussion focuses on both the participants' first-person accounts of their childbirth experiences as well as their challenges and travails of living with obstetric fistula. Embedded within the women's stories are details describing the socio-cultural and politico-economic conditions that allow the preventable problem of obstetric fistula to continue in Ghana (Ghana Health Service, 2015) and in other low- and middle-income countries (LMICs) when it is mostly eradicated elsewhere. It is to these themes that we turn for policy implications regarding the changes needed to at last eradicate obstetric fistula in Ghana, and everywhere.

Obstetric fistula remains a major public health issue in developing countries. Wall (2006) cited estimates that "*at least 3 million women in poor countries have unrepaired vesicovaginal fistulas, and that 30 000–130 000 new cases develop each year in Africa alone*" (p. 1201). Obstetric fistula is most prevalent and problematic in sub-Saharan Africa and the poor regions of Asia (Miller et al., 2005; Wall, 2006). To explain the prevalence of the problem in developing countries, Wall (2006) included a diagram from the Worldwide Fistula Fund (WFF) depicting "*the obstetric fistula pathway*," which involves "*a complex interplay of biological, social, and economic forces*" (p. 1205). As depicted in this diagram, the root cause of obstetric fistula is the "*low socio-economic status of women*," from which flows a cascade of factors culminating in "*obstructed labour injury complex*." The causal chain includes malnutrition, limited social roles, illiteracy and lack of formal education, early marriage, childbearing before pelvic growth is complete, cephalopelvic disproportion, lack of access to emergency services, and harmful traditional practices (Wall, 2006, p. 1205).

---

[1] Data presented in this chapter were originally collected for a Master's (Nursing) research study conducted in northeastern Ghana (Agana, 2010), and some of the findings of the study were previously published (Mwini-Nyaledzigbor et al., 2013).

F. B. Pilkington (✉)
School of Nursing, Faculty of Health, York University, Toronto, ON, Canada
e-mail: bpilking@yorku.ca

P. Mwini-Nyaledzigbor
Catholic University College, Fiapre, Sunyani, Ghana

A. A. Agana
Nursing and Midwifery Training College, Yeji, Bono East Region, Ghana

© Springer Nature Switzerland AG 2022
L. B. Drew et al. (eds.), *A Multidisciplinary Approach to Obstetric Fistula in Africa*, Global Maternal and Child Health, https://doi.org/10.1007/978-3-031-06314-5_9

At the time that the study on obstetric fistula that informs this chapter was conducted, data were lacking on the prevalence of obstetric fistula in Ghana (Agana, 2010). However, when the United Nations Population Fund (UNFPA) launched the global campaign to end fistula in 2003 (see http://www.endfistula.org/), the three northern regions (Upper East, Upper West, and Northern Region) were identified as having a high prevalence (Agana, 2010). The study was conducted in the Upper East Region. The Upper East Region is bordered on the east by Togo, on the north by Burkina Faso, on the south by the Northern Region, and on the west by Upper West Region.

Predominantly rural and very arid, the Upper East Region is approximately 1000 km away from Accra, the nation's capital. Temperatures range between 22 and 40 °C, with the hottest period occurring from March to May and the coolest in December and January. There is a brief rainy season (June to September) and severe water shortages in the dry season. The economy is based on subsistence farming (maize, groundnuts, and millet), and many people migrate to the southern part of the country to earn a living. The region does not have a good road network except in the business districts. Travel between communities is difficult, especially during the rainy season when roads become flooded and, often, impassable. People move about mostly by private transport including bicycles, motorcycles, and lorries.

The population of the Upper East Region comprises several ethnic groups that speak different languages. The common language spoken is *Kusaal*.[2] The dominant religions include Islam, Christianity, and traditional African religion. People are served by the District Hospital where the study was conducted and three government health centers, with the hospital serving as their referral point.

Clearly, the rural, remote locations in Upper East Region place the childbearing population at risk for obstetric fistula. Our study (Agana, 2010; Mwini-Nyaledzigbor et al., 2013) sought to answer questions regarding the emotional, social, psychological, and physical problems that women with obstetric fistulae experience; how long women live with the condition before receiving treatment; and the coping strategies they adopt to live with this condition. In this chapter, our purpose is to excavate participants' stories of their childbirth experiences and the experience of living with obstetric fistula as a case study of gender disparities in health. Drawing on the concept of intersectionality, we will expose the socio-cultural and politico-economic conditions that allow the preventable problem of obstetric fistula to continue in Ghana (Ghana Health Service, 2015) and in other low- and middle-income countries (LMICs). We argue that a lifespan view of women's health can inform the necessary policies and interventions to not only prevent obstetric fistula but improve the health of girl children and women.

We begin with a brief overview of the research methodology, followed by the presentation of women's accounts of their experiences with childbirth and of living with obstetric fistula, and their suggestions to improve the treatment of women with fistula. Next, in the discussion section, we explore the intersecting socio-cultural and politico-economic factors embedded in women's accounts that reflect the obstetric fistula pathway (Wall, 2006). We close with policy recommendations to reduce and eventually eradicate obstetric fistula in Ghana, and everywhere.

---

[2]The *Kusaal* language, also termed *Kusasi*, is a Gur language spoken by approximately 400,000 persons in northern Ghana. It takes its name from the *Kusasi* people, an ethnic group inhabiting northern Ghana and southern Burkina Faso.

9.2 Research Methodology

A qualitative descriptive-exploratory approach was employed to document the experiences of women living with obstetric fistula. Data collection took place between May 2009 and February 2010 through semi-structured interviews using mostly open-ended questions to encourage women to freely share their recollections, thoughts, and feelings regarding their experiences. The interviews focused on understanding the participants' perspectives on the pregnancy that resulted in the fistula; the personal, social, and economic impact of fistula on their lives; the coping strategies they used to deal with the impact of the fistula, and their recommendations for ways to prevent or treat fistula (Agana, 2010).

The study was approved by the ethics review board of the Noguchi Memorial Institute for Medical Research at the University of Ghana. Participants were recruited from a District Hospital and the Regional Hospital where fistula repairs are done. Interviews took place in a room in the hospital or in the participant's home, according to their preference. Before beginning the interviews, informed consent and permission to audio record the interviews were obtained. Participants were assured of anonymity and seemed appreciative of the opportunity to be interviewed. Most were interviewed in *Kusaal,* the native language of the area where the study was conducted, but three were interviewed in *Bisa.*[3] The recorded interviews were transcribed and translated into English by one of the authors (AA).

9.2.1 Profile of Research Participants

Participants were ten women who had sustained obstetric fistula and were residing in one of the districts in Upper East Region. Their ages ranged between 20 and 70 years, although most guessed their ages, as they had no documentation of their birth dates. None of the participants had any formal education. All participants were married before developing a fistula, but only five were still in the married at the time of the interview; of the remainder, two were widowed, two were divorced, and one was separated. All were gainfully employed prior to the fistula but when interviewed, only five were working: two were peasant farmers and three were petty traders. The rest depended on relatives or other supporters for their basic needs (Agana, 2010).

All participants except one were multiparous (i.e., had given birth to more than one child) and six had given birth five or more times (grandmulitparous). All participants had lost their baby during the labor that resulted in the fistula, and some had given birth to more than one stillborn baby (five, in the case of one woman). Only four of the mothers had attended antenatal care at least once; the remaining six women had never received antenatal care. All participants were in labor at home for three to four days before initially seeking medical care (Agana, 2010). Participants had been living with the fistula for at least two years and up to ten years.

9.3 Women's Accounts of Their Childbirth Experiences

Participants' accounts of their childbirth experiences revealed similar patterns. The following are selected excepts from the translated interview transcripts, with some editing to remove extraneous details (indicated with ellipsis points). Participants are anonymous and are identified by "P" and a number (e.g., P1, etc.).

---

[3] Bisa (or *Bissa*) is a Mande language spoken by approximately 600,000 persons in Ghana, Burkina Faso, and Togo.

9.3.1   Mother P1 (20 Years of Age; Had Delivered Three Babies, Two Stillborn)

My first born, I was in labour for two days and was later taken to … Hospital where surgery was done, but I lost the child.… For the third one, I was in labour from night to evening the following day but still did not deliver, then I was taken to … hospital where I delivered. It was this delivery that brought about this condition; meanwhile I did not get the child [i.e., it was stillborn].

When asked why she did not go to hospital when labor began, P1 replied:

It is the men who determine this, so I did not have a choice. Besides, you know from here to the hospital is very far and lorries only come here on market days [every three days], so when you are in labour someone will have to go to … town and hire a taxi cab to this place to take you which is very costly. So that was why it was deemed fit for me to try the labour at home. At home, when I was in labour, they gave me 'poateem[4]' to help me give birth. On reaching the hospital, I vomited, and they told me that I would have died if I did not come early.

9.3.2   Mother P3 (30 Years of Age; Had Delivered Five Babies; Four Living Children)

I delivered my first four children spontaneously at home. My fifth pregnancy was a miscarriage whilst the sixth baby died during delivery. During this labour, the baby blocked the birth passage and would not come out until I was taken to hospital where the baby was brought out dead.… I often gave birth alone. When I went into labour, the baby had died. I did not feel labour pains and was just lying down. The labour lasted from night to the next day in the evening before I was taken to hospital.… When I got to … [town], the doctor used instruments to pull the baby out immediately. I was told I would have died if I did not come now. As soon as the baby was removed, the urine started coming, then trees caught my legs [i.e., could not move her legs], so I was just lying down. I stayed at the hospital for some time and was told to go and treat myself with Kusaasi medicine to regain use of my legs since they did not have any here.

9.3.3   Mother P4 (40 Years Old; One Delivery, Baby Stillborn)

It was my first pregnancy that the condition occurred. I was healthy throughout the period of pregnancy but was in labour for about four days. When they could not make me deliver, I was taken to … hospital where they cut my genital area [episiotomy] and removed the baby but it was dead a long time.… I never had any prenatal care because any antenatal clinic is far from our place. Besides the pregnancy was not worrying me so I did not deem it necessary to have that.

Asked who attended to her when she was in labor, P4 replied:

They were elderly women from our family house and neighbours who have been assisting women in this regard previously. I was in labour for four days. They said it was a youthful pregnancy and for that matter not true labour as our people always say, so I was left there until my abdomen appeared to be divided into two. It was then that a certain man who visited us saw the state in which I was and insisted that they send me to hospital.… You know our people always say that young ladies often exaggerate labour pains prior to the actual labour so they thought I was not yet in labour, and the thing is also about to kill you. Before they realized, the abdomen was divided, with water on one side and the baby on the other side. It was that man who disagreed with them when he saw my condition at the time. That was what saved me.

---

[4] *Poateem* is a local analgesic medication used for abdominal pains

9.3.4 Mother P5 (Had Given Birth Twice; No Living Children)

My first born was a girl but died; the second one, I had a miscarriage. It was during my third delivery that I developed this condition after I was operated on in … [town]. I was in labour for three days, but nothing was done to me by the old ladies who attended to me, so I could not give birth. Later they went to …[another town] to bring nurses who took me in their car to … [that town] but there too they could not let me deliver. I was taken to … Hospital. When we got there, they injected me then I became unconscious and did not know what happened again but later I realized that they operated me.

When asked what they did during the three days she was in labor, P5 replied:

The old ladies gave me some herbal preparation called 'poateem' to take and only waited for this to take effect, but when the situation was not improving, they started questioning me about wrongdoing. They asked if when I visited my father's house I might have done something behind him, but my response was "no, I could never do such a thing," since we consider that as dirt, but they insisted that I confess to enable the baby to come out. Well, they thought that I had committed adultery and because of that the labour became difficult.… They gave up when they realized that I was getting weak and still insisted that I had nothing to confess, hence my being sent to hospital where I was operated upon but lost the baby. I believe it was because they delayed in taking me to hospital when I was in labour. If they had taken me to hospital promptly, I would have had my baby and been well also, but this is not a decision to be taken by me, the woman, as the men make such decisions since it involves money [transportation cost, hospital fees and so on]. The men on the other hand would not go in for hospital delivery like that until they are sure there is nothing fishy by consulting their gods.

When asked why her attendants did not take her to hospital as soon as she went into labor, Mother P5 reiterated:

You know such decisions are made by the men; so, if my husband did not ask them to send me, what could they as women do? What they could do was what they did.

Asked how long before she knew she had developed a fistula, P5 replied:

It took about 5 days before they told me that I lost my baby. They put a tube in me, then I was in the hospital for about 3 months before they removed it. When the catheter was eventually removed, the urine started coming in small quantities and I was told that it was because the wound was not completely healed, but that it will eventually stop when the wound heals completely; however, it did not.… I also got paralysed in one leg but recovered after undergoing some local treatment.

9.4 Women's Accounts of Their Experiences Living with Obstetric Fistula

After describing the circumstances in which they gave birth, the participants were asked about their experiences of living with an obstetric fistula. Because the data were voluminous, we have selected examples from several participants, omitting extraneous or repetitive details. Interviews with other participants were similar. Questions from the researcher are indicated with "R" and enclosed in brackets.

9.4.1 Mother P1 (20 Years of Age; Had Delivered Three Babies, Two Stillborn)

When you have this condition, you are bothered, all the time you are unhappy and confused. Some sympathize with me because sickness is from God, but others insult me. Sometimes they insult my children, they laugh and make fun of me. It disturbs me, but I cannot do anything about it.… You get fever, loss of appetite and abdominal pain. Sometimes I feel itchy inside me and when I scratch it becomes painful.

[R: How does it affect your urinary pattern and grooming?]

Sometimes when the urine is coming I become aware and go to urinate. Other times, I do not realize it.... I bathe frequently with soap and use perfumes to keep the odour down. I use pieces of old cloth as a pad and to keep these clean and odourless, I always ensure that I have soap and Dettol[5] which I use in washing the rags whenever they are soiled. As for the sores, each time I develop any, I treat them with warm water.

[R: How does it affect you in public or at gatherings?]

When you have this condition, embarrassment is always at your door. I say this because you know urine has a very strong scent; as such if you do not keep yourself well, anywhere you are should there be any pollution of the air by any one, all eyes will turn on you since they know of your problem. It is for this reason that I keep to myself without mingling with people. I used to farm onions and prepare rice to sell but now because of my condition, I cannot do these. I also sold my onions in markets of nearby towns and villages and buy rice to retail.... I don't sell again because when I go to the market and the people see the urine dripping like that, I become uncomfortable. It is very embarrassing and when your customers see you soiled like that, they will spread the news which would affect your sales. So, to avoid situations such as that, I decided not to do any trade again. I do not sit with people, when I go to the market; I buy my things and return home immediately.

[R: How does your husband relate with you since you got this condition? Does he support you?]

Initially my husband was helpful and caring. He tried to seek treatment for me but after a while, he neglected me. As at now he does not relate well with me. He does not even sleep with me again. For instance, when I was called to come back to ... hospital he did not see me off or even give me money to buy water on the way.... In the beginning he gave me money for treatment but later stopped. One time, I needed some money for medication in the hospital, but he told me to come home if I did not have money. Recently when I told him that I needed money to attend hospital for treatment, he told me he did not have money and if I had my own money I could go ahead.

[R: How do you cope with work and take care of yourself now that your husband does not support you?]

I fend for myself by doing menial jobs, sometimes others give me food to eat.

[R: Are you his eldest, second or third wife?]

I am the second wife. He married [third wife] after I developed this condition.

9.4.2 Mother P3 (30 Years of Age; Had Delivered Five Babies; Four Living Children)

I stayed in hospital for about one month. [Afterward] I was treated at home here and my legs healed. They used traditional medicine.

[R: What about the urine? Didn't they take you elsewhere for treatment?]

Nothing has been done about that. My husband has not got money to take me to the bigger hospitals which are very far away to treat me, so I have not sought any treatment for the urine problem. It was only last year a [health worker] came and wrote our names and invited us to go to [Hospital] for treatment. When the time came I went there with another woman, but we were told that we were too many. My friend was treated but I was not, then came home and have since not been called again.

[R: How long has it been since you developed the condition?]

It will be up to 8 years.

[R: Tell me how your condition has affected you.]

I used to brew pito[6] and sell, but ever since I developed this condition, I stopped doing that, so I will say it has crippled me financially. Now I only buy shea butter from the market and retail at home here.... Sometimes the urine leaks so profusely that it makes people avoid and stigmatise me. Sometimes ... they quickly ask me what I

---

[5]Dettol is a commercially manufactured liquid antiseptic disinfectant available in Ghana.

[6]*Pito* is a type of beer that is prepared from fermented sorghum or millet in northern Ghana, Nigeria, and other regions of West Africa. As an important income source for poor rural households, it is almost never obtainable in cans or bottles, instead being obtained from the person(s) who brew it.

want and even order me to leave the scene immediately if I have nothing to say. When I go to the market some people avoid me, … would remark that the smelly woman has arrived; such abusive comments make it difficult for me to continue with the trade.

It just flows like that [demonstrating].… It causes serious irritation; my genital area often gets so sore that I am not able to use the rags as a pad any longer but only hang some in front and some at the back to cover my nudity whilst allowing the urine to flow freely as well as allowing air to circulate so as to aid in the healing process.

[R: When you came home in this condition, what was your husband's reaction? Did he attempt to seek treatment for you?]

He has not done anything. He can't afford any orthodox treatment and the sickness is also not for the native doctors.

[R: How many wives does your husband have?]

Two, but one died leaving me.

[R: When your condition occurred did your husband sleep with you?]

We don't sleep together again.

[R: How do you feel about this?]

It definitely bothers me but what can I do? Sometimes I have sores and abdominal pains, other times it comes so profusely that I cannot go out, I can't mix with friends.…

I feel helpless and hopeless because I cannot do anything for myself.

[R: If you were called to come for treatment how will you go? Will your husband support you?]

The last time, they brought a vehicle from … [town] to take us to the hospital, but if they don't provide a vehicle, I will find my own money to go. My husband would have given me money to go if he had some, but he just does not have the money.

9.4.3 Participant P4 (40 Years Old; no Living Child)

As soon as the baby was out, the urine started coming.… They inserted a certain rubber and told me it will correct by itself with time. The correction was however never realized. I was just lying for about two months, but nothing was done for me until I was discharged.

[R: After discharge did you seek treatment any where again?]

My late husband who was old at the time could not afford any treatment for me, so I underwent local treatment for three consecutive years without any improvement. When he told friends and family members to take me to … [a city in another state] for treatment, they told him to bring money which he did not have. Eventually, my husband passed away and I continued suffering with it until recently when the health people took us to … [town] for operation. It is now better.

[R: What was your experience like with this native treatment?]

Hmm it wasn't easy, they used roots to treat me for three consecutive years. The herbalist came to prepare the herbs by boiling them in water then they used the solution to spray into me. I was also made to drink only the herbal concoction and use the same herbal preparation to cook my food for three years, but it was not effective because this is not a disease for traditional treatment. I only agreed to take because I was in pain. During the three years of herbal treatment, I did not go out to any place like the market; I did not eat fish or meat. I took only "dawadawa⁷" and nobody was allowed near me nor touch me including my husband, yet there was no improvement. They also used the solution to spray into me; whenever this was done, I got very weak. It also caused severe sores in my genital region, but I still had to use it on the sores even though it was very irritating. Each time this happened I only lay on my back and pat my thighs and cry. During the rainy season while every-

---

⁷*Dawadada* is a traditional aromatic seasoning used in Ghana that is prepared from the boiled and fermented locust bean. It is added to soups and stews.

body is busy working on their farms, I only lie in the room and cry. If I had my baby and then was subjected to this treatment it would not bother me.

[R: How did it affect your trade?]

I could no longer do any trade because when I am in public, people avoid and make fun of me, and it is only at such gatherings like funeral grounds and market squares that such trades are carried out.

[R: How do you feel about that?]

I feel pathetic and dirty everyday, you cannot mix with friends and other women anymore, and you can't work but only sit at one place. You cannot be like your fellow women again nor be able to play your role effectively as a woman; this is a very difficult and pathetic situation to bear…. You can't control the urine without using a pad. I used rags to pad myself but whenever I developed sores around my genital area I was unable to use the pads. During such periods, I just stay indoors and expose the sores for air to circulate thus aiding healing. Sometimes when the flow is less profuse I could go to the well to fetch water, market and back.

[R: How did you feel, losing your baby and developing this condition as well?]

I was disturbed and thought of it often. Apart from the double agony of losing my baby and becoming sick with urine dribbling from me all the time, people avoided and stigmatized me. I also lost my mother that same year and sometimes I sat alone in the house and cried from morning to evening without anyone to console me.

9.5 Participants' Suggestions to Improve Treatment for Women with Fistula

Participants' suggestions as to how to assist women living with fistula included the provision of fistula repairs for free and assistance in the form of food aid so that women could live their normal lives again. Some examples follow:

This is a condition that no woman should be allowed to suffer. If possible, it should be prevented, and in cases where women get it, they should be treated promptly and free of charge. It is not anything that one should be allowed to live with. There are too many problems associated with it. – Mother P4

More treatment centres should be opened to cater for women no matter where they come from, and treatment must be free so that no matter one's situation one can also get her repair. – Mother P6

Also, the men need to be educated so that no woman is left in labour for days and where it still occurs, free and prompt treatment should be given. – Mother P10

I think it would help us [fistula victims] a lot if we are given some food aid. The condition puts us out of a job thus making living so unbearable for us, especially when the victim is a breadwinner like myself—Mother P5

9.6 Discussion

In this section, we begin by comparing participants' accounts of their experiences to the obstetric fistula pathway described by Wall (2006). However, obstetric fistula is the outcome of a broad array of interrelated socio-cultural and politico-economic conditions that interact at the local, national, and global levels. In order to better understand the complex context in which obstetric fistula occurs so as to inform policy recommendations, we treat the problem as a case study of gender disparities in health, drawing upon the concepts of intersectionality, human rights, and a lifespan approach.

9.6.1   Tracing the Obstetric Fistula Pathway in Women's Stories

It is evident that participants' accounts of their childbirth experiences and experiences of living with fistula closely mirror the causal pathway of obstetric fistulae, its root cause being the "*low socio-economic status of women*" (Wall, 2006, p. 1205). The district in Upper East Region where participants lived is a remote, agricultural area and among the poorest in Ghana. Here, as elsewhere in the world, women are the poorest of the poor (Woods, 2009). Participants either worked as peasant farmers or petty traders, or they were unemployed.

Women's low socioeconomic status is associated with malnutrition, limited social roles, illiteracy, and lack of formal education (Wall, 2006). It was not determined whether any of the participants in the study were malnourished; however, it is possible and even likely, given the harsh geographic environment and the poverty in which they lived. If so, their growth would have been stunted, putting them at risk for obstructed labor due to cephalopelvic disproportion (CPD) (Wall, 2006). None of the participants had any formal education, and their social roles were restricted by their low income and female gender. The latter was apparent in references to decision-making about going to the hospital to give birth; for example:

"*You know such decisions are made by the men; so, if my husband did not ask them to send me, what could they as women do?*"—Mother P5

Moreover, once afflicted by a fistula,

"*You cannot be like your fellow women again nor be able to play your role effectively as a woman*"—Mother P4

All of the participants had developed obstetric fistula after prolonged labor, either due to CPD, multiparity, or both. All but one of the ten participants were multiparous; the latter were mature women who had developed a fistula after their third or fourth delivery. In this regard, the sample differed from fistula populations in other sub-Saharan African countries where over 25% had become pregnant before the age of 15 years, and over 50% had become pregnant before the age of 18 years (World Health Organization, 2006). However, the distribution of fistula occurrence is bimodal, peaking with the first pregnancy and in women with four or more pregnancies (Wall, 2006).

The obstetric fistula pathway also includes harmful traditional practices (Wall, 2006). While there was no evidence of such in the women's accounts, they did speak about harmful practices that seemed to be common, if not traditional. For instance, some recounted being given "*poateem*" a medication for stomach pains, when they were in labor. In addition, it was customary for women to give birth at home, either alone (e.g., "*I often gave birth alone,*"—Mother P3), or attended by "elderly women" and/or neighbors. Also, several participants related that they were pressured to confess to adultery when their labors were prolonged, because their birth attendants suspected that this was the cause. Another participant mentioned consulting the gods:

"*The men on the other hand would not go in for hospital delivery like that until they   are   sure there is nothing fishy by consulting their gods*" – Mother P4

These practices reflect ignorance about normal and abnormal labor and birth processes and contributed to the delay in transporting the women to hospital for an assisted delivery and ultimately, a stillborn baby and an obstetric fistula.

The women's accounts vividly illustrate various sequelae of "*obstructed labour injury complex*" (Wall, 2006), including fetal death, fistula formation, urinary incontinence, musculoskeletal injury, foot drop, chronic skin irritation, stigmatization, isolation and loss of social support, divorce or separation, worsening poverty, suffering, and illness (Mwini-Nyaledzigbor et al., 2013). Some participants recounted how they received treatments from "herbalists" or traditional healers, which involved elimination of meat and fish from their diet and ingestion of herbal concoctions. These treatments did not help and may have harmed the women, where they involved dietary restrictions.

Obstetric fistula is a double tragedy because it results in a stillborn baby. This loss is often brushed over in the literature on obstetric fistula; however, it likely contributes to negative psychological outcomes including depression. As Mother P4 said,

Apart from the double agony of losing my baby and becoming sick with urine dribbling from me all the time, people avoided and stigmatized me. I also lost my mother that same year and sometimes I sat alone in the house and cried from morning to evening without anyone to console me.

9.6.2   Obstetric Fistula: A Case Study of Gender Disparities in Health

In an important paper relevant to the issue of obstetric fistula, Nancy Fugate Woods (2009) examined how gender disparities in health are associated with the intersection of globalization and gender within various social, cultural, and political contexts. Woods' analysis of gender disparities in health is very relevant to understanding and responding to the issue of obstetric fistula, which is essentially an index of gendered health disparities in developing countries. To better understand how gender interacts with various social, cultural, and political contexts to produce health disparities, the concept of *intersectionality* is useful. Originating in critical feminist theory, it refers to coexisting identities or social locations (e.g., sex, gender, race, ethnicity, class, and age) that have a compounding effect on oppression and marginalization (McGibbon & McPherson, 2011). For instance, older women from a low social class and a minority racial or ethnic group would likely experience multiple forms of oppression and marginalization, and this would exacerbate health disparities. The issue of gender disparity is further discussed below, in relation to politico-economic and socio-cultural conditions that perpetuate the problem of obstetric fistula in Ghana.

9.6.2.1 Politico-Economic Conditions Contributing to the Fistula Problem

Globalization is important to consider when seeking to understand the context of health "*in countries undergoing changes related to economic development*" (Woods, 2009, p. 197). Globalization forces such as governance structures (e.g., International Monetary Fund, World Bank, World Trade Organization, etc.), global markets, the removal of cross-border trade barriers, and information and communication technologies act as distal determinants of health, because they shape and constrain what governments can do to address the needs of their populations, including those most vulnerable (Spiegel et al., 2004). For example, "*the challenges of debt repayment [distal determinant] constrain governments' abilities to invest in infrastructure for health and education*" (Woods, 2009, p. 198). Moreover, "*cultural, economic, environmental, political, and social processes … affect the proximal determinants of health [e.g., health services], in some cases amplifying health disparities*" (p. 197).

With respect to Ghana, an "*emerging market country*" (Schieber et al., 2012, p. 1), globalization exerts politico-economic influence on decisions around investment in the health system and transportation infrastructure, which, in turn, affects population health. In the case of obstetric fistula, participants' stories illustrate how the lack of such infrastructure in Upper East Region contributes to the prevalence of fistula; specifically, they had limited access to health facilities, in part, due to a poor road network and lack of transportation. As Mother P1 related,

"*from here to the hospital is very far and lorries only come here on market days, so   when   you are in labour someone will have to go to … town and hire a taxi cab to this place to take you which is very costly.*"

Ghana has a relatively well-developed health system and is one of the first countries in Africa to "*start implementing universal health insurance coverage by providing coverage to its vulnerable population groups*" (Schieber et al., 2012, p. 1). However, participants' stories reveal that they had limited access to antenatal and intrapartum care, let alone fistula repair. In a comprehensive study of Ghana's health system performance, Scheiber et al. (Scheiber et al., 2012, p.3) reported:

The performance of Ghana's health system is mixed. Consumer satisfaction is high, and access appears to have improved, including for the poor. Total health spending as a share of GDP is slightly below the global average for countries at the comparable level of income, however; Ghana has fewer hospital beds and health workers and worse under-five and maternal mortality outcomes than comparator countries; and health spending increased less rapidly than spending in most African counties between 1995 and 2009.

Governments make decisions around where to invest limited resources based on politico-economic considerations. Unfortunately, the most marginalized of peoples (e.g., those living in the northern regions of Ghana) often seem to have lower priority, and women are at the bottom of the heap. To shift priority setting, a human rights approach is needed, so that the needs of those most vulnerable are given higher priority (Wall, 2012; Crockett & Cooper, 2016). To solve the problem of obstetric fistula in Ghana (and other LMICs), all women must have access to primary health care (as prevention) and treatment (i.e., fistula repair) because this is their human right.

9.6.2.2 Socio-Cultural Conditions Contributing to the Fistula Problem

While social determinants of health (e.g., gender, income, education, employment, etc.) are well-recognized (World Health Organization, n.d.; McGibbon & McPherson, 2011), cultural influences may be less so. According to Woods (2009, p. 198),

Gender disparities in health are deeply rooted in the gender values of the culture, especially those in which males are valued more highly than females. From the time of birth, the meaning of being born female shapes the remainder of the life of a girl-child.

Gender values show up in differential gender role socialization, education and schooling, and social roles and occupations. Where girls are valued only for their reproductive capacity or as property, they are denied an education and married off early, which limits their options for the future (Woods, 2009). Other examples of gender disparity relevant to the problem of obstetric fistula include nutritional disparity and neglect of girls, overrepresentation of women and girls (70%) among the world's poorest; and lack of access to health care (Woods 2009; Levine et al., 2009).

Embedded in participants' accounts of their experiences of childbirth and living with obstetric fistula are striking examples of how, as mature and illiterate women, they were disadvantaged within the socio-cultural context of Upper East Region, one of the poorest areas of Ghana. For example, women described being excluded from decision-making about going to the hospital when labor was protracted, because this would cost money. Instead, they waited on men to make this decision for them, and the men were not necessarily available or amenable to helping. Also, polygamy was common, and most participants were the second or third wife of their husband, who was unable to financially support multiple wives. This meant that husbands, even if supportive, lacked the financial resources to help the women with their fistula predicament. Unable to work at their usual livelihood as peasant farmers or petty traders, women who were already poor became truly destitute and at risk of premature death.

9.6.3 A Lifespan View Is Needed to Tackle the Problem of Obstetric Fistula

Having examined the obstetric fistula pathway and the complex politico-economic and socio-cultural context of the problem, it is abundantly evident that obstetric fistula is not simply a reproductive health issue: It is a gender disparity issue. To counter the disparities arising from the intersection of globalization and gender within various social, cultural, and political contexts, and to inform the necessary interventions to improve the health of girl children and women, a lifespan view is needed (Woods, 2009). A lifespan view is comprehensive, encompassing the determinants of human development from birth to death. It acknowledges that early traumas and barriers to health and wellness will have a negative impact throughout women's life course (Crockett & Cooper, 2016; Woods, 2009). Moreover, it assumes that health is a basic human right (World Health Organization, 2017), and that, as stated in the Beijing Declaration and Platform for Action,[8] *"Women's right to the enjoyment of the highest standard of health must be secured throughout the whole life cycle in equality with men"* (United Nations, 1995, paragraph 92). Essentially, a lifespan view would entail a "Health in All Policies" approach (World Health Organization, 2013), but with particular attention to the gendered nature of health disparities (Crockett & Cooper, 2016) and the human rights of girls and women.

9.7   Policy Recommendations

The Ghana Health Service (2015) recently published a report on the burden of obstetric fistula in Ghana. It concluded (p. 138) as follows:

Obstetric fistula (OBF), which includes both vesico-vaginal fistula (VVF) and recto-vaginal fistula (RVF), represents a critically important but largely neglected problem in the field of reproductive health. Although fistula is preventable and curable, it will most likely remain a major public health problem for some more years to come, and this is because there is a lack of funding and infrastructure for adequate obstetric health care delivery throughout the country. Although health care at the primary level alone cannot resolve the problem of OBF, primary health care is integral for early detection of obstructed labor and to ensure that it is not prolonged by doing a C-section on time. Fistula is a problem of the developing world, unfortunately, our resources are limited. There is a need for national stakeholders and policy makers to partner with the industrialized world and benevolent organizations to tackle and eradicate OBF.

We endorse this conclusion, except to note that resource allocation is largely a political exercise; and so, if the women of Ghana were equally valued as men, the fistula problem would be given higher priority than it currently receives. Moreover, a mechanism would be found to fund not only *"infrastructure for adequate obstetric health care delivery throughout the country,"* but also educational and other programs and services needed to improve the life prospects for girls and women (Crockett & Cooper, 2016; Levine et al., 2009).

The participants in our study made modest and reasonable recommendations for improving treatment for obstetric fistula entailing social assistance in the form of food and fistula repairs for free. In addition, the Ghana Health Service (2015) made the following recommendations, which we endorse:

- **Information/Advocacy**: This would include "action-oriented research that directly involves patients who suffer from the condition" (p. 138). It would also entail development of a national database on the incidence and prevalence of fistula, in partnership with people and institutions committed to reproductive health research (p. 138).
- **Prevention**: "There should be large scale sensitization and awareness health education workshops for the general public about the importance of attending antenatal clinics and seeking skilled atten-

---

[8]The Fourth World Conference on Women held in Beijing in September 1995 produced the Beijing Declaration and Platform for Action, the most progressive blueprint ever for advancing women's rights. This Platform for Action created comprehensive commitments under 12 critical areas of concern, imagining a world where each woman and girl can exercise her freedoms and choices and realize all of her rights, such as to live free from violence, to go to school, to participate in decisions, and to earn equal pay for equal work. The Platform built upon consensus and progress that was made at earlier United Nations conferences, particularly the Conference on Women in held Nairobi in 1985.

dant care during childbirth" (p. 138). We would add that prevention should begin with universal education for girls and other measures to ensure that girls reach their full potential (Levine et al., 2009).

- **Treatment**: "More OBF repair units should be established across the country in primary healthcare facilities, especially in regions where OBF cases are prevalent.... The repair of fistula should also be free for patients" (p. 139).
- **Rehabilitation/Reintegration**: Patients and families should be provided with the necessary supports and counseling so that treated women can reintegrate into society. (p. 139).
- **Training**: "There is a pressing need to train more surgeons (especially gynecologists and urologists) to gain the skills for fistula repair" (p. 139).
- **Partner Organizations**: Due to the large scale of the problem, addressing it must involve partner organizations such as WHO, UNFPA, and the Worldwide Fistula Fund, whose global experience "can inform national strategies" (p. 139).

The Report on the Burden of Obstetric Fistula in Ghana (Ghana Health Service, 2015) ends with the statement, "Eradication of OBF has been achieved by some resource-poor countries, and this gives the hope that eradication could be achieved in Ghana as well. It is about time OBF is given some serious attention in Ghana" (p. 140). We echo that sentiment but would add: Where there is a (political) will, there is a way—and the way must be found!

9.8 Conclusions

In this chapter, we revisited first-person accounts of women living in the Upper East Region of Ghana of their childbirth experiences and experiences of living with obstetric fistula (Agana, 2010; Mwini-Nyaledzigbor et al., 2013), focusing on the politico-economic and socio-cultural conditions that allow this preventable problem to continue in Ghana. We treated the problem of obstetric fistula and the conditions under which it occurs as a case study of gender disparities in health, drawing on the concepts of intersectionality, human rights, and a lifespan approach—the latter being necessary if the problem is to be eradicated. Finally, we endorsed the recommendations in the recent Report on the Burden of Obstetric Fistula in Ghana (Ghana Health Service, 2015). Perhaps the most critical thing needed to make progress in eradicating obstetric fistula in Ghana is the political will to put these recommendations into action.

References

Agana, A. (2010). *Experiences of women with obstetric fistula in the Bawku East District of the upper east region (master's thesis)*. University of Ghana. Available from http://197.255.68.203/handle/123456789/7256 Accessed 18 May 2019

Crockett, C., & Cooper, B. (2016). Gender norms as health harms: Reclaiming a life course perspective on sexual and reproductive health and rights. *Reproductive Health Matters, 24*(48), 6–13. https://doi.org/10.1016/j.rhm.2016.11.003

Ghana Health Service. (2015). Report on the burden of obstetric fistula in Ghana... Available from: https://ghana.unfpa.org/en/publications/report-burden-obstetric-fistula-ghana Accessed 18 May 2019.

Levine, R., Lloyd, C. B., Greene, M., & Grown, C. (2009). *Girls count: A global action and investment agenda*. The Center for Global Development.

Miller, S., Lester, F., Webster, M., & Cowan, B. (2005). Obstetric fistula: A preventable tragedy. *Journal of Midwifery & Women's Health, 50*(4), 286–294. https://doi.org/10.1016/j.jmwh.2005.03.009

McGibbon, E., McPherson, C. (2011). Applying intersectionality and complexity theory to address the social determinants of women's health. *Women's Health and Urban Life, 10* (1), 59–86. Available from: https://pdfs.semanticscholar.org/ff37/233c2882e4b60a632456c983d37218531766.pdf Accessed 18 May 2019.

Mwini-Nyaledzigbor, P. P., Agana, A. A., & Pilkington, F. B. (2013). Lived experiences of Ghanaian women with obstetric fistula. *Healthcare for Women International, 34*, 440–460. https://doi.org/10.1080/07399332.2012.755981

Schieber, G., Cashin, C., Saleh, K., & Lavado, R. (2012). *Health financing in Ghana.* International Bank for Reconstruction and Development/The World Bank. Available from: http://apps.who.int/medicinedocs/en/m/abstract/Js20302en/

Spiegel, J. M., Labonte, R., & Ostry, A. S. (2004). Understanding "globalization" as a determinant of health determinants: A critical perspective. *International Journal of Occupational and Environmental Health, 10*(4), 360–367.

United Nations. (1995). *Beijing declaration and platform for action. Fourth world conference on women, Beijing, China, September 4–15.* Author. Available from: http://www.un.org/womenwatch/daw/beijing/pdf/BDPfA%20E.pdf

Wall, L. L. (2006). Obstetric vesicovaginal fistula as an international public-health problem. *Lancet, 368*, 1201–1209. https://doi.org/10.1016/S0140-6736(06)69476-2

Wall, L. L. (2012). A bill of rights for patients with obstetric fistula. *International Journal of Gynecology & Obstetrics, 127*(3), 301–304. https://doi.org/10.1016/j.ijgo.2014.06.024

Woods, N. J. (2009). Global imperative: Development, safety and health from girl-child to woman. *Health Care for Women International, 30*(3), 195–214. https://doi.org/10.1080/07399330802638465

World Health Organization. (2006). Integrated management of pregnancy and childbirth. Obstetric fistula: Guiding principles for clinical management and programme development. . Available from: http://apps.who.int/iris/handle/10665/43343.

World Health Organization. (2013). Health in all policies. Framework for country action. . . Available from: https://www.who.int/healthpromotion/frameworkforcountryaction/en/.

World Health Organization. (2017). *Human rights and health.* WHO. Retrieved from https://www.who.int/news-room/fact-sheets/detail/human-rights-and-health.

World Health Organization (n.d.). Social determinants of health. . . Available from: https://www.who.int/social_determinants/sdh_definition/en/.

Marie-Eve Paré, Julie Désalliers, Laurence Bernard, Salam Kouraogo, and Jacques Corcos

10.1 Introduction

Obstetric fistula is a devastating condition that affects the lives of sub-Saharan women and their families, causing both physical and social suffering. This important maternal health issue is the result of biological, social and economic factors. While rape, sexual trauma, premature marriage and the practice of female genital mutilation contribute to the phenomena, the majority of fistula cases are due to prolonged and obstructed childbirth (Semere & Nour, 2008; Wall, 2006). Risk factors for this condition include the woman's young age and immature pelvis, her early first pregnancy, small stature and poor nutritional state (Nour, 2006; Wall, 2006). Furthermore, such women usually have little education, belong to an underprivileged socio-economic group and have limited access to transportation (Harouna et al., 2001; Ndiaye, Amoul Kini, Abdoulaye, Diagne Camara, & Tal-Dia, 2009; Semere & Nour, 2008; Sombie, Conombo, Sankara, Ouedraogo, & Zoungrana, 2007; Tebeu, Bernis, Doh, Rochat, & Delvaux, 2009). Early marriage and the husband's occupation also contribute to the development of this condition (Onolemhemhen & Ekwempu, 1999). These social and demographic factors result in a lack of access to quality obstetric care, the main risk factor predisposing to the development of a fistula. The delay in reaching a healthcare centre can be explained by financial constraints, the lack of awareness, absence of available means of transportation or the husband's or in-law's refusal to act (Zheng & Anderson, 2009). One must also mention the insufficiency of the medical system where care is often inadequate, due to the lack of trained medical personnel and equipment, combined with logistical difficulties (Anoukouma, Attipou, Agoda-Koussema, Akpadza, & Ayite, 2010; Nathan,

M.-E. Paré (✉)
Department of Anthropology, College Professor at Cégep Edouard-Montpetit, Longueuil, QC, Canada
e-mail: marie-eve.pare@cegepmontpetit.ca

J. Désalliers
Espace Santé Nun's Island Clinical, Hôpital de LaSalle, Montréal, QC, Canada

L. Bernard
University of Ottawa, Ottawa, ON, Canada

S. Kouraogo
Department of Sociology, Université de Ouagadougou, Ouagadougou, Burkina Faso

J. Corcos
Department of Surgery (Division of Urology), McGill University, Jewish General Hospital, Montréal, QC, Canada

© Springer Nature Switzerland AG 2022
L. B. Drew et al. (eds.), *A Multidisciplinary Approach to Obstetric Fistula in Africa*, Global Maternal and Child Health, https://doi.org/10.1007/978-3-031-06314-5_10

Rochat, Grigorescu, & Banks, 2009; Ndiaye et al., 2009; Raassen, Verdaasdonk, & Vierhout, 2008; Sombie et al., 2007; Tebeu et al., 2009).

In West Africa, the unfortunate lack of infrastructure for gathering epidemiological data compromises the ability to precisely evaluate the incidence of obstetric fistula. A study conducted in Burkina Faso cites an incidence of 23.1 in 100,000, but it only covers women admitted to hospitals in that country (Sombie et al., 2007). Those figures definitely underestimate the real situation, but beyond the statistical portrait and the epidemiological causes of fistula, our objective is to better comprehend the general social impact of fistulas by studying specific cases of Burkinabe women and their families. To do so, we evaluated the role of families, communities and the medical system in protecting or endangering the situation of women who suffer from a fistula. For example, studies point to the increased risk of repudiation in this context.[1] But how does this phenomenon manifest in the Burkina Faso context and how do women experience it on a daily level? To answer these questions, we adopted an interdisciplinary approach, combining medical and anthropological expertise, in order to obtain a portrait based on the local experience of women living with a fistula.

To do so, we adapted the Arrowsmith, Hamlin, and Wall (1996) notion of the obstructed labour complex to analyse the physical and social harm resulting from obstructed labour and a lack of access to emergency obstetrical care. As well as being a sequel of obstructed labour, an obstetric fistula results in a physical and social injury for the women affected by it. Thus, the medical and social aspects of this condition are interdependent. From a medical standpoint, in addition to urinary or faecal incontinence, it can cause painful sores on the thighs, vaginal stenosis, infertility, amenorrhoea, kidney stones, kidney failure and infection (Ahmed & Holtz, 2007). Such physical complications prevent women from working and they consequently lose their autonomy. They sacrifice their ability to contribute to the livelihood of their group, which diminishes their status within their community. Furthermore, surgical treatment of obstetrical fistula is complex, and even when it is successful, 16% to 32% of women remain incontinent as a result of extensive fibrosis, reduced kidney function or lesions to the cervix, urethra or vaginal muscle (Lewis et al., 2009; Nardos, Browning, & Chen, 2009; Wall, 2006). From a social aspect, a fistula is a catalyst for social conflict since the condition is often not recognized. Marital, family and community relationships are greatly affected, at times leading to ostracism. The combined social and economic impact creates great psychological distress, the experience of women living with a fistula must therefore be considered in its totality.

In adopting a holistic perspective, this research study proposes to better understand the phenomenon as it occurs in Burkina Faso, combining anthropology and medicine to provide the women's perspective on their daily existence, specifically employing a longitudinal vision. Starting with their testimony, we attempted to determine the impact of fistulas on these women, particularly the role played by marital status, family and community in the social exclusion experienced by these women.

We also wanted to study the post-surgical period by focusing on the process of reinsertion and the various challenges encountered by these women. This second aspect is important, since few studies have examined the reinsertion process of marginalized West African women. Until now, the literature has primarily reported Eastern African experiences and demonstrates that after surgery, women experience progressive social reinsertion. Few obstacles exist, but most women manage to maintain a certain support system (Browning & Menber, 2008; Khisa, Wakasiaka, McGowan, & Campbell, 2017; Yeakey, Chipeta, Rijken, Taulo, & Tsui, 2011). Our research team therefore attempted to determine whether the same situation prevailed in Burkina Faso. We took the women's accounts into consideration in the form of participative action research. They expressed their concerns, shared their worries and proposed changes to the post-operative process and to the prevention of obstetric fistula.

---

[1] The percentage of women divorced or abandoned by their husbands due to fistula varies by study, but a meta-analysis compiled an average of 36% (Ahmed & Holtz, 2007).

10.2   Research and Methodological Context

This research was carried out in collaboration with the *Mères du Monde en Santé* Foundation (MMS) and the Boromo Medical Surgical Center (CMA), located in the Boucle du Mouhoun Region of Burkina Faso. The MMS Foundation is a Canadian organization working with women suffering from vesico-vaginal fistulas. From 2011 to 2016, two yearly surgical missions were conducted at the Boromo CMA in close collaboration with local healthcare personnel and various local and international organizations.[2] Since 2017, the MMS Foundation has continued its activity at the Ruhengeri Hospital in Rwanda. For this particular study, participants were recruited during MMS's surgical missions in 2012 to 2014, with the help of the Burkinabe association ARFOD (Association pour la Recherche la Formation et le Développement), recruitment took place across western Burkina Faso and some participants came from regions far removed from Boromo. Despite being open to women of all backgrounds, study participants were primarily rural women from underprivileged communities.[3]

The study aimed to obtain a longitudinal portrait of the experiences of women living with a fistula, and to do so, was conducted in two phases, a preparatory phase and a post-operative phase, which required seven separate data collection sessions in order to reach the saturation point. In reconstructing these women's life stories, several themes were discussed, namely the circumstances leading to the fistula, medical care and the various impacts on everyday life. We applied these themes during the second interviews in order to appreciate the progress of their situation. We will therefore respect this division of our result analysis in the following sections. A total of 39 women participated in an hour-long semi-structured interview prior to undergoing surgery at the Boromo CMA, from 2012 to 2014. In 2013 and 2015, one to two years after surgery, we conducted 29 h-long semi-structured follow-up interviews. Three patients had to be excluded, since they did not have an obstetric fistula, and seven patients could not be interviewed in person.[4] The 29 s phase interviews took place in the patients' villages, which was an essential aspect of the methodology specific to this research, in order to obtain a good follow-up rate, even among women living in very isolated communities. Our analysis further benefitted from direct observation of the women's living arrangements and socio-economic conditions. However, this aspect of our methodology prevented us from performing follow-up gynaecological exams. The surgical success was therefore clinically determined based on the women's report that they no longer had symptoms of urinary incontinence.

During the interviews, we opted for the dialogic method to promote an empathetic space for exchange. This participative action-research approach fosters the implementation of lasting change within the community. (Cargo & Mercer, 2008; Minkler & Wallerstein, 2008). In addition to recording life stories, interactive exchanges allowed women to propose suggestions for adapting surgical missions to local circumstances. Local and Canadian organizations were thus able to make adjustments during the research period, while others became long-term goals. Specifically, interviews included a basic socio-demographic questionnaire and a semi-structured discussion based on open questions from pre-established guidelines. Interviews were in Dioula or in Mooré, the two principal vernacular languages, and were directly translated into French on site by two local translators who were involved throughout this research. Interviews were recorded with the participants' consent and

---

[2] This research was supported and funded by the MMS Foundation to provide long-term medical and social follow-up to the women who had surgery, to identify obstacles to their reinsertion and to improve the intervention quality.

[3] This research received ethical approval from the Institutional Review Board of McGill University Faculty of Medicine and from the Director of the Boromo CMA and the Ministry of Health of Burkina Faso.

[4] During the second phase, seven patients were lost to follow-up: three were cured and joined their husbands in the Ivory Coast, one patient could not be contacted, but was not cured, according to her family, and three patients could not be located.

then transcribed verbatim. We processed to a cross-sectional qualitative analysis in which every verbatim was manually coded using clearly identified themes and subthemes. For the purpose of this chapter, we have grouped themes according to the stories of women living with a fistula. First, we will discuss the experience of obstructed labour and the trajectory of care until diagnosis. Subsequently, we will analyse the three main themes: economic consequences, the woman's conjugal situation and her relationship with her community. The latter greatly impacts the women's mental health, given the interconnectedness of their distress and their group relationships. These themes are developed in succession, taking into account the longitudinal perspective of the two study phases.

10.3   Living with a Fistula: From Childbirth to the Operating Table

In this first section, we will begin by presenting the circumstances that led to the fistula, based on the accounts of childbirth experiences and medical treatments of the women participating in the study. Subsequently, we will focus on all the socio-economic impacts that characterize the experience of women living with a fistula. First of all, we will start with a brief socio-demographic portrait of our participants. Although they are of various ethnic and religious backgrounds, they share numerous characteristics. They all belonged to the most vulnerable social categories of Burkinabe society. These were women between 22 and 65 years, mostly uneducated and from rural areas. The average age of marriage and first pregnancy was 18 years. Except for one, these women were all married prior to developing a fistula. Two thirds were in polygamous marriages with one or two co-wives and half of the women were in arranged marriages. On average, they had four pregnancies, which represent few children when compared to the national average of 6 or 7 in rural areas (INSD, 2012). They had a high rate of stillbirth (average of 1.7), which demonstrates a lack of access to quality obstetrical care. These women had suffered from fistulas for an average of nine years, some having occurred one year prior to surgery, while others had been suffering for more than twenty years.

10.3.1 The Experience of Obstructed Labour

Before discussing the women's birth experience, we must present a brief overview of the healthcare system in Burkina Faso. It is organized into sanitary districts, composed of two elements[5]: the Health Centre for Social Promotion (*Centre de Santé Promotion Sociale* or CSPS) and the Medical Centre with Surgical Antenna (*Centre Médical avec Antenne Chirurgicale* or CMA).[6] These are the two levels of primary care in the healthcare system. The CSPS provides basic medical services, such as medical, maternal and infant care, and disease control. It was the chosen birthing services establishment for many of the women interviewed. In Burkina Faso, the main issue seems to be the length of time labouring at home before leaving for obstetrical care. Nearly one-half of our respondents (16 of 33) reported a delay before going to the healthcare centre. Even with an imprecise time scale in some cases,[7] the baby is often stillborn long before caesarean section or extraction occurs. In an extreme

---

[5]A health district covers between 150,000 and 300,000 inhabitants. There is a CSPS in a radius of 10 km for about 10,000 inhabitants.

[6]There are other levels of health care. The Regional Hospital Center is a reference centre for the CMA and the National Hospital Center and University offers specialized treatment, training and research.

[7]Perception of time differs in Burkinabe society, and when past events are distant in time, it becomes even more difficult to pinpoint the exact deadline. As an illustration, some women do not know their age. We estimate the delay on circumstantial elements, such as their impression of what is long, the number of nights with the pains or the state of the child on arrival at the hospital.

case of shoulder dystocia, one woman remained nine days with her stillborn baby's head between her thighs, her in-laws refusing to take her to the hospital. Nafi,[8] who was 25 years old at the time, tells her story here:

> *"I had painful labour at home for three days. My stomach was swollen, my feet were numb. I asked my husband to give me money and he said he had no money to provide care. After three days the baby died. The head had crowned but I lay there for six days with the head emerged. My father realized what had happened and he brought me to the hospital."*

The family economic precariousness, which makes it difficult to find the funds for care and transportation, can partially explain the delay. In rural Burkina Faso, travel can be difficult, especially during the rainy season, when roads are completely submerged. Villages are isolated and health centres with the expertise to handle such cases are located in large urban area, sometimes hundreds of kilometres away. A relative or friend with a reliable vehicle must be enlisted to provide transportation.

The delay may also be explained by the husband or in-laws' refusal to evacuate the woman, either because they do not recognize the seriousness of the problem, or due to the social hierarchy structure.

> *"[…] I took a long time getting to the hospital because women are dependent on their husband or the men of the family. If the men aren't quick to decide to take us to the hospital, we have no say in the matter. He couldn't make up his mind to take me. They waited two days before evacuating me."* (Rachida, 25 years old).

As seen in this previous quote, the woman is not an isolated social agent, she belongs to a group whose influence is decisive in the care. According to Hassan and Ekele (2009), a significant proportion of women interviewed after surgery confirmed that they could not decide on care for a future pregnancy, revealing the unequal power relation in the household structure.

Some of the women who presented rapidly to the health centre, which represents one-half of the women in the study, did not receive adequate care, despite insisting, as was the case for Flora (29 years old):

> *"I was at the small hospital [CSPS]. When we arrived, they tried to intervene but weren't able to remove the baby. So, we remained there and for three days, nothing was done to help me. My husband went to see the nurses to ask them, 'If you can't help her, tell us and we will go elsewhere because my wife is suffering.'"*

As we have seen, the CSPS provides access to primary care for villagers, but since the staff often lacks necessary obstetrical training, we observed a delay recognizing and diagnosing obstructed labour, and as well transferring the patient to a healthcare centre with surgical facilities, in order to undergo caesarean section. Furthermore, there is often an additional delay in transferring the woman to the regional hospital due to the unavailability or high cost of transportation. These are aggravating structural elements that add to the delay at home. In this particular study, distant location of living was also a factor for cases of extreme delay. For 13 patients, obstructed labour occurred while the women were living in the Ivory Coast, with labour migration of Burkina Faso workers being an important phenomenon in this area. While we cannot judge the quality of Ivorian health care, we must mention that Burkinabe in this country generally work in plantations in the north of the country, far from urban centres. There is indeed a correlation between the non-proximity of service structures and the delay at home (8 of 33 cases).

---

[8]All names and other personal identifiers in the case studies (or chapter) have been changed to protect privacy and confidentiality.

To summarize, these women's testimonies reveal that daily barriers to receiving obstetrical care occur at several levels. Firstly, they have been socialized into a hierarchical community social organization where decision-making is done collectively and where family authority is based on a patriarchal ideology. Men are the ones responsible for the household's important expenses, such as travel and care. Thus, despite their influence in the area of reproduction and their economic involvement in the household, women have to comply with this patriarchal organization. In addition, chronic poverty and lack of education about maternal health interfere with the decision-making process and increase delays. Finally, the importance of structural problems, such as the reclusiveness of some villages, the challenges of transportation (incomplete or impractical roads, cost and lack of transportation), and the medical personnel that lacks resources and training, should be noted. In the next section, we will discuss the women's perspective on the postpartum care following their obstructed labour, specifically in the context of a diagnosis of the obstetric fistula.

10.3.2 The Process of Care

After obstructed childbirth and the development of an obstetric fistula, women's accounts allowed us to reconstruct their experiences with the Burkinabe healthcare system. Their chaotic trajectories contributed to the disruption of their lives. That is why, as part of our action-research project, we have recommended from the beginning to improve the identification of patients in order to provide them with earlier care, in the hope of reducing the social consequences of their condition. The common factor is the extent of the number of visits to healthcare centres, in a search for understanding and treatment for their disease. This was the case of Aisha (34 years old), who suffered from a simple fistula:

> *"When I realized [that I was incontinent], I returned to Koudougou to explain it to the nurses. They told me to come back in a month and they would treat me. So, I went and then came back. They made me pay for things, but nothing improved. These were simply visits to identify my condition. They made me come back and forth repeatedly. But ultimately, I never received any treatment."*

These women were waiting for treatment, often unaware of the cause or even the name of their disease. They unanimously complained about the lack of communication from the medical staff, saying that they never were diagnosed, given any explanation for the cause of their symptoms or given therapeutic options. They did not know how to handle their incontinence and its physical sequelae on a daily basis. This led them to disburse additional sums in the search for a treatment through traditional or allopathic medicine, but without any guarantee of success, which increased vulnerability. Furthermore, these women often found themselves isolated, feeling they were alone in the world. The lack of information contributed greatly to their psychological distress. However, when they finally got access to reconstructive surgery and entered the healthcare system, they seemed satisfied with the treatment received. The problem lies precisely in the difficulties integrating this system. The lack of qualified urologists and gynaecologists specialized[9] in repairing fistula in Burkina Faso, and the surgical complexity of fistula repair, means that despite consultation with local doctors, they must often await the arrival of foreign medical missions to access reconstructive surgery for their fistula.

---

[9] Surgeons capable of performing this surgery are few in West Africa. In Burkina Faso, among the 47 hospitals visited during the epidemiological survey of Sombie et al. (2007), only four had personnel qualified to perform fistula repair.

10.4 Disrupted Lives

The invasive nature of fistula symptoms greatly disrupts the daily lives of women in terms of their economic activities and social relationships. We observe that a fistula is a physically debilitating, thus forcing women to reduce or cease their economic activities. In addition, fistulas fuel relationship tensions at the level of the family and the community. These two interdependent dimensions contribute to psychological distress. In order to better understand the global repercussions of fistulas, we propose here an anthropological analysis of the socio-economic consequences on the women encountered during this study.

10.4.1 The Economic Impacts of Fistula

The physical consequences of fistulas profoundly disturb women's daily lives. The wounds on their thighs, the odour, the frequent and abundant flow of urine, in addition to generating numerous ancillary costs (medication, soap, clothes, water, etc.), impede their farming and commercial activities. A majority of the women (19 of 33) told us they were no longer able to provide similar effort in the fields, particularly during the rainy seasons, or even be totally unable to provide it.

> *"Before I used to sell things. I kept busy and was independent. But now I can't any longer. My husband doesn't have any money to give me, or else he would. So, I plant peanuts to sell and pay for my clothes, because each time I wash, it spoils my clothes. During the rainy season, it is cool, my sores hurt more and I can't work. It's really hard."* (Estelle, 35 years old).

The activities of those who sell food products (vegetables, peanuts, cakes, millet beer) are also compromised. For example, Marie (30 years old), from the Fulani ethnic group said:

> *"I used to prepare the Fulani porridge. But I can't any longer because of my condition. […] I considered that it wasn't hygienic with my illness. And if I go out to sell, people will insult me., […]."*

We observed that while these women recognize the social incompatibility of food preparation and incontinence in their culture, they also fear being the brunt of the community's criticism. Indeed, this type of discrimination is widespread and represents a major setback for their social integration and statutory progression. The capacity to contribute to her family's subsistence, specifically through her economic activities, partly determines a women's status (Badini, 1994). Finally, among many Burkinabe groups, the gendered division of labour defining the economic responsibilities for women and men involves a distinct separation of each spouse's budget. The men cover all necessities while women take care of their own and their children's needs (Antoine, 2002). When afflicted women lose their economic autonomy, they have to rely entirely on marital support (and the in-laws). However, as we will demonstrate in the next section, numerous husbands willingly support their wives in this ordeal. Despite this solidarity, which is not exceptional, economic dependence seriously affects a woman. She is no longer able to fulfil her customary obligations, defined by the gendered labour division. According to the virilocality[10] residency custom, she always remains an outsider within the in-law family; therefore, she risks losing status. She finds herself discriminated against and under pressure to return to her family. Aside from purely monetary considerations, some women are unable to accomplish their daily chores:

> *"When I became ill, I stopped everything, I live at home I can no longer do housework."* (Aida, 26 years old).

---

[10]Virilocality signifies that after marriage, the wife will come to live in her husband's home or with his family. In anthropology, this is also referred to as patrilocal residence or patrilocality.

In rural areas, gathering wood, cooking, drawing water, sweeping the courtyard and caring for children are demanding tasks that become almost impossible without the help of relatives. These women feel ashamed of their inability to fulfil their social obligations. In other terms, fistulas cause a rupture in the family unit's economic balance by (1) increasing household maintenance costs, (2) disabling women for domestic chores, (3) generating agricultural difficulties and (4) obliterating commercial alternatives. We therefore concluded that the majority of our respondents are in a situation of economic precariousness, some, although rare, having no choice but to resort to begging.[11]

10.4.2 The Impact on Marital Relationships

Before discussing marital relationships, it is important to briefly reconstruct a general portrait of the matrimonial system in Burkina Faso.[12] Marriage contributes to the social integration of women, to paternal lineage, reproduction, to agricultural mode production and to the gerontocratic organizational structure. In this sense, there is a high rate of polygamy, particularly in the rural regions, where 42% of women find themselves in a polygamous union during their lifetime (INSD, 2012). These figures are reflected in our study, since 21 out of the 33 patients live or have lived with co-wives. As with most Sub-Saharan populations, marriage is a family process involving political and economic alliances over several generations, and the partners' consent was not even mandatory until recently. This remains a contemporary practice, specifically in rural areas. Thus, among our respondents, more than half were enrolled in arranged marriages by relatives. This particularity allows us to infer that these women lived under a customary marriage when they developed their fistula. This type of union implies a distinct separation of the female and male social universe, a gendered division of labour and a polygamous patriarchal structure.[13]

Previous studies, specifically in East Africa, point to the increased risk of repudiation for women suffering from fistulas (Browning & Menber, 2008; Yeakey et al., 2011). This is consistent with our study, where one-third of the patients interviewed had been repudiated (11 out of 33). Such is the case of Fatim, 24 years old:

> "*Ever since I got a fistula, I have no support from my own family, my husband has repudiated me, and even own parents are in agreement. Since they said I smelled bad, they didn't want me in their house.*"

In some instances, the husband does not even bring his wife home, as was the case of Omela, who at age 20 years was abandoned by her husband on the road leading to her parents' village, when they returned from the hospital. Three others still lived in the husband's compound but in isolation, and seven women observed a substantial increase in conflict and tension with their spouse and co-wives. Awa (30 years old) explains how her relationship changed since the fistula:

> "*Even if my husband won't admit it, he has changed, we often fight for absolutely no reason! He picks up a fight with me for stupid little things. He even tells me that I can leave, he says 'I'll be happy if you leave.'*"

---

[11] Some studies indicate that women who had been repudiated by their husbands or abandoned by their community end up begging. (Ahmed & Holtz, 2007; Semere & Nour, 2008).

[12] We know that there are more than 63 ethnic groups in Burkina Faso with a diverse system of family relationship and matrimonial regimes. However, in spite of cultural differences, the majority of these ethnic group share the similar community and traditional ideology, which allows us to demonstrate general matrimonial trends.

[13] As a result, in the family compound, a hierarchy exists by which the husband rules as head of the household and under his authority his co-wives are ranked in order of their arrival in the home. This hierarchy becomes more complex if the compound is situated close to that of the in-laws. In that case, the senior generation of males (the father-in-law and his brothers) has more authority than does the husband (Badini, 1994).

Under these circumstances, we infer that fistulas have a deeply disruptive effect in marital relationships and, in some cases, engender violence. In societies in which marriage is an inevitable obligation, why such high rate of abandonment? Indeed, although separation is not exceptional in Burkina Faso (Gnoumou Thiombiano & Legrand, 2014), lineages can enact several mechanisms to avoid this final solution. Yet, none of our informants mentioned them. On the contrary, it seems that their respective families welcomed them back without issues. To understand this situation, we must refer to customary ideology of matrimonial arrangement. In Burkinabe marriages and in sub-Saharan Africa in general, certain expectations exist in terms of rights and duties the spouses must honour in order to be worthy and respectful of the prevalent social norms. (Kuyu Mwissa, 2005). As mentioned, women with fistula are no longer able to contribute sufficiently to community life (both economically and politically) and to comply with social expectations. (Badini, 1994). Moreover, as they experienced obstetrical failure, they usually have few or no children, while fearing and avoiding a new pregnancy (17 of 33 respondents), which is also against social norms. *"It's true that they insult me, but it's also because I have no children"* says Yasmine, 29 years old. Ultimately, fistulas are unknown and misunderstood by the population. The lack of awareness and communication issues often associate it with divine punishment or witchcraft (Hassan & Ekele, 2009). All these reasons, amplified by the lack of knowledge and access to treatment, can unfortunately explain discriminatory behaviours, which could lead to a form of repudiation.[14]

Nevertheless, we should not generalize these women's situations. While there is a significant increase in the risk of tension and rejection compared to the general population, the majority of our respondents, 19 out of 33, still live with their spouses and 16 of them assert that they receive some kind of support. In such cases, the husband and co-wives provide for their needs, protect them, contribute to additional expenses and accompany them when they travel, during surgical mission. For instance:

> *"I have no problem with my co-wives in the family. We get along well, they eat what I cook and vice versa. They even wash my dirty clothes" (Eveline, 31 years old).*

This example is meaningful because commensality is a sign of sharing, reconciliation and social harmony (Paré, 2017). On the other hand, in Mariam's case (45 years old), her co-wives prohibit her from sitting with them during meals, leaving her to eat by herself. This sharing rejection suggests a refusal to enter into a relationship, a highly outrageous and insulting social act in Burkinabe representations (Paré, 2017). Obviously, the relationship between co-wives is not always easy (Mason, 1988; Vinel, 2005). It could be described symbolically as either jealousy or solidarity. Our study reflects this social pattern. Samira, 27 years old, gives us an example of solidarity:

> *I have no issue with my co-wife. We really like each other. [...] When I came here, I asked her to please come with me [...]? She accepted without any intervention by our husband.*

However, the relationship may be harmful when co-wives gossip and spread rumours in the community. Such accounts reveal that polygamy is not an aggravating factor for women living with fistulas. In a polygamous situation (two-thirds of our respondents), the disengagement or the solicitude at the time of illness depends on the previous relationship state. In other words, if there was no harmony or if polygamy was poorly experienced beforehand, the fistula will become a catalyst that exacerbates tensions. Co-wives will take advantage of the vulnerability to try to evict their rival. On the contrary, if the agreement was well established, the co-wives will support each other as sisters through this

---

[14]We have seen that better awareness and information about fistulas can eliminate much discriminatory behaviour. By preventing the social association of madness and witchcraft with this disease, we observed an improvement in social relationships and community solidarity.

crisis. They will look after the affected woman's children, accompany her on her travels and help her with her daily chores. Since polygamy is a complex matrimonial structure, the appearance of fistula will tend to intensify pre-existing behaviour.

The matrimonial portrait described above inevitably has consequences on these women's sexuality. In our sample, among those who remained in relationship, only a minority,[15] (seven women) said they still had sex with their husband. Aside from these cases, the women stopped all forms of intimacy since contracting the disease: *"I told my husband: 'I am sick, so we can't have intimate relations, so wait until I am better.' (Eveline 31 years old)."* In addition to the fears of pregnancy, which seems to be the main element, the refusal justification is questions of hygiene and cleanliness. For example, her co-wife asked Mariam (45 years old) to stop sex on the pretext it would be dangerous:

> *"When a husband has several wives, each has her turn. My co-wife said she had no sex with our husband because it's forbidden, because a disease like that is harmful so it is not permitted."*

This refers to a sexual taboo related to bodily fluids prevalent in many Burkinabe ethnic groups. One could infer a fear of transmitting infection between co-wives following intimacy. These cultural prohibitions may mask rules of hygiene to avoid infectious consequences. In short, we observe a significant decline in the incidence of sexual relations, with a direct reduction in their fecundity, which contributes to increasing the risk of ostracism.

10.4.3 Community Rupture and its Effect on Mental Health

When considering all the facts discussed above, we can imagine the physiological distress experienced by the women. As mentioned earlier, the fact of being kept in ignorance of the causes, treatment and the proportion of women affected by fistulas discourages many of them. This reinforces their isolation. In addition, a phenomenon of social self-exclusion is developing since these women can no longer satisfy their social obligations and suffer from constant discrimination. The non-participation in social activities (wedding, ceremonies, funerals), that is necessary for maintaining local solidarity, illustrates the community rupture. This self-exclusion also appears daily since the women stay away from the marketplace and the *maquis* (local canteen). They fear judgement and prefer to confine themselves inside the compound. Thus, Samira (27 years old), who maintained a harmonious relationship with her husband and in-laws, spoke of her isolation:

> *What is certain is that things can't get worse because I already can't go out in public.   When I do, I realize I'm the only one with this condition. It bothers me.*

Despite these women's resilience, many of them have symptoms of depression, including sadness, loss of motivation, guilt and shame. Some unfortunately develop suicidal thoughts. The testimony of Larissa (31 years old) represents this distress:

> *"I was lonely, I felt isolated, At one time I thought of committing suicide, so I took a rope, I went into the woods, but once I was there, I thought about the fact that I have children. Why would I do this? I hang on for my children's sake."*

One must understand that suicide is a controversial and secret matter in these societies and clearly shows how deeply psychologically seared they are by the consequences of fistula.

---

[15]Of the 11 separated women, none mentioned that they still had sexual relationships. That said, it is a taboo subject and we did not insist on it in our interviews.

Community life is the norm in the Burkinabe villages; social activities also occur in a group. The marketplace, the field, the well, the local *maquis*, the various institutions and government services are all gathering spaces to chat, cooperate and socialize. As in other Sub-Saharan societies, all-important information is transmitted orally in the public place and by avoiding them, due to shame and fear of being insulted, the women cannot function properly in society. Emma, 37 years old, experienced this:

> *"When I go out in public like that, and when I get up after I've been sitting, I'm wet or I smell bad. People come up and insult me, When I walk by, people move away because of the odour. That sort of thing. Some say I must have done something wrong for which I'm being punished."*

The apprehension of being attacked publicly is genuine, since one-third of women reported having been gossiped about and insulted, as Emma's example demonstrates. Thus, even when family members display real support, the insults can come from the community itself. This explains why some women hide their condition. By protecting themselves from rumours and malevolence, they aggravate their exclusion. When this social rupture occurs, it amplifies the psychological effects and, unfortunately, encourages isolation behaviour. In short, in addition to the economic disequilibrium caused by fistula's physical attributes, it also acts as a catalyst for conflict and disrupts the entire sphere of women's living conditions and daily existence.

10.5 Getting over the Fistula: The Experience of Social Reinsertion

In the second phase of the study, our meetings were aimed at learning more about the status and attitudes of women with fistula towards convalescence after reconstructive surgery. By going to their respective villages, we wanted them to show us their living environment and tell us concretely about their return to daily life, one or two years after their operation. One of the purposes of this research was to better comprehend the social reintegration process and the obstacles encountered by these women. The analysis therefore focused exclusively on women who were cured (or those whose symptoms had improved considerably).

10.5.1 A Return to Health and Daily Activities

For the social reinsertion process to happen, surgery must be successful, or at least have substantially improved symptoms. Since one of the essential aspects of our methodology was to meet with the women directly in their village, this excluded the feasibility of a gynaecological examination during the follow-up visits. As a result, success in this study is defined as "clinical," meaning that during our follow-up, women reported that they no longer suffered from urinary incontinence.

In this regard, we already know the surgical outcome for 33 patients: 19 were cured, 6 showed definite improvement, and 8 had stable symptoms, for a clinical success rate of 58% (76% if we include women whose condition had somewhat improved), which conforms to national results. According to the studies and inclusion criteria, success rates vary considerably, ranging from 93% in East Africa to lower rates (44% in Niger and 60% in Burkina Faso) in West Africa (Raassen et al., 2008; Semere & Nour, 2008; Sombie et al., 2007). However, we must mention that the vast majority of the women (70%) in this study had complex obstetrical fistulas and had previously undergone surgery without success (from one to five operations). Physical convalescence was generally rapid and without post-operative complications. They noted a complete disappearance of wounds on their thighs and very few sexual issues or post-operatory dyspareunia. Nevertheless, we suspected that some women, who felt that their symptoms had greatly improved, still suffered from persistent urinary problems, such as stress incontinence or urinary urgency. This implied that they continued to have some residual symptoms, although they no longer had a constant flow of urine.

10.5.2 Regaining Economic Autonomy: A Gradual Journey

As we have just seen, surgical success allows for physical healing, and as a result all of the women had resumed their domestic activities. However, regaining economic autonomy is arduous. All of the cured women had also restarted their economic activities, which constitute a social obligation given their poverty state and the gendered division of labour. Yet, this a gradual journey. For example, for agricultural labour, the women waited several months or even a year before undertaking the heaviest tasks, for fear of recurrence of their fistula, although no such case was reported. Several limited their work to light chores, as in Awa's case:

"I haven't resumed farming work yet. I began with light work but since I suffered so much with the disease, I'm afraid to begin hard work. I don't want to fall sick again."

For commercial activities such as selling at the market, most women were able to resume their activities without difficulty. They were gradually able to rebuild their clientele, as is the case for Flora, 29 years old. At first, the people at the market were wary of her, but they all came back when rumours of her recovery spread. Some women even started new commercial activities in order to reimburse debts accumulated during the years they suffered from the fistula. Others had not yet acquired a stable source of income but were planning to do so.

In all cases, the women's economic situation remained very precarious, even a year or two after surgery. During the post-operatory path, they encountered many challenges to fulfil all their needs since most were already in a situation of chronic poverty. Every event threatens these families' economic stability. Relatives depend on a handful of individuals for basic support. In addition to the loss of income of one of its members, households, and often the women themselves, must assume all expenses related to the disease and its treatment. Under these circumstances, they accumulate considerable debt, proportional to the duration of the fistula. The debt cycle begins with expenses for hospitalization incurred during obstructed pregnancy (transportation, food, medicine, housing, the caesarean section), since the costs are being borne by the patient. We must also consider the multiple medical visits and the costs associated with their stay over the period of surgery. This is further increased by the loss of the women's productivity during their illness and convalescence, as well as accessory costs such as water, soap and clothing. The women must reimburse the institutions as well as relatives who have supported them, sometimes for years. All these factors imply that even if the women start working, they are in a catch-up situation; emerging from a cycle of debt is exacting. We deduce that the consequences of fistula last long after the recovery. The economic impact could be reduced or avoided if the fistulas were detected earlier and medical care offered more quickly, which would lighten the cost of stay at the hospital during surgical missions.[16] This aspect could be remedied concretely in order to improve the reinsertion process.

---

[16]This last point was brought up during our first round of interviews, and in the perspective of our action-research, the cost of transportation and food was later covered by the MMS Foundation in order to lighten the women's debt load.

10.5.3 A Return to Conjugal Harmony: A Family that Heals its Wounds

On the issue of conjugal relationships, once the cause of the social upheaval has been resolved, we observed a resolution of conflict with the husband and co-wives. For the women who lost marital support and faced a conflict situation, the couple seems to have re-established dialogue and cohesion.

> *"My husband provided no support while I was sick, we didn't get along. He never came near me, he didn't come to my room. Now we get along well. He comes to my room to talk, we have begun to have sex and all is well"* (Rama, 40 years old).

The same situation prevails for women such as Diane, 34 years old, who said that her husband supported her during the illness. He had remained present, but she always worried that he would leave her or take a second wife. There is a betterment for these women as well, since the fear of being repudiated had been a constant source of apprehension. The return of intimacy often accompanied the re-establishment of harmony. The majority of women who were cured (and those whose symptoms improved), waited six months to one year after their surgery to be certain of their recovery before starting sexual intercourse again. However, five of the them were still abstinent, for fear of recurring fistulas.

Accounts vary for women who had been repudiated by their husbands. Despite the disease, two of these women had remarried a new husband who supported them, whereas another remarried during her convalescence. One repudiated woman returned to live with her husband once cured, since they resolved their conflict. Three other women remained single, either waiting for their former husband to agree to return, or because they were still marked by the bad treatment to which they had been subjected in their marriage. Larissa, 31 years old, spoke about this:

> *"My husband didn't want to take me back after the operation, even though I was cured. It doesn't bother me because I don't want anything to do with him. Since he rejected me and treated me badly beforehand, I am still angry and I don't want him to come to my room. I don't want another husband either; I prefer to stay like this with my children."*

The improvement of marital relationships leads to a corollary reduction of conflicts and rivalries with co-wives. Indeed, women retrieved their place and their safety within the household and were no longer rejected. When the cause of disagreement disappears, members of the family at large will consider gossips and insults unacceptable. In other words, social harmony is restored on its own according to the conflict resolution process (Bidima, 1997).

10.5.4 Social Reinsertion, Physical and Psychological Healing

This form of social dynamics is also effective on a community level and promotes women's reinsertion into daily life. The women's social relationships change significantly after surgery since they resume their public activities and attend events; healing itself is a source of celebration. Even those who are not completely healed, but whose condition has improved, participate more in the social life because it is easier to handle the physical repercussions of their disease. The exclusion process that includes gossips, insults and hurtful comments fade. Given that this recurrent discrimination was one of the main factors of their isolation, the women feel liberated from that burden and are able to reintegrate the circle of social relationships.

> *"In my courtyard, they found out I was no longer sick, so the family spread the news outside the home and people knew that I was better. People don't gossip about me anymore. I am not resentful about those who said negative things about me."* (Asséta, 26 years old).

Similar to Asséta, most of them had no resentment and chose the option of social reconciliation. This attitude goes hand-in-hand with the psychological healing observed during our meetings with the women in their villages, in which symptoms of depression and suicidal thoughts had subsided. There was no more sadness, shame, loneliness and self-exclusion, and all the women expressed their happiness and gratitude during the interviews. It is also the case for those who were not cured, but whose symptoms had improved. This is partly due to the creation of an informal solidarity network among the women through surgical missions. Without any involvement of the MMS Foundation, the women banded together around their common condition. Aside from feeling less lonely in their personal tribulations, in the course of their hospitalization, they helped each other out, confided and exchanged advice and information. This gave them the confidence to face the consequences of their fistula and they gained newfound hope from the cure of their friends. Nevertheless, some psychological sequelae are lasting, particularly anxiety about fistula recurrence. This was demonstrated by excessive precautions taken, such as the avoidance of fieldwork or prolonging sexual abstinence beyond the prescribed period. There were also significant concerns regarding a future pregnancy, which will be discussed in the next section. In short, while we can say that the women are in better psychological state a year after their operation, they remain fragile.

Notwithstanding this nuance, based on their experience and in a demonstration of resilience, some healed women wished to provide advice and raise their community's awareness of the disease. This desire was highlighted through the five-year research period, as the last cohorts of women were much more knowledgeable about the medical problem, thanks to the efforts that our Foundation's local partner association, ARFOD, which contributed to the village awareness campaign. However, many women still considered this disease shameful and did not dare advocate about it, even when they had been cured. Several of them agreed with the idea of group discussion and information sessions on the subject, either with specialists or with women who have already experienced the condition. In light of this, perhaps such groups should be a part of surgical missions and patient treatment, in order to develop an approach coherent with local practices.

10.5.5 The Obstetrical Future, Between Fear and Conforming to Social Norms

During the interviews, there was a great ambivalence towards their obstetrical future. As we saw earlier, they feared a return of the fistula and its consequences. They wanted to rest and explicitly mentioned their heavy debt load to justify their indecisiveness. Twelve of the nineteen women who were cured chose to avoid pregnancy. Birth control methods varied: four were using Norplant,[17] one used Dépo-Provera,[18] one used the contraceptive pill, and six were abstaining from sex.

> "I don't want any more children, but if I have one, I will keep it. It is the disease that is the problem. When I married my new husband, we went together to implant the Norplant. I decided to do that because I am afraid of becoming pregnant again." (Albertine, 26 years old).

This choice can have serious consequences, especially for women with few or no children. Most are disappointed with their situation and sad about their obstetrical failure. Statutory progression depends on their fertility and their matrimonial situation (Gruénais, 1985; Hannequin, 1990), and offspring provide a form of safety net. Despite their desire for more children, they were worrying about the risks of a new pregnancy. They felt that they lacked information on this topic, which increased their anxiety.

---

[17]Implant contraceptive that lasts for 5 years.

[18]Contraceptive injected every 3 months.

Furthermore, secondary infertility is known to be a complication of fistulas and surgery, due to various causes such as severe injury to the cervix, hypophysis or hypothalamic dysfunction, inter-uterine scarring and Asherman's syndrome (Abrams et al., 2012). Like Flora, 29 years old, who desperately hoped for another pregnancy but was not successful after a year, two other participants were also amenorrhoeic at the time of our follow-up. According to a 6-months post-operative study conducted in Ethiopia, there is a 29% rate of amenorrhoea among such women (Browning & Menber, 2008). The risk of miscarriage and premature birth due to an injured cervix is also high among these patients. (Abrams et al., 2012; Browning, 2009). During our follow-up phase, three participants had become pregnant since surgery: one was 2 months pregnant on our visit, another had a stillbirth at 7 months, and the third had experienced a difficult at-term birth at home, which resulted in a stillborn. The women who manage to become pregnant after surgery are at high risk of developing the obstetrical problems that caused their fistula. Few studies exist on this subject, but research by Browning (2009) showed a good success rate for pregnancies among women operated for fistulas if a planned caesarean section was performed. Success rates are much lower for women who give birth vaginally, with a high incidence of infant mortality.

10.6 Conclusions

This study proposed to describe and analyse the experience of women living with a fistula and their post-operatory reinsertion in Burkina Faso, combining medical and anthropological expertise. Our interdisciplinary methodology considered the physical and psychological effects of this disease, as well as the challenges that diagnosis and treatment present. These aspects were associated with an anthropological analysis of the society since women suffering from fistulas are not isolated social agents, but belong to a global social network which influences the way they experience their fistula on a daily basis. Thus, it was essential to comprehend their testimonies through a contextual analysis that considers the local matrimonial dynamics, hierarchal structures, gendered division of labour and community networks. In other terms, we wanted to draw a nuanced portrait of these women's reality and their milieu by showing in a transversal manner the influence of various individual, social and structural factors within the context of Burkina Faso.

Firstly, using birthing narratives and the treatment journey, we highlighted the factors leading to the development of obstetric fistulas and the lack of services for referral and care. Major delays before going to health centres during obstructed labour were reported, due to poverty, difficult road conditions, lack of education and the household power relations. We must also point out the structural challenges of the Burkinabe healthcare system, specifically in the area of available information and communication about diagnosis and treatment of obstetric fistula. As a corollary, this has delayed treatment, sometimes for many years, evidenced here by the chaotic journey of women to access restorative surgery. Our results are consistent with the existing literature on the subject and confirm that it is indeed a major healthcare issue.

In terms of the daily impacts of fistulas, three interdependent spheres have emerged: economic, matrimonial and community/psychological. We have seen that the physical sequelae of fistulas make women economically more precarious, rendering them dependent on their entourage. A disequilibrium set in for the couple as well as a cycle of debt that lasts even after recovery. Their loss of autonomy and their inability to assume their economic roles, as determined by the gendered division of labour, are a source of tension and conflict in the household. There is an increased risk for conjugal rejection. Since most women were welcomed in their home village, the conflict dimension is therefore restricted to the marital family. Polygamy does not appear to be an additional risk factor, but rather reflects relationships between co-wives prior to the fistula. Indeed, in several cases, co-wives even provided support and accompanied the women on surgical missions. Despite their isolation and rejection from the community, it was interesting to note that many women still received some support either from their spouse, a co-wife, or another family member, and were therefore not completely abandoned. Shame and self-exclusion were also generally shown to be mechanisms of exclusion that were even more powerful than rumours or gossip in the community. Our interviews explored the links between a rupture with the community and the serious psychological impacts of the disease, leading women to isolate themselves from their milieu and to sink into depression.

As for social reinsertion, we observed a resolution of household conflict, a return to normal activities, an improvement in the relationship with the husband (except for the women who had been repudiated), as well as a complete disappearance of depression symptoms. The phenomenon of solidarity observed during our surgical missions appears to alleviate these women's suffering. Some repudiated women were able to remarry or return to their husband, but others remained single, at times harbouring painful memories of their former relationship and with no desire to find a new partner. Despite significant betterment of their daily lives, some psychological symptoms remained, particularly anxiety about a relapse, which led many women to avoid farm work and intimacy with their husband. Furthermore, they demonstrated great ambivalence and lacked information about their childbearing future. Lastly, financial reintegration is laborious due to accumulated debts, loss of productivity during the illness and pre-existing conditions of chronic poverty. Subsistence economy practised by these women before their illness makes it difficult for them to reimburse their debts. Many had to be imaginative and engage in new business ventures in order to regain some economic stability, while others continued to be in an extremely precarious financial situation.

The participation-action research approach proved to be relevant in our case, as the women's implication allowed us to include suggestions to help their reintegration process and our collaboration with the local association ARFOD. Thanks to a more intensive recruitment of women with fistulas, they were referred earlier for surgery, which attenuates their indebtedness and psychosocial consequences. Expenses associated with the surgery (food and transportation) are now also covered. Other ideas were discussed to assist the women's economic reinsertion, such as micro-credit or technical training during their stay at the hospital. It is crucial not to favour former fistula patients financially in relationship to other members of the community by creating imbalances, especially in monetary terms, which might cause negative perception of the patients in the community. Unfortunately, even a year after their surgery, many women were still in a very unstable financial condition and had not yet managed to regain their previous economic situation. These issues require further reflection, particularly at the level of humanitarian project planning.

This brings us to address some of the shortcomings of this study. The methodological choices of the life stories and post-operative visits to the villages allowed us to collect rich and locally contextualized data. However, these methods also have their limitations. First, we could not conduct gynaecological examinations during the second interview; the success of surgery therefore had to be based on clinical discussion with the patients. Moreover, by focusing on women's testimonies and observations of their living environment, we only obtained the reflection of their personal perception. It would have been preferable to include visits to health centres and interviews with healthcare professions in the study in order to gather a complete picture of their work. Interviews with individuals from these women's entourage would have acknowledged the daily consequences as experienced by the families. This would have significantly contributed to the holistic perspective of the research.

In conclusion, we would like to encourage a reflection on the aspect of prevention. Although this research emphasized mainly the follow-up and reinsertion of women already suffering from fistulas, prevention of obstetrical complications must be paramount. Training of traditional midwives and healthcare personal, access to adequate follow-up during pregnancy and emergency obstetrical care, as well as popular education campaigns that target not only women but the authority figures responsible for decisions, notably men and elders, are key aspects in preventing obstetric fistula. This research has shed light on the importance women attach to information about their reproductive health, and on their wish for involving their husbands and families in these matters. Ideally, healthcare personnel and women in the community who have lived similar experiences should conduct education sessions jointly. If local involvement is key, it is not sufficient. Improvements of public health policies at a governmental level must also take place. It is not only about fistulas, but about improving the health of an entire population.

Acknowledgements Thanks to the following research assistants and translators: Stéphanie Breton, Alessandro Carini, Maria Cherba, Catherine Coulombe, Marie-Charlotte De Koninck, Célia Ido, Safiatou Ouédraogo.

References

Abrams, P., Ridder, D., DeVries, C., Elneil, S., Esegbona, G., Mourad, S., et al. (2012). *Obstetric fistula in the developing world*. Société Internationale d'Urologie (SIU). Available from: https://www.siu-urology.org/themes/web/assets/files/ICUD/pdf/ICUD_Vesicovaginal%20Fistula_2010.pdf Accessed 1 July 2019

Ahmed, S., & Holtz, S. (2007). Social and economic consequences of obstetric fistula: Life changed forever? *International Journal of Gynaecology and Obstetrics, 99*(Suppl 1), S10–S15. https://doi.org/10.1016/j.ijgo.2007.06.011

Anoukouma, T., Attipou, K. K., Agoda-Koussema, L. K., Akpadza, K., & Ayite, E. A. (2010). Epidemiological, aetiological and treatment aspects of obstetrical fistula in Togo. *Progrès en Urologie, 20*(1), 71–76. https://doi.org/10.1016/j.purol.2009.08.038

Antoine, P. (2002). Les complexités de la nuptialité: de la précocité des unions féminines à la polygamie masculine en Afrique. In G. Caselli, J. Vellin, & G. Wunsch (Eds.), *Démographie : analyse et synthèses. Volume II : Les déterminants de la fécondité*. Available from: https://core.ac.uk/download/pdf/39845400.pdf Accessed 5 July 2019

Arrowsmith, S., Hamlin, E., & Wall, L. (1996). Obstructed labour injury complex: Obstetric fistula formation and the multifaceted morbidity of maternal birth trauma in the developing world. *Obstetrical & Gynecological Survey, 51*(9), 568–574.

Badini, A. (1994). *Naître et grandir chez les Moosé traditionnels*. Ouagadougou Sépia.

Bidima, J. G. (1997). *La palabre: Une juridiction de la parole*. Éditions Michalon.

Browning, A. (2009). Pregnancy following obstetric fistula repair, the management of delivery. *An International Journal of Obstetrics and Gynaecology, 116*(9), 1265–1267. Available from: https://obgyn.onlinelibrary.wiley.com/doi/full/10.1111/j.1471-0528.2009.02182.x. Accessed 29 July 2019

Browning, A., & Menber, B. (2008). Women with obstetric fistula patients in Ethiopia: A 6-month follow-up after surgical treatment. *An International Journal of Obstetrics and Gynaecology, 115*(12), 1564–1568. Available from: https://obgyn.onlinelibrary.wiley.com/doi/full/10.1111/j.1471-0528.2008.01900.x. Accessed 29 July 2019

Cargo, M., & Mercer, S. (2008). The value and challenges of participatory research : Strengthening its practice. *Annual Review of Public Health, 2*, 325–350. https://doi.org/10.1146/annurev.publhealth.29.091307.083824

Gruénais, M.-É. (1985). Aîné, aînées; cadets, cadettes. Les relations aînés/cadets chez les Mossi du centre (Burkina Faso). In M. Abéles & C. Collard (Eds.), *Age, pouvoir et société en Afrique Noire* (pp. 219–245). Karthala.

Hannequin, B. (1990). Etat, patriarcat et développement: le cas d'un village mossi du Burkina Faso. *Revue canadienne des études africaines, 24*(1). https://doi.org/10.1080/00083968.1990.10803851

Harouna, Y., Seibou, A., Maikano, S., Djambeidou, J., Sangare, A., & Bilan, E. S. S. (2001). La fistulevesico-vaginale de cause obstetricale: Enquête auprès de 52 femmes admises au village des fistuleuses. *Médecine d'Afrique Noire, 48*(2), 55–59. Available from: http://www.santetropicale.com/Resume/24802.pdf. Accessed 30 July 2019

Hassan, M., & Ekele, B. (2009). Vesicovaginal fistula: Do the patients know the cause? *Annals of African Medicine, 8*(2), 122–126. https://doi.org/10.4103/1596-3519.56241

Institut National de la Statistique et de la Démographie (2012). Enquête Démographique et de Santé à Indicateurs Multiples 2010. Available from: https://dhsprogram.com/pubs/pdf/FR256/FR256.pdf. Accessed 30 July 2019.

Khisa, W., Wakasiaka, S., McGowan, L., & Campbell, M. (2017). Understanding the lived experience of women before and after fistula repair: A qualitative study in Kenya. *BJOG. An International Journal of Obstetrics and Gynaecology, 124*(3), 503–510. https://doi.org/10.1111/1471-0528.13902. Available from: https://obgyn.onlinelibrary.wiley.com/doi/full/10.1111/1471-0528.13902. Accessed 10 August 2019

Kuyu Mwissa, C. (2005). *Parenté et famille dans les cultures africaines*. Karthala.

Lewis, A., Kaufman, M. R., Wolter, C. E., Phillips, S. E., Maggi, D., Condry, L., et al. (2009). Genitourinary fistula experience in Sierra Leone: Review of 505 cases. *Journal of Urology, 181*(4), 1725–1731. https://doi.org/10.1016/j.juro.2008.11.106

Mason, K. F. (1988). Co-wife relationships can be amicable as well as conflictual: The case of the moose of Burkina Faso. *Canadian journal of African studies, 22*(3), 615–624. https://doi.org/10.2307/485958

Minkler, M., & Wallerstein, N. (2008). *Community-based participatory research for health: From process to outcomes.* Josey-Bass.

Nardos, R., Browning, A., & Chen, C. C. (2009). Risk factors that predict failure after vaginal repair of obstetric vesi-covaginal fistula. *American Journal of Obstetrics and Gynecology, 200*(5), 578.e1–578.e4. https://doi.org/10.1016/j.ajog.2008.12.008

Nathan, L., Rochat, C., Grigorescu, B., & Banks, E. (2009). Obstetric fistulae in West Africa: Patient perspectives. *American Journal of Obstetrics and Gynecology, 200*(5), 40–42. https://doi.org/10.1016/j.ajog.2008.10.014

Ndiaye, P., Amoul Kini, G., Abdoulaye, I., Diagne Camara, M., & Tal-Dia, A. (2009). Epidemiology of women suffering from obstetric fistula in Niger. *Médecine Tropicale, 69*(1), 61–65.

Nour, N. (2006). Health consequences of child marriage in Africa. *Emerging Infectious Disease, 2*(11), 1644–1649. Available from: https://www.ncbi.nlm.nih.gov/pmc/articles/PMC3372345/. Accessed 30 July 2019

Onolemhemhen, D., & Ekwempu, C. (1999). An investigation of sociomedical risk factors associated with vaginal fistula in northern Nigeria. *Women & Health, 28*(3), 103–116. https://doi.org/10.1300/J013v28n03_07

Paré, M.-E. (2017). *Le pluralisme des systèmes juridiques et les perceptions de la justice. Une ethnographie des conflits matrimoniaux chez les Mossi de Koudougou, Burkina Faso.* Université de Montréal.

Raassen, T., Verdaasdonk, E., & Vierhout, M. (2008). Prospective results after first-time surgery for obstetric fistulas in east African women. *International Urogynecology Journal and Pelvic Floor Dysfunction, 19*(1), 73–79. https://doi.org/10.1007/s00192-007-0389-6

Semere, L., & Nour, M. (2008). Obstetric fistula: Living with incontinence and shame. *Reviews in Obstetrics and Gynecology, 1*(4), 193–197. Available from: https://www.ncbi.nlm.nih.gov/pmc/articles/PMC2621054/. Accessed 30 July 2019

Sombie, I., Kambou ,T., Conombo, S., Sankara, O., Ouedraogo, L., Zoungrana, T. (2007). Retrospective study of uro-genital fistula in Burkina Faso from 2001 to 2003. Médecine Tropicale, 67(1), 48–52.

Tebeu, P., Bernis, L., Doh, A., Rochat, C., & Delvaux, T. (2009). Risk factors for obstetric fistula in the far North Province of Cameroon. *International Journal of Gynecology & Obstetrics, 107*(1), 12–15. https://doi.org/10.1016/j.ijgo.2009.05.019

Thiombiano, B. G., & Legrand, T. K. (2014). Niveau et facteurs de ruptures des premières unions conjugales au Burkina Faso. *African Population Studies, 23*(8), 1432–1446. Available from: http://aps.journals.ac.za/pub/article/view/641/540. Accessed July 29 2019

Vinel, V. (2005). *Des femmes et des lignages : ethnologie des relations féminines au Burkina Faso (Moose-Sikoomse).* L'Harmattan.

Wall, L. (2006). Obstetric vesico-vaginal fistula as an international public-health problem. *Lancet, 368*(9542), 1201–1209. https://doi.org/10.1016/S0140-6736(06)69476-2

Yeakey, M., Chipeta, E., Rijken, Y., Taulo, F., & Tsui, A. (2011). Experiences with fistula repair surgery among women and families in Malawi. *Global Public Health, 6*(2), 153–167. https://doi.org/10.1080/17441692.2010.491833

Zheng, A., & Anderson, F. (2009). Obstetric fistula in low-income countries. *International Journal of Gynecology & Obstetrics, 104*(2), 85–89. https://doi.org/10.1016/j.ijgo.2008.09.011

Girls' and Women's Social Experiences with Obstetric Fistula in Tanzania: A Public Health Problem

Stella Masala Mpanda and Lilian Teddy Mselle

11.1   Introduction

Obstetric fistula is one of the most neglected issues impacting girls and women's health and the quality of their lives. Despite international and national efforts, millions of girls and women still die in childbirth or live with maternal morbidities such as fistula (Wall et al., 2005). In Tanzania, approximately 2500–3000 new cases of fistula are estimated to occur each year (Bangser, 2006; Raassen, 2005). In Tanzania, it is estimated that ~46,000 women are living with obstetric fistula in 2010 (National Bureau of Statistics of Tanzania; ICF Macro, 2011). These numbers will likely have increased by approximately 2000–3000 each year since 2010. It is expected that there will be approximately 62,000–70,000 girls and women suffering from fistula by 2018 in Tanzania.

The most common type of fistula in Tanzania is obstetric fistula. This results from obstructed labor causing either vesicovaginal fistula (VVF) or rectovaginal fistula (RVF), or both (VVF+RVF); depending on what bodily organs are affected, urine or stool can pass through the vagina (Arrowsmith et al., 1996; Capes et al., 2011). Apart from obstetric causes, fistula may also occur as an iatrogenic injury during surgical procedures related to child delivery. A third group of causes of vaginal fistula includes accidents, sexual abuse, and rape in war or conflict areas (Raassen et al., 2014).

The continuing widespread occurrence of obstetric fistula in Tanzania is an indicator that health and social systems are failing to meet the basic needs of girls and women in the country (World Health Organization, 2018). The root causes are deeply embedded in social, cultural, and economic determinants that underlie poverty and social inequity. Obstetric fistula largely affects girls and women living in rural areas with difficult terrain, poor infrastructure, and who suffer severe poverty (Mselle & Kohi, 2016). They often lack access to adequate health services and information, cannot afford transport to health facility in cases of obstetric emergency, and are poorly educated. Moreover, fistula inhibits

S. M. Mpanda
Childbirth Survival International,
Dar es Salaam, Tanzania

L. T. Mselle (✉)
Department of Clinical Nursing, Muhimbili
University of Health and Allied Sciences,
Dar es Salaam, Tanzania
e-mail: lmselle@muhas.ac.tz

© Springer Nature Switzerland AG 2022
L. B. Drew et al. (eds.), *A Multidisciplinary Approach to Obstetric Fistula in Africa*, Global
Maternal and Child Health, https://doi.org/10.1007/978-3-031-06314-5_11

women's ability to work and to interact with other people, driving them deeper into poverty and further undermining their economic and social position (Women's Dignity Project and EngenderHealth, 2006). Despite these challenges, however, girls and women with fistula are typically strong and resourceful, continuing to support their families and themselves (Wall et al., 2005; Women's Dignity Project and EngenderHealth, 2006).

It is a well-documented fact that obstetric fistula destroys the lives of many young women in Tanzania (Women's Dignity Project and EngenderHealth, 2006). Obstetric fistula has disappeared from the industrialized world but exists in developing countries. The number of vesico-vaginal fistulas occurring in a country reflects the quality and the level of maternal health care delivered by the local health systems (World Health Organization, 2018).

Fistula happens to young girls and older women alike. While there are often reports of young girls getting fistula, two separate studies in Tanzania indicate that the median age of fistula patients was 22 and 24 years old, respectively (UNFPA & EngenderHealth, 2003; Women's Dignity Project, 2003). Regardless of age, however, girls and women with obstetric fistula typically come from poor families. They are often undernourished, lack access to adequate health services and information, and cannot pay for medical treatment (Bangser et al., 2011; Mselle & Kohi, 2016; Tuncalp et al., 2015).

One study in Tanzania by Women's Dignity Project and EngenderHealth (2006) observed that there was a significant range in the length of time the girls and women had lived with fistula, spanning from one month to 50 years. The majority of women had lived with fistula for two years or more at the time of the study; a minority of the women had lived with fistula for more than ten years.

The following sections will explain in detail the social experiences of obstetric fistula among girls and women in Tanzania using the Social Injustice Model. The model will first discuss social injustice as root cause of fistula leading to severe social consequences to the girls and woman in Tanzania (Fig. 11.1).

11.2   Social Injustice

In Tanzania, obstetric fistula commonly develops as a result of prolonged labor due to lack of access to quality and appropriate obstetric emergency care. Social, political, and economic causes are factors that indirectly lead to the development of obstetric fistula. Issues of poverty, malnutrition, lack of education, early marriage and childbirth, status of women in the family and community, and lack of good quality or accessible maternal health care are the major contributing factors (Wall et al., 2005).

11.2.1 Poverty

Poverty is the main indirect cause of obstetric fistula in Tanzania. Tanzania is among those poor sub-Saharan countries with low income, but it also lacks adequate infrastructure, trained healthcare personnel, and adequate medical equipment and supplies, which contribute greatly to the occurrence of fistulae (World Health Organization, 2018). Obstetric fistula affects girls and women from poor families and mostly from resource-limited remote areas. Poverty contributes to malnutrition, which in turn causes inadequate and delayed pelvic development among adolescent and teenage girls for the effective passage of the fetus during birth (Mselle & Kohi, 2016; Wall et al., 2005). This inadequate pelvis can result in an obstructed labor, and when the baby becomes stuck in the pelvis during birth, it compresses maternal circulation and leads to tissue necrosis and fistula. Poverty hinders women from being able to access normal and emergency obstetric care because of long distances and lack of transport. In Tanzania, rural areas are characterized by difficult terrain (especially during the rainy season

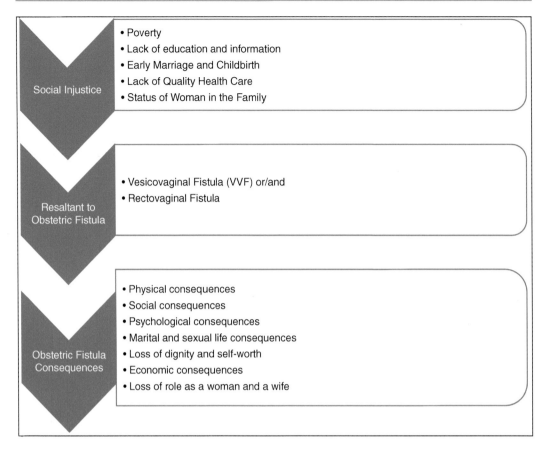

Fig. 11.1 The social injustice model (Credit: Stella Mpanda)

when roads and bridges can be washed out and impassable), long distances to health facilities, and societal preferences for delivery with a traditional birth attendant—all of these contribute to delays in accessing necessary obstetric care.

11.2.2 Lack of Education and Information

Widespread and severe poverty also lead to low levels of education among disadvantaged girls and women concerning reproductive and maternal health. Poor education is associated with low use of health services and family planning services. In addition, the lack of information, in combination with obstacles preventing rural women to easily travel to and from hospitals, lead many to arrive at the health facility without adequate prenatal care (Mselle & Kohi, 2016). This leads to women being assisted by traditional birth attendants at home who may not identify the signs of an obstetric emergency on time.

11.2.3 Early Marriage and Childbirth

In Tanzania like any other sub-Saharan countries, many girls enter into arranged marriages soon after menarche, usually below 15 years of age. Social factors and economic factors contribute to this practice of early marriages. Socially, some grooms want to ensure their brides are virgins when they get married, so an earlier marriage is desirable (Women's Dignity Project and EngenderHealth, 2006). Poverty contributes to early marriages; a girl child will be prevented to go to school or to go to higher classes in order to be married and bring income to the family—this is a common practice in rural areas of Tanzania. Early marriages lead to early childbirth, which increases the risk of obstructed labor, since young mothers who are poor and malnourished may have underdeveloped pelvises. In a survey conducted by the Ministry of Health, Community Development, Gender, Elderly and Children (MOHCDGEC), Tanzania Mainland, Ministry of Health Zanzibar, National Bureau of Statistics (NBS), Office of the Chief Government Statistician (OCGS) and ICF (2016) between 2015 to 2016 found that among respondents ages 15–49 years, 50% of women and 48% of men in Tanzania have completed primary school (and did not continue on to secondary school). Twenty-three percent (23%) of women and 28% of men had attended secondary school or beyond. That indicates that almost one-half of girls and women are not continuing to higher education, becoming married at 15 years of age or younger.

11.2.4 Lack of Quality Health Care

Some women who develop an obstetric emergency are able to access a health facility on time but do not get proper health care once they arrive due to lack of skilled attendants, resources, medical equipment and supplies ("stuff"), poor infrastructure, and overburdened healthcare system from endemic diseases such as malaria, HIV/AIDS, and tuberculosis, leading to healthcare system breakdowns at multiple levels (Schwartz, 2015). This breakdown puts many people at risk, specifically women (Mselle & Kohi, 2016). The survey by the Ministry of Health, Community Development, Gender, Elderly and Children (MOHCDGEC), Tanzania Mainland, Ministry of Health Zanzibar, National Bureau of Statistics (NBS), Office of the Chief Government Statistician (OCGS) and ICF (2016) also found that the problems most often reported by women as barriers to health care were failure to get money to pay for treatment and distance to the health facility, as well as women not wanting to go alone to the health facility.

11.2.5 Status of Women in the Family

In Tanzania, women who are affected by obstetric fistula do not have decision-making powers over their health and that of their children. Rather, their husbands and other family members such as the mother-in-law and sisters-in-law have control in determining the healthcare needs. The survey done by Ministry of Health, Community Development, Gender, Elderly and Children (MOHCDGEC), Tanzania Mainland, Ministry of Health Zanzibar, National Bureau of Statistics (NBS), Office of the Chief Government Statistician (OCGS) and ICF (2016) found that one of the barriers to accessing health care is that the spouse makes the decision for the woman to go or not to go to the health facility.

11.3 The Consequences of Obstetric Fistula

In Tanzania like elsewhere, women with obstetric fistula live a challenging life and face rejection and isolation. These women live both a changed and challenging life and suffer physical (continuous leakage of urine and or feces), social, psychological, sexual, and economic challenges. They are socially isolated and rejected, stigmatized and depressed, and with no joy in their sexual life. Therefore, living with a fistula presents multidimensional consequences affecting women, their families and communities. Most girls and women experience isolation and discrimination hindering reintegration in family and community. Quality of life is diminished for those who remaining incontinent for a long period of time (Ahmed & Holtz, 2007; Bala Baba, 2014; Mselle, Kohi, et al., 2011; Mselle, Moland, et al., 2011; Roush, 2009; Siddle et al., 2013; Wilson et al., 2015; Women's Dignity Project, 2003; Women's Dignity Project and EngenderHealth, 2006).

11.3.1 Physical Consequences

The most immediate consequence of fistula is leaking of urine and/or feces continuously through the vagina, resulting in constant wetness and smell. Fistula can also cause ulceration of the genital area from the leaking. In some cases, neurological damage to the legs caused by prolonged labor results in "foot drop," a condition which may completely impair one's ability to walk. For many women, their menstrual pattern is also disrupted (Goh & Browning, 2005).

The women's lives are generally disrupted the moment they realize that they are leaking urine continuously. They are wet all the time, a challenge they have to cope with by devising ways of passing less urine and avoiding being noticed by those around them (Mselle & Kohi, 2015). One woman said that

> When I sleep and wake up all clothes are wet, when I work up, urine flows on its own.

In response to the leakage, women decide to drink less to reduce being constantly wet. On the other hand, drinking less make them produce concentrated and smelly urine, which causes irritation to the skin leading to sores on the external genital area and thighs and may lead to kidney stones. In order to prevent wetting clothes, which can be an embarrassment, women put on locally made pads which are made from old pieces of clothes wrapped in a plastic sheet to prevent wetting—this creates irritation and pealing of the skin causing sores to the external genitalia and the thighs. Women with obstetric fistula are constantly occupied with ways to prevent wetting their clothes and to prevent being noticed by the public (Mselle et al., 2012; Mselle, Kohi, et al., 2011; Mselle, Moland, et al., 2011).

These women face a dramatically altered life as they force themselves to drink less water, believing that drinking much water will increase the urine flow and less water will reduce urine flow, but the consequence of this is that the urine becomes more concentrated. The continuous leakage of urine, the home-made padding, and the concentrated urine cause irritation to the skin of the genitalia and the thighs causing sores. This situation makes it very difficult to pad themselves because of the sores and pain, resulting to difficulties in body movements. One woman said that:

> I have been with the condition for 2 years and life has been very difficult. I use pieces of cloth as pads. The pads burn my private parts and I am full of wounds due to padding myself all day long. These wounds do not allow me to walk properly. I walk like a lame woman.

It is difficult for women to conceal the leakage, causing them to change the way they pad themselves. The locally made special pad has many layers of old cloth plus a plastic sheet to contain the continuous leakage of urine and feces. Women must frequently wash their clothing to avoid the smell and the rash around the genitalia and thighs. One woman commented that

> The most difficult situation I have passed through is washing myself and my clothes frequently; I wash every day. You have to keep washing to avoid smelling. You can't put on the same cloth twice. Then the sores I get in my private parts as a result of heat and urine is awful.

11.3.2 Social Consequences: Isolation, Rejection, and Stigma

The social consequences of these complications of obstetric fistula are severe. Girls and women living with fistula are often forced to live a life of shame and humiliation. Many are abandoned by their husbands, families, and the society around them. They are often forced to work, eat, and sleep alone (Mselle & Kohi, 2015). Most of these girls and women feel ashamed of themselves and their lives are seriously impaired by the stigmatization of their leaking (Mselle et al., 2012; Mselle, Kohi, et al., 2011; Mselle, Moland, et al., 2011; Pope et al., 2011; Women's Dignity Project and EngenderHealth, 2006). They isolate themselves or are isolated by relatives and friends. They feel they are rejected by family, friends, neighbors, and relatives as a result of the leakage and the smell, and self-isolation can become a coping mechanism for most of the women.

11.3.3 Self-Isolation

In studies by Bangser et al. (2011) and Mselle, Moland, et al. (2011), women reported the awful situation of living with constant leakage and the offensive smell or urine. The women themselves experienced the strong smell of strong urine and frequently felt ashamed. This situation causes self-isolation as women are afraid to sit near other people, afraid of the shame from the urine smell, and not wanting others to know their intimate problems. And for obvious reasons, some women feel like outcasts in the company of other people, including friends and even family.

The experience of the bad smell is worse when a woman leaks feces in addition to urine. The women feel the situation of the foul smell of urine and excrement would drive away anybody they come in contact with. These women often take long time to clean themselves, in an attempt to reduce the smell. One study (Mselle, Moland, et al., 2011) even found that one woman was using antiseptics (Dettol) thinking that the smell will go away; unfortunately, it made the situation worse. She said

> I tried using water mixed with Dettol to clean the vagina (douching), but eventually I ended up developing bruises and sores. I could not even walk.

Several additional women commented

- Where I pass, they say, she smells urine. This makes my life to be very difficult. I cannot go to village meetings or to church or visit friends or attend to visitors due to the smell. Also, I fear that I will wet myself in front of people.
- I always stay in my room due to strong smell from urine.
- I fear to drink when I want to go somewhere so that urine flow is not much. But, the urine that comes out when I have not taken any thing, the smell is very bad.

Women with fistula hide from the public—they cannot socialize because of being afraid to be seen they are wet and leaking urine and smelling from urine and feces. These women cannot socialize, nor can they attend any public gathering. They choose to isolate themselves from friends, as they cannot afford to sit for a long time and chat and, hence, they eventually decide to abandon their former peers and friends. As a result of all of these things, they lose social support network (Mselle, Kohi, et al., 2011; Mselle, Moland, et al., 2011; Population Council, 2004; Roush, 2009; Women's Dignity Project and EngenderHealth, 2006). One woman commented

> Friends changed! They are not like how they used to be. For those whom I used to sit and chat with for a long time, it can't happen anymore. This is because; if she overstays, you will leave her there and you hide yourself to change pads and from there, she will say you no longer love her. Therefore, I just hide my problem from most of them and I have decided to chuck out most of them.

Also, other reason why the women isolate themselves from relatives is because relatives are speaking badly about them, and they cannot continue with such relationships. One woman said that;

> When my sister in law visited me in hospital, she found out that I was leaking. She spread the news about my condition that I was leaking urine. I decided to remain alone and cut off all of them. I do not invite them nor visit them so am at home with no friends.

Leaking urine affects a woman's social interactions to such a degree that they prefer to remain alone and isolated as a coping response. Affected women cannot participate in activities that they were culturally supposed to enjoy, such as entertainment and cooking for visitors, for they fear of wetting or soiling themselves as they participate. One woman shared her experience

> Ever since I got the problem, I felt so bad. All the time you are in fear of not wetting yourself in front of others. You are invited to weddings but you cannot attend due to fear and also changing the pads all the time. I became very shy and feared hanging around with my people. Even when I got visitors, I felt I could not prepare them food because I was afraid of their attitudes towards my condition. I leave a pool wherever I sit. I therefore avoid gatherings.

Some women shared their experiences of avoiding public functions such as funerals and attending church because of the leakage and smell of urine, and worse. Those who attended social and religious functions had to develop some behavior modifications; for example, women avoid standing up, or raising their voices when singing. They sit still until all people have left the room. One woman shared her experience;

> Life has been very difficult for me. I hate myself and cannot mix with people. I cannot attend any party, social function or even go to church. If I am to go anywhere I have to tie bundles of clothes around me and when they get wet they burn my thighs and private parts. If I am at church and praising, I don't dance and jump because if I do, a lot of urine and feces will come out. I even sing at a low tone because of the same reason. I would never enjoy the service or anything for I would be preoccupied with how to avoid my outer clothes being wet.

11.3.4 Rejection

These women are socially excluded, as they cannot perform their culturally expected normal duties, such as preparing food. They cannot touch anything; they are considered unclean, and if they do, whatever they touch can be thrown away. It is no surprise that this way of moving through life makes women with fistulas feel socially rejected. One woman shared her experiences saying that

> Nobody wants to associate with me because am smelling urine. I was denied of everything. I could neither touch on anything nor prepare food for the family. Whenever I prepare food or touch a utensil some of my family members would not eat or take that food.

Another woman said that

> The neighbours feel bad when I give food to their children; as a result, they stop their children from coming to my place or playing at my premises.

One woman expressed her feelings as follows:

> I do not have friends anymore; even members of my family do not want to associate with me. I cannot talk to anybody for they are pushed off by the smell of urine. I am alone and isolated.

Women with fistula lose their friends, because no friend would tolerate their toilet habits and think that their friends would feel ashamed to be in their company when in public. As related by another woman

> Those who used to go out with me have cut off the relationship because of the condition. When I go out with a friend, and she notices that I go out to the toilet all the time, she changes her minds and the next step is to drop you by giving excuses. They don't want to go with you because they feel ashamed to be with you in public.

These women suffer rejection and abandonment by relatives upon realizing that they have been continuously leaking urine. This rejection is across all age groups. Children and close relatives laugh and mock the women, which worsens the rejection and prompts the women with obstetric fistula to isolate themselves as a form of coping (Mselle & Kohi, 2015).

Furthermore, these women often conceal, or attempt to hide, the fact that they are leaking urine. Women feel that it is helpful to never disclose their illness to relatives and neighbors. The rejection that these women experience worsens as time goes by. In the early stage, husbands hope that the woman will heal, but as the condition continues for months to years, their partners abandon them. The majority of these women are abandoned by their husbands after realizing that their wife's condition is continuing and will not be cured.

The experience of being excluded by relatives, friends and the community causes tremendous harm to the social and psychological well-being of the affected girls and women. The majority of the women are being scorned and abused both verbally and non-verbally. Women are hurt mostly when the abuse come from relatives and parents who voice that the women with fistula are a disgrace and deserve to suffer.

In a study by Mselle, Moland, et al. (2011), some women reported that it was better for them to live in a separate house or room away from their husbands in order to spare their husbands from similar discrimination by the community. Furthermore, it is not uncommon for families and friends to persuade husbands to break up with their affected wives and marry a new woman who can give birth to children. One woman shared her ordeal

> When I returned from the hospital, my sisters-in-law started saying; our sister-in-law is damaged and smells. They used to tell my husband; ... how could you live with a woman who is leaking urine? Later on, they called a family meeting and a decision was made that my husband should divorce me. They called my grandma, and told her ... grandmother, we do not want your granddaughter because she has this problem of leaking urine. We want our son to marry another woman...

The husband of one woman affected with fistula commented that

> My wife could never stay with me for more than 15 min or so ...at times even sitting with her children is difficult. She has turned into one who hides and runs away from others, sits on one end of the house, alone.

11.3.5 Stigma

A study by Mselle, Moland, et al. (2011) found that discrimination resulting from fistula affects not only the individual woman living with obstetric fistula, but also the whole family. Similar to other regions in Africa, sharing and getting involved in other people's life events such as weddings and funerals is culturally important and essential in maintaining social networks in rural Tanzania. Too often situations have occurred in which neighbors have avoided asking the family of a woman suffering from fistula to share anything including household items and vice versa, since the entire family is regarded as unclean and contaminated. The family is commonly not invited to take part in social events, and is thus excluded from forums where social relations are established, confirmed, and reinforced. Families become practically ostracized from the society.

The family feel ashamed in their community because they have a young girl or a woman leaking and smelling urine or/and feces. One woman commented that

My friends and my relatives are irritated and they don't want to come to my place anymore. I also don't go to their places because I feel like a burden to them. We both fear each other. The neighbours feel bad when I give food to their children; as a result, they stop their children from coming to my place or playing from there.

Obstetric fistula is a very painful experience; women face discrimination and rejection; both the women and family suffer stigma.

11.3.6 Psychological Consequences

Women with fistula are depressed by the condition of leaking urine and or feces. The stress of living with a fistula is compounded by worries that there may be no cure for the condition. To make matters worse, many affected women fear the condition is for life. On some occasions, this anxiety and depression lead to suicidal ideation, thinking that their life is not worthwhile (Bala Baba, 2014; Mselle, Kohi, et al., 2011; Mselle, Moland, et al., 2011; Wilson et al., 2015; Zeleke et al., 2013). One woman shared her experience and said that;

People were saying that the condition could never be treated, so I will have to die with it. I started fearing to live with the problem the rest of my life. They said that I would never be well. So if am wise, I should just get a rope to hang and kill myself! I was going to do it but my mother stopped me.

These women are constantly worried that others will notice their problems. Many of the women with vaginal fistula have to deal with shame, embarrassment, and humiliation (Semere & Nour, 2008); the psychological impact of this condition should never be underestimated. Women experience low self-esteem; feelings of shame, loneliness, rejection, stress, anxiety, loss of sexual pleasure, and even depression are some psychological consequences that can follow this morbidity. These women suffer rejection from society, from husband and/or divorce and isolation. Most women have lost their social network and support as a result of their fistula (Mselle, Moland, et al., 2011; Roush, 2009). They are deemed unworthy, and their illness is often attributed to some fault of their own (Bala Baba, 2014; Mselle, Moland, et al., 2011; Population Council, 2004; Wilson et al., 2015; Zeleke et al., 2013).

11.3.7 Marital and Sexual Life Consequences

Most women feel their marital and sexual lives frustrating, while others feel that they have lost their marital and sexual rights altogether. Their bodies have changed, and they are no longer like other women, missing the happiness they formerly enjoyed. Women describe their sexual lives have been negatively impacted because of the leakage of urine, which is hateful to both the women and their partners and having sexual relations becomes a major challenge. Sex is no longer as it used to be, and there are many difficulties to overcome. One woman who suffered fistula for 12 years (Mselle, Moland, et al., 2011) shared her experience by saying that

Because I am leaking urine, I am useless, I have no value. If I did not have this problem, my husband would not have abandoned me. But my husband left me because I am leaking urine and I would not bear a child for him.

In the same study, one husband commented that

I had to have another woman. Given the situation she was in, of leaking urine, she agreed; saying it is ok, just look for one to be with...yes she had to accept. If she refused, I could have left her.

In some cases, women with fistula face divorce and rejection as they fail to satisfy their husband's sexual needs and/or fail to bear children. As the women become incapable of performing the family and gender roles expected of them, they are perceived as "useless" beings. Therefore, they became neglected and abandoned. A woman reported that she was mistreated by her spouse after the fistula incident

> He left me and threw out all of my belongings; ever since I developed the condition, and we have not been together as husband and wife. I have been left out here to care for the old lady (mother-in-law).

It also appears that the rates of separation or divorce increase the longer a woman lives with a fistula, particularly if she remains childless (Mselle et al., 2012; Mselle & Kohi, 2015; Mselle, Kohi, et al., 2011; Mselle, Moland, et al., 2011).

Women experience feeling of a changed vagina. Some women report that their partners felt that sex was different now compared to the period before the development of the fistula. In addition, some partners tell their wives that sex with them is different from sex with women without a fistula. Furthermore, women feel that their vagina has physically changed, and as a consequence, their feeling for sex has decreased. One woman said that

> I hate myself because, when am cleaning myself… I feel my vagina is widened … I feel pain in the vagina and sores all over so this reduces my appetite for sex. When I squat to urinate, it becomes worse and air just blows into me. Even the man I got, at first he did not know but afterwards, he came and asked me, what is the problem? As you are different (sexually) from other women!

It can occur that when these women remain in the hospital for a long time during treatment, after returning home they find their husbands already remarried. Some husbands did not hesitate to say openly (Mselle, Moland, et al., 2011) that they left their wives because of the leaking; commenting that;

> Yes I left her for good...we had to separate, I have two houses, she has her bed and her house and I have my bed and my house (laughs). We are like a brother and sister now.

These women feel that their right to sex is denied because their partners, as a strategy to cope with the changed sexual experience, looked for other "normal" women and left their wives with fistula sexually unattended. On the other hand, some women are forced into sex even when they have pain, and most of them no longer enjoy sexual relations anymore.

There are few women who still want to have sex but they are challenged by the fact that husbands have divorced them to marry other wives. Women report that in these settings, men are culturally the initiators of sex. Therefore, the women felt that being divorced and yet being unable to initiate new sexual relationships is a violation of their sexual rights. The women thought a fistula had stood in their way, even when they still had a desire for sex. Most women have completely abstained from sex. Others think that almost all women with a fistula were not having sex. Some women fear being talked about if their sexual relations did not go right and, hence, decide to avoid it altogether.

The majority of these women decide to continue life without sex after facing sexual challenges. Others often stay away from their partners to avoid abuse and neglect, and separation or divorce is very common among them. Most of these women either left their abusive partners or their partners just abandoned them or sent them away to their parents. One husband (Mselle, Moland, et al., 2011) commented that

> Firstly is the discomfort of leaking urine, the smell, and the soaked clothes which burns... yes...burns her genitalia, resulting in her developing wounds. ...again, as a man, trying to have sex with her; on the first day I did not feel well, it was distasteful and unpleasant all the way through.

11.3.8 Loss of Dignity and Self-Worth

Women with fistula experience loss of dignity and self-worth due to lack of power and feelings of dependency. These are a result of multifactorial factors such as lack of support and family care, physical or economical incapability to access care, and lack of information or knowledge about fistula care and treatment (Mehta et al., 2007; Mehta & Bangser, 2006; Mselle & Kohi, 2016; Mselle, Kohi, et al., 2011; Mselle, Moland, et al., 2011; Women's Dignity Project and EngenderHealth, 2006). These feelings of loss are also a result of the reactions and comments of family members as well as other people with a poor understanding of the condition that they suffer from.

The failures of the women to control urine and/or feces, maintain their marriages, bear children, or participate in social economic activities make them lose their identity as women, wives, friends, and community members. They tend to see themselves as worthless, incomplete, and compare themselves with children. Adulthood is marked largely by not only managing one's emotions but also through being able to control body functions. Losing control of bodily functions is embarrassing as an adult. With an awful smell from the leakage of urine or feces, women are unable to keep themselves clean and attractive. In Tanzania, a woman's beauty is associated with not only body cleanliness, neatness, and aromatic smell, but also with the capacity to assume domestic, marital, and social roles. Women living with obstetric fistula are deprived of all these attributes. Many studies have shown that most of these women suffering fistula live in rural areas with limited or no water supply, no sanitary pads or pampers which can hold urine for a while indicating that it is extremely difficult to maintain personal hygiene and smell good. Moreover, because they cannot work and earn a living by themselves, they are unable to get cash to buy scented soap and lotion that could help control the smell. As one woman put it

How can you be a woman with this condition of leaking urine and smell?

Nearly all women isolate themselves, staying away even from their families, friends, and the community. This tendency of isolating themselves from others and services has a profound impact on their quality of life, their dignity, and self-worthiness.

11.3.9 Economic Consequences

It is unfortunate that in addition to family, community and social functions, some women have their economic activities affected. Women with fistula are unable to continue with income-generating activities to support themselves. The main reason is that they feel they are unprepared to continue working because of pre-occupation with how to cope with effects of leakage and smell. Also, they feel that they will be rejected by co-workers. Those doing petty business fear that nobody will buy from them if they try to take their goods to the market (Mselle, Moland, et al., 2011). Moreover, these women feel that no one is willing to employ a woman leaking urine, as demonstrated by a woman who have suffered fistula for 19 years:

I had a petty business stall. I was selling doughnuts, but now I cannot live that kind of life...I cannot sit for long... again, if you prepare doughnuts while leaking urine who will buy and eat them?

Another one who suffered fistula for 10 years said that;

Before, I was able to earn a living on my own. I was working in other people's houses as a maid. For now I cannot work for anybody because I am afraid of staying in people's houses...I am just afraid... I am afraid of soaking other people's beds.

The reasons cited by these women for not being able to work, or working less than before, include suffering poor health or feeling pain due to the fistula and/or needing to clean themselves constantly and change clothes (Mselle et al., 2012; Mselle, Moland, et al., 2011; Roush, 2009; Women's Dignity Project and EngenderHealth, 2006).

Women living with obstetric fistula also experience lack of invitation to income-generating activities in the community because of the leaking and the bad smell, which prohibits interaction with other people. Most of these women lost their jobs, especially those that require strict adherence to hygiene such as selling foodstuffs. One woman shares her experience saying that

> I used to sell cooked rice but my condition has obliged me to stop. My sales started dwindling as the news of my urine incontinence spread.

Therefore, they can fall deeper into poverty and start to beg for survival (Ahmed & Holtz, 2007; Mselle, Moland, et al., 2011; Women's Dignity Project and EngenderHealth, 2006). One woman reported that prior to her fistula she had engaged in petty trade and made 3000 Tanzanian shillings (Tsh.) profit every week (approximately USD$3.00). Since she sustained fistula and paralysis of her legs, she had been unable to work. As a result, sometimes she was unable to meet the basic needs of herself and her baby. She also became an economic burden to her family (Women's Dignity Project and EngenderHealth, 2006).

Families and parents of women with fistula spend most of their resources to support the woman cost of medical interventions. Families and parents have been forced to sell their crops and even take loans to pay for treatment expenses. In some cases, the money that was to be used for sending children to school is instead spent for medical treatment for fistula. As a result, children are forced to postpone school for lack of money for fees. Some families have not been able to cultivate their farms because of the time they spend caring for the daughter with fistula.

11.3.10   Loss of Role as a Woman and a Wife

A woman's role in the community includes being a wife, a mother of children and a beauty in the house. A woman in the family and community is expected to have children, to prepare food for the family, take care of children, perform house chores, and provide care for her husband; this is African beauty. But when a woman suffers fistula, she will not be able to carry out all of her roles because of stigma, isolation, rejection, and abandonment from the family and community.

Studies by Mselle, Moland, et al. (2011) and Mselle, Kohi, et al., 2011 found that women were unable to attend to their daily commitments as women, wives, and mothers. They found that in addition to the leakage, pain, and discomforts of the wounds, women tended to experience general body weakness or malaise, which reduced their capacity to carry out their day-to-day responsibilities. Because of this experience, some women did not have the courage to go back to their homes after they developed fistula. One woman commented that

> I could not return to my husband because I am unable to carry out my daily duties. I have just been staying at my mother's house. ...I have not been able to work, so if I went to live with my husband that could have caused problems I would not have been able to wash his clothes nor mine. Until now, I only clean my toilet rags. My sister's daughter washes my clothes. Misunderstandings could have arisen, that is why I did not return.

Many women have spoken of their inability to carry out domestic chores, farming, business, or employment. Some women were not allowed to cook for the family as they were judged as dirty or unclean. Another woman suffering fistula for 20 years said that

> I am not cooking, yes, because when I cook, others, including my husband do not eat. They see it as dirt.... if I prepared food, he (husband) would not eat, and thereafter he started to cook food himself.

In our experience in nearly every case of obstetric fistula, the baby has died, aggravating the situation faced by these girls and women. In communities where childbearing is essential to women's social status and dignity, childlessness resulting from fistula can be damaging (Mselle et al., 2012; Mselle, Kohi, et al., 2011; Mselle, Moland, et al., 2011).

11.4 Conclusion

Living with fistula is associated with multiple prejudicial social experiences that impact the quality of life, and too often even the survival, of the affected girls and women in Tanzania. Obstetric fistula predisposes individuals living with the condition to social stigmatization that can only be addressed through improved access to social and economic development for girls and women in general, with ensuing better access to quality and timely obstetric care. Most of the affected women are poor, uneducated, and young, who marry early, and who live in remote, rural, and poor resource areas with little or no access to emergency obstetric care. In addition, women who live with obstetric fistula typically cannot easily travel to hospital facilities because of long distances, high costs of transportation, or lack of decision-making power within their family.

These experiences of living with obstetric fistula have a tremendously negative impact on women's dignity and self-worthiness. Women suffer the day-to-day social discrimination and loss of independent income that results from the condition. Women who live with fistula are not able to assume their expected socio-cultural roles and responsibilities.

Fistula reduces women's ability to work, and if they do not get support of their husbands and relatives, can be driven deeper into poverty. They can become a burden to the family because they cannot contribute to the family earnings, cannot satisfy their husband's needs, nor bear children. Therefore, in the eyes of the society they are of less value due to failure to carry out social and marital roles.

References

Ahmed, S., & Holtz, S. (2007). Social and economic consequences of obstetric fistula: life changed forever? *International Journal of Gynecology & Obstetrics, 99*, 510–515. https://doi.org/10.1016/j.ijgo.2007.06.011

Arrowsmith, S., Hamlin, E. C., & Wall, L. L. (1996). Obstructed labor injury complex: Obstetric fistula formation and the multifaceted morbidity of maternal birth trauma in the developing world. *Obstetrics and Gynecological Survey, 51*(9), 568–574.

Bala Baba, S. (2014). Birth and sorrow: The psychological and medical consequences of obstetric fistula. *International Journal of Medical Sociology and Anthropology, 2*(2), 55–65.

Bangser, M. (2006). Obstetric fistula and stigma. *Lancet, 367*(9509), 535–536. https://doi.org/10.1016/S0140-6736(06)68188-9

Bangser, M., Manisha, M., Janet, S., Chris, D., Catherine, K., et al. (2011). Childbirth experiences of women with obstetric fistula in Tanzania and Uganda and their implications for fistula program development. *International Urogynecology Journal, 22*, 91–98. https://doi.org/10.1007/s00192-010-1236-8

Capes, T., Ascher-Walsh, A. C., & Brodman, M. (2011). Obstetric fistula in low and middle income countries. *Mount Sinai Journal of Medicine, 78*(3), 352–361. https://doi.org/10.1002/msj.20265

Goh, J. T., & Browning, A. (2005). Use of urethral plugs for urinary incontinence following fistula repair Australian. *New Zealand Journal Obstetrics Gynaecology, 45*(3), 237–238.

Mehta, M., & Bangser, M. (2006). *Risks and resilience: Obstetric Fistula in Tanzania*. Women's Dignity Project and Engender Health.

Mehta, M., Bangser, M., Barber, N., & Lindsay, J. (2007). *Sharing the Burden: Ugandan women speak about obstetric fistula*. Women's Dignity Project and Engender Health.

Ministry of Health, Community Development, Gender, Elderly and Children (MOHCDGEC), Tanzania Mainland, Ministry of Health Zanzibar, National Bureau of Statistics (NBS), Office of the Chief Government Statistician (OCGS) and ICF. (2016). *Tanzania demographic and health survey and malaria indicator survey (DDHS-MIS) 2015-2016*. MoHCDGEC.

Mselle, L., Moland, K., Evjen-Olsen, B., Mvungi, A., & Kohi, T. (2011). "I am nothing": Experiences of loss among women suffering from severe birth injuries in Tanzania. *BMC, 11*(1), 49. https://doi.org/10.1186/1472-6874-11-49

Mselle, L. T., Evjen-Olsen, B., Moland, K. M., Polit, C., Mvungi, A., & Kohi, T. W. (2012). Hoping for a normal life again: Reintegration after fistula repair in rural Tanzania. *Journal of Obstetrics and Gynaecology Canada, 34*(10), 927–938.

Mselle, L. T., & Kohi, T. W. (2015). Living with constant leaking of urine and odour: Thematic analysis of socio-cultural experiences of women affected by obstetric fistula in rural Tanzania. *BMC Women's Health, 15*, 107. https://doi.org/10.1186/s12905-015-0267-1

Mselle, L. T., & Kohi, T. W. (2016). Healthcare access and quality of birth care: Narratives of women living with obstetric fistula in rural Tanzania. *Reproductive Health, 13*, 87. https://doi.org/10.1186/s12978-016-0189-x

Mselle, L. T., Kohi, T. W., Mvungi, A., Evjen-Olsen, B., & Moland, K. (2011). Waiting for attention and care: birthing accounts of women in rural Tanzania who developed obstetric fistula as an outcome of labour. *BMC, 11*(75), 1471–2393. https://doi.org/10.1186/1471-2393-11-75

National Bureau of Statistics of Tanzania; ICF Macro. (2011). *Tanzania demographic and health survey 2010*. NBC and ICF Macro.

Pope, R., Bangser, M., & Requejo, J. H. (2011). Restoring dignity: Social reintegration after obstetric fistula repair in Ukerewe, Tanzania. *Global Public Health, 6*(8), 859–873.

Population Council. (2004). *Healing wounds. Instilling hope. The Tanzanian partnership against obstetric fistula. Qualit/Qalidad/Qualite*. One Dag Hammerskjold Plaza.

Raassen, T. (2005). *Personal communication based on international estimates and local conditions. Cited in Risk and Resilience: obstetric fistula in Tanzania: An overview of findings and recommendations from the study*. Women's Dignity Project and Engender Health.

Raassen, T. J., Ngongo, C. J., & Mahendeka, M. M. (2014). Iatrogenic genitourinary fistula: An 18-year retrospective review of 805 injuries. *International Urogynecological Journal, 25*(12), 1699–1706.

Roush, K. M. (2009). Social implications of obstetric fistula: An integrative review. *Journal of Midwifery and Women's Health, 54*(2), 21–33. https://doi.org/10.1016/j.jmwh.2008.09.005

Schwartz, D. A. (2015). Interface of epidemiology, anthropology and health care in maternal death prevention in resource-poor nations. In D. A. Schwartz (Ed.), *Maternal mortality: Risk factors, anthropological perspectives, prevalence in developing countries and preventive strategies for pregnancy-related death* (pp. ix–xiv). Nova Science Publishers, Inc.

Semere, L., & Nour, N. M. (2008). Obstetric fistula: Living with incontinence and shame. *Reviews in Obstetrics and Gynecology, 1*(4), 193–197.

Siddle, K., Mwambingu, S., Malinga, T., & Fiander, A. (2013). Psychosocial impact of obstetric fistula in women presenting for surgical care in Tanzania. *International Urogynecological Journal, 24*(7), 1215–1220.

Tuncalp, O., Tripathi, V., Landry, E., Stanton, C. K., & Ahmed, S. (2015). Measuring the incidence and prevalence of obstetric fistula: Approaches, needs and recommendations. *Bulletin of the World Health Organization, 93*(1), 60–62.

UNFPA and EngenderHealth. (2003). *Obstetric fistula needs assessment report: Findings from nine African countries*. Retrieved 5 May, 2019, from https://www.unfpa.org/sites/default/files/pub-pdf/fistula-needs-assessment.pdf

Wall, L. L., Arrowsmith, S. D., Briggs, N. D., Browning, A., & Lassey, A. (2005). The obstetric vesicovaginal fistula in the developing world. *Obstetrical and Gynecological Survey, 60*(7), 3–51.

Wilson, S. M., Sikkema, K. J., Watt, M. H., & Masenga, G. (2015). Psychological symptoms among obstetric fistula patients compared to gynecology outpatients in Tanzania. *International Journal of Behavioral Medicine, 22*(5), 605–613.

Women's Dignity Project. (2003). *Faces of dignity. Seven stories of girls & women with fistula*. Women's Dignity Project.

Women's Dignity Project and EngenderHealth. (2006). *Risk and resilience: Obstetric fistula in Tanzania*. Women's Dignity Project and EngenderHealth. Retrieved 5 May, 2019, from https://www.engenderhealth.org/wp-content/uploads/imports/files/pubs/maternal-health/obstetric_fistula_brief_overview.pdf

World Health Organization. (2018). *10 facts on obstetric fistula*. WHO.

Zeleke, B. M., Ayele, T. A., Woldetsaddik, M. A., Bisefegn, T. A., & Adane, A. A. (2013). Depression among women with obstetric fistula and pelvic organ prolapse in northwest Ethiopia. *BMC Psychiatry, 13*, 236. https://doi.org/10.1186/1471-244X

Physical, Psychological, and Social Assessments of Fistula Recovery Among Women in Nigeria and Uganda

12

Beth S. Phillips, Justus K. Barageine,
Dorothy N. Ononokpono, and Alison M. El Ayadi

12.1 Introduction

Female genital fistula resulting in chronic leakage of urine and/or feces most commonly results from prolonged obstructed labor in low-resource settings and may also be caused by iatrogenic and traumatic etiologies. Numerous challenges to estimating the global prevalence of obstetric fistula exist (Stanton et al., 2007; Tunçalp et al., 2015), but available metrics suggest that as many as two million women are living with female genital fistula, mostly in sub-Saharan Africa and South Asia, with an annual incidence of up to 100,000 (Adler et al., 2013; de Bernis, 2007). Self-reported lifetime prevalence of fistula-related symptoms among women of reproductive age in sub-Saharan Africa ranges from 0.04% in Burkina Faso to 4.1% in Guinea, with important regional variation within countries (Institut National de la Statistique, République de Guinée, 2019; Maheu-Giroux et al., 2015).

Significant international efforts over the last two decades have resulted in increased surgical capacity for treating female genital fistula worldwide. Training programs have increased the number of certified surgeons and support staff capable of fistula care provision (Elneil, 2015; Slinger et al., 2018), and 25,000 women are now surgically operated annually (Direct Relief, 2016). Surgical success rates are good, with most studies reporting rates of fistula closure at hospital discharge at approximately 90% (Browning & Whiteside, 2015; Creanga & Genadry, 2007; Delamou et al., 2016; Muleta

B. S. Phillips
Institute for Global Health Sciences, University of
California San Francisco, San Francisco, CA, USA

J. K. Barageine
Department of Obstetrics and Gynaecology,
Makerere University College of Health Sciences,
Kampala, Uganda

D. N. Ononokpono
Department of Sociology and Anthropology,
University of Uyo, Uyo, Nigeria

A. M. El Ayadi (✉)
Department of Obstetrics, Gynecology and
Reproductive Sciences, University of California San
Francisco, San Francisco, CA, USA
e-mail: alison.elayadi@ucsf.edu

© Springer Nature Switzerland AG 2022
L. B. Drew et al. (eds.), *A Multidisciplinary Approach to Obstetric Fistula in Africa*, Global Maternal and Child Health, https://doi.org/10.1007/978-3-031-06314-5_12

et al., 2010; Sori et al., 2016). However, surgical closure is less likely to be achieved with more complex fistula (Frajzyngier et al., 2012).

Fistula closure is an important surgical metric; however, it remains an inadequate representation of patient outcome. Recent research has highlighted the importance of moving beyond clinical outcomes to incorporate patient-reported outcomes in fistula care, as fistula outcomes are not reducible to surgical closure due to the array of other physical and psychosocial correlates of fistula (Ahmed et al., 2016; Ahmed & Holtz, 2007; Delamou et al., 2017; El Ayadi et al., 2017; El Ayadi, Barageine, Korn, et al., 2019; Goh et al., 2005; Goh et al., 2016; Krause et al., 2019). Novel assessment of the burden of fistula has included econometric assessment. McFarland et al. estimated that 111,570 disability-adjusted life years (58.56 DALYs per fistula case) could be attributed to obstructed labor and fistula, with the cost per DALY averted by cesarean section estimated at US $1.11 (McFarland, 2010). Health interventions for preventing the development of obstetric fistula, namely cesarean section, have been estimated to cost $251 to $3462 for each disability-adjusted life year by country (Alkire et al., 2012). Fistula surgery alone has been estimated to be a highly cost-effective intervention, with cost per DALY ranging from $40 in Ethiopia to $54 in Uganda (Epiu et al., 2018; Johnson et al., 2015). While this broader measurement attention represents an important extension beyond surgical numbers, further development of relevant patient-reported outcomes for fistula care is necessary. This work requires a nuanced understanding of women's perspectives of recovery and reintegration. Research on reintegration and recovery in Uganda found that beyond incontinence, major domains of interest for recovery and reintegration among this study population included mobility and social engagement, meeting family needs, comfort with relationships, and general life satisfaction (El Ayadi et al., 2017).

Further research is necessary to understand women's perspectives of recovery and reintegration across the varied socioeconomic and cultural contexts within which fistula occurs. Female genital fistula can occur wherever women face inadequate access to high-quality emergency obstetric care; thus, it is most commonly reported within sub-Saharan African and South Asian countries (Wall et al., 2005). Data from surgical providers also demonstrate its occurrence in broader geographies including the Caribbean, South East Asia, and the South Pacific (Direct Relief, 2016). Thus, women affected by fistula live within countries and regions with extremely diverse sociocultural, environmental, and political norms and opportunities which structure women's individual and collective experiences across the full continuum of fistula-related experiences, from fistula development, living with fistula, accessing surgical and other supportive care, and recovering from fistula (Hannig, 2017; Heller & Hannig, 2017; Maheu-Giroux et al., 2015; Maheu-Giroux et al., 2016). The experience of obstetric fistula, both its occurrence, recovery potential and process, is intersectional (Bauer, 2014). For example, fistula development and treatment opportunities follow a social gradient, where women with greater social vulnerabilities face increased risk of fistula and more severe consequences from fistula compared to their colleagues with greater individual and community resources (Keya et al., 2018; Maheu-Giroux et al., 2015). While stigma is a common experience among women with fistula, any one individual may experience stigma resulting from their multiple social identities (e.g., health condition, ethnicity, and socioeconomic status). Given the social gradient of this condition, women with fistula not only face the physical and psychosocial consequences of the fistula, but also the conditions that placed them at higher risk of fistula which continue to persist after fistula occurrence and increase the likelihood of their exposure to other sources of trauma and stress (Turan et al., 2019). Integration of the multiple vulnerabilities experienced by many women who develop fistula into the broader fistula prevention, rehabilitation, and advocacy efforts is paramount.

Thus, the purpose of this analysis was to compare and contrast women's perspectives of recovery from female genital fistula in two higher prevalence countries: Nigeria and Uganda. We sought to understand women's primary recovery-related concerns and their experiences of recovery and reintegration across a variety of life domains.

12.2 Study Contexts

12.2.1 Nigeria

During 2014 when the Nigeria research commenced, nearly half a million people were displaced in North East Nigeria due to Boko Haram insurgencies. The ensuing conflict over the subsequent 5 years between Boko Haram and government and other armed forces now accounts for an estimated 2.2 million internally displaced Nigerians in Nigeria and Cameroon (Omole et al., 2015; United Nations High Commissioner for Refugees 2019). Maternal health in Nigeria was already poor and has been considerably affected by this regional violence, terrorism, and resulting displacement. Boko Haram has had important impacts on other health conditions as well, exacerbating child malnutrition and malaria outbreaks, among others (Nigeria Ministry of Health, 2019). Weak clinical infrastructure and continued shortages of skilled providers continue to challenge comprehensive and accessible quality maternal healthcare services in Nigeria (UNFPA, 2017). While lifetime fertility rate has decreased in the last decade, it remains high at 5.3 with regional variation 4.5–5.9 in urban and rural areas, respectively (National Population Commission and IPC, 2019). Modern contraceptive use remains very low (12%).

Regional variation in reproductive and maternal health is substantial in Nigeria, most notably in terms of maternal death. Nigeria has one of the highest maternal mortality ratios (MMR) in the world, with an estimated 814 maternal deaths per 100,000 live births, and as many of 1549 women dying per 100,000 live births in North East region of the country (WHO, UNICEF, UNFPA, World Bank Group, and United Nations Population Division, 2015). The 2018 Demographic Health Survey (DHS) reports that 19% of teenagers in Nigeria have been pregnant or had a child, with urban teens being less likely than rural to have started childbearing (8% compared to 27%). Antenatal care (ANC) coverage is not universal; during their most recent pregnancy preceding the 2018 DHS survey, 67% of women reported having attended any ANC, with 57% having four or more ANC contacts (National Population Commission and IPC, 2019). Home-based childbirth remains common, particularly in rural areas where 78% of deliveries occur at home compared to 38% in urban areas (Adewuyi et al., 2017). Nationally, fewer than half of women (39%) delivered in a health facility (National Population Commission and IPC, 2019). Emergency obstetric care (EmOC) services are suboptimal in Nigeria ranging from 2.2% to 4.4% of deliveries taking place in EmOC facilities and few facilities meeting the minimum requirement of four or more midwives for 24-hour EmOC service (Abegunde et al., 2015; Mezie-Okoye et al., 2012; Saidu et al., 2013). Where EmOC is available, reported knowledge and skills among providers are often low (Ameh et al., 2012; Okonofua et al., 2019). Current estimates reflect roughly 15,000 cases of obstetric fistula in Nigeria with an estimated 12,000 new cases occurring every year (Nigeria Ministry of Health, 2019). There are 22 fistula surgeons permanently associated with facilities in Nigeria (Direct Relief, 2016).

12.2.2 Uganda

Indicators of maternal health have improved over time in Uganda, although challenges remain in achieving optimal coverage for population health, including chronic shortage of qualified physicians and nurses and poor clinical infrastructure, particularly in rural areas (UNFPA, 2011). Ugandan women also experience early marriage, low prevalence of modern contraceptive use (39%), high total fertility rate of 5.4, and high maternal mortality at 336 maternal deaths per 100,000 live births (Uganda Bureau of Statistics and ICF, 2018). From 2011 to 2016, 25% of births in Uganda occurred at home. Among Ugandan women reporting a recent live birth in the 2016 DHS, ANC attendance was nearly universal; however, only 2% of women achieved the WHO's recommendation of 8 ANC contacts, with mean ANC contacts ranging from 3.2 to 4.3 by region (Uganda Bureau of Statistics and ICF,

2018). Facility delivery has doubled over the past two decades, increasing from 37% to 73% from 2000–2015; however, regional variation is substantial (56–94%). Access to comprehensive emergency obstetric care is limited: only 9% of facilities offer all 7 signal functions (life-saving services), 47% of facilities had emergency transport, and only 6% of births were delivered by cesarean section (Uganda Bureau of Statistics and Macro International, 2007). In Uganda, approximately 200,000 women are living with fistula and there are 2000 incident cases annually (Uganda Ministry of Health, 2011). Self-report of lifetime fistula-related symptoms among women of reproductive age is 1.4%, ranging from 0.5% to 4.3% regionally (Uganda Bureau of Statistics and ICF, 2018). Fistula surgery is available at 20 centers of excellence in Uganda, with 25-trained surgeons at various levels of experience employed by national and regional referral hospitals (Uganda Ministry of Health, 2011). Increases in treatment availability have been facilitated by the Ugandan National Fistula Technical Working Group, established with the United Nations Population Fund's (UNFPA) Global Campaign to End Fistula (Uganda Ministry of Health, 2011). Over the period 2010 to 2015, the annual number of fistula surgeries in Uganda increased from 1377 to 2065 (Direct Relief, 2016).

12.3 Methods

12.3.1 Nigeria

Findings from Nigeria are based on a cross-sectional, qualitative-focused study conducted at four obstetric fistula treatment facilities in Akwa Ibom, Ebonyi, Plateau, and Sokoto States of Nigeria during 2014 and 2015. Research methods included participant observation, in-depth interviews, and focus group discussions. Respondents were pre/post-operative fistula patients, clinicians, policymakers, and health professionals. For this paper, we report only findings from the in-depth interviews with women ($n = 86$). The methods and primary results from this study are reported elsewhere (Phillips et al., 2016). The interview guide for obstetric fistula patients was developed and translated into four languages (Hausa, Ibibio, Igbo, and Tiv), field tested among small groups of patients at each site, and revised accordingly. Interview questions covered the woman's experiences and opinions about pregnancy, childbirth, obstetric fistula, family, work, fistula surgery, rehabilitation, and experiences within the Nigerian's healthcare system generally. Half of the women were interviewed by the first author in English. The remaining patients were interviewed in one of the local languages by the research team or by a facility-based social worker. All interviewers received basic training on research protocols, aims, and ethics. The average interview lasted 40 min, with the shortest being 15 min and the longest, 1 h and 20 min. All interviews were audio-recorded, and then translated and transcribed by graduate students at the University of Calabar in South-South Nigeria. Data analysis was completed using a thematic framework with specific analytic codes developed and refined under the general study themes through iterative process between the first and third authors, another study investigator and two research assistants. Research ethics review boards at the National Fistula Centre in Abakaliki, Ebonyi State, the Mbreibit Itam VVF Hospital in Uyo, Akwa Ibom State, the Evangel Hospital in Jos, Plateau State, and the Maryam Abacha Women and Children Hospital in Sokoto, Sokoto State each approved the study.

12.3.2 Uganda

Findings from Uganda are based on two qualitative samples of women ($n = 63$) who underwent obstetric fistula surgery at Mulago Hospital in Kampala, Uganda (Byamugisha et al., 2015). Women in the first sample ($n = 33$) were eligible if they had obstetric fistula surgery 6–24 months previously, spoke Luganda or English, resided within 100 km of Mulago Hospital, and provided a telephone contact at surgery. Their data were collected from June 2014 to August 2014 (first phase) through in-depth interviews ($n = 16$) and focus group discussions ($n = 4$; 17 participants). Interviews and focus groups focused on women's perspectives and priorities for reintegration. Women in the second sample were a nested group of participants from a larger longitudinal cohort study which had been followed for one year following fistula surgery at interview ($n = 30$). These women were eligible for participation in the longitudinal cohort if they spoke Luganda or English and resided in a community with cellular telephone coverage. Their qualitative data were collected from November 2016 to December 2016 (second phase). Women in this sample were queried around their perspectives of recovery and reintegration and probed in detail on their criteria for fistula recovery. In-depth interviews and focus group discussions were audio-recorded with the explicit permission of participants and concurrently translated and transcribed into English for analysis by an experienced translator. Transcripts from in-depth interviews and focus group discussions were coded using inductive and deductive codes within Atlas.ti software and analyzed for domains most relevant to family and community integration by two researchers, one Ugandan and one American. Coding disagreements were resolved by discussion. Thematic analysis was concurrent with data collection to assist in determining achievement of data saturation (Marks & Yardley, 2004). Coded data were analyzed thematically to describe the different dimensions and commonalities of each theme and the patterns and linkages between themes. The study protocol was approved by the Makerere University College of Health Sciences Research and Ethics Committee, the Ugandan National Council on Science and Technology, and the University of California, San Francisco Human Research Protection Program, Committee on Human Research.

12.3.3 Joint Analysis

To understand the range of women's perspectives on recovery and reintegration across the two contexts, the first and last author re-reviewed the transcripts and related thematic frameworks from both studies. After this review, they discussed their findings from each sample and developed an initial set of themes. Each author returned to her data and conducted additional coding as necessary using the original study transcripts and coded them afresh using these initial themes to refine and build out others where necessary. Then, each reviewed the others' coding and together they refined their thematic framework for this analysis, using an iterative process. All authors reviewed the final analysis and interpretation.

12.4 Results

12.4.1 Participant Characteristics

Participant characteristics are presented in Table 12.1 and Fig. 12.1. Nigerian participants averaged 29 years when interviewed with mean age of first fistula onset at 24 years, ranging from 2 months to 14 years living with fistula. Over two thirds (66%) were married or cohabitating and 13% had no formal education. The majority (55%) had no living child, with the remaining 45% having 1–8 children living. Most (93%) had vesicovaginal fistula only. Current employment was reported at 58%, although 81% of women reported being employed before developing fistula. Women from Southern sites in Nigeria were commonly employed in formal work sectors, such as human resources and store manag-

Table 12.1 Participant characteristics

	Nigeria ($n = 86$) n (%)	Uganda ($n = 63$) n (%)
Current age[a]	29.1 (10.7)	31.6 (9.5)
Age at fistula development[a]	24.1 (8.5)	24.7 (7.8)
Time lived with fistula		
<1 year	41 (47.7)	33 (52.4)
1–2 year	13 (15.1)	3 (5.8)
3–5 years	9 (10.5)	3 (5.8)
5+ years	23 (26.7)	24 (38.1)
Married/living together	57 (66.3)	42 (66.7)
Completed primary education	52 (60.5)	27 (42.8)
Any living children	38 (45.2)	40 (63.5)
VVF only	80 (93.0)	62 (98.4)
RVF only	5 (5.8)	–
VVF and RVF together	1 (1.2)	1 (1.6)

[a] Notes: mean (SD)

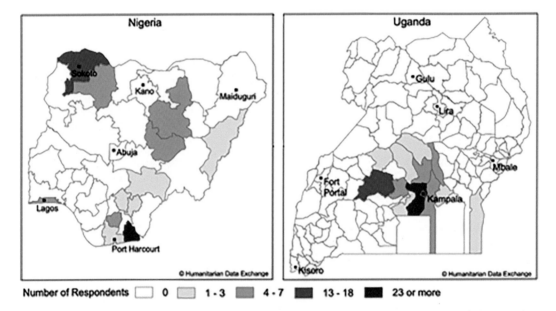

Fig. 12.1 Location of study participant residence, Nigeria and Uganda (Source: The Humanitarian Data Exchange. United Nations Office for the Coordination of Humanitarian Affairs (OCHA). https://data.humdata.org/, licensed under the terms of the Creative Commons Attribution 4.0 International License (http://creativecommons.org/licenses/by/4.0/))

ers, police officers, and schoolteachers, while in Northern Nigeria, women were most often local market vendors and/or small-scale farmers.

Ugandan participants were 32 years on average and had developed fistula at mean age 25 years; the range of time lived with fistula was several weeks through 38 years. Most were married (67%) and 64% had living children. Nearly two-thirds had not completed primary education (57%). Most participants had had vesicovaginal fistula only (95%). Women were also most commonly agricultural workers or ran informal small businesses such as selling prepared food at the market; slightly more than half (54%) reported working outside the household.

12.4.2 "I Mean to Be Out of this Urine"[1]: Urinary Incontinence Is the Overarching Challenge to Physical, Psychological, and Social Reintegration

Unsurprisingly, urinary leakage was the main physical experience that both Nigerian and Ugandan women associated with the condition of fistula. Most of the women equated being recovered from their fistula as being dry. This link was consistent across narratives of women whose leakage had resolved and among those who continued to leak. One woman shared *"I healed completely, [laughs] I healed. What I base [my healing] on is not leaking anymore"* (31-year-old Ugandan interviewee), while another stated *"My problem is to get healed; I mean to be out of this urine."* (27-year-old Nigerian interviewee).

While achieving continence was primary in most women's narratives about recovery, it often manifested differently in their recovery experiences. Women often described the actual leaking of urine by framing their incontinence in terms of its impacts on their physical, psychological, and social recovery. In the following sections, we present key examples where women from our two samples described how their recovery and reintegration is impacted by their leaking and associated impacts on their work and social lives and also explore other prominent physical, psychological, and social aspects featured in their recovery and reintegration narratives.

12.4.3 "The Leg Is Still Paining; It Has Never Improved…"[2]: The Role of Other Physical Symptoms in Fistula Recovery

Physical assessment factored into many women's narratives about their perspectives on recovery and rehabilitation from fistula and any repair surgeries. Despite the prevalent discussion around healing and recovery focused on achievement of incontinence, women's assessment of recovery intersected with a variety of other physical symptoms. Women shared specific examples of pain, weakness, coldness, sexual intimacy concerns, and other physical experiences that they perceived to be associated with their fistula recovery. Many of the concerns mentioned were considered direct consequences of the physical or psychosocial effects of incontinence, including pain, skin irritation from urine exposure, sleep quality, and the influence of depression on energy and appetite. Other concerns represented the impact of fistula-related physical conditions on other aspects of women's lives. The experience of physical symptoms affected all facets of women's recovery, including the physical, psychological, and social.

Across both countries, pain and functional disability featured heavily within the discussions of physical experiences that were relevant to women's recovery perceptions. For example, one woman described the pain and mobility symptoms she was experiencing,

> Since [being at the] hospital I [am] using a walking stick because I cannot walk […] the feeling and the pain is too much for me. You know when I'm eating I'm not feeling good. You know this pain. […] I just leave the food. It's very hard to cope with all these things. (32-year-old Nigerian interviewee)

Women discussed experiencing pain from a variety of different sources, including general pain, pain from skin irritation due to urine exposure, pain during urination, and pain during sex, some of which eventually resolved over time. The relationship between women's experiences of physical pain and perspectives on their recovery varied. For example, one woman reported feeling healed despite continued pain,

---

[1] 27-year-old Nigerian interviewee.

[2] 16-year-old Ugandan interviewee.

I healed. Ever since I was repaired last year, I no longer leak. [However,] the bladder that still pains, headache and backache.... I even don't want to merely touch it because it hurts.... I go through a lot of pain. (38-year-old Ugandan interviewee)

Conversely, another woman described the significant leg pain overshadowing her continued leaking due to its severity, *"My main problem was the legs because it pains me though I leak but that was not as painful as my legs. I wanted the leaking to be over as well." (21-year-old Nigerian interviewee).*

While fewer women reported symptoms of peroneal nerve damage as a result of obstructed labor, those who did had mixed experiences with persistent leg problems following fistula surgery. One young woman described the leg pain and difficulty walking she continued to experience, sharing: *"The leg is still paining; it has never improved. In fact, I don't want anyone to touch it." (16-year-old Ugandan interviewee).* Another woman chronicled the "sickness" created by her fistula and failed surgeries: *"Because the sickness that has made me to be like this. I get that I cannot walk right, and I've gone down … my weight has gone down wey wey." (18-year-old Nigerian interviewee).* Another woman also described experiencing intense pain, cold, and functional impairment:

I pass through this pain, cold, you know, wow… Since last year, I was having that pain anytime I see my menses. It was another thing entirely. But since March this year, 2014, it has released me a bit, doesn't give me cold and shivering. It's only the pains below my belly here. As I'm holding this phone my hand [is] paining me. It's very stiff. People say it is caused by the same problem. Because I'm always cold down here and my hand looks as if [I] touched a naked [electrical] wire; [I] now have pains and shakes all around. I can't squat down to urinate I have to stand. So it's very uncomfortable" (34-year-old Nigerian interviewee)

Relatedly, women's mobility challenges while living with fistula also surface in their excitement over a return to mobility and resumption of social and economic roles, further elaborated in the social recovery section below. One woman shared, *"I felt so excited and wanted to move all the time!" (26-year-old Ugandan interviewee).* Others described the experience of returning to mobility as being able to do a range of activities, *"Yeah, [I healed]. I am fine because I can do everything freely, be it jumping dancing, sitting, sleeping and any other thing that I can do." (46-year-old Ugandan interviewee).* Meanwhile another woman shared her perspective that she had finally recovered because her pain was gone: *"I healed. [I say that I am healed] because I don't feel any pain anywhere." (29-year-old Ugandan interviewee).*

Some women also noted that their appetite and energy improved with physical recovery, sharing how they did not eat well and had low energy while they were still leaking, but that these changed after restoration of continence with surgery. One Ugandan woman discussed being able to resume her prior household work,

"I can do now all the things I used not to do when I was sick.... I can now dig and wash my clothes plus my husband's, I can cook food, fetch water from the well and cook some of it for drinking, I can now go and gather firewood and more others." (20-year-old Ugandan interviewee). Another Ugandan woman echoed this sentiment: "I feel that I have the energy because I can now work, something I couldn't do in the past.... In fact [my mother] couldn't allow me to fetch water! However I can now fetch it myself and then prepare food." (21-year-old Ugandan interviewee).

Other women's narratives emphasized how significantly their sleep was impacted by incontinence and conversely, for some, on their continence return. For example, one woman shared about how sleeping makes her leak more:

So yeah if I want to sleep the urine will be worry my body. I'll get up quick quick before I will go to toilet it will come...when I sleep, sha! I cannot enjoy the sleep. Because the bladder is weak, just leaking. (40-year-old Nigerian interviewee).

Being continent appeared to allow women to sleep more soundly and thereby feel more recovered or healed as shared by one Ugandan woman,

Yes, I feel healed and fine now…. My life went back to normal, I am fine and don't have any problem. What I saw is that I am able to sleep and wake up on a dry bed and I don't pad myself anymore. (32-year-old Ugandan interviewee).

Another woman appreciated that her leaking was less compared to some women who were constantly awake at night changing their bedding or pads due to their incessant leaking subsequent: "*You see some women, they don't even sleep in the night, changing, changing, changing. It doesn't do me like that. I sleep, I change pad, not less than two pads in a day. Or once." (35-year-old Nigerian interviewee).*

Among those women who mentioned their relationships in the context of their physical recovery from fistula and repair, many shared they had urged their husbands to leave them to focus on their recovery. Many felt so consumed by their recovery they could not fathom being with their husbands intimately. They felt they needed to focus all their recovery fully on getting well physically. One Nigerian woman recalled what she had told her ex-husband:

For myself I say he should go and marry another wife, I will stay my own. I don't want problems. If he insists I go do, otherwise I want to stay my house. I want to stay my father's house I don't want to marry again. Because this problem too much for me! (32-year-old Nigerian interviewee).

A similar sentiment was shared by a Ugandan woman who said, "*I am not even interested [in sex] because whenever I think about my condition, I lose interest…. Even when I heal completely, it will take me a long time…." (16-year-old Ugandan interviewee).*

A few women also explicated that their lack of physical recovery negatively impacted their sexual life with their partners in other ways. For instance, one woman shared that "*My husband is always afraid so since I had this problem, we have not had any sexual intimacy. Whenever he feels like being intimate with me, I would be afraid it is not as it was before." (28-year-old Nigerian interviewee).* She feared having sex might cause her to develop another fistula, so she avoided having sex even though she and her husband desired to be intimate again. Another woman explained that her husband felt hesitant to engage in sex because of her chronic leakage: "*The most worst is that if I want to have sex, urine will be coming out from my body. So that is the big problem. The man will feel bad." (39-year-old Nigerian interviewee).* In other words, while both partners wanted to have sex, these women's incontinence placed limits on their comfort with sexual intimacy.

Concerns around fertility and childbearing spanned both physical and psychological themes and we discuss these concerns in both sections. Some women conceptualized the physical conditions of their recovery in terms of impact on their future fertility. One Ugandan woman discussed how she did not feel fully healed until after giving birth to another child with no consequence:

I think [I felt healed] within the past months. You see since I gave birth to that child (after the fistula repair) and yet they say that one is not supposed to give birth normally, it means that I had fewer chances for that baby to come out. So I think I am healed…. [That fear] has just stopped recently like I have said, after giving birth to that child and realizing that I was not leaking again. (28-year-old Ugandan interviewee)

Despite not leaking anymore, another Ugandan woman's fears of not being able to have another child also continued to impact her, "*I healed … I no longer leak… it is just that I worry a lot. I have spent almost one year and two months without getting my periods." (21-year-old Ugandan interviewee).* These women's narratives evidenced concern around their ability to become pregnant again and to give birth without fistula recurrence.

In summary, women across both countries most often assessed their physical state of recovery from their fistula, perhaps unsurprisingly, around their continued or chronic leakage; however, they notably also shared other physical health symptoms that challenged their physical recovery.

12.4.4 "I Eat Food, But I Don't Enjoy It Because I Think Much[3]": Intersections of Mental Health with Physical Symptoms

Being dry or getting dry was paramount among the women who shared mental health challenges in relation to their fistula recovery, and the majority assessed themselves as unwell mentally because of their chronic leakage. Women described feeling hopelessness, loneliness, uncertainty, and depression, among other mental health issues. Given the importance they placed on being dry, when women became continent they typically felt great joy, relief, and peace. Other physical health symptoms, including pain, sleeplessness, or fertility, also sometimes weighed on women more emotionally than physically. Though women typically brought up psychological aspects related to their continence status, some also situated these other physical symptoms, concerns about children or relationships as psychologically impacting their recovery from fistula.

Negative mental health impacts of unresolved urine leakage were common across both countries. Women shared feeling depressed, anxious, and frustrated as a result of fistula-related symptoms and their consequences. For example, one woman from Nigeria stated that *"I pity my life with this problem" (24-year-old Nigerian interviewee)* while another lamented, *"it makes me worried all the time. Everything has changed for the worse." (30-year-old Nigerian interviewee)* A Ugandan woman who remained incontinent of urine shared, *"I am not so proud of myself because any person would only be proud about themselves when they are healthy…. I don't feel [worthy] because when you are not feeling fine in the heart, you don't feel any worth." (28-year-old Ugandan interviewee).* A Nigerian woman explained through her tears *"Thinking, thinking. The thoughts are too much. The thoughts are too much," (29-year-old Nigerian interviewee)* and another woman explained the physical sensation of her sadness as a result of her chronic leakage: *"Sadness swept me as I see myself always leaking in urine." (21-year-old Nigerian interviewee).*

Meanwhile other women talked about repeated failed fistula surgeries that left them incontinent and caused them great angst. For instance, the woman in the following discussion delayed returning for another surgery because her first repair failed to completely close her fistula and she feared being disappointed again.

> I then know that I can be treated through surgery but since the first time I had the surgery and never got dry I lost hope and never returned, until now… It's paining me about this leaking that I got in to, since last weeks when the catheter was removed from me. (27-year-old Nigerian interviewee).

Conversely, becoming continent brought dramatic changes, especially to women's mental health and their outlook on the future. *"Right now, I feel valuable" (28-year-old Ugandan interviewee)*, a woman explained after her successful surgery when she was no longer leaking urine. Women discussed such changes in their thought orientation with successful surgery. In particular, reduction in anxiety and depression seemed the paramount psychological improvements among women who became dry. A woman explained, *"I am now feeling fine, I don't wish to die anymore because I recovered my life. I am [happy]. I stopped [feeling sorry for myself, and] I stopped crying." (28-year-old Ugandan interviewee).* Women's self-perceptions appeared significantly altered when they were no longer leaking, with many women talking about how good they felt. Their self-esteem improved. A Ugandan woman shared being able to socialize with her family and friends again: *"I felt so good; I went to visit my aunties, uncles and friends and told them that I healed and everyone would wonder how I did it and I would tell them." (22-year-old Ugandan interviewee).*

---

[3] 29-year-old Nigerian interviewee.

As noted in the physical recovery section above, achievement of continence also allowed some women to sleep more which provided mental relief. "*I thought I will never recover but I am getting there, as the urine no longer leaks on my bed. That is why I am happy*" remarked a 45-year-old Nigerian woman several months after her surgery. This intersection of physical with psychological is not unique to fistula recovery. Sleep may fall under both psychological and physical themes due to the multiple potential mechanisms, including anxiety around fistula and through the physical discomfort of urine leakage interrupting sleep. Regardless of mechanism, several women discussed improvements in the quality of their sleep as associated with recovery that made them feel better. A Ugandan woman who was no longer leaking recalled: "I felt so good. I would wake up at night and touch around to feel if there was any urine [on the mattress] and indeed there wasn't!" *(22-year-old Ugandan interviewee)*. Another Ugandan woman similarly stated: "*I feel completely healed; I have a nice restful sleep [now].*" *(32-year-old Ugandan interviewee)*.

In addition to sleep or lack thereof, other physical symptoms impacted women's mental health, in particular their changing appetite. A woman from Nigeria stated "*I don't even eat food that I like (crying). How then am I going to be okay?!*" *(50-year-old Nigerian interviewee)*. Women noted other symptoms that contributed to their poor mental health as they tried to recover from their fistulas. Most shared about not wanting to eat food and having no appetite or having heightened blood pressure, such as this woman from Nigeria,

> But fear's in my heart. My in-law said make [sure] I don't worry because [if the health providers] see my [blood pressure] rise they will not do it [her second repair attempt], that let me calm my temper and I feel free. (35-year-old Nigerian interviewee).

The variance among the mental health impacts during women's fistula recovery also revealed nuances between not leaking versus leaking just a little. Women whose incontinence had improved despite complete resolution were hopeful about their condition. A Ugandan woman described,

> I used to be so worried all the time and I was leaking a lot. It would be too much that sometimes whenever I wore a cloth you would think someone poured water on me! But am now starting to get better…. I am still leaking, [but] it's not much…. I feel a very big difference. (40-year-old Ugandan interviewee)

Another Ugandan commented that she felt nearly recovered from her fistula because she barely leaked, "*I feel like I healed completely except in times after drinking a lot when it leaks a few drops. Otherwise I can walk properly wearing only my knickers and nothing else.*" *(23-year-old Ugandan interviewee)*.

Other stressors peripheral to their leakage also weighed on some women's mental health, namely concerns related to marriage and children. Akin to physical intimacy discussed in previous section, relationship themes surfaced in some women's narratives of their mental health state during the aftermath of their fistula surgery. Women described feeling unfit or incapable of being a wife or caring for their husband's needs. For example, one woman from Nigeria recalled that "*I had told him [her husband] to go and marry another wife. Since I could no longer be counted among the living.*" *(33-year-old Nigerian interviewee)*. Others, however, wished their husbands were around and with them during their recovery and suggested that their mental health was worse because their husbands were not supportive, as shared a Nigerian woman: "*How will I feel happy despite I am ill, he [her husband] never asks after me nor follow me here.*" *(30-year-old Nigerian interviewee)*.

Persistent worries about the ability to have a child or the impact of secondary infertility on women's marriages also weighed on women's minds. For instance, in Uganda,

> The thing which stresses me is sometimes the man and the children mostly. Not being with him, because I don't have him since we separated; we have not lived together again. Secondly, it is the children; there is a problem living with children. It is paying their school fees. (42-year-old Ugandan interviewee)

Another woman similarly summarized that if only she could give her husband a child, things would be better for their marriage:

> I want to have children for him because [not having a child] is the only thing that can bring misunderstanding.... That if you come from work, he will not answer your greeting... You will cook, he will not eat because someone has abused him outside. He'll be feeling bad, that is the only thing. But what if I can have children for him, I believe that my future is bright. (38-year-old Nigerian interviewee)

These concerns around children also emerged as mental health stressors outside of marriage discussions. One Ugandan woman discussed how worried she was about her children who were staying at their father's house while she was being cared for by her parents,

> Of course during that time while I was sick my children were still at their father's place, so I would think about them... My parents wouldn't allow me to bring them in either and yet the condition at their father's home where they were was not good. So, my mind was always on my children but after bringing them in, I am now very fine. (28-year-old Ugandan interviewee)

Unlike this woman, however, the majority of those interviewed in both countries did not have children. For many, their childlessness brought them considerable grief and stress. One Nigerian woman put it *"if you marry now, without no child, you are nothing in Nigeria." (37-year-old Nigerian interviewee)*. Another woman self-diagnosed her major depression as due to, *"No marriage, no healing, no child. I've been thinking so much, I will end my life like this."* (40-year-old Nigerian interviewee). Women explained that they could better deal with ongoing pain, community rejection or incontinence if only they had a child.

Several women described stillbirths, miscarriages, and newborn deaths and that these experiences contributed to their poor mental health and fistula recovery process. For instance, one woman shared that *"if the baby has survived I could have lived with the problem, without ever bothering and just be taking care of the baby. What is annoying me is that each time I give birth the child dies, that is why I am not happy!"* (45-year-old Nigerian interviewee). A woman from Uganda underscored this point, *"What stresses me most are the children that are dying, first they get out even before the pregnancy is old enough; this puzzles me a lot." (26-year-old Ugandan interviewee)*

Other women in our two samples, however, prioritized their physical recovery, being dry, as paramount to having (more) children to further emphasize the strength of their desire for full recovery. A woman stated that *"I just want to be dry again. Don't even need more children. I'm okay with that two. Just for me to be healthy again." (34-year-old Nigerian interviewee)*. Another woman did not want to risk opening her fistula if she conceived again, so instructed the doctors to also perform a hysterectomy during her recent fistula surgery, *"No, I am now okay, dry, and asked the doctors to help make me barren so that I will not give birth again, so now my womb is removed."* (40-year-old Nigerian woman). Here, similar to the tensions with their husbands and marriages, we see the tensions between bearing children and bearing another fistula that exists in women's decisions about fertility and relationships. Some share that they do not even want children, they only desire to be "dried" as evidenced in the following comment form a Nigerian woman: *"These complications are more than what I thought. If I become dried I don't mind if I never give birth again (laughing)."* (25-year-old Nigerian interviewee)

Importance of faith and God played into some women's mental health narratives about their fistula recovery, more so in Nigeria. Generally, women whom cited God or their faith were those who felt hopeless that anything more could be done for them. For example, a Nigerian woman lamented *"However, there was nothing I could do other than crying daily. I resigned my fate in God for allowing something like that to befall me" (21-year-old Nigerian interviewee)* while another woman explained *"I go to farm and that time I told God to take my life as I see my life as useless as anything." (35-year-old Nigerian interviewee)*. Other women framed their faith as an important source of strength that could help them get them through their struggles, as shared in the following excerpt from a Nigerian woman:

> Now that I am sick I cannot do anything for myself because of the disgrace and shame. But if God stands by me and I become normal, I would either go to school or do anything to better my situation in life. (33-year-old Nigerian woman)

In Uganda, multiple women described their faith as an important source of support and hope, as seen in the following quotation: *"I am hopeful that if it God's plan, I will get healed even if I am called for a second repair.... it just lies with God. You just have to pray to God for his intervention into your situation."* (46-year-old Ugandan interviewee).

To summarize, across both countries, many women experienced considerable stress and anxiety related to their recovery, often in relation to their incontinence and other physical disabilities. Unsurprisingly, they commonly found great joy and relief when they become less or completely continent or more able-bodied again. Others, however, also shared that partnerships, family relationships, children, and/or fertility concerns contributed to worsening their mental health during their fistula recovery.

12.4.5 "Now I Am Useful to My Home"[4]: Social Reengagement During Fistula Recovery

Fistula-related incontinence placed extreme limitations on women's social participation including their physical, social, and economic mobility opportunities. Where women were no longer leaking, their narratives of recovery focused on resuming the social roles and activities that they had held prior to developing fistula, whereas those who had not yet achieved continence emphasized the continuing challenges they faced in social participation. Multiple intersecting mechanisms were at play in this process, including challenges managing incontinence, physical pain or discomfort, and stigma. In particular, fistula-related stigma influenced the way women were talked to and treated, how they felt about themselves, and the extent to which they chose to engage with others.

Women's assessment of social recovery from obstetric fistula frequently occurred within the context of stigma in both Nigeria and Uganda. Anticipated and internalized stigma resulted in restricting time with family members and friends, significantly limiting social participation and was an important source of stress. In both countries, women preferred to remain alone at home or at the fistula repair center[5] in order to avoid stigmatizing behaviors from community and family members. Ugandan women often described limiting their interactions with others due to their incontinence and incontinence-related odor:

> I could no longer do anything on my own.... I wasn't moving. I couldn't even move out of my bedroom. There were times when I felt like going out of my bedroom and going out to my neighbors and conversing, but it was impossible because I would all get wet. (32-year-old Ugandan interviewee)

> In the past I wouldn't even sit with my own husband because I would suspect that my stench was inconveniencing him. In fact, I would also feel that I am releasing a bad smell. Even when I went to visit friends I wouldn't feel free. (19-year-old Ugandan interviewee)

Experiences with stigma and isolation were prominently featured in many Nigerian women's narratives from all four sites. For example, a Nigerian woman stated *"Because of this sickness I cannot*

---

[4] 37-year-old Nigerian interviewee.

[5] In Nigeria, in the North West site of Sokoto, some women interviewed had moved to live in informal settlements in and around the health center.

do what I am supposed to do. I cannot work, I cannot go to church, I cannot attend public functions." *(22-year-old Nigerian interviewee).* A young Nigerian woman who had undergone multiple surgeries without success explained,

> Since I met many people with this problem [at the fistula health center], I decided to remain here with them. I think to stay here is better because no one will see me as a person with strange condition. […] When I was at home even my sister will not sleep with me in the same room because of the problem. (18-year-old Nigerian interviewee)

Resumption of social engagement was consistently mentioned as a top priority of women following successful surgery. Several participants highlighted the social support that community engagement facilitated and the recovered sense of belonging with others, contrary to the alienation they had experienced during the time they suffered from fistula-related incontinence. Such sentiments were expressed by two Ugandan women who shared,

> Now I have hope because I feel good, I can go anywhere, and I also enjoy life because I can be with my friends and even my family which keeps me happy. (24-year-old Ugandan interviewee).

> Now you easily sit beside your friend when they have invited you somewhere but back [when you had fistula], you would sit and you yourself you could feel the cloth you used to pamper yourself really smelling. Now you can sit with people and you feel like a human being too. (33-year-old Ugandan interviewee).

Women whose urinary incontinence persisted felt not yet fully recovered because of continued limitations on their socialization. Incontinence challenged their ability to recover socially, interact, or to feel back to their normal social selves. Incontinent women often emphasized that the risk of urine soaking through their padding was too high to warrant them interacting socially again: *"It can disgrace you at any time, don't you understand?! Even though you pack, the thing can soak at any time"* one Nigerian woman explained (25-year-old Nigerian interviewee). However, some women were able to engage in social situations while still leaking through creatively concealing their incontinence. Such women put significant preparation into ensuring leakage management while interacting with community and family members, attending social functions and going about their work routine with careful management using cloths, pads, or adult diapers. In Nigeria, a few women were able to continue attending church services and other important gatherings, without their incontinence being revealed, through their attentive leakage management as described by this Nigerian woman: *"If I go to church, I will be sitting and timing myself. I use pieces of clothes to pack myself."* *(22-year-old Nigerian interviewee).*

Recovering within a marriage and family context brought challenges to some women and reassurance to others. While the intensity of women's experiences with enacted stigma varied, nearly all perceived their ability to get back into normal social and household routines as a marker of their recovery. However, entering the process of getting back to normal often required social support. For example, one woman who had recently undergone fistula surgery explained that while *"I will like to go back to my husband's place but no one will help me with house chores and as you know after operation I need rest."* *(20-year-old Nigerian interviewee).* Having even a few supportive family or partners could help their social reintegration substantially. Some women from both contexts had stronger support of their husbands and/or other family members. A Ugandan woman, for instance, discussed her happiness in resuming her household chores after a successful surgery,

> It is much better because all the responsibilities I had for everyone I can meet them unlike before …. For example, before, my husband would wake up and prepare the kids for school but now, I wake up and prepare [them] or sometimes prepare something to eat for him before going to garden and when he is back, he finds that I have prepared everything and I have cleaned the whole home. This was not the case during the time when I had a fistula; then he was responsible for all that. (28-year-old Ugandan interviewee)

For this woman and others in both samples, being able to help with (or take back over responsibility for) household chores marked social assessment of their recovery from fistula as much as physical.

Overlapping with women's narratives on social participation and also physical recovery from fistula was the importance of economic participation. The ability to work played a distinct role in altering women's perceptions of their self-value through their ability to participate in their previous work activities, achieve their previous roles, and allow them to potentially meet their own needs and the needs of their dependents. Achieving continence seemed to free some women to think more broadly after their surgery, allowing them to pay attention to future needs, including economic survival. A woman from Uganda described that she could support herself again:

> I buy my own clothes, except for the food and hospital bills, it is that lady (boss) that supports me…. [My financial status] has changed because I can now move and do other work to get more money; I can now travel. (28-year-old Ugandan interviewee)

Women who described their inability to work all cited their struggles with incontinence. Similar to socialization, most women seemed to equate their ability to work with incontinence management. However, some women worked despite continued leakage or other related symptoms, where appropriate coping was possible or support available. For example, a Nigerian petty trader was able to maintain her market stall due to access to a local toilet for frequent changing and help from other vendors to watch her store while she changed. Maintaining economic engagement also had a powerful effect on women's self-esteem, as described by a Ugandan woman:

> [Now] I can now cultivate food which is enough for my children so that they don't live a needy life apart from need for money. Food, I can offer that very well to my children, they can eat, and all be happy. Now I am useful to my home. (47-year-old Ugandan interviewee)

This perspective was echoed by another Ugandan woman who after becoming dry reported,

> I felt so valuable. I even got a hotel job and made some money and I decided to go for more training in hairdressing, but the money wasn't enough. So, I was told to return when I raise more money. (22-year-old Ugandan interviewee)

In summary, the physical effects of fistula resulted in significant limitations for women with broad impacts on mental health and mobility through challenges managing incontinence, physical pain or discomfort, and stigma. While resumption of social engagement was a top priority of women, for most women, it required resolution of incontinence. Resuming work and/or household responsibilities was also emphasized as a powerful marker of getting back to normal and mattered economically.

12.5 Discussion

Across both samples, women shared specific examples of weaknesses, leakage, coldness, pain and other physical conditions that they perceived as part of their recovery. Leakage resolution or partial resolution was most common physical assessment women used of their recovery status. Issues with pain, mobility, energy, and loss of appetite also significantly bothered many women, and for some was more debilitating than their continued incontinence.

These experiences of bodily symptoms affected all aspects of their recovery, including physical, psychological, and social. As evidenced in the results section, it was not possible to parse apart the physical and psychological components, due to the strong reinforcing relationships between these two domains. Many women linked feelings of hopelessness, despair, and fear to their leakage, and this was a primary cause of various types of stigma. Importantly, continence or the lack thereof was not the only factor that psychologically disturbed the women we interviewed in Uganda and Nigeria. Some posited that if only they could have a child or be with their children, they would feel happy or normal. Others shared feelings of inadequacy and anxiety about their familial and marital relationships. Concerns around childbearing and return to fertility also worried some. Along the same line, feeling renewed hope and energy and general improved mental health were often related to women noticing that they were leaking less, having less pain, experiencing better mobility, or feeling improvement in other physical symptoms they had associated with their obstetric fistula.

Our analysis also identified some notable differences between the two samples. Issues with sleep appeared to feature more heavily in Ugandan interviews. Experiences of continued leakage and resulting severe psychological sequalae appeared more pronounced in Nigeria, likely partially because some women were interviewed pre-operation and many more women in Nigeria had multiple unsuccessful repairs compared to the Ugandan sample. Social-related assessment of their recovery and reintegration after having fistula also surfaced in women's narratives across both groups though with differences. Importance of participating in household chores, being about to work or earn a living, and contribute back to their home and family came up for some women, though especially in Nigeria where many more women shared about returning to employment even if they were still not completely dry. Variability in socioeconomic and employment status across the two sites was also evident and likely impacted how work featured into women's narratives about their fistula recovery and reintegration processes. In the Nigerian sample, women were more educated with a larger proportion reporting employment after their fistula compared to the Ugandan sample. Much of the Ugandan sample worked in subsistence agriculture; thus, their work activities were likely differentially impacted.

Differences between the two samples in stigma experiences also emerged in the narratives. Enacted stigma and anticipated stigma, including concern of being caught leaking, were prevalent themes in women's discussions about managing or returning to social situations. Prior working and health status, familial support, one's social identity, and other individual and structural level factors intersect and frame the psychosocial contexts of living with incontinence and recovering from fistula. These contexts, in turn, may influence also the cultural meaning of incontinence and fistula in each setting and thereby impact women's narratives about stigma. Stigma was a pervasive experience and important theme among Ugandan women, which we have written about previously (El Ayadi, Barageine, et al., 2020; El Ayadi, Barageine, Miller, et al., 2019), and compared to the Nigerian sample, it appeared that Ugandan women experienced somewhat less severe enacted stigma and often had at least one strong source of social support which may have buffered their experience. In contrast, women in Nigeria, particularly those in the North, experienced significant enacted stigma to the point of ostracism from the community, as evidenced by multiple women choosing to move to live in settlements near the fistula hospitals with other women like them. In both countries, religion was brought up as important; however, in women's narratives, it appeared to function more as social support in Uganda whereas it was more fatalistic in Nigeria.

Our research shows that physical recovery from fistula is paramount, but this analysis supports extending the current biomedical perspective that sole repair of the fistula is primary. Our findings suggest that fistula recovery includes a constellation of fistula-related symptoms, including but not limited to incontinence, that are particular to each woman. This specificity and breadth are critical to building holistic support systems for women dealing with and recovering from fistula. For some women in our samples, the experience of fistula-related symptoms overshadows the importance of incontinence. Our analysis emphasizes the important intersecting relationships between the physical, psychological, and social domains involved in the fistula experience, and the difficulty of parsing apart primary versus secondary influences and consequences across these domains. Beyond only physical recovery, investment is needed on mental health and social reintegration as evidenced by our study. Indeed, one critical implication of the current research is how the concept of women's reintegration relative to fistula extends across the full continuum of physical health, incorporating support for symptom and stigma management throughout. Intervention and assistance within not-solely-physical areas, including support for mental health and employment-related consequences of physical symptoms, represent an important strategy for improving women's quality of life.

Currently, it appears that few women are recipients of additional programming to support their supplementary physical, psychological, and social needs. In the Nigeria data, six women reported getting additional care from local non-profit organizations associated with the fistula centers and three other women mentioned getting support from church groups in their community. Only a couple of women in the Ugandan sample reported receiving some additional support from a local non-profit organization. A recent scoping review of the literature identified a limited evidence base for reintegration programming globally, but reported the existence of dedicated yet small reintegration programming in both Nigeria and Uganda including support from governments (Nigeria) and non-profit organizations (Nigeria and Uganda) (El Ayadi, Painter, et al., 2020).

Several limitations to our analysis exist. First and foremost, the interpretation and implications of our findings are the result of qualitative research designed to understand the range of women's experiences, but which did not seek to provide findings generalizable to the national or regional level in either country. Additionally, our cross-context comparison was conducted across different settings using data collected at different time points with different samples, recruitment strategies, and interview instruments. Initial analyses were conducted separately, with the first and last author jointly reading each other's codebooks and transcripts. Because the initial study purposes for both projects were not solely fistula recovery and reintegration, interview probing may not have adequately captured all being important for this inquiry. Sample characteristics seemed particularly different in terms of regional and religious variation in Nigeria. Additionally, in North West Nigerian site of Sokoto, some women interviewed lived in informal settlements in and around the health center. Staying at or around the fistula repair center for purposes other than treatment was not discussed in Uganda and is not a commonly known experience in this setting. Lastly, women were interviewed at different points along their recovery experience, some before surgery (only Nigeria), some after (all for Uganda), and others after many repairs (most prevalent in Nigeria sample).

12.6   Conclusions

Our chapter underscores the growing call in fistula care and research to move beyond surgical genital fistula closure as metric of treatment success to incorporate patient-reported outcomes into fistula care to comprehensively meet women's recovery needs from this condition. Our findings from nearly 150 women in Nigeria and Uganda demonstrate the importance of broadly conceptualizing recovery, and the physical, psychological, and social components for recovery, and highlights the interrelationships between these domains. Additionally, we observe the different experiences of Nigerian versus Ugandan women affected by fistula within diverse structural and sociocultural contexts which configure their individual and collective experiences. As we work to improve the evidence base on how to best support women affected by fistula, we must prioritize holistic support systems to address the constellation of fistula-related symptoms and consequences affecting women's lives.

Acknowledgments We want to sincerely acknowledge the women who shared time with us to recount their experiences living with and recovering from obstetric fistula. We also thank the field and study teams who contributed to the data collection and data transcription and translation for these projects, and the hospital staff and government officials who allowed our teams space to interview the women. We also thank Jia Nocon for developing our participant residence map.

Funding This research was supported by the US Fulbright Scholars Program 2014-2015 (Nigeria) and the Eunice Kennedy Shriver National Institute on Child Health and Human Development (Grants: R21HD075008 and K99HD086232, Uganda)

References

Abegunde, D., Kabo, I. A., Sambisa, W., Akomolafe, T., Orobaton, N., Abdulkarim, M., et al. (2015). Availability, utilization, and quality of emergency obstetric care services in Bauchi State, Nigeria. *International Journal of Gynaecology and Obstetrics, 128*(3), 251–255. https://doi.org/10.1016/j.ijgo.2014.09.029

Adewuyi, E. O., Zhao, Y., Auta, A., & Lamichhane, R. (2017). Prevalence and factors associated with non-utilization of healthcare facility for childbirth in rural and urban Nigeria: Analysis of a national population-based survey. *Scandinavian Journal of Public Health, 45*(6), 675–682. https://doi.org/10.1177/1403494817705562

Adler, A. J., Ronsmans, C., Calvert, C., & Filippi, V. (2013). Estimating the prevalence of obstetric fistula: a systematic review and meta-analysis. *BMC Pregnancy and Childbirth, 13*, 246. https://doi.org/10.1186/1471-2393-13-246

Ahmed, S., Anastasi, E., & Laski, L. (2016). Double burden of tragedy: Stillbirth and obstetric fistula. *The Lancet Global Health, 4*(2), e80. https://doi.org/10.1016/s2214-109x(15)00290-9

Ahmed, S., & Holtz, S. A. (2007). Social and economic consequences of obstetric fistula: Life changed forever? *International Journal of Gynaecology and Obstetrics, 99*(Suppl 1), 10–15.

Alkire, B. C., Vincent, J. R., Burns, C. T., Metzler, I. S., Farmer, P. E., & Meara, J. G. (2012). Obstructed labor and caesarean delivery: The cost and benefit of surgical intervention. *PLoS ONE, 7*(4), e34595. https://doi.org/10.1371/journal.pone.0034595

Ameh, C., Msuya, S., Hofman, J., Raven, J., Mathai, M., & van den Broek, N. (2012). Status of emergency obstetric care in six developing countries five years before the MDG targets for maternal and newborn health. *PLoS ONE, 7*(12), 49938. https://doi.org/10.1371/journal.pone.0049938

Bauer, G. R. (2014). Incorporating intersectionality theory into population health research methodology: Challenges and the potential to advance health equity. *Social Science and Medicine, 110*, 10–17. https://doi.org/10.1016/j.socscimed.2014.03.022

Browning, A., & Whiteside, S. (2015). Characteristics, management, and outcomes of repair of rectovaginal fistula among 1100 consecutive cases of female genital tract fistula in Ethiopia. *International Journal of Gynaecology and Obstetrics, 131*(1), 70–73. https://doi.org/10.1016/j.ijgo.2015.05.012

Byamugisha, J., El Ayadi, A., Obore, S., Mwanje, H., Kakaire, O., Barageine, J., et al. (2015). Beyond repair - Family and community reintegration after obstetric fistula surgery: Study protocol. *Reproductive Health, 12*(1), 115. https://doi.org/10.1186/s12978-015-0100-1

Creanga, A., & Genadry, R. (2007). Obstetric fistulas: A clinical review. *International Journal of Gynaecology and Obstetrics, 99*(Suppl 1), S40–S46.

de Bernis, L. (2007). Obstetric fistula: Guiding principles for clinical management and programme development, a new WHO guideline. *International Journal of Gynaecology and Obstetrics, 99*(Suppl 1), 117–121.

Delamou, A., Delvaux, T., Beavogui, A. H., Toure, A., Kolie, D., Sidibe, S., et al. (2016). Factors associated with the failure of obstetric fistula repair in Guinea: Implications for practice. *Reproductive Health Journal, 13*(1), 135. https://doi.org/10.1186/s12978-016-0248-3

Delamou, A., Delvaux, T., El Ayadi, A. M., Tripathi, V., Camara, B. S., Beavogui, A. H., et al. (2017). Fistula recurrence, pregnancy, and childbirth following successful closure of female genital fistula in Guinea: A longitudinal study. *The Lancet Global Health.* https://doi.org/10.1016/s2214-109x(17)30366-2

Direct Relief. (2016). *Global Fistula Map.* Retrieved 1 August, 2019, from http://www.globalfistulamap.org/

El Ayadi, A., Barageine, J., Korn, A., Kakaire, O., Turan, J., Obore, S., et al. (2019). Trajectories of women's physical and psychosocial health following obstetric fistula repair in Uganda: A longitudinal study. *Tropical Medicine and International Health, 24*(1), 53–64. https://doi.org/10.1111/tmi.13178

El Ayadi, A., Byamugisha, J., Obore, S., Mwanje, H., Kakaire, O., Barageine, J., et al. (2017). Development and preliminary validation of a post-fistula repair reintegration instrument among Ugandan women. *Reproductive Health Journal, 14*(1), 109. https://doi.org/10.1186/s12978-017-0372-8

El Ayadi, A. M., Barageine, J. K., Miller, S., Byamugisha, J., Nalubwama, H., Obore, S., et al. (2019). Women's experiences of fistula-related stigma in Uganda: A conceptual framework to inform stigma-reduction interventions. *Culture, Health & Sexuality, 2019*, 1–16. https://doi.org/10.1080/13691058.2019.1600721

El Ayadi, A. M., Barageine, J. K., Miller, S., Byamugisha, J., Nalubwama, H., Obore, S., et al. (2020). Women's experiences of fistula-related stigma in Uganda: A conceptual framework to inform stigma-reduction interventions. *Culture, Health & Sexuality, 22*(3), 352–367. https://doi.org/10.1080/13691058.2019.1600721

El Ayadi, A. M., Painter, C. P., Delamou, A., Barr-Walker, J., Obore, S., Byamugisha, J. K., et al. (2020). Rehabilitation and reintegration programming adjunct to female genital fistula surgery: A systematic scoping review. *International Journal of Gynaecology and Obstetrics, 148*(1), 42–58.

Elneil, S. (2015). Global efforts for effective training in fistula surgery. *International Journal of Gynaecology and Obstetrics, 131*(1), 64–66. https://doi.org/10.1016/j.ijgo.2015.02.003

Epiu, I., Alia, G., Mukisa, J., Tavrow, P., Lamorde, M., & Kuznik, A. (2018). Estimating the cost and cost-effectiveness for obstetric fistula repair in hospitals in Uganda: A low income country. *Health Policy and Planning, 33*(9), 999–1008. https://doi.org/10.1093/heapol/czy078

Frajzyngier, V., Ruminjo, J., & Barone, M. A. (2012). Factors influencing urinary fistula repair outcomes in developing countries: A systematic review. *American Journal of Obstetrics and Gynecology, 207*(4), 248–258.

Goh, J. T., Sloane, K. M., Krause, H. G., Browning, A., & Akhter, S. (2005). Mental health screening in women with genital tract fistulae. *British Journal of Obstetrics and Gynaecology, 112*(9), 1328–1330. https://doi.org/10.1111/j.1471-0528.2005.00712.x

Goh, J. T., Tan, S. B., Natukunda, H., Singasi, I., & Krause, H. G. (2016). Outcomes following surgical repair using layered closure of unrepaired 4th degree perineal tear in rural western Uganda. *International Urogynecology Journal, 27*(11), 1661–1666. https://doi.org/10.1007/s00192-016-3024-6

Hannig, A. (2017). *Injury, healing, and religion at an Ethiopian hospital.* University of Chicago Press.

Heller, A., & Hannig, A. (2017). Unsettling the fistula narrative: Cultural pathology, biomedical redemption, and inequities of health access in Niger and Ethiopia. *Anthropology & Medicine, 2017*, 1–15. https://doi.org/10.1080/13648470.2016.1249252

Institut National de la Statistique, République de Guinée. (2019). *Enquête Démographique et de Santé 2018 (EDSG V).* Institut National de la Statistique, Ministère du Plan et du Développement Economique, République de Guinée.

Johnson, C., Johnson, T., & Adanu, R. (2015). *Gawande essential surgery: Disease control priorities* (Vol. 1, 3rd ed., p. 5). The International Bank for Reconstruction and Development.

Keya, K. T., Sripad, P., Nwala, E., & Warren, C. E. (2018). "Poverty is the big thing": Exploring financial, transportation, and opportunity costs associated with fistula management and repair in Nigeria and Uganda. *International Journal for Equity in Health, 17*(1), 70. https://doi.org/10.1186/s12939-018-0777-1

Krause, H., Ng, S. K., Singasi, I., Kabugho, E., Natukunda, H., & Goh, J. (2019). Incidence of intimate partner violence among Ugandan women with pelvic floor dysfunction. *International Journal of Gynaecology and Obstetrics, 144*(3), 309–313. https://doi.org/10.1002/ijgo.12748

Maheu-Giroux, M., Filippi, V., Maulet, N., Samadoulougou, S., Castro, M. C., Meda, N., et al. (2016). Risk factors for vaginal fistula symptoms in Sub-Saharan Africa: A pooled analysis of national household survey data. *BMC Pregnancy and Childbirth, 16*, 82. https://doi.org/10.1186/s12884-016-0871-6

Maheu-Giroux, M., Filippi, V., Samadoulougou, S., Castro, M. C., Maulet, N., Meda, N., et al. (2015). Prevalence of symptoms of vaginal fistula in 19 sub-Saharan Africa countries: A meta-analysis of national household survey data. *The Lancet Global Health, 3*(5), 271–278. https://doi.org/10.1016/s2214-109x(14)70348-1

Marks, D. F., & Yardley, L. (Eds.). (2004). *Research methods for clinical and health psychology.* SAGE Publications, Inc..

McFarland, D. (2010). 'The economics of obstetric fistula and current research. In *Meeting report: Obstetric fistula prevention as a catalyst for safe motherhood: Success and opportunities.* The Carter Center.

Mezie-Okoye, M. M., Adeniji, F. O., Tobin-West, C. I., & Babatunde, S. (2012). Status of emergency obstetric care in a local government area in south-south Nigeria. *African Journal of Reproductive Health, 16*(3), 171–179.

Muleta, M., Rasmussen, S., & Kiserud, T. (2010). Obstetric fistula in 14,928 Ethiopian women. *Acta Obstetricia et Gynecologica Scandinavica, 89*(7), 945–951. https://doi.org/10.3109/00016341003801698

National Population Commission & IPC. (2019). *Nigeria demographic and health survey 2018 - key indicators report.* NPC and ICF.

Nigeria Ministry of Health. (2019). *National strategic framework for the elimination of obstetric fistula in Nigeria, 2019–2023.*

Okonofua, F., Ntoimo, L. F. C., Ogu, R., Galadanci, H., Gana, M., Adetoye, D., et al. (2019). Assessing the knowledge and skills on emergency obstetric care among health providers: Implications for health systems strengthening in Nigeria. *PLoS ONE, 14*(4), e0213719. https://doi.org/10.1371/journal.pone.0213719

Omole, O., Welye, H., & Abimbola, S. (2015). Boko Haram insurgency: Implications for public health. *The Lancet, 385*(9972), 941. https://doi.org/10.1016/S0140-6736(15)60207-0

Phillips, B. S., Ononokpono, D. N., & Udofia, N. W. (2016). Complicating causality: Patient and professional perspectives on obstetric fistula in Nigeria. *Culture, Health & Sexuality, 18*(9), 996–1009. https://doi.org/10.1080/13691058.2016.1148198

Saidu, R., August, E. M., Alio, A. P., Salihu, H. M., Saka, M. J., & Jimoh, A. A. G. (2013). An assessment of essential maternal health services in Kwara State, Nigeria. *African Journal of Reproductive Health, 17*(1), 41–48.

Slinger, G., Trautvetter, L., Browning, A., & Rane, A. (2018). Out of the shadows and 6000 reasons to celebrate: An update from FIGO's fistula surgery training initiative. *International Journal of Gynaecology and Obstetrics, 141*(3), 280–283. https://doi.org/10.1002/ijgo.12482

Sori, D. A., Azale, A. W., & Gemeda, D. H. (2016). Characteristics and repair outcome of patients with Vesicovaginal fistula managed in Jimma University teaching Hospital, Ethiopia. *BMC Urolology, 16*(1), 41. https://doi.org/10.1186/s12894-016-0152-8

Stanton, C., Holtz, S. A., & Ahmed, S. (2007). Challenges in measuring obstetric fistula. *International Journal of Gynaecology and Obstetrics, 99*(Suppl 1), S4–S9.

Tunçalp, O., Tripathi, V., Landry, E., Stanton, C. K., & Ahmed, S. (2015). Measuring the incidence and prevalence of obstetric fistula: Approaches, needs and recommendations. *Bulletin of the World Health Organization, 93*(1), 60–62. https://doi.org/10.2471/blt.14.141473

Turan, J. M., Elafros, M. A., Logie, C. H., Banik, S., Turan, B., Crockett, K. B., et al. (2019). Challenges and opportunities in examining and addressing intersectional stigma and health. *BMC Medicine, 17*(1), 7. https://doi.org/10.1186/s12916-018-1246-9

Uganda Bureau of Statistics, & ICF. (2018). *Uganda demographic and health survey 2016*. UBOS and ICF.

Uganda Bureau of Statistics and Macro International. (2007). *Uganda demographic and health survey 2005/2006*.

Uganda Ministry of Health. (2011). *National obstetric fistula strategy 2011/2012-2015/2016*. Uganda Ministry of Health.

UNFPA (2011) 'The state of the world population'. UNFPA.

United Nations High Commissioner for Refugees. (2019). *As Boko Haram violence surges, UNHCR seeks US$135 million to aid displaced.*

UNFPA. (2017). *Country programme document for Nigeria*. 2017. UNFPA – Country programmes and related matters.

Wall, L. L., Arrowsmith, S. D., Briggs, N. D., Browning, A., & Lassey, A. (2005). The obstetric vesicovaginal fistula in the developing world. *Obstetrical and Gynecological Survey, 60*(7), S3–S51.

WHO, UNICEF, UNFPA, World Bank Group, and United Nations Population Division. (2015). *Trends in maternal mortality: 1990 to 2015*. WHO, UNICEF, UNFPA, World Bank Group, and United Nations Population Division.

Socioeconomic and Healthcare Causes of Obstetric Fistula in Tanzania: Perspectives from the Affected Women

13

Lilian Teddy Mselle and Stella Masala Mpanda

13.1 Introduction

Obstetric fistula is a major public health problem which occurs during the birthing process among women in low- and middle-income countries (Hill et al., 2007; Wall, 2006). It is one of the most severe childbirth injuries that can occur when labor is allowed to progress for a period lasting from several days to a week without timely medical intervention, usually a cesarean section (Danso et al., 2007; Wall et al., 2006). Following a prolonged obstructed labor, the compressed surrounding soft tissues are subject to necrosis, thus creating open communication between the bladder and vagina (vesicle-vaginal fistula (VVF) or vagina and rectum (recto-vaginal fistula (RVF)), through which urine and/or feces leak (Danso et al., 1996; Donnay & Ramsey, 2006). It is an acquired defect in the genital tract connecting the vaginal or uterine cavity to the bladder, urethra, ureters, rectum, or colon. Obstetric fistula develops after many days or more of obstructed labor, when the pressure of the baby's head against the mother's pelvis cuts off blood supply to delicate tissues until it causes necrosis and leaves a communicating defect, or hole (Hilton, 2003). Women affected by obstetric fistula suffer not only from physical problems, but also from social exclusion and economic decline (Cook et al., 2004; Gharoro & Agholor, 2009; INFO Project, 2004; UNFPA, 2006; Women's Dignity Project, Engender Health, 2006; Yeakey et al., 2009). Other types of fistula may occur due to cervical cancer, radiation therapy, or injuries following surgery (Wall et al., 2004).

Estimates indicate that about 2–3.5 million or more women worldwide live with vesico-vaginal fistula (VVF) or rectal vaginal fistula (RVF), and the majority of these reside in Africa and Asia (Opara et al., 2012; Suellen et al., 2005; Wall, 2006). Recent institutional-based data on obstetric fistula in Tanzania indicate that there are between 2500 and 3000 new cases of fistula each year, which is higher than earlier estimates of about 1200 obstetric fistulas per year (Bangser, 2002; Women's

L. T. Mselle (✉)
Department of Clinical Nursing, Muhimbili
University of Health and Allied Sciences,
Dar es Salaam, Tanzania
e-mail: lmselle@muhas.ac.tz

S. M. Mpanda
Childbirth Survival International,
Dar es Salaam, Tanzania
e-mail: mpandas@yahoo.com

© Springer Nature Switzerland AG 2022
L. B. Drew et al. (eds.), *A Multidisciplinary Approach to Obstetric Fistula in Africa*, Global Maternal and Child Health, https://doi.org/10.1007/978-3-031-06314-5_13

Dignity Project, Engender Health, 2006), indicating a possible increase in the magnitude of problem. However, because these estimates are institutional-based, it is likely that the increase is due to an increased influx of women affected by obstetric fistula to the health facilities for treatment. At the present time, the number of cases may be increasing as a result of an increased influx of women with obstetric fistula to the health facilities for treatment following active case finding programmes and advocacy for free fistula treatment (UNFPA, 2010).

Studies on women affected by obstetric fistula in resource-poor countries have shown that biological, social-cultural, environmental, and health system factors contribute to the occurrences of obstetric fistula (Hassan & Ekele, 2009; Mselle, Kohi, et al., 2011). These factors include cultural beliefs and practices, limited decision-making power by women, illiteracy, low status of women, sexual inequality, malnutrition, and the lack of emergency obstetric care (Elneil & Browning, 2009; Nour, 2006; UNFPA, 2002). Universal access to emergency obstetric care for women suffering from prolonged obstructed labor could dramatically reduce the prevalence of obstetric fistula (Graham & Hussein, 2007). However, in Tanzania, access to emergency obstetric care is still limited, which makes timely intervention in cases of obstetric fistula a major challenge (Olsen et al., 2005).

Studies on obstetric fistula in Tanzania primarily have assessed the availability of fistula treatment (Bangser, 2002), prevention, treatment, and repair (Majinge, 1995; Mteta et al., 2006). Other studies have focused on dimensions of living with fistula and the associated social vulnerability of affected women (Bangser, 2006; Mselle, Moland, et al., 2011; Women's Dignity Project, Engender Health, 2006), explored experiences of living with a fistula (Mselle & Kohi, 2015; Mselle, Kohi, et al., 2011), or have assessed reintegration and quality of life following fistula surgery (Mselle et al., 2012; Pope et al., 2011). There is only one fistula study that was conducted in Tanzania describing perceived causes of fistula (Kazaura et al., 2011). In this study, participants came from the general population and included women of reproductive age, men, health providers, birth attendants, and community leaders. This study describes socioeconomic and healthcare causes of obstetric fistula from the perspectives of women affected by it in Tanzania. Among other findings, this study found that people still hold misconceptions about obstetric fistula.

13.2   Conceptual Framework

In this study, the availability, accessibility, acceptability, and quality of care (AAAQ) concept and the three delays model were used to understand the causes of obstetric fistula from the perspectives of women affected by it in Tanzania.

The "three delays" model (Thadeus & Maine, 1994) illustrate levels of delay where barriers block women from getting timely and appropriate obstetric care. This model identifies barriers that can delay access in the different phases of birth care to effective interventions that prevent maternal mortality. These barriers include delay in individual decision-making to seek care, delay in identifying and getting to a health facility, and delay in obtaining adequate care after arriving at the facility. According to Thaddeus and Maine, delay in seeking care focuses on the individual, the family, or both. The factors that shape the decision-making process at the household level include the actors involved in decision-making, the health status of the woman, the distance from the health facility, the financial and opportunity costs, previous experiences with the healthcare system, and the perceived quality of care. Delay in reaching an appropriate and adequate health facility, on the other hand, focuses on physical accessibility factors. These include the way in which health facilities are distributed in the area (distance), the travel distance from the home to a health facility, the availability and cost of transportation, and the infrastructure (i.e., road condition). Delay in receiving adequate care at the health facility, the third form of delay, focuses on shortages of supplies and equipment, lack of trained and competent personnel, and inadequacy of the referral system. The three phases of delay are closely connected. The barriers and poor care encountered in reaching and receiving care feed back into subsequent decision-making in regard to seeking care, producing a series of potentially life-threatening delays. The three delays model was used in the present study to explore social economic and healthcare experiences that women perceived to cause the occurrence of fistula in the three phases of seeking birth care. There was a specific focus on decision-making before arrival at a health facility, the barriers to reaching health facilities, and the barriers to getting access to adequate care in health facilities.

The concept of *availability, accessibility, acceptability,* and *quality of care* (AAAQ) (UN Committee on Economic. Social and Cultural Rights (CESCR), 2000) was used to explore the birth care experiences of women who developed obstetric fistula after prolonged labor. The AAAQ concept operationalizes the right to health in terms of the concept's four components. It asserts that if the right to health is to be realized, AAAQ must be ensured at all levels of care. Adequate health infrastructure and services must be *available* within a geographic area. Health facilities should be *accessible* physically and economically, especially for members of the most vulnerable and disadvantaged sections of the population, such as women and children. *Acceptability* requires health facilities to be respectful of medical ethics, culturally appropriate, and gender-sensitive. Therefore, healthcare workers need to be aware of cultural sensitivities in the provision of health care. The *quality of health care* is a decisive factor. Health facilities must be scientifically and medically appropriate and be of adequate medical quality. Failure to ensure AAAQ of emergency obstetric care (EmOC) will result in delays in getting access to adequate health care, which can be fatal (Physicians for Human Rights, 2007).

13.3 The Context and Design

The study was conducted at the Comprehensive Community Based Rehabilitation Tanzania (CCBRT) hospital in Dar es Salaam and Bugando Medical Centre (BMC) in Mwanza regions (Fig. 13.1). The choice to conduct the study in these areas was influenced by both ethical and practical considerations. The BMC and CCBRT hospitals are the major service points for fistula surgery, with higher fistula repair rates than are found at health facilities elsewhere in the country (Bangser, 2002). Selection of these settings ensured access to an adequate number of women affected by fistula. The CCRBT hospital is a private non-governmental organization (NGO) and a major service delivery point for obstetric fistula repair, and about 200 VVF and RVF operations are performed there each year. BMC is a consultant and teaching hospital that has 900 beds and a special ward dedicated to fistula repair and recovery, with a capacity of 70 beds. On average, more than 300 women with obstetric fistula are treated annually at BMC.

A mixed-method research design (Creswell, 2003; Leech & Onwuegbuzie, 2009) was used. A mixed-method research design involves collecting, analyzing, and interpreting both qualitative and quantitative data in a single study. Specifically, a *partial mixed concurrent dominant status design* (Fig. 13.2) was used (Leech & Onwuegbuzie, 2009). In this type of design, both qualitative and quantitative data are collected at approximately the same time. The dominant method in the present study was qualitative. The challenges of obstetric fistula are highly complex, and a combination of qualitative and quantitative methods was considered appropriate to gaining an understanding of the perceptions and experiences of girls and women affected by fistula. This approach offered several advantages, not the least of which was that it would generate different perspectives on the causes of obstetric fistula from the women affected by obstetric fistula that had both depth and breadth.

A qualitative triangulation research design was used to enhance the validity of the data by triangulating various approaches to form a more complete picture of the issue under study. Ascertaining the complementarity of various data sources can enable researchers to expose multiple dimensions of the same research issue and thereby increase their level of understanding (Leech & Onwuegbuzie, 2009).

Fig. 13.1 Map of
Tanzania showing
Mwanza and Dar es
Salaam. (Source: Central
Intelligence Agency,
2021)

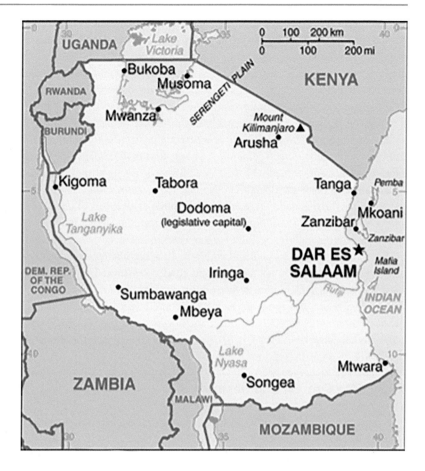

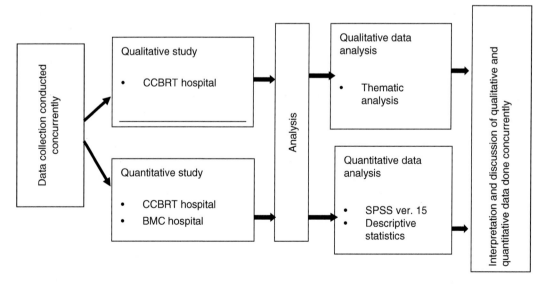

Fig. 13.2 Partial mixed concurrent dominant status design

13.4   Participants and Data Collection

Following the ethical approval from the Institutional Review Board of Muhimbili University of Health and Allied Sciences (MUHAS) and permission to conduct the study in the CCBRT and BMC, all women affected by obstetric fistula admitted to hospitals were asked to participate in the study. Participants were informed about the purpose of the study, voluntary nature of participation, and about issues of confidentiality. Those who met the inclusion criteria, agreed to take part in the study and gave written consent, were enrolled. The inclusion criteria to participate in the study were girls and women who were: (a) affected by obstetric fistula, (b) had been admitted to hospital for fistula repair either before or after an initial surgical fistula repair, (c) were Kiswahili speakers, and (d) and had agreed to participate in the study. With recognition of the potential bias of convenience sampling (Buetow, 2010), this strategy was nonetheless chosen for time and cost reasons. The strategy made it possible to obtain an adequate number of participants during the study period, and thus obtain useful data and information. Senior nurses with experience in health research assisted in the identification of the women who met the inclusion criteria. Before the study, the researchers explained to the participants the purpose, method, and procedures of the study including the aspect of confidentiality.

Semi-structured individual interviews (Kvale, 1996) were conducted with 16 women affected by obstetric fistula, either before or after surgical fistula repair. This permitted face-to-face interviews with women affected by obstetric fistula that was conducted to explore their perceptions of what caused their fistula. Given the exploratory nature of the present study, semi-structured interviews helped to draw out contextual and descriptive information and allowed informants to identify issues they encountered during labor and birth from their own perspectives. The individual face-to-face interviews were conducted in Kiswahili, the national language of Tanzania. The semi-structured interview guide based on pre-prepared topics (Dahlgren et al., 2004) was used, in which questions were revised through several rounds during the interview process to ensure that emergent themes are captured. The interview guide explored the details of the problem of fistula in relation to participants' perceptions of the causes of obstetric fistula. In each interview, the informant was the major speaker, and the researcher was mainly a guide and a facilitator. The level of openness of the interviewees varied but was generally good. Field notes on signs of emotion and interactions during the interviews were taken and were considered during the analysis phase. All interviews were audio-recorded with the permission of the participants and the duration of the interview ranged from 45 to 120 min.

A semi-structured questionnaire was used to assess the sociodemographic characteristics of the women, as well as the women's experiences pertaining to the pregnancy, labor, and delivery that led to fistula. Prior to the main study, the questionnaire was translated from English to Kiswahili and pilot-tested at Muhimbili National Hospital; questions that seemed ambiguous were revised accordingly. For the main study, all women admitted to the fistula wards at the CCBRT and BMC hospitals during the quantitative data collection period were asked to participate in the study. Only those who provided written informed consent were recruited, and there were no women who refused to participate. As a result, 151 women were enrolled. Two trained research assistants (a senior nurse midwife and a nurse teacher), both with experience in health research, collected data using closed-ended questionnaires.

13.5   Data Analysis

Thematic analysis (Braun & Clarke, 2006) was employed during the analysis of data acquired through semi-structured interviews. The actual process did not emerge as different from qualitative content analysis frameworks; it involved the grouping of data into themes created from recurring codes, which were similar or connected to each other (Buetow, 2010). The analysis involved five major steps:

becoming familiar with the data, generating initial codes, searching for themes, revising the themes, and defining and naming themes. This method of analysis does not consider salient codes that do not recur; however, as recently documented by Buetow (2010), the mere recurrence of codes is not necessarily a sufficient indication of their importance. In the present study, all codes and themes that captured important aspects in relation to the overall research question were considered. The thematic analysis followed specific steps, as described in the sections that follow.

Familiarization with the Data This stage started during data collection. It was important to become familiar with the material while working in the field; questions that did not seem to explore much information from the informants were revised, and new questions that emerged from the data were added for further exploration. Details of the content of the material were discussed with the research team after each interview. Therefore, post-field analysis involved reading repeatedly through the field notes of the collected material. A research assistant was hired to transcribe the 16 audio-recorded interviews. The researcher (the present author) read all 16 transcripts while comparing them with the audio-recorded interviews. This was an important step for a systematic immersion in the data.

Generating Initial Codes This stage of analysis began with familiarization of the data as described in the previous stage. This stage entailed re-reading the text and coding the material. In each transcript, a column was created where codes identified in the transcript were recorded regardless of how many times these codes emerged. All codes identified from the interview transcripts of the women affected by obstetric fistula on their perceived causes of obstetric fistula were then listed. Although this list of initial codes was long and unorganized, it was a first attempt at noting the main topics and themes that had emerged from the interviews with the women and the discussions with husbands and community members.

Searching for Themes The list of codes was revised and organized, and furthermore nuanced lists were created. A table that had three columns was created in which the left column had a list of codes that were organized according to how the codes connected to each other. In the middle column was a list of major themes and in the right column the relevant quotes. During the process, related pieces of text were highlighted, and then pasted under relevant themes. This stage involved both creating and increasing the number of nuanced codes and collating those that were considered similar.

Reviewing and Defining the Themes The objective of this stage was to have each theme explain perception and to identify the essence of what each identified theme was all about (interpretation). This process involved all members of the research team, who read the themes to generate concise and clear names for each theme.

The Statistical Package for the Social Sciences (SPSS) version 15 for Microsoft Windows was used to analyze the quantitative data. Descriptive analysis was performed where frequencies and proportions were used to summarize results. Findings from the quantitative data were used for triangulation and to broaden understanding of the perceptions of causes of obstetric fistula from the affected women.

13.6 Findings and Discussions

13.6.1 Characteristics of the Participants

The sixteen women who were interviewed about their perceptions of the causes of their fistula described themselves as peasants ($n = 13$), petty business persons ($n = 2$), or homemakers ($n = 1$). They varied between 18 and 43 years of age; seven were either divorced or separated; five were married and four were single. Fourteen (88%) of the participants were from remote rural areas, seven (44%) lived with fistula for more than 6 years, four were illiterate, and only two (12.5%) had education beyond primary school. The age distribution of the 151 hospitalized women affected by obstetric fistula recruited in a survey ranged from 16 to 72. Descriptive statistics of the sample is presented in Table 13.1.

Table 13.1 Characteristics of the study participants in the survey

Factors	Number	Frequencies (%)
Age at interview		
<18	21	13.9
18–20	25	16.6
21–30	59	39.1
31–40	32	21.2
>40	14	9.3
Total	151	100.0
Education level		
Illiterate	48	31.8
Primary school	99	65.6
Secondary school and above	4	2.6
Total	151	100.0
Marital status		
Married	98	64.9
Single	24	15.9
Divorced	27	17.9
Widowed	2	1.3
Total	151	100.0
With whom do you live		
Husband/partner	90	42.7
Parents	35	16.6
In-laws	11	5.2
Children	33	15.6
Relatives	35	16.6
Alone	7	3.3
Total	211	100.0
Age at first delivery		
<18	62	41.1
18–20	40	26.5
21–30	44	29.1
>30	1	0.7
Missing data	4	2.6
Total	151	100.0
Parity when fistula occurred		
First	84	55.6
Second	18	11.9
Third	13	8.6
Fourth	14	9.3
Fifth and above	22	14.6
Total	151	100.0
Lived with fistula		
<1 year	86	57.0
1–2 years	28	18.5
3–6 years	17	11.3
>6 years	20	13.2
Total	151	100.0

Fig. 13.3 Themes of socioeconomic and healthcare causes of obstetric fistula

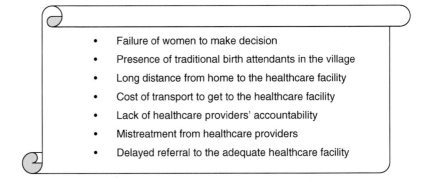

- Failure of women to make decision
- Presence of traditional birth attendants in the village
- Long distance from home to the healthcare facility
- Cost of transport to get to the healthcare facility
- Lack of healthcare providers' accountability
- Mistreatment from healthcare providers
- Delayed referral to the adequate healthcare facility

In the analysis of the perception and views of women affected by obstetric fistula about the cause of their fistula, it was realized that women could not identify the real cause of their fistulas, but attributed their experiences of labor and delivery as the reason for the fistula occurrence. From their descriptions, 7 themes emerged (Fig. 13.3).

13.6.2 Failure of Women to Make Decisions

There are cultural restrictions that prevent women from taking full advantage of the reproductive health services that are available. Sociocultural aspects may contribute to women's lack of power to make decisions about their reproductive health concerns (Chapagain, 2006). For example, decisions such as when a woman should start bearing children, when to seek medical care, and where to go in times of illness and childbirth are often made by husbands or other family members, not by the woman herself (Chapagain, 2006; Kuponiyi & Alade, 2007). Women are less likely to make independent decisions on family size, child spacing, family planning, and childbirth, especially if they are first-time mothers or pregnant teenagers who already have one or more children. Most of the women would like to give birth in a health facility. However, because of their economic and social power, decisions concerning where to go to seek birth care are commonly made by others and not by the woman herself. These findings are similar to the study done in Zambia (Sialubanje et al., 2015), in which 70% of the decisions on where birth care should be sought were made by husbands. Among 151 women affected by obstetric fistula surveyed in this study, only 7% of the women decided by themselves, while the husband and in-laws, mostly mothers-in-law made the decision in 60% of the cases. Women also reported that their husbands and mothers-in-law were inclined to prefer home delivery for a number of reasons including convenience, custom, and cost. Many of the women had to accept giving birth at home because they did not have money of their own to cover the expenses for a health facility delivery. Women who depended on their husband's consent to deliver in a health facility had to wait for him to return from other chores before a final decision on the birthplace could be reached. If he was not available, no one could make the decision. As one of the women explained:

> I planned to deliver at the hospital, but it was not possible because I did not have cash and I did not know where I will get money from. It was January, during the farming season, I did not go to the field, my husband went, I did not go, and it was then that I got these problems.

13.6.3 Presence of Traditional Birth Attendants in the Village

In many places, home birth is customary. Participants' grandmothers and mothers had given birth at home and considered home birth to be normal and safe. Furthermore, their close kin commonly knew traditional birth attendants (TBAs) and had great faith in their delivery skills. The World Health

Organization (WHO) has defined TBAs as persons who assist the mothers during childbirth and learns their skills through apprenticeship that involves both observation and imitation, and are often highly regarded by the community that chooses them to assist women in childbirth (World Health Organization, UNICEF,, and United Nations Population Fund, 1992). Studies in developing countries have reported that women commonly give birth in homes because of the effectiveness and acceptability of TBAs in the community provided the impetus for many women to give birth at home (Central Statistics Office, Ministry of Health, Tropical Disease Research Centre, Univerity of Zambia, Macro International Inc, 2009; Miller et al., 2012; Ministry of Health and Social Welfare, 2011; Nyamtema et al., 2011; Titaley et al., 2010). Shortages of skilled personnel in the health facilities may contribute to home deliveries by TBAs. For example, in Tanzania, the proportion of births attended by skilled attendants is still low—only 51% (National Bureau of Statistics and ICF Macro, 2011), indicating that many women give birth at home with the assistance of TBAs or relatives. In this present study 15% of women gave birth at home, and of these 5% were assisted by TBAs. Despite the faith women have on traditional birth attendants some blamed the TBAs for their birth injuries:

> My parents said I should wait as I could deliver at home. (…) you know in the village people do deliver in homes (…) in our village, there is a TBA, she is the one who harmed us.

> (…) my mother told my uncle that I am sick, and then he said that she (mother) has to call the traditional birth attendant

Many women preferred to be assisted by TBAs for a variety of reasons that were not available in the healthcare facilities. For example, women reported that TBAs do more than providing delivery services—they support and relate with women in the community long before, during, and after their pregnancies. TBAs provide women with information on contraceptives as well as regarding postnatal care. They assist in obtaining a birth certificate for their babies (Izugbara et al., 2009). Other studies have confirmed that mothers felt that TBA services were useful (Moindi et al., 2016). Traditional birth attendants provide psychosocial support and, important in multilingual societies, speak the local language (Sparks, 1990). Therefore, the presence of TBAs, the great faith that women had in these attendants, and the combined experiences of grandmothers and mothers with home delivery all appeared to be important factors that influenced the decision to have a home delivery. Many women did not seek adequate birth care in the health facilities because they resented the humiliation to which they were being subjected by healthcare providers. To prevent obstetric fistula, the WHO recommends the use of the partograph to monitor women's progress of labor and timely decision-making in case of an obstructed labor (Mwangi & Warren, 2008). This is not possible if women choose to labor at home (WHO, 1994). When women try to labor at home unsuccessfully, they are more likely to come to the hospital at a late stage because of the long distance they must travel to get to the equipped health facility.

13.6.4 Long Distance from Home to the Healthcare Facility

Consistent with the study in Southern Tanzania by Kazaura et al. (2011) and other investigators (Moindi et al., 2016; Pettersson et al., 2004), many people lived far from where health facilities were located. Therefore, once the decision to seek care for a delivery in a health facility was made, many women were delayed in getting there because of long distances to travel, unavailability of public transport, and failure to meet transportation cost, causing the laboring women to spend a long time on the road (Kulmala, 2000; Shrestha et al., 2012). In this study, only 49% of women affected by obstetric fistula arrived at the healthcare facility where they had a delivery within 2 days; one-half of them (51%) arrived after two or more days of laboring at home. Among the 151 women who were affected by obstetric fistula, 43% reported to have been traveling by public transport while 20% reported that they had walked or been carried to the health facility. Most of the women affected by obstetric fistula lived in remote rural areas, and not all villages were privileged to have a health facility nearby:

> In our village there is no dispensary and there was no transport, we had to walk for three hours to get to the Hospital. I had very strong labor pains and after about two hours walk, I felt like something had ruptured in the womb. I started bleeding and we had to stop and rest before I could manage to continue walking.

Other women were stuck at home because there was no transport available:

> (…) from our village to hospital is 24 km, is very far, and there was no means of transport. Therefore, when labor pains started, everybody was confused because I could not walk, and there was no means of transport to take me to the Hospital. I therefore remained at home.

Interventions such as "waiting homes" to accommodate the expectant mothers residing far from the nearest health facilities for days leading up to their labor can be helpful in ensuring that women get timely skilled assistance (Abebe et al., 2012). Although the Tanzanian Government provides birth care free of charge at all public and private healthcare facilities at all levels (Ministry of Health and Social Welfare, 2006), having access to these facilities by women can be limited.

13.6.5 Cost of Transport to the Healthcare Facilities

Public transport in many rural areas of Tanzania is limited, and where available, women have to pay to reach the antenatal clinic (ANC) or hospital for obstetric services. In these rural settings, transportation expenses are too costly for an ordinary peasant family to afford. Studies have shown that all women wished to give birth in a health facility, but had to accept giving birth at home because they did not have money to cover transportation cost. Sometimes women and/or their families had raised the necessary cash by obtaining donations, selling family property, or borrowing money. Therefore, women needed cash to be able to travel to access both ANC and obstetric services.

> (...) you cannot walk, you have to take a bus, and the bus fare is 5500 shillings (3 USD) and if you are two it will be 11,000/ = (6 USD)

> I planned to give birth in the facility but because of cash, fare I was unable. (…) not only that, because for food (…) I had pounded and was waiting to mill (…) then my spouse said he did not secured money

> I was asked to deliver at the hospital, but it was not possible because I did not have cash and I did not know where I would get the money to go there. As peasants, our income as you know are very little (…) we did not have money

> (…) labor pains started while I was at home which is far, (…) there were no means of transport, even bicycles or push carts. (…) it was not possible for me to walk to the hospital when the baby's head was already protruding out

13.6.6 Lack of Healthcare Provider Accountability

Immediate and skilled care during labor and delivery is crucial for the safety of future mothers and their newborns, because life-threatening obstetrical complications are largely unpredictable and can occur very quickly (Schwartz, 2015). In Tanzania, health system utilization for essential maternal health services is still low, with the very lowest coverage among the poor. Estimates indicate that around 50% of births in Tanzania occur in health facilities; among these only 51% receive skilled care (National Bureau of Statistics and ICF Macro, 2011). Studies in Tanzania (Mrisho et al., 2007; Women's Dignity Project, Engender Health, 2006) and elsewhere (Bell et al., 2003; Nathan et al., 2009; Schwartz, 2015) have demonstrated that even after women arrive early in the health facility, still they are not assured of receiving adequate obstetric care. This is due to institutional factors including staff competence and lack of staff managerial support. Women affected by obstetric fistula attributed their fistula problem to the nonaccountability of nurses because they were not available to monitor the progress of their labor. Women felt that had nurses been attentive and had they received the necessary help, they would not have ended up developing fistula.

> (…) the day when I had labor pains, a nurse was not there (…) the baby's head was already out (…). I think if a nurse was around I would not have ended with this problem, and if they would have failed, they could have taken me to theatre many hours earlier

Women perceived that their fistula was a result of nurses' negligence. They believed that if a nurse did not personally know them, or if they were unable to give money to health providers they would not receive better treatment and prompt assistance. The following accounts from women illustrate this:

> If a nurse or a doctor knows you, or if you have money to give them, you will receive very good service but if you do not, you suffer (…). They need to take care of patients without nepotism…I think this is the result of negligence

Another woman lamented:

> (…) the reason I got fistula I see is nurses' negligence

The experience of women with healthcare provider's negligence and nepotism reported in this study corroborates findings from other researchers (Asuquo et al., 2000; Bangser et al., 2011). In these studies, a large number of women reported experiences of neglect by doctors and nurses who were on duty, who only gave their attention to friends and relatives or those they had seen privately. During interviews the perception of nurses' negligence was reiterated when one woman said:

> I think nurses contribute to the development of fistula. (...) they keep you waiting for so long in labor without making any decision of taking you to theatre for operation.

13.6.7 Mistreatment by the Healthcare Provider

Skilled attendance at birth is considered to be the most critical intervention for ensuring safety of both the baby and the expectant mother. It helps to ensure the timely delivery of emergency obstetric and new-born care when life-threatening complications arise. Skilled attendance denotes not only the presence of skilled midwives with right attitude to perform midwifery work, but also an enabling environment (Graham & Hussein, 2007). Women in the study did not describe these qualities to be present among midwives who provided their care. Poor assessment of the progress of labor and lack of supportive care were among the experiences that women encountered during labor. Women reported being left alone screaming with pain and without consistent assessment of their progress of labor. Other women reported being left alone halfway through labor, and some were left to give birth unaided and unsupervised. Other women reported experiences of being beaten by the midwives who were assisting them during delivery. For these women, such unethical and unprofessional acts were responsible for the development of their fistula:

> (…) I think it is because of torture from nurses while they were trying to assist me during delivery, they beat me around the waist while others were pulling my legs and I was tired

A study in Tanzania has reported that midwives had to sometimes scold and slap women during delivery to "pressurize" them through labor and ensure that the baby was delivered safely—they performed these acts to avoid punishment from the administration over the birth of the dead baby (Mselle et al., 2013). This example illustrates the poor access to quality obstetric care for women in Tanzania. This is of critical importance, as having access to skilled obstetric care has been identified as a major condition to lower maternal morbidity and mortality (WHO, UNFPA, UNICEF,, & AMDD, 2009). It is commonly expected that upon reaching a health facility, women will receive quality and safe obstetric care from skilled providers (Graham et al., 2001; World Health Organization, 2005). When these expectations are unmet, women usually lose trust in the healthcare system and resort to seeking unskilled obstetric care (Mrisho et al., 2007). Women may avoid a nearby health facility and instead seek care at one that is far away if it is perceived to provide better services (Olsen et al., 2005; Physicians for Human Rights, 2007), contributing to delays. The actions of healthcare providers are often more important for patient satisfaction than is the hospital's physical environment. The experiences of women with negligence, nepotism, delays, and torture by healthcare providers contribute to poor access of skilled obstetric care in the health facility (Otis & Brett, 2008), thus denying women their rights to obstetric care (Physicians for Human Rights, 2007).

13.6.8 Delayed Referral to an Adequate Healthcare Facility

The availability and access to emergence obstetric care (EmOC) is important in ensuring prompt treatment of pregnancy- and labor-related complications, and is key in both improving maternal outcome (Graham & Hussein, 2007), attaining Sustainable Development Goals (SDG) 3 and 5 to ensure healthy lives and promote well-being for all at all ages, and to achieve gender equality and empower all girls and women (Switzerland Government, 2018; United Nations, 2015). To facilitate access to quality primary and reproductive health care for all Tanzanians as stipulated in its national health policy (Ministry of Health, 2003), the Government has extended basic healthcare infrastructure into peripheral rural areas, where the majority of people reside. The health system is organized in a referral pyramid, starting from dispensaries at the bottom and rural health centers (RHCs) that provide Basic Emergency Obstetric Care (BEmOC) and treatment of minor conditions. At the district level, there are district hospitals at the first referral level where necessary drugs, equipment, and skilled staff are available to provide comprehensive emergency obstetric care (CEmOC) that includes basic emergence care (parenteral antibiotics, oxytocic drugs and anticonvulsants for pregnancy-induced hypertension) and also performing cesarean section and blood transfusion. There are also regional hospitals in each region, with the highest level being national and specialized hospitals (Ministry of Health and Social Welfare, 2006). Obstetric care is provided at all levels of health facilities depending on the needs (i.e., BEmOC or CEmOC) of the woman. In 2008 as much as 72% of the Tanzanian population lived within 5 km, and 93% within 10 km, of a healthcare facility (Ministry of Health and Social Welfare, 2008).

WHO estimates indicate that approximately 15% of all pregnant women will develop pregnancy- and childbirth-related complications that require access to first referral care (WHO, 1996). The use of partograph could facilitate timely detection of difficult labor and an early referral decision to a facility providing EmOC, thus preventing obstructed labor and thereby preventing obstetric fistula (Mwangi & Warren, 2008). In Africa, unfortunately, lack of knowledge on the use of partograph, non-availability of a partograph, and shortage of midwives with the appropriate attitude (Qureshi et al., 2010; Yisma et al., 2013) prevent many women from accessing adequate obstetric care.

A woman with prolonged obstructed labor due to cephalo-pelvic disproportion (CPD) will definitely require immediate cesarean section (Neilson et al., 2003) in a health facility offering CEmOC. In such situations, accessing a health facility providing EmOC is critical. However, to evaluate an obstructed labor that would require surgical intervention, midwives must provide close and skillful monitoring of a woman's progress of labor. In our study, women perceived a failure to foresee obstacles to normal delivery and late referral that extended from dispensaries to health facilities providing CEmOC as major causes of their fistulas:

> I was in labor for a long time while in the hospital. Labor pains comes and goes and each time when you call nurses tells you that you should wait though I had very strong pains. I didnt see the reason as to why I could not be sent for operation early (…). I think nurses contributed to my problem.

Another woman had this to say:

> (…) I was delayed to be transferred to the main hospital. If I was referred early perhaps, they could have done an operation and get my baby and I would not have ended up with all these problems

Effective communication between patients and healthcare providers is key to all clinical care, particularly in the case of maternity services. It becomes effective only if the relevant information is made available to, and understood by, those who need to act on it (The King's Fund, 2008). Therefore, each healthcare provider should possess the skills necessary to promote effective communications. Failure of healthcare providers to communicate the poor progress of labor to pregnant women so that they could reallocate to an adequate healthcare facility was perceived as a cause of fistula:

> If I was informed early about the problem, my family could take me to a big hospital for operation (…).

> (…) the problem was that doctors did not tell me early about the problem I was having for me to move on to another hospital.

Other women who stayed in labor for a long time without being referred for adequate care commented:

> I went to the dispensary early in the morning just after labor started. I was in labor until at around 2 pm when the membranes ruptured, still I was told to wait. Until on the next day at 2 am is when they tranfered me to another hospital for operation! That is how I lost my baby and got fistula.

Even women who had been previously informed of the importance of having a cesarean section in their subsequent pregnancy because of a history of CPD were unnecessarily made to wait for treatment by healthcare providers:

> I was already in hospital for 9 days when labor started. I was previously told that since I had rupture of uterus, in the next pregnancy I should attend to the health facility early for operation. I was in labor for 12 h and each time I reminded nurses to send me for operation. However, 'They kept on telling me that there was no problem'. When the doctor came the next day, he asked nurses, 'why didn't you call me early?' You have delayed this woman, and now the baby is already dead.

In a study by Kazaura et al. (2011), perceived health system causes of obstetric fistula reported perforation of the urinary bladder when doctors performed delivery by operation or nurses when removing the urinary catheter. Women in this study did not report these findings. Similar findings were noted elsewhere (Hassan & Ekele, 2009; Neilson et al., 2003; Suellen et al., 2005), where prolonged labor due to big babies was perceived by women to cause fistula:

> The delivery was difficulty because the baby was big, and that was the cause for this problem (…)

13.7 Conclusions

In this study, women's perceptions on the socioeconomic and healthcare-related causes of obstetric fistula reflect their experiences of delays in not only receiving adequate and timely birth care, but also receiving poor quality obstetric care from healthcare providers at multiple levels of healthcare facilities. Women's limited decision-making power, lack of money, long distances to the health facilities, and provision of incompetent care all contribute to delays in accessing and receiving adequate maternity care. This study highlights significant gaps in the healthcare provisions as illustrated by birth care experiences of Tanzanian women affected by obstetric fistula, and it calls for a policy that will consider realistic local deficiencies in the provision of timely and competent maternal health care. One such measure would possibly be the training of community midwives to work in the community and support the available dispensaries and health centers that are close to the majority of people in the rural areas. Although the Tanzanian government is striving to bring many women to give birth in health facilities, there is a need for the government to ensure that women who manage to get to the health facility for obstetric care receive adequate care consistent with their expectations. With the governmental efforts to provide health facilities with equipment, materials, and supplies and increasing staffing levels, it should also implement mechanisms that will make health providers accountable for their work and also to assume personal responsibility in case of fault. Improper conduct by healthcare providers during the provision of obstetric care and the occurrence of acts of obstetric violence breach the code of ethical conduct, grounded in the philosophical ethical principle of fidelity and respect for dignity, worth, and self-determination of persons. Feedback mechanisms by women, through exit reflections or others, should be a requirement. Such feedback would assist the health facility in improving the quality of obstetric care, and consequently assist the Government to meet its national health policy on improving access to reproductive and maternal health care and make a necessary step toward the achievement of the Sustainable Development Goals (SDG) 3 and 5 of ensuring healthy lives and promoting well-being for all at all ages and to achieve gender equality and empowering all girls and women.

Acknowledgments This study was supported by Gender, Generation and Social Mobilization (GeSoMo) – NUFU Project.

References

Abebe, F., Berhane, Y., & Girma, B. (2012). Factors associated with home delivery in Bahirdar, Ethiopia: A case control study. *BMC Research Notes, 5*, 653. https://doi.org/10.1186/1756-0500-5-653

Asuquo, E., Etuk, S., & Duke, F. (2000). Staff attitude as a barrier to the utilisation of University of Calabar Teaching Hospital for obstetric care. *African Journal of Reproductive Health, 4*(2), 69–73. https://doi.org/10.4314/ajrh.v4i2.7711

Bangser, M. (2002). Tanzania fistula survey 2001. Ministry of Health.

Bangser, M. (2006). Obstetric fistula and stigma. *Lancet, 367*(9509), 535–536. https://doi.org/10.1016/S0140-6736(06)68188-9

Bangser, M., Mehta, M., Singer, J., Daly, C., Kamugumya, C., & Mwangomale, A. (2011). Childbirth experiences of women with obstetric fistula in Tanzania and Uganda and their implications for fistula program development. *International Urogynecology Journal and Pelvic Floor Dysfunction, 22*(1), 91–98. https://doi.org/10.1007/s00192-010-1236-8

Bell, J., Hussein, J., Jentsch, B., Scotland, G., Bullough, C., & Graham, W. (2003). Improving skilled attendance at delivery: A preliminary report of the SAFE strategy development tool. *Birth, 30*(4), 227–234. https://doi.org/10.1046/j.1523-536X.2003.00252.x

Braun, V., & Clarke, V. (2006). Using thematic analysis in psychology. *Qualitative Research in Psychology, 3*(2), 77–101. https://doi.org/10.1191/1478088706qp063oa

Buetow, S. (2010). Thematic analysis and its reconceptualization as "saliency analysis". *Journal of Health Services Research & Policy, 15*(2), 123–125. https://doi.org/10.1258/jhsrp.2009.009081

Central Intelligence Agency. (2021). *Tanzania map showing major cities as well as parts of surrounding countries and the Indian Ocean. The World Factbook.* Central Intelligence Agency.

Central Statistics Office, Ministry of Health, Tropical Disease Research Centre, Univerity of Zambia, Macro International Inc. (2009). *Zambia demographic and health survey, 2007.* CSO and Macro International Inc.

Chapagain, M. (2006). Conjugal power relations and couples' participation in reproductive health decision-making: Exploring the links in Nepal. *Gender, Technology and Development, 10*(2), 159–189. https://doi.org/10.1177/097185240601000201

Cook, R. J., Dickens, B. M., & Syed, S. (2004). Obstetric fistula: The challenge to human rights. *International Journal of Gynecology & Obstetrics, 87*(1), 72–77. https://doi.org/10.1016/j.ijgo.2004.07.005

Creswell, J. W. (2003). *Research design: Qualitative, quantitative and mixed methods approaches.* Sage.

Dahlgren, L., Emmelin, M., & Winkvist, A. (2004). *Qualitative methodology for international public health.* Umeå University.

Danso, K. A., Martey, J. O., Wall, L. L., & Elkins, T. E. (1996). The epidemiology of genitourinary fistulae in Kumasi, Ghana, 1977-1992. *International Urogynecology Journal and Pelvic Floor Dysfunction, 7*(3), 117–120. https://doi.org/10.1007/BF01894198

Danso, K. A., Opare-Addo, H. S., & Turpin, C. A. (2007). Obstetric fistula admissions at Komfo Anokye Teaching Hospital, Kumasi, Ghana. *International Journal of Gynecology & Obstetrics, 99*(1), 69–70. https://doi.org/10.1016/j.ijgo.2007.06.029

Donnay, F., & Ramsey, K. (2006). Eliminating obstetric fistula: Progress in partnerships. *International Journal of Gynecology & Obstetrics, 94*(3), 254–261. https://doi.org/10.1016/j.ijgo.2006.04.005

Elneil, S., & Browning, A. (2009). Obstetric fistula- A new way forward. *BJOG : An International Journal of Obstetrics and Gynaecology, 116*(1), 30–32. https://doi.org/10.1111/j.1471-0528.2009.02309.x

Gharoro, E. P., & Agholor, K. N. (2009). Aspects of psychosocial problems of patients with vesico-vaginal fistula. *Journal of Obstetrics and Gynaecology: The Journal of the Institute of Obstetrics and Gynaecology, 29*(7), 644–647. https://doi.org/10.1080/01443610903100609

Graham, W. J., Bell, J. S., & Bullough, C. H. W. (2001). Can skilled attendance at delivery reduce maternal mortality in developing countries ? In V. De Brouwere & W. Van Lerberghe (Eds.), *Safe motherhood strategies: A review of the evidence* (pp. 97–129). University of Aberdeen. https://doi.org/10.1186/s12939-016-0408-7

Graham, W. J., & Hussein, J. (2007). Minding the gaps: A reassessment of the challenges to safe motherhood. *American Journal of Public Health, 97*(6), 978–983. https://doi.org/10.2105/AJPH.2005.073692

Hassan, M. A., & Ekele, B. A. (2009). Vesicovaginal fistula: Do the patients know the cause? *Annals of African Medicine, 8*(2), 122–126. https://doi.org/10.4103/1596-3519.56241

Hill, K., Thomas, K., AbouZahr, C., Walker, N., Say, L., Inoue, M., & Suzuki, E. (2007). Estimates of maternal mortality worldwide between 1990 and 2005: An assessment of available data. *Lancet, 370*(9595), 1311–1319. https://doi.org/10.1016/S0140-6736(07)61572-4

Hilton, P. (2003). Vesico-vaginal fistulas in developing countries. *International Journal of Gynecology & Obstetrics, 82*(3), 285–295.

INFO Project. (2004). *Obstetric fistula: Ending the silence, easing the suffering.* INFO Project.

Izugbara, C., Ezeh, A., & Fotso, J. C. (2009). The persistence and challenges of homebirths: Perspectives of traditional birth attendants in urban Kenya. *Health Policy and Planning, 24*(1), 36–45. https://doi.org/10.1093/heapol/czn042

Kazaura, M. R., Kamazima, R. S., & Mangi, E. J. (2011). Perceived causes of obstetric fistulae from rural southern Tanzania. *African Health Sciences, 11*(3), 377–382.

Kulmala, T. (2000). *Maternal health and pregnancy outcomes in rural malawi maternal health and pregnancy outcomes in rural malawi.* University of Tampere.

Kuponiyi, F. A., & Alade, O. A. (2007). Gender dynamics and reproduction decision making among rural families in Orire Local Government Area of Oyo State, Nigeria. *Journal of Social Sciences, 15*(2), 101–104. https://doi.org/10.1080/09718923.2007.11892568

Kvale, S. (1996). *Interviews: An introduction to qualitative research interviews* (2nd ed.). Longman.

Leech, N. L., & Onwuegbuzie, A. J. (2009). A typology of mixed methods research designs. *Quality and Quantity, 43*(2), 265–275. https://doi.org/10.1007/s11135-007-9105-3

Majinge, C. R. (1995). Successful management of vesicovaginal fistula at St Gaspar Hospital Itigi, Singida, Tanzania: A preliminary report. *East African Medical Journal, 72,* 121–123.

Miller, P. C., Rashida, G., Tasneem, Z., & Haque, M. U. (2012). The effect of traditional birth attendant training on maternal and neonatal care. *International Journal of Gynecology & Obstetrics, 117*(2), 148–152. https://doi.org/10.1016/j.ijgo.2011.12.020

Ministry of Health. (2003). *National health policy.* Ministry of Health.

Ministry of Health and Social Welfare. (2006). *Tanzania service availability mapping 2005-2006.* Ministry of Health and Social Welfare.

Ministry of Health and Social Welfare. (2008). *Human resource for health strategic plan 2008 – 2013.* Ministry of Health and Social Welfare.

Ministry of Health and Social Welfare. (2011). *National postpartum care guideline.* Ministry of Health and Social Welfare.

Moindi, R. O., Ngari, M. M., Nyambati, V. C. S., & Mbakaya, C. (2016). Why mothers still deliver at home: Understanding factors associated with home deliveries and cultural practices in rural coastal Kenya, a cross-section study Global health. *BMC Public Health, 16*(1), 1–8. https://doi.org/10.1186/s12889-016-2780-z

Mrisho, M., Schellenberg, J. A., Mushi, A. K., Obrist, B., Mshinda, H., Tanner, M., & Schellenberg, D. (2007). Factors affecting home delivery in rural Tanzania. *Tropical Medicine and International Health, 12*(7), 862–872. https://doi.org/10.1111/j.1365-3156.2007.01855.x

Mselle, L. T., Evjen-Olsen, B., Moland, K. M., Mvungi, A., & Kohi, T. W. (2012). "Hoping for a normal life again": Reintegration after fistula repair in rural Tanzania. *Journal of Obstetrics and Gynaecology Canada, 34*(10), 927–938.

Mselle, L. T., & Kohi, T. W. (2015). Living with constant leaking of urine and odour: Thematic analysis of socio-cultural experiences of women affected by obstetric fistula in rural Tanzania. *BMC Women's Health, 15*(1), 107. https://doi.org/10.1186/s12905-015-0267-1

Mselle, L. T., Kohi, T. W., Mvungi, A., Evjen-Olsen, B., & Moland, K. (2011). Waiting for attention and care: Birthing accounts of women in rural Tanzania who developed obstetric fistula as an outcome of labor. *BMC Pregnancy and Childbirth, 11*(1), 75. https://doi.org/10.1186/1471-2393-11-75

Mselle, L. T., Moland, K., Evjen-Olsen, B., Mvungi, A., & Kohi, T. W. (2011). "I am nothing": Experiences of loss among women suffering from severe birth injuries in Tanzania. *BMC Women's Health, 11*(1), 49. https://doi.org/10.1186/1472-6874-11-49

Mselle, L. T., Moland, K. M., Mvungi, A., Evjen-Olsen, B., & Kohi, T. W. (2013). Why give birth in health facility? Users' and providers' accounts of poor quality of birth care in Tanzania. *BMC Health Services Research, 13*, 174. https://doi.org/10.1186/1472-6963-13-174

Mteta, K., Mbwambo, J., & Mvungi, M. (2006). Iatrogenic ureteric and bladder injuries in obstetric and gynaecologic surgeries. *East African Medical Journal, 83*, 79–85.

Mwangi, A., & Warren, C. (2008). Taking critical services to the home: Scaling-up home-based maternal and post-natal care, including family planning, through Community midwifery in Kenya Frontiers in Reproductive Health. *Population Council, 2008*, 1–43.

Nathan, L. M., Rochat, C. H., Grigorescu, B., & Banks, E. (2009). Obstetric fistulae in West Africa: Patient perspectives. *American Journal of Obstetrics and Gynecology, 200*(5), 40–42. https://doi.org/10.1016/j.ajog.2008.10.014

National Bureau of Statistics and ICF Macro. (2011). Tanzania demographic and health survey 2010. Tanzania Demographic and Health Survey. .

Neilson, J. P., Lavender, T., Quenby, S., & Wray, S. (2003). Obstructed labor. *British Medical Bulletin, 67*, 191–204. https://doi.org/10.1093/bmb/ldg018

Nour, N. M. (2006). Health consequences of child marriage in Africa. *Emerging Infectious Diseases, 12*(11), 1644–1649. https://doi.org/10.3201/eid1211.060510

Nyamtema, A. S., Urassa, D. P., & van Roosmalen, J. (2011). Maternal health interventions in resource limited countries: A systematic review of packages, impacts and factors for change. *BMC Pregnancy and Childbirth, 11*(1), 30. https://doi.org/10.1186/1471-2393-11-30

Olsen, Ø. E., Ndeki, S. S., & Norheim, O. F. (2005). Availability, distribution and use of emergency obstetric care in northern Tanzania. *Health Policy and Planning, 20*(3), 167–175. https://doi.org/10.1093/heapol/czi022

Opara, P. I., Jaja, T., Dotimi, D. A., & Alex-hart, B. A. (2012). Newborn cord care practices amongst mothers in yenagoa local government area, Bayelsa State, Nigeria. *International Journal of Clinical Medicine, 3*(1), 22–27.

Otis, K. E., & Brett, J. A. (2008). Barriers to hospital births: Why do many Bolivian women give birth at home? *Revista Panamericana de Salud Publica - Pan American Journal of Public Health, 24*(1), 46–53. https://doi.org/10.1590/S1020-49892008000700006

Pettersson, K. O., Christensson, K., de Freitas, E. D. G. G., & Johansson, E. (2004). Adaptation of health care seeking behavior during childbirth: Focus group discussions with women living in the suburban areas of Luanda, Angola. *Health Care for Women International, 25*(3), 255–280. https://doi.org/10.1080/07399330490272750

Physicians for Human Rights. (2007). *Deadly delays: Maternal mortality in Peru. A rights-based approach to safe motherhood.* Physicians for Human Rights.

Pope, R., Bangser, M., & Requejo, J. H. (2011). Restoring dignity: Social reintegration after obstetric fistula repair in Ukerewe, Tanzania. *Global Public Health, 6*(8), 859–873. https://doi.org/10.1080/17441692.2010.551519

Qureshi, Z. P., Sekadde-Kigondu, C., & Mutiso, S. M. (2010). Rapid assessment of partograph utilisation in selected maternity units in Kenya. *East African Medical Journal, 87*, 235–241.

Schwartz, D. A. (2015). Interface of epidemiology, anthropology and health care in maternal death prevention in resource-poor nations. In D. A. Schwartz (Ed.), *Maternal mortality: Risk factors, anthropological perspectives, prevalence in developing countries and preventive strategies for pregnancy-related death* (pp. ix–xiv). Nova Science Publishers, Inc.

Shrestha, S. K., Banu, B., Khanom, K., Ali, L., Thapa, N., Stray-Pedersen, B., et al. (2012). Changing trends on the place of delivery: Why do Nepali women give birth at home? *Reproductive Health, 9*(1), 25. https://doi.org/10.1186/1742-4755-9-25

Sialubanje, C., Massar, K., Hamer, D. H., & Ruiter, R. A. C. (2015). Reasons for home delivery and use of traditional birth attendants in rural Zambia: A qualitative study. *BMC Pregnancy and Childbirth, 15*(1), 1–12. https://doi.org/10.1186/s12884-015-0652-7

Sparks, B. T. (1990). A descriptive study of the changing roles and practices of traditional birth attendants in Zimbabwe. *Journal of Nurse-Midwifery, 35*(3), 150–161.

Suellen, M., Felicia, L., Monique, W., & Cowan, B. (2005). Obstetric fistula: A preventable tragedy. *Journal of Midwifery and Women's Health, 50*(4), 286–294. https://doi.org/10.1016/j.jmwh.2005.03.009

Switzerland Government. (2018). *The 2030 agenda: 17 sustainable development goals.* Retrieved 5 May, 2019, from https://www.eda.admin.ch/post2015/en/home/agenda-2030/die-17-ziele-fuer-eine-nachhaltige-entwicklung.html

Thadeus, S., & Maine, D. (1994). Too far to walk: Maternal mortality in context. *Social Science & Medicine, 38*(8), 1091–1110.

The King's Fund. (2008). *Improving safety in maternity services: Communication.* Retrieved 2 May, 2019, from https://www.kingsfund.org.uk/sites/default/files/field/field_related_document/Improving-safety-in-maternity-services-communication1.pdf

Titaley, C. R., Hunter, C. L., Dibley, M. J., & Heywood, P. (2010). Why do some women still prefer traditional birth attendants and home delivery? A qualitative study on delivery care services in West Java Province, Indonesia. *BMC Pregnancy and Childbirth, 10*, 43.

UN Committee on Economic. Social and Cultural Rights (CESCR). (2000). *General Comment No. 14: The right to the highest attainable standard of health (Art. 12 of the covenant).* Retrieved 4 May, 2019, from https://www.refworld.org/pdfid/4538838d0.pdf

UNFPA. (2002). *Second meeting of the working group for the prevention and treatment of obstetric fistula.*

UNFPA. (2006). *Reproductive health and safe motherhood.* UNFPA.

UNFPA. (2010). *Campaign to end fistula. The challenge of living with fistula.* Retrieved 4 May, 2019, from http://www.endfistula.org/sites/default/files/pub-pdf/sep-chap_fistula-may24.pdf

United Nations. (2015). *Sustainable development goals kick off with start of new year.* Retrieved 4 May, 2019, from https://www.un.org/sustainabledevelopment/blog/2015/12/sustainable-development-goals-kick-off-with-start-of-new-year/

Wall, L. L. (2006). Obstetric vesicovaginal fistula as an international public-health problem. *Lancet, 368*(9542), 1201–1209. https://doi.org/10.1016/S0140-6736(06)69476-2

Wall, L. L., Arrowsmith, S. D., Lassey, A. T., & Danso, K. (2006). Humanitarian ventures or "fistula tourism?": The ethical perils of pelvic surgery in the developing world. *International Urogynecology Journal and Pelvic Floor Dysfunction, 17*(6), 559–562. https://doi.org/10.1007/s00192-005-0056-8

Wall, L. L., Karshima, J. A., Kirschner, C., Arrowsmith, S. D., & Polan, M. L. (2004). The obstetric vesicovaginal fistula: Characteristics of 899 patients from Jos, Nigeria. *American Journal of Obstetrics and Gynecology, 190*(4), 1011–1019. https://doi.org/10.1016/j.ajog.2004.02.007

WHO. (1994). World Health Organization partograph in management of labor. World Health Organization Maternal Health and Safe Motherhood Programme. *Lancet, 994*(343), 1399–1404.

WHO. (1996). *Mother-baby package: Implementing safe motherhood in countries: Practical guide.* Retrieved 5 May, 2019, from https://apps.who.int/iris/bitstream/handle/10665/63268/WHO_FHE_MSM_94.11_Rev.1.pdf?sequence=1&isAllowed=y

WHO, UNFPA, UNICEF, & AMDD. (2009). *Monitoring emergency obstetric care: A handbook.* World Health Organization.

Women's Dignity Project, Engender Health. (2006). *Risk and resilience: Obstetric fistula in Tanzania.* Retrieved 3 May, 2019, from https://www.engenderhealth.org/wp-content/uploads/imports/files/pubs/maternal-health/obstetric_fistula_brief_overview.pdf

World Health Organization. (2005). *Making pregnancy safer (MPR): Skilled attendants.* WHO.

World Health Organization, UNICEF, & United Nations Population Fund. (1992). *Traditional birth attendants: a joint WHO/UNPA/UNICEF statement.* http://www.who.int/iris/handle/10665/38994

Yeakey, M. P., Chipeta, E., Taulo, F., & Tsui, A. O. (2009). The lived experience of Malawian women with obstetric fistula. *Culture, Health & Sexuality, 11*(5), 499–513. https://doi.org/10.1080/13691050902874777

Yisma, E., Dessalegn, B., Astatkie, A., & Fesseha, N. (2013). Knowledge and utilization of partograph among obstetric care givers in public health institutions of Addis Ababa, Ethiopia. *BMC Pregnancy and Childbirth, 13*(1), 17. https://doi.org/10.1186/1471-2393-13-17

Health-Seeking Behavior Among Women with Obstetric Fistula in Ethiopia

14

Jordann Loehr, Heather Lytle, and Mulat Adefris

14.1 Introduction

An obstetric fistula is an abnormal connection between the vagina, cervix, or uterus and the urinary system, digestive system, or both. This abnormal connection leads to incontinence of urine and/or stool. Obstetric fistulas are considered a sequela of obstructed labor, occurring when the fetus cannot pass through the mother's pelvis, although they also occur as a complication of episiotomies, poorly repaired vaginal lacerations, forceps or vacuum-assisted deliveries, symphysiotomies, and cesarean sections.

During labor, the tissues of the woman's pelvic organs are compressed between the presenting part of the fetus and the woman's pelvic bones. The longer and harder these tissues are compressed, the more likely they will lose blood flow and ultimately die. When these devitalized tissues heal, a hole can remain and a fistula is created. Symptoms of an obstetric fistula typically present between the third and tenth postpartum day (Hilton, 2003). If the labor forces were compressing the fetal head against the symphysis pubis, in the area of the lower urinary tract, a vesicovaginal fistula forms with subsequent continuous urinary incontinence. If the labor forces were compressing the fetal head against the sacrum near the rectum, a rectovaginal fistula forms, allowing flatus or stool to pass from the rectum into and out of the vagina, resulting in fecal incontinence. Prolonged compression can also result in nerve damage which can manifest, for example, as lower extremity weakness or difficulty walking (Browning & Whiteside, 2015).

To understand the relationship between obstetric fistula and health-seeking behaviors, obstetric fistula is divided simply into three categories as depicted in Fig. 14.1. This schematic does not include

All potentially identifying information in this chapter has been changed for confidentiality.

J. Loehr (✉)
University of Gondar, Gondar, Ethiopia
e-mail: jordannloehr@gmail.com

H. Lytle
Department of Obstetrics and Gynecology, University of Utah Health, Salt Lake City, UT, USA

M. Adefris
Department of Obstetrics and Gynecology, University of Gondar, Gondar, Ethiopia

© Springer Nature Switzerland AG 2022
L. B. Drew et al. (eds.), *A Multidisciplinary Approach to Obstetric Fistula in Africa*, Global Maternal and Child Health, https://doi.org/10.1007/978-3-031-06314-5_14

Fig. 14.1 Types of obstetric fistula as used in this chapter (Credit: H. Lytle)

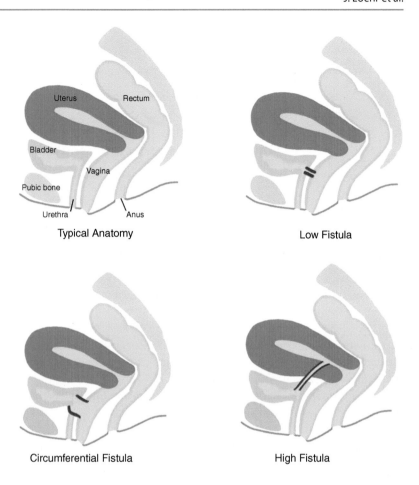

Typical Anatomy   Low Fistula

Circumferential Fistula   High Fistula

rectovaginal fistula, though rectovaginal fistula is considered to be similar in severity and complexity as circumferential fistula, and often complicated by nerve damage.

Low Obstetric Fistula The result of obstructed labor, typically involving the anterior vaginal wall, underlying bladder neck, and/or urethra. This type of obstetric fistula is caused by tissue compression, and therefore a delay in the interval from obstruction to delivery is critical in the formation of low obstetric fistula (Wall, 2012).

Circumferential Fistula

Has similar etiology to the low obstetric fistula, and the damage is greater. Instead of a fistula forming through one side of the bladder or urethra, a larger area of tissue is damaged, and the urinary system is transected completely in two: a circumferential defect in the middle of the urinary system. Women who suffer circumferential fistula typically have a worse obstetric history. These women are more likely to be primiparous, have a history of stillbirth, and have labored for longer prior to delivery. Additionally, women with a circumferential fistula have a worse prognosis even with accessing fistula treatment. Once a circumferential fistula is present, the chances of ever achieving complete continence are poor (Wright et al., 2016).

High Obstetric Fistula

Often the result of obstetric intervention. The damage leading to high fistula can occur at the time of cesarean section or surgical repair from uterine rupture. High obstetric fistula is more common in multiparous women than in primiparous women. These fistulae represent a different behavior pattern than the other obstetric fistula. High obstetric fistula has a good prognosis after surgical repair.

There is not one simple solution that can prevent obstetric fistula and the entire obstructed labor injury complex. Due to the multifactorial nature of fistula development, there are no definitive "cut off" times which can prevent every fistula. Even when cesarean delivery is available, it cannot prevent all cases of fistula from developing. Indeed, a high percentage of women with a low obstetric fistula following prolonged labor ultimately had a cesarean section during the incident birth (Wright et al., 2016). Therefore, fistula prevention requires a multifactorial response which reaches far beyond the healthcare setting. Changing behaviors in order to end fistula requires government recognition of fistula as a major public health concern, improvement in transportation and infrastructure, improvement in the societal status of women, increase in the number of girls accessing primary school education, and increased provision of affordable, accessible, and acceptable services for family planning and pregnancy, in addition to the required early intervention in cases of obstructed labor (Hilton, 2003; Wall, 2012). This is a massive undertaking, and one that Ethiopia has been addressing.

14.2 Health-Seeking Behaviors

Health-seeking behaviors have been defined as, "any action undertaken by individuals who perceive themselves to have a health problem or to be ill for the purpose of finding an appropriate remedy" (Olenja, 2003). The study of health-seeking behaviors is vital in the field of maternal health as well as fistula care, as prompt health-seeking is critical to mitigate the morbidity and mortality associated with obstetric emergencies and to facilitate restoration of health and reintegration for women suffering with obstetric fistula.

The decision-making processes that govern health-seeking behavior are complex. The interaction of each individual's health beliefs and her own unique context and characteristics mean that health behaviors will be heterogeneous and may not always be understandable or categorizable. The health of women is a social and economic phenomenon, far beyond our clinical and biomedical framework (Filippi et al., 2018), and yet we can only know the health behaviors of the women we have encountered (Heller & Hannig, 2017). However, health-seeking behaviors are malleable and can be influenced and altered. Therefore, to make progress toward ending fistula there is value in increasing understanding in the complexities involved with seeking maternity and fistula care (Olenja, 2003).

14.3 Ethiopian Women at Home

In order to understand the health behaviors of women with obstetric fistula we must understand the context in which they live. In rural Ethiopia, women typically live with their families in basic houses without running water, electricity, or refrigeration. They have had limited formal education and identify with strongly ingrained gender roles. Culturally, women are responsible for collecting water, gathering fuel, preparing food, preparing coffee, washing, cleaning, as well as significant social responsibilities. Ethiopian women have additional responsibilities as both a wife and a mother. These domestic activities are physically intense and time-consuming. For example, without refrigeration, most foods must be prepared fresh daily. In addition, coffee in Ethiopia is purchased green and roasted, ground, and prepared daily. If a woman is unavailable to do this essential work due to medical illness, childbirth, or otherwise, her entire household will be affected by her absence. A solution for her inability to work is to bring some of the children out of school such that the children assist in the running of the household. This absence of the woman can cost a family their children's education.

Currently, only ten percent of women in the Amhara region are literate. Keeping children in school as much as possible is vital for the future. Additionally, there is an inverse relationship between literacy and obstetric fistula, so keeping girls in school has the long-term effect of decreasing maternal morbidity and mortality (Gjerde et al., 2017).

The marital relationship is in the center of most Ethiopian families. Ethiopia has a strong patriarchal tradition (Gjerde et al., 2018) and a majority of the women in Ethiopia are economically dependent on their husbands (Adefris et al., 2017). Ethiopian men depend on their wives for food and water; there can be equality in these gendered relationships. In mutually respectful relationships, this arrangement can be functional and successful. Yet, without economic independence, a woman's options to leave her relationship are constrained. Even if she were financially able to leave for medical care or for her own well-being, the burden and guilt of leaving her family without food and water can be as prohibitive as the lack of economic independence.

Men in Ethiopia, as in the rest of the world, may be good, supportive husbands, or they may not be. In Orthodox Ethiopian culture and belief, when a man and a woman get married, they become the same person. This belief is ingrained in Ethiopian law and can be seen, for example, by the absence of statistics of intermarital rape. According to Ethiopian law it is impossible to rape ones' wife, as husband and wife are one person, and it is impossible to rape ones' self. This law exemplifies the patriarchal structures that influence reproductive decision-making in some Ethiopian relationships. There are men in the Ethiopian context who understand this relationship system and, in turn, deeply respect their wives. These men cannot imagine harming their wife, having sex with her when she does not consent, or depriving her of her needs. We intersect with these husbands when they willingly bring their wives to Addis Ababa, a city that feels like "the ends of the earth" to many rural Ethiopians. Unfortunately, there are also men who understand this belief about marriage and who treat their wives as disposable, expendable, and property. This can leave a woman feeling as if she does not matter, is insignificant, and has no voice; these feelings complicate health and health-seeking behaviors.

Young age at marriage is a known risk factor for fistula. Women who are married young are more likely to have limited autonomy, with a negative impact on their health-seeking behaviors (Gjerde et al., 2017). "Child brides" have historically been prevalent in Ethiopia, although the average age of marriage is increasing. Child marriage, under the age of 18 years, has been banned in Ethiopia, and several steps have been taken to enforce this ban. In 2007, the median female age at first marriage in Ethiopia was 16 years old, with 31% of women married by age 15 years old, and 12% of the total fertility rate derived from births to women aged 15–19 years old (Muleta et al., 2007). In the Amhara region, where young age at first marriage remains common, the median age at first marriage is 15.1 years. One must note, however, that young age at the time of pregnancy does not necessarily portend obstetric fistula formation; one sees teenage pregnancies worldwide that occur without obstetric fistula. Fundamentally, it is a lack of access to and/or use of quality obstetric care which results in obstetric fistula (Biadgilign et al., 2013; Fleck & Hamlin, 2013; Heller & Hannig, 2017; Wall et al., 2017).

Interpersonal dynamics in Ethiopia are further impacted by a strong culture of silence. Traditionally, the Ethiopian people do not openly discuss what is bothering them. It is hard to listen to the voices of others when the voices of others are silent. Women may find it challenging to break this cultural norm even when they find themselves in an extreme circumstance, such as suffering from an obstructed labor or leaking urine continuously. A woman is likely unable to seek help if she is unable to make her problems known.

Cultural, familial, financial, and interpersonal relationship factors all impact a woman's autonomy and decision-making. When a woman's autonomy and freedom to make decisions are inhibited her health care-seeking behaviors are negatively impacted and thus may contribute to risk, recognition, and treatment of obstetric fistulas (Gjerde et al., 2018).

14.4   Orthodox Christianity and Health Beliefs in Ethiopia

Both inside and outside of the Ethiopian home, religion is present. An estimated 45% of Ethiopians identify as Ethiopian Orthodox Christian, 20% as Protestant Christian, and 33% as Muslim—these are the majority religions in the country. The strong cultural and spiritual beliefs associated with religion generate health beliefs that fall outside of the biomedical realm. This results in health-seeking behavior outside of the Westernized infrastructure (Gjerde et al., 2018; Wall, 2012). Additional research on the effect of non-Orthodox Christian religions on health behaviors of women with obstetric fistula is welcome.

The belief in metaphysical causes of biomedical problems is common, though the extent of these is hard to discern as they are shrouded by secrecy (Gjerde et al., 2018). In one Ethiopian example, a man with impotence is believed to have committed adultery. Therefore, if a man becomes impotent, he will likely never report this, even to his wife, choosing instead to avoid her for fear of being accused of infidelity. In addition, in Ethiopia, there are some people who, by simply looking at another, are believed to make others disabled, ill, or die (Gjerde et al., 2017). There are deeds and rituals that are routinely carried out to maintain a good relation to the evil spirits and to avoid these "bad eyes" (Gjerde et al., 2018). Similar examples of beliefs can be true with obstructed labor and with obstetric fistula. Some believe that obstructed labor is caused by infidelity, and a plethora of sins can be responsible for obstetric fistula. Although we do not know all of the specifics around the metaphysical causes of obstetric fistula, we can see the consequences of these beliefs. Women report being afraid to disclose their condition (Adefris et al., 2017; Bashah et al., 2018; Gjerde et al., 2017), and women, when returning from fistula repair, often are afraid to discuss why they were gone, even though they received adequate and satisfactory treatment (Neilsen et al., 2009). In several studies, a majority of women had not discussed their problem even with their husbands (Zeleke et al., 2013).

14.5   Ethiopian Infrastructure and Health System

In rural Ethiopia, the primary means of transportation is walking. There are few roads, few vehicles, and limited access to fuel. Figure 14.2 shows an example of rural infrastructure. These limitations severely impact a woman's options and decision-making. A woman cannot choose to take an ambu-

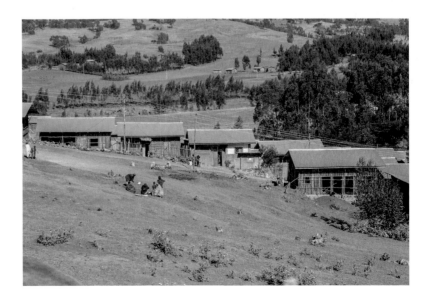

Fig. 14.2 Government-built housing in rural Ethiopia (Photo Credit: Davidson Loehr)

lance to a hospital for birth, or take a ride to a fistula hospital, if there are no ambulances, vehicles, or if the terrain is impassible. Along this line, a woman cannot choose to birth in a health facility if there are no health facilities, if the health facilities do not have appropriately trained clinicians, and if there are no supplies.

The public healthcare system in Ethiopia consists of community health workers, health posts, health centers, primary hospitals, district hospitals, and referral hospitals. There are also private, NGO, mission, and faith-based healthcare services. Although this is a health system with numerous players, overall, there is still a large unmet need for healthcare services for the population.

This inadequacy has been, and continues to be, actively improved. Improvements in maternal services were prioritized in the fourth and final phase of the 20-year Ethiopian Health Sector Development plan, culminating in an increased provision of maternal care. In the past decade, the number of community-based health centers increased by almost 50%. There are also substantial increases in physician training, midwifery training, road improvements, ambulance procurement, and prioritization of ambulance use for laboring women in each district (Ballard et al., 2016). The government also introduced a targeted training program in emergency surgery and obstetrics for health officers, mid-level health workers, who are to be based in rural health facilities and capable of performing a cesarean section. In addition, the Ethiopian health authorities educate and deploy 7500 new health extension workers each year to survey and educate the community (Muleta et al., 2010).

These priorities and subsequent improvements have decreased the incidence and changed the presenting types of new obstetric fistulas. In a health survey in 2016, 22% of Ethiopian women had heard of obstetric fistula, and the prevalence of obstetric fistula was 6:10,000 with the prevalence of untreated fistula being 2:10,000. This is a substantial reduction from 2005 when the estimated prevalence of obstetric fistula was 22:10,000 (Ballard et al., 2016). The prevention of fistula includes access to family planning information and services, as well as access to quality maternal care, therefore the incidence and severity of fistula can be used as a proxy for gauging the adequacy of maternal health programs (Donnay & Weil, 2004).

If a woman has even one antenatal care appointment, it means that she has accessed the limited healthcare system during her pregnancy and established a health behavior that is likely to be reproduced if a complication arises (Yismaw et al., 2019). Several studies have shown that women who do not attend antenatal care have higher rates of maternal morbidity and mortality than women who have accessed antenatal care even once. The "unbooked" women suffer, on average, longer labors, more stillbirths, and more urethral damage if they develop obstetric fistula (Muleta et al., 2010; Wall et al., 2017). Despite aforementioned improvements, at this point in Ethiopia, there are not enough health posts, centers, or hospitals for every pregnant woman to receive even one antenatal appointment.

14.6   Demographics of Women with Obstetric Fistula

The demographics of women presenting with obstetric fistula have changed over time, and demographic studies in the past show different overall results (Adefris et al., 2017; Muleta et al., 2010; Neilsen et al., 2009; Tebeu et al., 2012; Wall et al., 2017). Historically, women with obstetric fistula have been referred to as "girls" (Heller & Hannig, 2017), and have been presented as young, divorced, abandoned, childless, and economically dependent (Neilsen et al., 2009; Wall et al., 2017). No study has shown the demographics to be as concordant with the media portrayal of these women. A close examination of the women who present for care shows that the story is more complex.

Figure 14.3 shows characteristics of women presenting with fistula in 2019. Overall, the majority had a vaginal delivery (74.4%) of a living infant (57.6%). About half accessed antenatal care services at least once (50.4%) and just over half delivered within the health system (52%). About half were

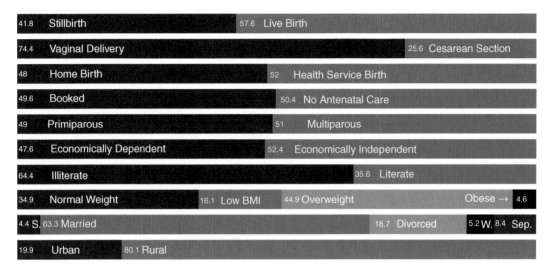

Fig. 14.3 Demographic characteristics of women presenting with obstetric fistula, 2019. *BMI* body mass index, *S* single, *W* widowed, *Sep* separated. (Source: Yismaw et al., 2019)

primiparous (49%) but the other half had had children previously (51%). The majority were married (63.3%) and were considered economically independent (52.4%). The overwhelming majority (80.1%) live rurally and are illiterate (64.4%) (Yismaw et al., 2019).

There are four significant risk factors which are independently associated with obstetric fistula: age at marriage (relative risk [RR] 1.23), history of an operative vaginal delivery (RR 3.44), lack of adequate antenatal care (RR 4.43), and labor lasting longer than 1 day (RR 14.84) (Wall et al., 2017). As can be seen, protracted labor lasting longer than 1 day has the highest relative risk. In Ethiopia, any pregnant woman could suffer a protracted labor; therefore, every woman is at risk.

As discussed previously, low fistula, circumferential fistula, and high fistula have different etiologies and the demographics and health behaviors of women with different types of fistulas seem to be different. Those with low circumferential fistula, the most severe form of fistula, are typically young, with a third being under 20 years old (Wright et al., 2016). High fistula is more common in women who have protracted labor and access health centers and have cesarean delivery. Cesarean sections after obstructed labor or uterine rupture are far more complicated than routine cesarean sections, and have higher risk of fistula occurrence, even in a relatively resource-rich context.

14.7   History of Obstetric Fistula in Ethiopia

The struggle to end obstetric fistula has many chapters throughout Ethiopian history. Although we can presume obstetric fistula has been affecting women throughout history, the first biomedical interventions in Ethiopia were implemented by Reginald and Catherine Hamlin who started this process in the 1950s. They established the first dedicated fistula hospital in Africa in 1975 and have been paramount in the struggle to end obstetric fistula. Since that time, Ethiopia has also participated in several governmental, non-governmental, and international initiatives that have brought us to where we are today. The Hamlin Fistula Center reports that throughout its history, it has treated over 50,000 women for obstetric fistula with a 95% closure rate.

The number of new fistula cases is dropping. A decrease of 20% per year over 4 years, from 2011 until 2015 (Wright et al., 2016) was noted at the two main organizations that provide the majority of fistula treatments in Ethiopia. A recent study revealed a 0.06% prevalence rate of obstetric fistula in three rural zones, compared to the prior estimates of 0.3% or 0.22%. The same study also showed a prevalence of symptomatic pelvic organ prolapse of 100:10,000 (1%) (Ballard et al., 2016), a condition similar in its signs, symptoms, consequences, and surgical resolution to obstetric fistula.

The prevalence of obstetric fistula may be decreasing due to the diligent work of those that treat fistula. However, the diminishing incidence of new obstetric fistula cases over the last decade likely points to a general improvement in the availability and uptake of maternal health services and emergency obstetric services. Thanks to these interventions, the number of women who develop fistula is decreasing. Concerningly, the relative percentage of those presenting who have a high obstetric fistula is increasing. The concomitant increase of high fistula suggests that women may be presenting late at health facilities and require complex cesarean sections. Although surgical training for health officers and midwives, as has occurred in Ethiopia, is a possible solution, these health professionals may still not have the extensive training and experience that is necessary to safely perform a complex cesarean in difficult surgical circumstances such as in protracted, obstructed labor or after uterine rupture (Wright et al., 2016).

14.8   Incorporating Pelvic Organ Prolapse into Fistula Initiatives in Ethiopia

Ethiopian gynecologic surgeons are highly motivated and compassionate toward the struggles of their patients and have seen numerous women who present for treatment of fistula who actually suffer from pelvic organ prolapse. Pelvic organ prolapse is a surgically correctable condition whose symptoms of urinary and/or fecal incontinence, voiding difficulties, vaginal heaviness, and painful sex overlap with those of obstetric fistula. It is also treated by gynecologic surgeons. Women with pelvic organ prolapse are generally illiterate, economically dependent, live far from the health centers, and have difficulties leaving their home due to responsibilities for their children and household chores (Gjerde et al., 2018). Like fistula, prolapse is associated with prolonged labor and birth. It leads to severe difficulties and pain while carrying out daily chores which, as discussed previously, for Ethiopian women involves hard manual labor (Gjerde et al., 2017). In Ethiopia, the women will carry their children on their backs and continue their work and responsibilities. The heavier the weight carried, whether a child, water, or materials, the more pressure is on the pelvis which can worsen pelvic organ prolapse. Prolapse severely affects a woman's well-being and relationship with her husband—not the least because of the inability to perform chores expected of them (Gjerde et al., 2017). Ninety-seven percent of women with obstetric fistula and 67.7% of women with stage 3 and 4 pelvic organ prolapse (the most severe forms in which the pelvic organs may protrude from the vagina) have symptoms of depression (Zeleke et al., 2013). Currently, women with pelvic organ prolapse are typically ineligible for services at the fistula hospitals because of the nature and funding sources of fistula hospitals. It has been stated in Gondar that for every 1 woman with an obstetric fistula there are 20 women with pelvic organ prolapse. There is will and passion from the biomedical workers to incorporate the care of women with pelvic organ prolapse into the mission of fistula centers. As one British gynecologist reported, "It is easier to get funding for fistula treatment than it is to raise money for more hospitals with maternity wards" (Heller & Hannig, 2017).

14.9   Health-Seeking Behavior of Women with Obstetric Fistula in Ethiopia

The framework used in understanding the development and treatment of obstetric fistula is the "Three Delay" framework laid out by Thaddeus and Maine (1994). The first delay is in deciding to seek care. The factors that affect this delay are often more vague, intangible, and difficult to influence or control than the other delays (Wall, 2012). The second delay is associated with transport and arrival at a suitable facility. The third delay is a delay in receiving appropriate care once at that facility. The second and third delays are largely political problems and can be overcome even in low-resource countries (Wall, 2012). We will first discuss these delays as they relate to emergency and comprehensive obstetric care in Ethiopia, as this is the cause of obstetric fistula. We will then look again at these delays and how they relate to women suffering from fistula. In addition, we will discuss the fourth delay of fistula, the delay of reintegration into society.

14.9.1 Obstetric Delays

14.9.1.1 Delay #1: Delay in Deciding to Seek Care

Initial delays in seeking hospital care during obstructed labor are caused by failure to recognize that labor is prolonged, confusion about what should be done, the lack of women's agency, unfamiliarity with, and fear of, hospitals and the treatments they offer (often surgery) and economic constraints. A woman and her community must also understand that the consequences of not intervening quickly within the biomedical system during obstructed labor can be devastating and deadly. Concurrently, the care that patients expect to receive must be perceived to be both effective and high quality in order for them to want to seek care (Wall, 2012).

During labor, many women in Ethiopia will deliver without trained supervision at their family home. If labor is being supervised by trained personnel, the diagnosis of obstructed labor is typically not difficult. When delivering alone, with family members, or with traditional birth attendants, what is regarded as the "normal" length of labor differs from obstetric norms (Wall, 2012). The mean duration of labor among fistula patients ranged from 2.5 to 4 days, markedly longer than normal labor (Muleta et al., 2010; Tebeu et al., 2012).

Ethiopia has a pluralistic medical system. In Ethiopia, it is estimated that about 80% of people regularly seek care and cure outside of the biomedical system. In Amhara, the most common means of healing are local remedies, medicinal plants, or spiritual guidance (Gjerde et al., 2018). The healthcare options sought for obstetric labor in Ethiopia include holy water, local healers, clinics, or a hospital that can perform surgery. Some Ethiopians believe that obstructed labor is punishment for sins. Within this framework, a woman and family seek cure from a priest in order for these sins to be forgiven (Gjerde et al., 2018). Within this understanding of obstructed labor, this is a logical course of action. However, it is clear that these beliefs compound the first delay: first, a woman's identification of the problem is delayed by the shame of knowing that her complication comes from a sin. Then, her time and resources are utilized to seek care from a priest and she has yet to take a step toward gaining successful medical treatment for her labor. Finally, after seeking care from a priest, she may then turn to a traditional healer, which continues to use time and resources and delay the decision to seek biomedical care. In the biomedical framework, this diagnostic and treatment logic is both ineffective and harmful for treating obstructed labor and preventing obstetric fistula.

14.9.1.2 Delay #2: Accessing Care

Accessing care involves a combination of social support, infrastructure, transportation, and money. Government health professionals, communities, religious leaders, families, and husbands play a role in reducing delays in accessing care.

In the public health system, the health posts in villages are run by health extension workers trained in basic maternal care (Ballard et al., 2016). Basic and emergency obstetric care (BEmOC) is reported to be available in only 53% of these centers. Comprehensive EmOC, which includes cesarean delivery, is only an option in some hospitals, typically only at the level of a regional hospital. Accessing

Fig. 14.4 Simien mountains with villages in the distance. No vehicular access. (Photo Credit: Davidson Loehr)

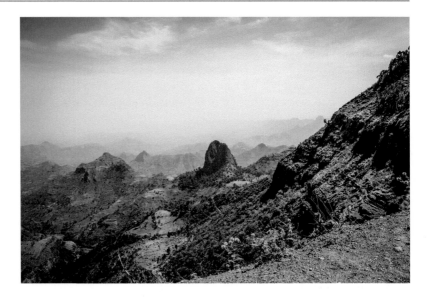

comprehensive emergency obstetric care from rural Ethiopia requires transportation from home to the health post or community health center, then from the health center to the district hospital, and then from the district hospital to a regional hospital capable of cesarean section (Muleta et al., 2007). Figure 14.4 depicts a rural region with villages in Amhara, Ethiopia without access to vehicular transportation. Sixty-two percent of government facilities charge routine user fees for general health services. There are exemptions for obstetric and gynecologic emergencies, and maternal health care is reported to be "free" in the public health system. Still, there are often fees for medications and supplies, for example, the IV tubing required for a safe cesarean section (Gjerde et al., 2018). One also needs to pay for food, transportation of the family member going with the woman, and consider the opportunity costs for being absent from one's family and other children. The cost of transportation to reach care may cost more than the care itself.

Even if willing, one may not be able to access care as these barriers may be insurmountable (Wall, 2012). The population of Ethiopia is approximately 100 million and there are 144 regional hospitals. Fifty-two of these regional hospitals are located in Addis Ababa. At times, women may make it to the local health center and not ever reach the referral center because of lack of additional transportation, lack of funds, fear, conflict, road blockades, and other geopolitical barriers (Wright et al., 2016). Ethiopia is mitigating this by having designated ambulances reserved for maternal use. Still, there are times when regions will run out of fuel, when the ambulance is otherwise busy, or when the woman feels it is insurmountable to go further from home than the health center. Women who have obstetric fistula are "near misses" for maternal mortality, their knowledge and lived experience can augment the verbal autopsies and records currently relied upon for understanding delays in accessing obstetric care (Donnay & Weil, 2004).

14.9.1.3   Delay #3: Receiving Care at the Hospital

In Ethiopia, there have been numerous campaigns to increase in-hospital births. Yet, the major hospitals in Ethiopia can be so crowded that no support person is permitted to accompany a laboring woman. There is often minimal privacy: labor words can be open bays with no divisions between women. Hospitals are frequently short staffed. Many organizations and initiatives are working on increasing in-hospital births and far too few are working on improving the quality of hospitals or care within them. This causes the governmental healthcare system to be overwhelmed, understaffed, undersupplied, uncomfortable, unclean, and unsafe. Women report being abused, mistreated, and having unnecessary interventions (Wall, 2012). Women know that accessing care is not the same as accessing quality care and increasing efforts for in-hospital births without increasing the safety and dignity associated with hospital birthing is destructive. Furthermore, the number of fistulas created by biomedical error appears to be on the rise, and women's perceptions of biomedically caused fistulas may be even higher, fueling fear of seeking timely care during obstetric complications (Heller & Hannig, 2017). What is striking are the ways in which all three phases of delay are linked—the decision to get care is directly related to the difficulty in accessing care and the perceived quality of care that will be obtained at the final destination (Wall, 2012).

14.9.2 Obstetric Fistula Delays

14.9.2.1 Delay #1: Deciding to Seek Care

The decision to seek care by an Ethiopian woman with an obstetric fistula is a complex decision as depicted by the framework in Figs. 14.5 and 14.6.

At any point in the above framework, a woman can change course and choose different health-seeking behaviors. Some of the decisions can be reversed, some cannot. A woman can always choose to disclose her fistula; once she has disclosed it, that decision is final. The delay in seeking care for obstetric fistula has been cited to be anywhere from months to decades after the incident of pregnancy occurred (Donnay & Weil, 2004; Muleta et al., 2010; Zeleke et al., 2013). During this time the woman is navigating life with obstetric fistula and its sequelae through various coping behaviors. Walking through this framework allows us to better understand the health-seeking behaviors of Ethiopian women with obstetric fistula.

Women with obstetric fistula leak urine, feces, or both which can cause a foul odor to surround the woman. The leakage of urine or stool begins between the third and tenth day after birth, at a time

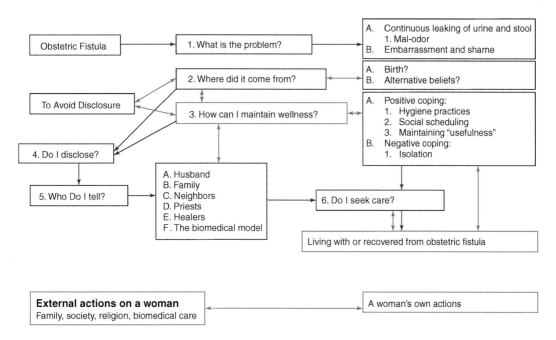

Fig. 14.5 Health-seeking behavior framework 1, related to obstetric fistula in Ethiopia (Credit: J. Loehr)

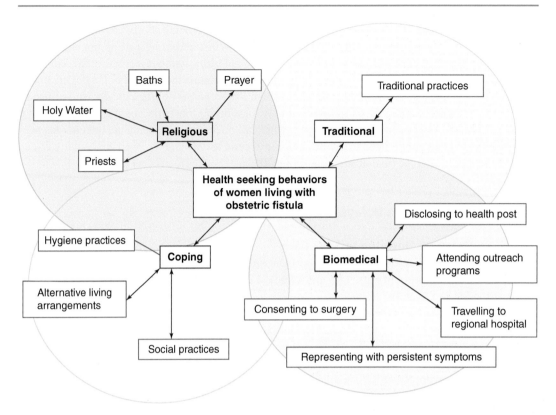

Fig. 14.6 Health-seeking behavior framework 2, related to obstetric fistula in Ethiopia (Credit: J. Loehr)

when the woman is still bleeding from birth, and either caring for a newborn or mourning a stillbirth. Common first reactions of a woman who develops fistula symptoms include crying, feelings of frustration, and wanting to die. Suicidal ideation is common (Muleta et al., 2007). Other feelings include a loss of dignity, lack of support, lack of power to seek care, loss of hope, fear of the future, and feelings of dependency (Bashah et al., 2018). Typically, Ethiopian women stay at their parent's home in the peripartum period. Women are often reluctant to return to their marital home until they convalesce. The full extent of the problem may not be completely understood until after the postpartum period has passed. Postpartum absences of up to several months are not unusual (Heller & Hannig, 2017).

In a culture shrouded in shame and secrecy, where most women have a limited formal education and where strong cultural and religious beliefs are present, there are diverse beliefs regarding the etiology of incontinence after delivery. An Ethiopian woman may believe her symptoms are caused by obstructed labor, by adultery or other sins, due to punishment for wrong behavior, from an evil spirit, or even due to a fault of their husbands (Heller & Hannig, 2017; Muleta et al., 2007). In a survey of women with obstetric fistula, 27% of them were aware that obstetric fistula came from obstructed labor, and only 16% of them had shared this with their community (Neilsen et al., 2009). There is hope that the campaigns against fistula have increased awareness of the obstructed labor cause and helped to eliminate the stigma that results from beliefs outside of the biomedical model.

Once a fistula is present a woman must decide how she will maintain her wellness, or seek health, and if she is going to disclose her situation.

Wellness with undisclosed, untreated fistula can be achieved. The number of women in this state is unknown (Zeleke et al., 2013) although it has been reported that 68% or "most" women in Ethiopia do not seek treatment for obstetric fistula or pelvic organ prolapse, despite the availability of treatment facilities for both conditions in the country (Adefris et al., 2017; Biadgilign et al., 2013; Zeleke et al., 2013). To avoid discrimination women will work hard to hide their problems from others. To successfully hide their condition, women living with fistula must overcome hygiene problems, social isolation, and maintain their essential responsibilities and social roles. Women with incontinence will compensate by wearing and frequently changing cotton towels in their underwear, wearing several pairs of undershorts and changing them frequently, and by increasing laundering. Perfumed soaps and scented herbs are also used to conceal the odor associated with incontinence (Bashah et al., 2018). Women use countless strategies to manage their work while avoiding disclosure. Some women cope with fistula by delegating more work to other family members including their children, which may keep children from school. Other women will find alternate excuses to avoid work in order to conceal their condition successfully. All women interviewed strove to continue with their lives, their daily chores, and to work despite discomfort and pain (Gjerde et al., 2017). However, women with fistula cannot work in sectors that require strict hygiene like making food or coffee. Some women are required to enter the informal economy such as petty trading, work where a sustainable income is difficult to achieve (Bashah et al., 2018). Sleeping arrangements can also be healthily adjusted so that women do not soil the family's sleeping area. This can be done by using a plastic sheet, wearing several undershorts, or sleeping elsewhere. Though fistula complicates relationships, it is not always a curse to become a social pariah.

Having incontinence makes it difficult to sit for long coffee ceremonies, a three-cup process, and participate in longer responsibilities such as a wake for a friend, family, or neighborhood member's death. Individual women report overcoming these losses by only drinking the first cup of coffee or arriving late for functions and leaving early. If one has cleaned immediately prior to arrival for coffee, there is typically time to stay for an hour or so before possible exposure as a woman with incontinence. These are all attempts to "pass" as continent. If successful, a woman is able to remain integrated in her social circle. If the desire to "pass" requires more effort and strength than the success of passing, these women can suffer greatly. Staying social is paramount to wellness, and most women make significant effort to maintain control over the information others have about their condition. Ethiopian women are adept at transforming their fistula into a socially invisible condition (Heller & Hannig, 2017).

There are also unhealthy ways of maintaining wellness, or of not being well at all, as obstetric fistula is an extraordinary challenge to a woman's coping abilities (Bashah et al., 2018). On a physical level, a woman might decrease the amount of water she consumes in order to reduce the amount of urine she leaks (Browning & Whiteside, 2015). This is intuitive. Unfortunately, this causes a hyperconcentrated urine that smells worse and can cause skin damage because of the highly concentrated urea. Drinking more water, a non-intuitive action, dilutes the urine and helps avoid these complications. Along this line, women with fecal incontinence will often reduce their food intake, which can lead to malnutrition and anemia. Women who do not eat with their families because of their symptoms, eating only what remains of the food after the family has finished, will also suffer malnutrition and anemia (Hilton, 2003).

Socially, women may feel ashamed and alienate themselves from friends and family (Andargie & Debu, 2017; Heller & Hannig, 2017; Muleta et al., 2007; Neilsen et al., 2009). Reduction of stigma remains a major challenge for public health programs. Virtually every study of obstetric fistula mentions that the social stigma associated with this condition and states that women with fistulas are often ostracized (Biadgilign et al., 2013). When a community is unsupportive, when the beliefs that an obstetric fistula is a punishment for sinning are strong, if prior women with incontinence have been rejected by the community, a woman is torn between exposing herself outright and being abandoned or suffering in isolation with extreme efforts to avoid exposure (Ballard et al., 2016; Muleta et al., 2007). In Ethiopia, social isolation and abandonment often lead to low self-esteem, depression, a deep sense of loss, and prolonged emotional trauma (Andargie & Debu, 2017; Zeleke et al., 2013). Ninety-seven percent of women with obstetric fistula screen positive for depression (Browning & Menber, 2008). Within this, there are high levels of mental distress, with 14% of women reporting attempting suicide. The issue causing the greatest distress and frustration was the lack of social life. Nearly all women encountered by biomedical researchers suffered isolation, shame, and stigma, and would not go into public places due to the risk of being insulted or simply ignored (Gjerde et al., 2017; Neilsen et al., 2009). Although women with obstetric fistula feel apprehensive about placing themselves in close proximity to others unaware of their condition, it is overcoming this apprehension and entering back into society that offers protection from non-physical negative consequences of fistula (Heller & Hannig, 2017).

Women with obstetric fistula also have the pressure to remain "useful." In Ethiopian culture, being considered "useless" is a great fear (Bashah et al., 2018). Usefulness seems to mean an ability to complete socially determined responsibilities, typically within the home. This involves the previously mentioned responsibilities of cooking, cleaning, mothering, being a spouse, and having a sexual relationship with her partner. With a fistula, the relationship between a woman and her husband can become complicated. Even if a woman manages to pass as continent for all of her other responsibilities, having a successful sexual relationship with an obstetric fistula is difficult (Zeleke et al., 2013). Most women remember their first sexual encounter following the development of an obstetric fistula with sadness, sorrow, pain, and/or trauma (Muleta et al., 2007). A woman who has not disclosed her condition will often attempt to avoid sex for prolonged periods by staying where she delivered (usually her parents' house), telling her husband she is menstruating, or refusing him outright (Gjerde et al., 2017). Many women with obstetric fistula find themselves in a liminal phase of sorts—not technically divorced, but often not living with their husbands either. Some women use fistula as an opportunity to avoid returning to an abusive partner (Gjerde et al., 2018; Heller & Hannig, 2017).

If a woman decides to disclose her condition, overcoming fears of embarrassment, abandonment, and other social consequences, she must also decide to whom she discloses. She can choose to tell her family, parents, friends, neighbors, husband, or to disclose to priests, healers, or the biomedical system. The choice about who a woman first discloses to cannot be generalized. Most women experience substantial support from relatives, friends, and at times from their husbands after disclosing their condition (Gjerde et al., 2017). About half of the women with obstetric fistula remained married, and generally their husbands were supportive. Some husbands will think, "how could I dare to leave her during a bad time?" Some will rent cars, an extraordinary financial commitment, and drive their wives or daughters to Addis Ababa (Muleta et al., 2007). When presenting to the fistula centers, unmarried women were more depressed than married ones, likely because being married implies that there is a caring partner, and a married woman also avoids the social stigma associated with being alone or divorced (Zeleke et al., 2013). Social stigma, money, old age, and divorce all contribute to delays in seeking treatment by negatively impacting the woman's economic status and by having no friend or community that supports and encourages a woman to overcome the barriers in accessing care (Adefris et al., 2017). The support of a woman's husband and or community contributes to restoring health and well-being (Muleta et al., 2007), as delays in seeking treatment are 16 times higher if a woman is divorced than if she were never married (Adefris et al., 2017). Still, 72% of women had never discussed with anyone about their pelvic floor symptoms before coming to the hospital (Zeleke et al., 2013).

A woman then decides to seek care for her symptoms or avoids seeking care. Women have reported deciding against seeking biomedical care because of perceiving obstetric fistula to be a permanent irreparable condition and fear that the treatment is too expensive (Ballard et al., 2016). When women decide to seek care, it is more complex than "doing nothing" or "going to the hospital." There are many competing therapeutic options. Women will seek care from where she believes the solution is for what she believes the problem is, what she can safely access, afford, and when the act of seeking care is less costly, less risky, than the symptoms from which she suffers. Some women go to a local healer and perform ceremonies, some adhere to the spiritual healing rituals—fasting, baptism, prayers, and consumption of holy water—that are needed in collaboration with surgery, both of which cost money (Wall, 2012). Although seeking care from priests or healers, women often do not disclose the reason that they seek care. This is due to shame and the fear of being ostracized from the church for having obstetric fistula. Sometimes, though seeking baptism for cure, the women do not participate in baptism because it requires being naked, which is embarrassing with pelvic conditions (Gjerde et al., 2018). Risk depends on local perceptions and assumptions, values, and cultural constructs (Wall, 2012). There is substantial disagreement over what is risky, how risky it is, and what to do about it. Disclosing fistula to one's husband carries substantially different risks in different relationships, as does disclosing fistula to one's community, or traveling to seek care.

14.9.2.2 Delay #2: Accessing Care

There are similarities between accessing care with obstetric emergencies in the distance to care facilities, the terrain one must traverse, and the expense of the journey and time away from home, and then there are vast differences.

Obstructed labor is an emergency, obstetric fistula and pelvic organ prolapse are not. Pregnancy and labor are common, fistula is not. There are more hospitals with comprehensive obstetric care services than there are fistula centers in Ethiopia. With obstetric fistula one will likely need to go further for care, and one can save money, arrange more affordable or safe transport, arrange for childcare or wait until your children are older or out of school, and also wait for mobile campaigns to come to your region. Of the women who delayed biomedical care, they reported that the unavailability of roads, lack of transportation, greater than two days of travel to the nearest health facility, and walking as the only means of transportation were the main barriers that prevented women from arriving at a fistula treatment center earlier. The majority of women who underwent surgery at a regional hospital reported that they would not have traveled to Addis Ababa for treatment because the journey seemed more terrifying than living with a fistula, they could not leave their dependents for weeks or months, and they could not afford travel expenses (Neilsen et al., 2009).

The Story of Merhawit, a woman living with an obstetric fistula in Gondar, Ethiopia

Merhawit is a young woman who was brought in from the countryside by a family member to live with a distant cousin who now lives and works at the University of Gondar. The father of the family absorbing this cousin is a professor at the University and the mother owns a small grocery and coffee shop. They have three school-aged children of their own, their middle child won the math award during middle school. This family lives in university provided faculty housing, a one-bedroom apartment with a kitchen, front room, balcony, laundry and storage room and intermittent electricity and running water. The water reliably comes once a week, providing opportunities to refill the storage barrels within the home.

Merhawit joined this family because of her fistula and because of the proximity of the family to the Fistula center of Gondar. Merhawit was treated at the fistula center and went through the recovery process. She had a complicated fistula and the first surgery was unsuccessful. She has stayed with her extended family for years, as she has subsequently undergone five attempts at surgical repair. Within the family she does the washing and some of the cooking, as the mother also cooks, and Merhawit makes the injera. She is also home to care for the children when both parents are working. Family meals are shared from the same plate and eaten without cutlery. Oftentimes she eats after the family has finished eating. She doesn't get paid, and she is not required to pay rent. She sets up a bed in the laundry / storage room off of the balcony as the rest of the family shares the single bedroom.

She reached out to us, as foreigners, to get help with her persistent fistula symptoms, and we brought her back to the Fistula Center in Gondar, where she was evaluated by staff who know her well. Merhawit has been operated on by one of the most experienced fistula surgeons in the world, more than once, and she has only the vaginal mucosa present that has successfully closed the anatomic defect of her fistula. There is no muscle or nerve tissue remaining to prevent incontinence, and she still leaks continuously. Doing additional surgery on her would cause damage. She has been told this several times through the fistula center in Gondar, and she was told again by us. Her plan now is to save up money and resources in order to travel to the fistula center in Addis Ababa. Because of the network of fistula sites across the country the surgeons who work in Addis Ababa, the same surgeons she is saving up to see, have already operated on her more than once. The fistula site discussed this with her, and her family, and yet she persists.

These women with obstetric fistula and pelvic organ prolapse are unlikely to receive treatment or supportive counseling at routine outpatient clinics in the way that a pregnant woman who has accessed prenatal care would get counseling on labor (Zeleke et al., 2013). The government needs to increase the number and accessibility of services, the health extension workers need to address the cognitive accessibility to the community and families about the problems, to identify cases, and to facilitate referrals such that communities living in rural areas can choose the biomedical model and access it (Adefris et al., 2017; Gjerde et al., 2018).

14.9.2.3 Delay #3: Receiving Care at the Hospital

Ethiopian fistula surgeons are well trained and work at a network of coordinated fistula centers throughout the country. Women arrive at the centers on their own, through a referral system, or after a campaign. The women wait at the center until a sufficient volume of women needing surgery are present and a well-trained fistula surgeon from Addis Ababa will arrive at the center and provide surgery while working with and training Ethiopian urogynecologists and Ethiopian gynecologists. Women do not report the same abuses and poor treatment from the fistula centers that they report from obstetric units.

Fistula treatment has become more efficient in Ethiopia. Recovery now takes between 3 and 6 weeks at most of the fistula hospitals (Heller & Hannig, 2017; Yismaw et al., 2019). Fistula surgery is an individualized surgery, as each defect can be different, and the health status of each individual woman is also different. The recovery period also varies due to several factors, as listed in Fig. 14.7.

Fig. 14.7 Factors that shorten the recovery time of women with obstetric fistula (Yismaw et al., 2019)

Factors that Shorten Recovery Time
Small width and length of fistula
Multiparous
Treatment within 3 months of antecedent birth
Literacy
Havingantenatal visits
Birth at a health facility
Labor lasting less than two days
Vaginal delivery
Height equal or greater than 150cm
Weight less than 50kg
Economic independence

Factors that increase the likelihood of a low fistula or a high fistula, both easier to surgically repair, also decrease the likelihood of a circumferential fistula (Browning & Menber, 2008; Yismaw et al., 2019). The health-seeking behaviors that decrease the likelihood of a circumferential fistula also increase the likelihood of a shorter and more continent recovery, reinforcing the value of understanding the behaviors, and motivations behind the behaviors, that women have both in labor and with fistula.

Repair of a fistula is a three-step process. The first is the anatomic closure of the fistula by surgery. Anatomic closure can occur in 85–89% of fistula surgeries with well-trained, experienced hands. The Ethiopian urogynecologists at the Gondar site will not begin even what appears to be a low fistula repair without a fistula subspecialist present because of the law of diminishing returns and the reality that even a simple fistula can be deceptively complicated. Up to 15% of women who undergo fistula surgery have a persistent fistula after surgery (Goh, 2004; Yismaw et al., 2019). The second arm of repair is the functional return to continence. The occurrence of stress incontinence in patients following successful repair of obstetric VVF is well known, estimated to range from 10% to 12%, with urge incontinence and mixed incontinence occurring in an additional 15–20% of women, and efforts to improve surgical techniques or offer non-surgical options that might lead to improvements in quality of life with these failures of surgical repair need to be considered (Ballard et al., 2016). This intermittent incontinence is reported as an improved quality of life from the continuous incontinence of fistula, and it facilitated the possibility of social reintegration (Neilsen et al., 2009). The third arm is the return of the woman to successful urinary health, reproductive health, sexual health, psychological health, and quality of life (Goh, 2004; Neilsen et al., 2009).

Comprehensive treatment and rehabilitation include mental health services. Special care is needed and provided to tend to the social and psychological trauma associated with obstetric fistula (Donnay & Ramsey, 2006). This is done both prior to and following the surgery while the women wait and recover in the fistula centers. Additionally, health education for women and their families is critical to prevent the recurrence of the fistula in subsequent pregnancies. Patients with obstetric fistula are at high risk of obstruction, ruptured uterus, and possible maternal and fetal death when they become pregnant again. During the hospitalization, both preoperatively and in the recovery period, multiple programs are in place for patients and their families to receive advice and education regarding future pregnancies and the need to deliver near a hospital with capacity for cesarean section. Yet, when studied, 40% of the women heavily counseled on these topics did not remember these instructions (Neilsen et al., 2009). Fistula patients' long postoperative period also provides an opportunity to improve women's socioeconomic status through literacy programs and skills training which can help them upon their return to society (Donnay & Ramsey, 2006). Women who get training tend to accept the reality in order to cope in a better way and keep themselves busy doing handcrafts (Bashah et al., 2018).

After the immediate post-surgical period there can be persistent fistulas that spontaneously close over time, and there can be persistent incontinence that improves over time. Additionally, an immediate appearance of continence can progress into urge, stress, or continuous incontinence over the postsurgical weeks and sometimes surgically repaired fistula reappear after the woman returns to work, sex, or even during transportation home (Browning & Menber, 2008). After surgical closure 33–50% of women may continue to suffer from any form of incontinence—stress, urge, or persistent (Ballard et al., 2016; Browning & Menber, 2008). As in many other forms of surgery, a law of diminishing returns is evident in fistula repair (Hilton, 2003). If the first surgery does not work, it is less likely that the second will work, and still less likely that any further surgical repair will resolve the incontinence. Persistent incontinence after surgical repair of the fistula is 25% for women whose fistula occurred after the birth of their first child, and 10% for women whose fistula was after a second or subsequent birth (Muleta et al., 2010). There is also greater risk of persistent incontinence after a complicated or circumferential fistula than after a low fistula.

14.9.2.4   Delay #4: Reintegrating Into Society

Returning home after fistula surgery repair can be complicated. Some women left for fistula surgery without telling anyone where they were going, and some women do not go home (Biadgilign et al., 2013). Of women who had their obstetric fistula repaired: 95% remained married and 30–71% remained married and sexually active (Browning & Menber, 2008; Neilsen et al., 2009). At least moderate improvement with sex was reported by 82.9% of women, though the reports of sex ran the gamut from intolerable to terrifying for fear of recurrence to fine (Muleta et al., 2007). Forty-one percent of the women who were sexually active were using contraception, and 26% were amenorrheic and subsequently infertile (Neilsen et al., 2009). Of those who were sexually active, a third had become pregnant. Of those who had become pregnant there was a marked recurrence of obstetric catastrophe. Despite weeks of advice while recovering from fistula and vouchers for free transportation and care, it is difficult to have a successful obstetric outcome in the community after fistula repair. When women don't present to a hospital with comprehensive obstetric care capacities for birth, they die from obstructed labor, suffer fetal deaths, and some have fistula recurrence (Browning & Menber, 2008; Wall et al., 2017). There are thoughts that women don't present to the hospital because of hope for the current pregnancy despite the history, and concern that the woman may not have told her new husband of her history with a fistula (Neilsen et al., 2009). Finding women to interview after fistula repair is difficult, so numbers from these studies in Ethiopia have been small (Browning & Menber, 2008; Donnay & Ramsey, 2006).

Restoration after surgical repair of a fistula includes the ability to return to work. Prior to development of a fistula, 92% of the women who developed obstetric fistula and presented for surgery were farmers, 5% were domestic workers, and 3% were potters. Once they had a fistula 22% stopped working. After surgery 75% of those who had stopped working returned to work, leaving a total of women who do not work after fistula surgery at 5.5% (Neilsen et al., 2009). Socially, only 15% of women with a fistula attended social gatherings prior to surgery, and after surgery 79% attended social gatherings (Browning & Menber, 2008). It is notable that at 6 months, the woman's living arrangements had not necessarily changed from where she lived prior to surgery—some continued to live alone, live with her parents, or live with her husband—though the situation inside of the homes had changed (Browning & Menber, 2008). Prior to surgery many of the women were not allowed to eat with their family members, after treatment virtually all were able to eat together with their families (Muleta et al., 2007). Treatment of fistula was generally helpful in improving the status of individual women in their family and community. However, it was still difficult for some women to fully enjoy family and community life after treatment, and most women complained of at least one persistent health problem (Muleta et al., 2007).

Women who choose to disclose that they recovered from an obstetric fistula serve as ambassadors to their communities. Women who have disclosed raise awareness of the dangers of obstructed labor, the causes of fistula, and the biomedical option for healing. They are examples of women who have overcome fistula and are accepted back into their communities which provides visualized hope for other women with fistula in their communities. Particularly interesting is, moreover, the manner in which access to successful healing of shameful maternal health conditions was shown to be followed by a rapid decrease in the shame and secrecy surrounding the condition (Gjerde et al., 2018). As a result of newly gained awareness, previous perceptions of surgery were also said to be transforming (Gjerde et al., 2018).

14.10 Conclusions

The health behaviors of women with fistula in Ethiopia are complicated, complex, and do not occur in a vacuum. As we have expanded upon in this chapter, Ethiopian women act within their cultural, religious, economic, familial, and personal contexts. Behaviors which may seem counterproductive from an outside context can be logical when approached from the perspective of these women. Unfortunately, Ethiopian women face many challenges when approaching and accessing health care, both to prevent and then to treat fistula. Many women, either through choice or through lack of options, adapt to life with fistula and the challenges it brings and don't ever seek biomedical care. Those that do access surgical repair then face the challenges of reintegration. Ultimately, it is testament to the strength of Ethiopian women that they meet these challenges with such dignity.

References

Adefris, M., Abebe, S. M., Terefe, K., Gelagay, A. A., et al. (2017). Reasons for delay in decision making and reaching health facility among obstetric fistula and pelvic organ prolapse patients in Gondar University hospital, Northwest Ethiopia. *BMC Women's Health, 17*, 64. https://doi.org/10.1186/s12905-017-041609

Andargie, A. A., & Debu, A. (2017). Determinants of obstetric fistula in Ethiopia. *African Health Sciences, 17*(3), 671–680.

Ballard, K., Ayenachew, F., Wright, J., & Atnafu, H. (2016). Prevalence of obstetric fistula and symptomatic pelvic organ prolapse in rural Ethiopia. *International Urogynecology Journal, 27*, 1063–1067. https://doi.org/10.1007/s00192-015-2933-0

Bashah, D. T., Worku, A. G., & Mengistu, M. Y. (2018). Consequences of obstetric fistula in sub Sahara African countries, from patients' perspective: A systematic review of qualitative studies. *BMC Women's Health, 18*, 106. https://doi.org/10.1186/s12905-018-0605-1

Biadgilign, S., Lakew, Y., Reda, A. A., & Deribe, K. (2013). A population based survey in Ethiopia using questionnaire as proxy to estimate obstetric fistula prevalence: Results from demographic and health survey. *Reproductive Health, 10*, 14.

Browning, A., & Menber, B. (2008). Women with obstetric fistula in Ethiopia: a 6-month follow up after surgical treatment. *BJOG, 2008*(115), 1564–1569. https://doi.org/10.1111/j.1471-0528.2008.01911.x

Browning, A., & Whiteside, S. (2015). Characteristics, management, and outcomes of repair of rectovaginal fistula among 1100 consecutive cases of female genital tract fistula in Ethiopia. *International Journal of Gynecology & Obstetrics, 131*, 70–73.

Donnay, F., & Ramsey, K. (2006). Eliminating obstetric fistula: Progress in partnerships. *International Journal of Gynecology & Obstetrics, 94*, 254–261.

Donnay, F., & Weil, L. (2004). Obstetric fistula: The international response. *Lancet, 363*, 71–72.

Filippi, V., Chou, D., Barreix, M., Say, L., et al. (2018). A new conceptual framework for maternal morbidity. *International Journal of Gynecology & Obstetrics, 141*(1), 4–9. https://doi.org/10.1001/ijgo.12463

Fleck, F., & Hamlin, C. (2013). Giving hope to rural women with obstetric fistula in Ethiopia. *Bulletin of the World Health Organization, 91*, 724–725. https://doi.org/10.2471/BLT.13.031013

Gjerde, J. L., Rortveit, G., Adefris, M., Mekonnen, H., Belayneh, T., & Blystad, A. (2018). The lucky ones get cured: Health care seeking among women with pelvic organ prolapse in Amhara Region, Ethiopia. *PLoS ONE, 13*(11), e0207651. https://doi.org/10.1371/journal.pone.0207651

Gjerde, J. L., Rortveit, G., Muleta, M., Adefris, M., et al. (2017). Living with pelvic organ prolapse: Voices of women from Amhara region, Ethiopia. *International Urogynecology Journal, 28*, 361–366. https://doi.org/10.1007/s00192-016-3077-6

Goh, J. T. W. (2004). A new classification for female genital tract fistula. *Australian and New Zealand Journal of Obstetrics and Gynaecology, 44*, 502–504.

Heller, A., & Hannig, A. (2017). Unsettling the fistula narrative: Cultural pathology, biomedical redemption, and inequalities of health access in Niger and Ethiopia. *Anthropology & Medicine*. https://doi.org/10.1080/13648470.2016.1249252

Hilton, P. (2003). Vesico-vaginal fistulas in developing countries. *International Journal of Gynecology & Obstetrics, 82*, 285–295. https://doi.org/10.1016/S0020-7292(03)00222-4

Muleta, M., Hamlin, E. C., Fentahun, M., Kennedy, R. C., et al. (2007). Health and social problems encountered by treated and untreated obstetric fistula patients in rural Ethiopia. *Journal of Obsteterics and Gynaecology Canada, 30*(1), 44–50.

Muleta, M., Rasmussen, S., & Kiserud, T. (2010). Obstetric fistula in 14,928 Ethiopian women. *Acta Obstetricia et Gynecologica Scandinavica, 2010*, 1–7.

Neilsen, H. S., Lundberg, L., Nygaard, U., Aytenfisu, H., et al. (2009). A community-based long-term follow up of women undergoing obstetric fistula repair in rural Ethiopia. *BJOG, 116*, 1258–1264.

Olenja, J. (2003). Health seeking behavior in context. *East African Medical Journal, 2003*, 61–62. https://doi.org/10.4314/eamj.v80i2.8689

Tebeu, P. M., Fomulu, J. N., Khaddaj, S., de Bernis, L., et al. (2012). Risk factors for obstetric fistula: A clinical review. *International Urogynecology Journal, 23*, 387–394. https://doi.org/10.1007/s00192-011-1622-x

Thaddeus, S., & Maine, D. (1994). Too far to walk: Maternal mortality in context. *Social Science & Medicine, 38*(8), 1091–1110.

Wall, L. L. (2012). Overcoming phase 1 delays: The critical component of obstetric fistula prevention programs in resource-poor countries. *BMC Pregnancy and Childbirth, 12*, 68.

Wall, L. L., Belay, S., Heregot, T., Dukes, J., Berhan, E., & Abreha, M. (2017). A case-control study of the risk factors for obstetric fistula in Tigray, Ethiopia. *International Urogynecology Journal, 28*, 1817–1824. https://doi.org/10.1007/s00192-017-3368-6

Wright, J., Ayenachew, F., & Ballard, K. D. (2016). The changing face of obstetric fistula surgery in Ethiopia. *International Journal of Women's Health, 8*, 243–248.

Yismaw, L., Alemu, K., Addis, A., & Alene, M. (2019). Time to recovery from obstetric fistula and determinants in Gondar university teaching and referral hospital, northwest Ethiopia. *BMC Women's Health, 19*, 5.

Zeleke, B. M., Ayele, T. A., Woldetsadik, M. A., Bisetegn, T. A., et al. (2013). Depression among women with obstetric fistula, and pelvic organ prolapse in northwest Ethiopia. *BMC Psychiatry, 13*, 236.

Part III

Fistula Treatment, Management, and Models of Care

Classification of Female Genital Tract Fistulas

15

Judith Goh and Hannah G. Krause

15.1 Introduction

Obstetric fistula (OF) is the most common fistula worldwide and is mainly due to sub-optimal obstetric care. Most obstetric fistulas occur from pressure necrosis of maternal structures (vagina, lower urinary tract, anorectum) from prolonged compression of the foetal presenting part (usually head) in the maternal pelvis. However, with increasing caesarean section rates, these may also contribute to fistula formation or more maternal injuries whilst delivering the baby (usually not alive) through compromised and necrotic maternal tissue (Beltman et al., 2011; Loposso et al., 2015). Forceps delivery has been advocated to reduce caesarean section rates (Ayala-Yanez et al., 2015) and this may be extrapolated to the delivery of a dead foetus during prolonged obstructed labour to reduce maternal injuries.

OF is usually due to prolonged obstructed labour and/or operative deliveries (Fig. 15.1). In Uganda, 1.4% of women aged 15–49 years have symptoms of fistula (Uganda Demographic and Health Survey, 2016). Most obstetric fistulas occur in sub-Saharan Africa. At present, there is no internationally accepted system to classify female genital tract fistulas. A standardised fistula classification system would enable better communication and comparisons published in the literature (Goh, Krause, et al., 2009a; Goh, Stanford et al., 2009).

Classifications are used as a means of communication, to relay and retrieve information. A classification is a structured arrangement of similar objects/individuals/conditions which are grouped based on specific characteristics. Classification systems are generally not used as predictors, for example, in botanical taxonomy, the genus of one plant may not predict the height of the plant or its lifespan. Prediction is associated with data mining.

J. Goh (✉)
Griffith University, Gold Coast, QLD, Australia

Greenslopes Hospital, QEII Hospital,
Brisbane, QLD, Australia
e-mail: judith@qpfs.com.au

H. G. Krause
Greenslopes Hospital, QEII Hospital,
Brisbane, QLD, Australia

Fig. 15.1 Obstructed labour compressing vagina/urethra/bladder to the pubic symphysis and rectum to the sacrum. Illustration by Creative Studio, The Royal Children's Hospital Melbourne. Published with permission from © Judith Goh. All Rights Reserved

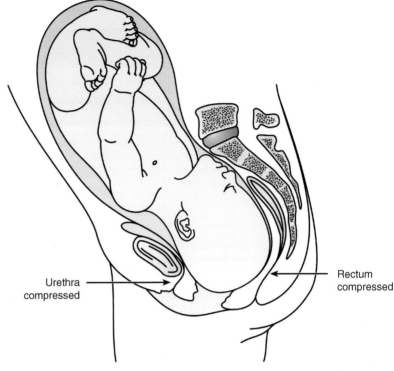

Urethra compressed

Rectum compressed

Fig. 15.2 Descriptive anatomical classification of genito-urinary fistulas. Illustration by Creative Studio, The Royal Children's Hospital Melbourne. Published with permission from © Judith Goh. All Rights Reserved

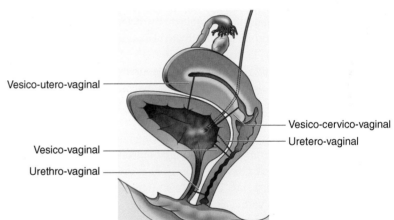

Vesico-utero-vaginal

Vesico-cervico-vaginal

Uretero-vaginal

Vesico-vaginal

Urethro-vaginal

Classifications of female genital tract fistulas have been proposed for over 150 years. Most are descriptive, utilising characteristics such as fistula size, location, vaginal scarring and involvement of structures (e.g., urethra, bladder, ureter, rectum, anus, cervix, uterus) (Fig. 15.2). The aims of this chapter are to provide an overview of classification systems and describe more recent applications of some of these systems to predict outcomes.

15.2   Historical Aspects of Classification Systems for Genito-Urinary Fistula

Sims opened the first hospital dedicated to women with fistula in New York in 1855. Reginald and Catherine Hamlin (Fig. 15.3) opened the second fistula hospital in Addis Ababa. Sims classification system (Sims, 1852) was based on the anatomical position of the fistula—Urethro-vaginal, Bladder neck, Vesico-vaginal and Utero-vaginal.

Mahfouz (1929) expanded Sims' classification to include fistulas that involved more than one anatomical site, e.g., vesico-urethro-vaginal fistula and vesico-cervico-vaginal fistula. Moir (1956) was also anatomically descriptive in his classification but introduced the concept of the circumferential fistula in his book on vesico-vaginal fistula (Moir, 1967). Most OFs of the urinary tract involve the anterior vaginal wall and the posterior aspects of the urethra and/or bladder. There are circumstances where the posterior and anterior portions of the lower urinary tract are affected by pressure necrosis. It is believed that with severe obstruction and pressure necrosis, the maternal structures are compressed on the pubic bone (especially pubic symphysis). This severe obstruction would then cause necrosis not only of the anterior vaginal wall and posterior urethra/bladder but also involve the anterior portion of the urethra/bladder. In other words, a total segment (circumference) of the urethra/bladder is necrosed off and this results in a gap or complete separation of the distal urethra from the proximal portions of the urethra/bladder (Fig. 15.4).

Fig. 15.3 Dr E Catherine Hamlin, cofounder of the Addis Ababa Fistula Hospital. http://resource.nlm.nih.gov/101428981

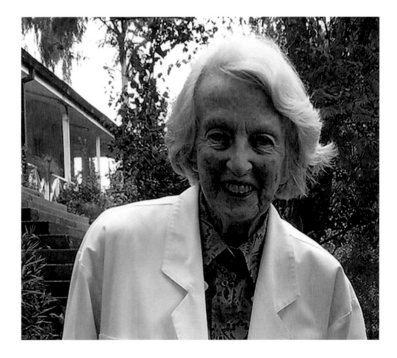

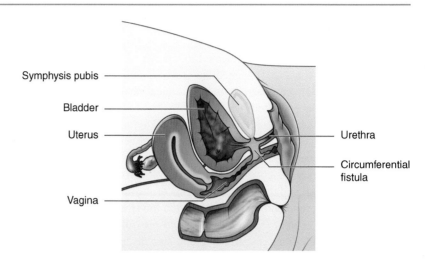

Fig. 15.4 Circumferential fistula with loss of anterior and posterior segments of the urethra and anterior vaginal wall. Illustration by Creative Studio, The Royal Children's Hospital Melbourne. Published with permission from © Judith Goh. All Rights Reserved

McConnachie (1958) had the insight to realise that there was no standardised universal classification to interpret the published literature and hence one could not compare techniques and results. He proposed a classification system that not only utilised the site and size of the fistula but also the conditions that would affect the surgery such as scarring and access to the fistula. McConnachie used two parameters for his classification and integrated the grade of fistula and type of fistula as follows:

- The grade of the fistula related to the status of the tissues, whether or not the 'sphincters' are affected and access to the fistula site.
  - Grade I: Normal healthy tissues, sphincters present, easy access
  - Grade II: Similar to Grade 1 but mild scar tissue
  - Grade III: Similar to Grade II with more scarring and poor access vaginally
- Type of fistula is related to the size of the fistula
  - Type A: Less than 1 cm diameter
  - Type B: 1 cm but less than 2 cm diameter
  - Type C: Over 2 cm
  - Type D: Any of the above plus recto-vaginal fistula

For example, a Grade 1, Type C fistula is more than 2 cm in diameter, with healthy tissues, normal sphincters and easy access to the fistula via the vaginal route. McConnachie also used his classification to correlate with surgical closure of the fistula and post-fistula urinary incontinence. Unlike many fistula surgeons who considered 'cure' as surgical closure, McConnachie only considered cure of the fistula if the fistula was closed and the woman was continent of urine. He also used 'muscle cross-strut slings' (from levator ani muscle, bulbo-cavernosus muscle) to improve stress urinary incontinence rates.

Bird (1967) combined the anatomical aspects of Mahfouz's (1929) classification with Moir's (1956) circumferential fistula but also added the description of fixation of the fistula to the pubic bone. Bird used his classification to assess fistula closure and urinary incontinence rates. Lawson (1968) employed the word 'juxta' and 'massive' in his classification. Gray (1970) in a small series suggested using only 4 Grades of classification and assessed for risk of post-operative urinary incontinence following surgery.

Genital tract fistulas, both urinary and anorectal, were incorporated into classification by Hamlin and Nicholson (1969). The six categories of the classification were as follows:

- Simple vesicovaginal fistula
- Simple rectovaginal fistula
- Simple urethrovaginal fistula
- Difficult high rectovaginal fistula
- Vesicouterine fistula
- Difficult urinary fistula

Hamlin and Nicholson (1969) categorised complete urethral destruction as 'difficult urinary fistula' and suggested a reconstructive method to improve surgical closure and urinary continence after surgery.

Waaldijk (1995) suggested another classification because although there are other classifications, 'all are based on the anatomic location of the fistula without surgical implications'. This is obviously not correct as reflected by the literature already presented. Waaldijk utilised a classification based on the involvement of urethra, closing mechanism, circumferential defect and fistula size. The classification is divided based on Types I–III and Types A, B, a and b as follows:

- Type I: not involving closing mechanism
- Type II: involving closing mechanism
- Type III: ureter and other exceptional fistulas
- Type A: without total urethra involvement
- Type B: with total urethra involvement
- Type a: without circumferential defect
- Type b: with circumferential defect

Goh (2004) proposed fixed reference points to describe and classify fistulas to allow comparisons between different observers. Goh also recognised that previous classifications could be ambiguous as there were no definitions for terminology such as 'simple' fistula or 'closing mechanism'. Other terminology could also be very subjective such as 'big' or 'high' fistula. An inexperienced vaginal fistula surgeon may classify a fistula as 'big and high' whereas an experienced vaginal fistula surgeon may classify the same fistula as 'small and mid-vagina'. Goh's classification uses 3 subclassifications to classify each fistula: Types 1–4; Types a–c and Types i–iii as follows:

- Types 1–4 of fistula—anatomical position in relation to a fixed reference point. For genito-urinary fistula, the external urinary meatus is that point.
  - Type 1: Distal edge of the fistula is >3.5 cm from external urinary meatus
  - Type 2: Distal edge of the fistula is 2.5–3.5 cm from external urinary meatus
  - Type 3: Distal edge is 1.5 to <2.5 cm from external urinary meatus
  - Type 4: Distal edge is <1.5 cm from external urinary meatus
- Types a–c of the fistula—size of the fistula
  - Type a: Size <1.5 cm, in largest diameter
  - Type b: Size 1.5–3 cm, in largest diameter
  - Type c: Size >3 cm in largest diameter

- Types i–iii: other considerations

  - Type i: None or only mild fibrosis and/or vaginal length >6 cm, normal capacity
  - Type ii: Moderate or severe fibrosis and/or reduced vaginal length and/or capacity
  - Type iii: Others—post-radiation, ureteric involvement, circumferential fistula, previous repair

Goh's classification has also been used to confirm good inter-observer correlations and good intra-observer correlations (in outpatient clinic and in operating theatre) (Goh, Krause, et al., 2009b). This classification has also been utilised to predict the risk of surgical closure and residual post-operative urinary incontinence (Goh et al., 2008).

Tafesse (2008) proposed another classification system based on whether or not the fistula is circumferential, urethral involvement, bladder size and vaginal length.

- Types I–IV: circumferential fistula or not
  - Type I: Non-circumferential new fistula (not previously operated)
  - Type II: Non-circumferential old fistula (previously operated)
  - Type III: Circumferential new fistula
  - Type IV: Circumferential old fistula
- Types I–IV: urethral involvement
  - Type I: No involvement of urethra (urethral length ≥4 cm)
  - Type II: Urethra involved but not middle third (urethral length 2.7–3.9 cm)
  - Type III: Middle one-third partly involved (urethral length 1.4–2.6 cm)
  - Type IV: Middle one-third completely involved but some urethral tissue remains (urethral length <1.4 cm but some urethral tissue remains)
  - Type V: No urethra
- Types a–c: bladder size
  - Type a: Longitudinal diameter >7 cm
  - Type b: Longitudinal diameter 4–7 cm
  - Type c: Longitudinal diameter <4 cm
- Types 1–3: Anterior vaginal tissue loss

  - Type 1: Less than 50% of anterior vagina is involved (≥3.5 cm healthy vagina remains)
  - Type 2: More than 50% of anterior vaginal wall is involved (<3.5 cm vagina remains)
  - Type 3: Obliterated vagina (vagina can't admit more than a finger)

Tafesse (2008) classification does have some specific anatomical assumptions – that the female urethra is 4 cm long and vaginal length of 7 cm. It also uses very specific measurements which may not be practical in the clinical setting such as urethral length in Type II of 2.7–3.9 cm. This classification also does not indicate whether it is total urethral length remaining, that is, whether the length involves the portions of urethra proximal and distal to the fistula. In this classification, there is no description of the method to measure the bladder size. Is it done with a measuring device inserted into the urethra and how much pressure to exert on the device as this will alter the length measured? In addition, if the fistula is circumferential in nature, is the bladder size measured before or after re-anastomosis of the fistula?

Browning and Williams (2009), as medical directors of the BahirDar Fistula Centre, Ethiopia and Addis Ababa Fistula Hospital, challenged Tafessa's premise the classification was based on research performed at the Fistula Hospitals. Browning and Williams wanted to clarify that the parameters proposed in the classification were not based on research as suggested by the author.

15.3   Anorectal-Vaginal Fistula

Less has been published on anorectal-vaginal fistula (Fig. 15.5). In limited-resource areas, true recto-vaginal fistula from obstructed labour is less common than the genito-urinary fistula. It may be that the rectum is more protected as it is more distensible, more easily evacuated and the curve of the sacrum provides more protection from pressure necrosis than the pubic symphysis, anteriorly, for the bladder and urethra. Unrepaired 4th degree perineal trauma or total perineal defect (Goh et al., 2020) is, however, quite common in some areas (Goh et al., 2016).

Mahfouz (1929) classified anorectal-vaginal fistulas into three types as the type would influence the route of surgery, that is, abdominal approach for Type 3 and vaginal for Types 1 and 2.

- Type 1: fistula situated at or near the perineum
- Type 2: Fistula situated in the middle third of the vagina
- Type 3: Fistula situated at the vault

Lawson (1968) proposed a classification based on two types of fistula as follows:

- Type 1: Involving the lower half of the vagina
  - Type A: Low rectovaginal fistula
  - Type B: Perineal trauma.
- Type 2: Involving the upper half of the vagina

  - Type A: High rectovaginal fistula
  - Type B: Massive perineal trauma

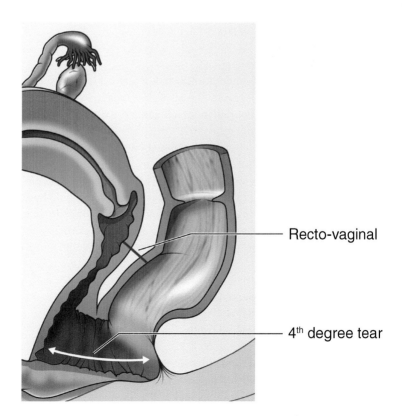

Fig. 15.5 Descriptive locations of ano-rectal vaginal fistulas. Illustration by Creative Studio, The Royal Children's Hospital Melbourne. Published with permission from © Judith Goh. All Rights Reserved

Recto-vaginal

4th degree tear

Rosenshein et al. (1980) proposed an anatomical classification in women who have had obstetric or surgical fistulas:

- Type I: Loss of perineal body, not associated with an identifiable fistulous tract
- Type II: Loss of perineal body associated with a fistulous tract involving lower third of vagina
- Type III: Fistula involving lower third of vaginal with an intact or attenuated perineal body
- Type IV: Fistula involving middle third of vagina
- Type V: Fistula involving upper third of vagina

Rothenberger and Goldberg (1983) suggested either 'simple' or 'complex' fistulas:

- Simple: Low or mid-vaginal fistula, ≤2.5 cm in diameter, due to traumatic or infectious cause
- Complex: High vaginal fistula, >2.5 cm in diameter, due to inflammatory bowel disease, irradiation or neoplastic cause

Goh (2004) extrapolated the fixed reference point classification to include ano-rectal vaginal fistulas as follows:

- Type 1: Distal edge of the fistula is >3.5 cm from hymen
- Type 2: Distal edge of the fistula is 2.5–3.5 cm from hymen
- Type 3: Distal edge is 1.5 to <2.5 cm from hymen
- Type 4: Distal edge is <1.5 cm from hymen

1. Types a–c of the fistula—size of the fistula
   a. Type a: Size <1.5 cm, in largest diameter
   b. Type b: Size 1.5–3 cm, in largest diameter
   c. Type c: Size >3 cm in largest diameter

- Types i–iii: Other considerations
  - Type i: None or only mild fibrosis and/or vaginal length >6 cm, normal capacity
  - Type ii: Moderate or severe fibrosis and/or reduced vaginal length and/or capacity
  - Type iii: Others—post-radiation, inflammatory disease, malignancy, previous repair

Tafesse (2008) classification is again based on whether or not the fistula is circumferential, and the amount of vaginal tissue loss and sphincter involvement. There is the assumption that the posterior vaginal length is 9 cm in length. There is also a significant potential for inter-observer variation in determining whether or not the edges of the fistula are reachable by the examining finger. There may also be intra-observer incongruity during clinic and operating theatre classification of the accessibility of the fistula edge in the presence of pain or discomfort during examination. In other words, it may not be possible to reach the edge of the fistula in the outpatient clinic due to pain/discomfort.

- Type I: Non-circumferential new fistula (not previously operated)
- Type II: Non-circumferential old fistula (previously operated)
- Type III: Circumferential new fistula
- Type IV: Circumferential old fistula

1. Type: posterior vaginal tissue loss and involvement
   a. Type a: Less than 50% of the posterior vagina is involved (≥4.5 cm of healthy vagina remains)
   b. Type b: More than 50% of vaginal wall is involved (<4.5 cm health vagina remains)
   c. Type c: Obliterated vagina

- Type: accessibility of proximal edge

  - Proximal edge of fistula reachable by examining finger and distal edge of fistula >3 cm from the anus
  - Proximal edge not reachable by examining finger but distal edge >3 cm from anus
  - Proximal edge of fistula reachable by examining finger but distal edge ≤3 cm from the anus
  - Proximal edge not reachable by examining finger and distal edge ≤3 cm from anus

15.4   Classification Systems, Clinical Outcomes and the Future

Earlier classification systems such as that of Sims (1852) and Mahfouz (1929) were used as a means to describe and communicate clinical findings. Moir (1956) eluded to fistula characteristics and outcomes. Moir suggested previous repairs and urethral destruction as having poorer outcomes. However, Moir believed that extensive loss of tissue of the bladder neck and extensive dense fibrosis with the fistula adherent to surrounding bony pelvis as significant factors for fistula closure and post-surgical urinary incontinence.

Assessing outcomes of surgery in a new classification system was accomplished by McConnachie (1958). McConnachie also suggested that fistulas from higher resource areas cannot be compared to obstetric fistulas as the former fistulas are usually smaller with less scar and more easily repaired surgically. Contrary to many other fistula surgeons, McConnachie understood that a 'cure' resulting from fistula surgery entailed closure of the 'hole' plus functional aspects. In other words, fistula surgeons often cited anatomical closure of the fistula as success or cure but McConnachie defined success/cure as continence and anatomical closure. In McConnachie's paper, 298 women had surgery for genito-urinary fistula. A higher rate of surgical failure to close the fistula was associated with increasing presence of vaginal scarring, repeat surgery and presence of a rectovaginal fistula. The amount of scarring also had an impact on post-fistula urinary incontinence.

Although Bird (1967) reported results in 70 women with genital tract fistulas using the classification system that was described in the manuscript, the correlation between classification and outcomes was not performed.

A larger series of 987 women with obstetric genito-urinary fistulas were classified using Goh (2004) system and correlated with outcomes in terms of failure to anatomically close the fistula and residual urinary incontinence (Goh et al., 2008). The Type 1–4 fistula (location of fistula from external urethral meatus) and size of the fistula did not significantly affect rates of successful closure of the fistula. The presence of significant vaginal scarring and the circumferential fistula were significant risk factors for failure of surgical closure of the fistula. The risk of residual urinary incontinence after fistula closure was affected by the Type of fistula. Type 1 fistulas (distal fistula edge >3.5 cm from external urethral meatus) were more likely to be continent. There was a tendency towards worsening urinary incontinence from Type 2 to Type 4 fistulas. In other words, the closer the distal edge is to the external urethral meatus, the higher the risk of ongoing urinary incontinence even after successful closure of the fistula. Other significant risk factors for residual urinary incontinence were the circumferential fistula, presence of significant vaginal scarring and larger size fistula.

Comparisons on the different classification systems are uncommon in literature. In general, classification systems are primarily used to communicate, describe or categorise similar conditions by employing specific features/properties. In more recent times, comparisons of genito-urinary fistula classification systems and/or use of various categories of classification systems have been used to attempt to predict outcomes following surgery. There are no comparisons of anorectal-vaginal fistula classification systems published in the English literature. Capes et al. (2012) conducted the first comparative study on two different genito-urinary fistula classification systems. It was a prospective study on women with obstetric genito-urinary fistulas utilising the Goh (2004) and Waaldijk (1995) classification systems. The Goh classification was significantly superior in predicting successful surgical closure of the fistula (Capes et al., 2012).

Arrowsmith (2007) suggested using a fistula score rather than classification to predict the risk of urinary incontinence after genito-urinary fistula closure as it may be unethical to attempt a repair if the prognosis is known to be very poor. This system scored two conditions, vaginal scarring and urethral status, based on clinical findings. The Panzi score (Mukwege et al., 2018) for genito-urinary fistula was introduced at the Panzi Hospital, Democratic Republic of the Congo. Data were retrospectively analysed for features of surgical failure using the Goh and Waaldjik classification systems. Mukwege et al. (2018) stated that the Tafesse classification was not used as it is a descriptive classification and was not able to be reduced to a single numerical score. The authors explored characteristics that were associated with failure and attempted to combine parameters such as Goh classification Types 1–4 into 2 types—2.5 cm or more from external urinary meatus or less than 2.5 cm from external urinary meatus. A scoring system was then created by extrapolating the data obtained. The Panzi score utilised a scoring system based on location of the fistula, size of the fistula and whether or not the fistula was a circumferential defect based on the findings that a fistula less than 2.5 cm from the external urinary meatus, larger than 3 cm in diameter and was circumferential had a higher risk of surgical failure.

Frajzyngier et al. (2012) performed a systematic review on factors which may affect genito-urinary fistula surgery outcomes (closure and subsequent incontinence) in low resource areas and thereby attempted to assess the possibility of developing a prognostic scoring/classification system. Factors that did not predict surgical outcomes included age of the woman at the time of fistula repair and age at occurrence of fistula. There were other factors that did not consistently correlate with surgical outcomes, such as the parity of the woman, mode of delivery and duration of fistula. This study (Frajzyngier et al., 2012) did find an association of surgical outcomes with presence of vaginal scarring and amount of urethral involvement. There was insufficient data to comment on the relationship of previous repairs, combined anorectal/genito-urinary fistulas, ureteric involvement, use of flaps and antibiotics to surgical outcomes. In a subsequent publication, Frajzyngier et al. (2013) also suggested that prediction of fistula classification systems may not solely depend on clinical findings as surgeon skill/experience, and peri-operative management such as catheter care are as important (or more important) in influencing surgical closure of the fistula.

In conclusion, classification systems have been primarily used to describe, compartmentalise and communicate. Objective terminology-based classification systems, such as measurement of the size of fistula, may provide better inter-observer concordance. However, some clinical findings may be difficult to objectively measure as there may be no standardised method to describe a finding, for example, amount of scarring in the vagina. Some have suggested a prognostic based classification system. However, as Frajzyngier et al. (2013) had pointed out, other factors apart from the characteristics of the fistula may be equally or more important in determining successful fistula closure, such as surgical skill and post-operative care.

References

Arrowsmith, S. (2007). The classification of obstetric vesico-vaginal fistulas: An evidence-based approach. *International Journal of Gynecology & Obstetrics, 9*, 25–27. https://doi.org/10.1016/j.ijgo.2007.06.018

Ayala-Yanez, R., Bayona-Soriano, P., Hernandez-Jimenez, A., Contreras-Rendon, A., Chabat-Manzanera, P., & Nevarez-Bernal, R. (2015). Forceps, actual use, and potential caesarean section prevention: Study in a select Mexican population. *Journal of Pregnancy*. https://doi.org/10.1155/2015/489267

Beltman, J., Van Den Akker, T., Van Lonkhuijzen, L., Schmidt, A., Chidakwani, R., & Van Roosmalen, J. (2011). Beyond maternal mortality: Obstetric haemorrhage in a Malawian district. *Acta Obstetricia et Gynecologica Scandinavica, 90*(12), 1423–1427. https://doi.org/10.1111/j.1600-0412.2011.01219.x

Bird, G. C. (1967). Obstetric vesico-vaginal and allied fistulae. *The Journal of Obstetrics and Gynaecology of the British Commonwealth, 74*, 749–752. https://doi.org/10.1111/j.1471-0528.1967.tb03791.x

Browning, A., & Williams, G. (2009). A new classification of female genital fistula: Letter to editor. *Journal of Obstetrics and Gynecology of Canada, 31*(4), 303. https://doi.org/10.1016/S1701-2163(16)34144-5

Capes, T., Stanford, E. J., Romanzi, L., Foma, Y., & Moshier, E. (2012). Comparison of two classification systems for vesicovaginal fistula. *International Urogynecology Journal, 23*(12), 1679–1685. https://doi.org/10.1007/s00192-012-1671-9

Frajzyngier, V., Li, G., Larson, E., Ruminjo, J., & Barone, M. A. (2013). Development and comparison of prognostic scoring systems for surgical closure of genitourinary fistula. *American Journal of Obstetrics and Gynecology, 208*(2), 112. https://doi.org/10.1016/j.ajog.2012.11.040

Frajzyngier, V., Ruminjo, J., & Barone, M. A. (2012). Factors influencing urinary fistula outcomes in developing countries: A systematic review. *American Journal of Obstetrics and Gynecology, 207*(4), 248–258. https://doi.org/10.1016/j.ajog.2012.02.006

Goh, J., Romanzi, L., Elneil, S., Haylen, B., et al. (2020). An International Continence Society (ICS) report on terminology for female pelvic floor fistulas. *Neurol Urodybam.* https://doi.org/10.1002/nau.24508

Goh, J., Stanford, E. J., & Genadry, R. (2009). Classification of female genito-urinary fistula: A comprehensive review. *International Urogynecology Journal, 20*, 605–610. https://doi.org/10.1007/s00192-009-0804-2

Goh, J. T. W. (2004). A new classification for female genital tract fistula. *Australian and New Zealand Journal of Obstetrics and Gynaecology, 44*, 502–504. https://doi.org/10.1111/j.1479-828X.2004.00315.x

Goh, J. T. W., Browning, A., Berhan, B., & Chang, A. (2008). Predicting the risk of failure of closure of obstetric fistula and residual urinary incontinence using a classification system. *International Urogynecology Journal, 19*, 1659–1662. https://doi.org/10.1007/s00192-008-0693-9

Goh, J. T. W., Krause, H., Browning, A., & Chang, A. (2009b). Classification of female genitor-urinary fistula: Inter- and intra-observer correlations. *Journal of Obstetrics and Gynaecology Research, 35*, 160–164. https://doi.org/10.1111/j.1447-0756.2008.00831.x

Goh, J. T. W., Krause, H. G., Browning, A., & Chang, A. (2009a). Classification of female genito-urinary tract fistula: Inter- and intra-observer correlations. *Journal of Obstetrics and Gynaecology Research, 35*, 160–164. https://doi.org/10.1111/j.1447-0756.2008.00831.x

Goh, J. T. W., Tan, S. B. M., Natukunda, H., Singasi, I., & Krause, H. G. (2016). Outcomes following surgical repair using layered closure of unrepaired 4th degree perineal tear in rural western Uganda. *International Urogynecology Journal, 27*(11), 1661–1666. https://doi.org/10.1007/s00192-016-3024-6

Gray, P. H. (1970). Obstetric vesicovaginal fistulas. *American Journal of Obstetrics and Gynecology, 107*, 898–901. https://doi.org/10.1016/S0002-9378(16)34043-1

Hamlin, R. H., & Nicholson, E. C. (1969). Reconstruction of urethra totally destroyed in labour. *British Medical Journal, 2*, 147–150. https://doi.org/10.1136/bmj.2.5650.147

Lawson, J. B. (1968). Birth-canal injuries. *Proceedings of the Royal Society of Medicine, 61*, 22–24.

Loposso, M. K., Ndundu, J., De Win, G., Ost, D., Puga, A. M., & De Ridder, D. (2015). Obstetric fistula in a district hospital in DR Congo: Fistula still occur despite access to caesarean section. *Neurourology and Urodynamics, 34*, 343–347. https://doi.org/10.1002/nau.22601

Mahfouz, N. (1929). Urinary and recto-vaginal fistulae in women. *The Journal of Obstetrics and Gynaecology of the British Empire, 36*, 581–589. https://doi.org/10.1111/j.1471-0528.1929.tb06705.x

McConnachie, E. L. F. (1958). Fistulae of the urinary tract in the female. *South African Medical Journal, 32*, 524–527.

Moir, J. C. (1956). Personal experience in the treatment of vesicovaginal fistulas. *American Journal of Obstetrics and Gynecology, 71*, 476–491. https://doi.org/10.1016/0002-9378(56)90476-8

Moir, J. C. (1967). *The vesico-vaginal fistula. Chapter 11: The circumferential vesico-vaginal fistula* (pp. 134–144). Bailliere Tindall and Cassell.

Mukwege, D., Peters, L., Amisi, C., Mukwege, A., Smith, A. R., & Miller, J. M. (2018). Panzi score as parsimonious indicator of urogenital fistula severity derived from Goh and Waaldijk classifications. *International Journal of Obstetrics and Gynecology, 142*, 187–193. https://doi.org/10.1002/ijgo.12514

Rosenshein, N., Genadry, R., & Woodruff, J. D. (1980). An anatomic classification of rectovaginal septal defects. *American Journal of Obstetrics and Gynecology, 137*, 439–442. https://doi.org/10.1016/0002-9378(80)91124-2

Rothenberger, D. A., & Goldberg, S. M. (1983). The management of rectovaginal fistulae. *Surgical Clinics of North America, 63*, 61–73. https://doi.org/10.1016/S0039-6109(16)42930-0

Sims, J. M. (1852). On the treatment of vesico-vaginal fistula. *The American Journal of the Medical Sciences, 23*, 59–82. https://doi.org/10.1097/00000441-185201000-00004

Sims, J. M. (n.d.). *U.S. National Library of Medicine Digital Collections.* http://resource.nlm.nih.gov/101428981

Tafesse, B. (2008). New classification of female genital fistula. *Journal of Obstetrics and Gynaecology Canada, 30*, 394–395. https://doi.org/10.1016/S1701-2163(16)32823-7

Uganda Demographic and Health Survey. 2016. https://dhsprogram.com/pubs/pdf/FR333/FR333.pdf

Waaldijk, K. (1995). Surgical classification of obstetric fistula. *International Journal of Gynecology & Obstetrics, 49*, 161–163. https://doi.org/10.1016/0020-7292(95)02350-L

Surgical Treatment for Obstetric Fistula: Not an Easy Option

16

Andrew Browning

16.1 Introduction

Over the course of human history and in particular the history of childbirth and its complications, the surgical management for obstetric fistula is a relatively recent innovation. There are mummified records of obstetric fistula dating back some 4000 years and papyrus writings describing obstetric fistula dating back 3500 years. However, the first known cure of an obstetric fistula patient was a relatively recent event, dating back less than 350 years ago to 1675 AD (Zacharin, 1988). Many obstacles had to be overcome, catheter drainage, surgical principles, methods of dissection, suture materials, anesthesia, and antibiotics. All of which took time and progress was slow, taking place over generations. James Marion Sims was credited with developing the flap splitting method of fistula repair and built a Women's Hospital in New York in 1855, primarily to care for patients suffering from obstetric fistula (Wall, 2017). This hospital later closed and obstetric fistula has been eradicated in the western world thanks to the advent of safe obstetric care for all women.

Since the days of Sims in the mid-nineteenth century, surgery has been the mainstay of treatment for women suffering from obstetric fistula. The principles pioneered by Sims have continued to be refined and built upon. There have been many exciting surgical innovations in the last couple of decades that have vastly improved the physiological and clinical outcomes with regard to regaining continence. Indeed, the methods of restorative surgery offered to women with obstetric fistula in the last few years would be barely recognizable to Sims, but there is still room for improvement. This in itself tells the reader that the perfect solution for the problem still has not been found, and that further research and refinements are needed.

Despite these advancements, surgery has its limitations. The obstetric fistula is described as a "field injury", meaning that the ischemic insult affects all the tissues in the pelvis. As a consequence, the bladder, vagina, bowel, ureter, urethra, cervix, uterus, levator complex, nerves, and bones can all be injured to varying degrees of severity, varying from a minor insult to complete necrosis and sloughing away (Arrowsmith et al., 1996). This results in tissue loss and/or injury, which despite the body's heal-

A. Browning (✉)
Maternity Africa, Arusha, Tanzania

Barbara May Foundation, Bowral, NSW, Australia

Bahir Dar Fistula Centre, Bahir Dar, Ethiopia
e-mail: andrew_browning@hotmail.com

© Springer Nature Switzerland AG 2022
L. B. Drew et al. (eds.), *A Multidisciplinary Approach to Obstetric Fistula in Africa*, Global Maternal and Child Health, https://doi.org/10.1007/978-3-031-06314-5_16

ing and regenerating properties, tissues still need surgical intervention (Figs. 16.1, 16.2, and 16.3). Surgery can only repair tissues anatomically and sometimes help symptoms physiologically. The overriding symptom of the obstructed labor field injury is the bladder fistula leading to incontinence, but there are also other pathologies resulting from the "field injury" that range from immobility caused by nerve damage (Fig. 16.4), muscle loss in the pelvis, and renal damage including damaged ureters (Fig. 16.5). As a result of the incontinence associated with obstetric fistula, there can exist neglect, social ostracism, spousal and familial isolation, stigmatization, depression, and suicide. Restoring continence and function can indeed affect the array of other complaints, but not entirely.

Fig. 16.1 Small fistula in the urethra. (Photo Credit: Andrew Browning)

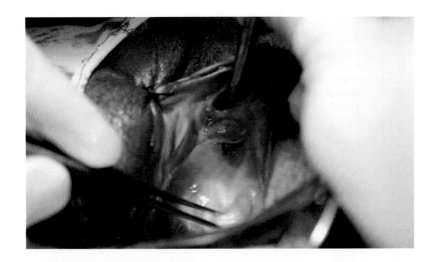

Fig. 16.2 A medium-to-large vesicovaginal fistula. Most of the anterior vagina is missing. (Photo Credit: Andrew Browning)

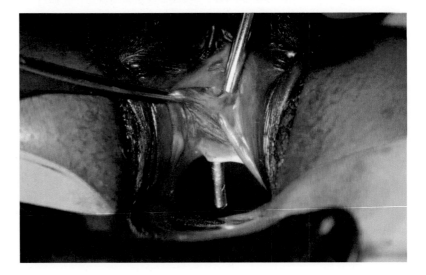

Fig. 16.3 Rectovaginal fistula. Note the bowel mucosa seen on the posterior vagina. The urethra is torn and almost absent. (Photo Credit: Andrew Browning)

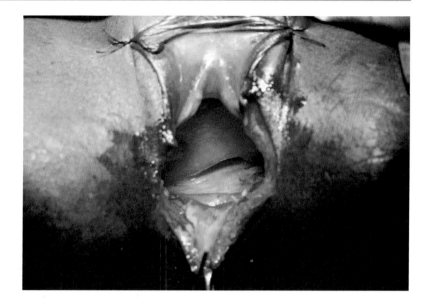

Fig. 16.4 Foot drop in a woman with nerve damage and obstetric fistula. (Photo Credit: Andrew Browning)

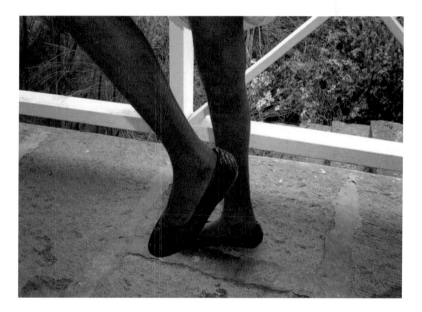

Fig. 16.5 Radiograph of the pelvis demonstrating hydroureters and hydronephrosis in a woman with obstetric fistula. (Photo Credit: Andrew Browning)

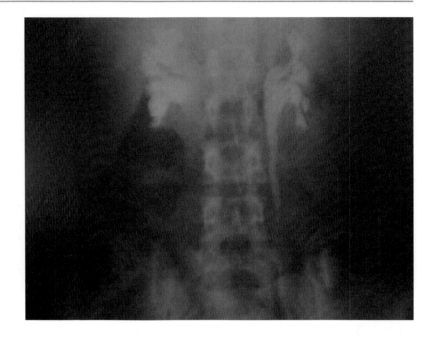

16.2   Urinary Incontinence

For years surgery has focused on just closing the hole between the bladder and the vagina, or if there is a rectal fistula present, closing the hole in the bowel. Over time surgical techniques improved, sutures improved, and methods of grafting came and went. It became quite easy to close the fistula, or hole, but doing so didn't necessarily mean that the patient would be continent. In many women, the urethra is involved in the ischemic process, meaning that all the structures that provide the physiological closure of the urethra are either damaged or destroyed. The surgeon might feel pleased for repairing the defect in the bladder and urethra and so obtaining a good anatomical result, but the patient remained wet. The now- anatomically-repaired bladder and urethra has no physiological function, the muscles and ligaments that normally produce continence were no longer, and if they are not reconstructed it will leave the patient still leaking, disappointed and ostracized (Figs. 16.6 and 16.7). She would go home wondering if anything had actually been done for her and despite counseling, doubting whether any further treatment would ever be able to help her.

Thirty years ago, the published ongoing incontinence rate was some 6%, but this was misleading (Kelly & Kwast, 1993). The paper cited the number of women returning to one particular hospital some time after surgery, but they were still complaining of incontinence despite a closed fistula. It was assumed that if they didn't return, then, despite leaving the hospital still leaking, they had improved with time and were now cured.

There is still no standardized method of assessing ongoing incontinence after a fistula repair, and often the patient is recorded as being "'cured" if the fistula is closed but she is still wet. Closer examination revealed that between 33% and 45% of patients had incontinence after the removal of the catheter. Some did indeed improve with time, but this was not the rule (Browning, 2004, 2006).

The nature of this incontinence is poorly understood. From up to 7–8% of these patients will have urinary retention with overflow which is easily managed with clean intermittent self-catheterization. Nearly all of the patients with retention and overflow in the short term will be dry and voiding nor-

Fig. 16.6 Fistula
repaired, but the urethra
is short, open, and no
physiological function.
(Photo Credit: Andrew
Browning)

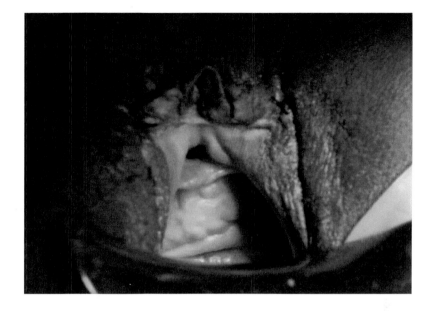

Fig. 16.7 Ostracized
with obstetric fistula.
(Photo Credit: Andrew
Browning)

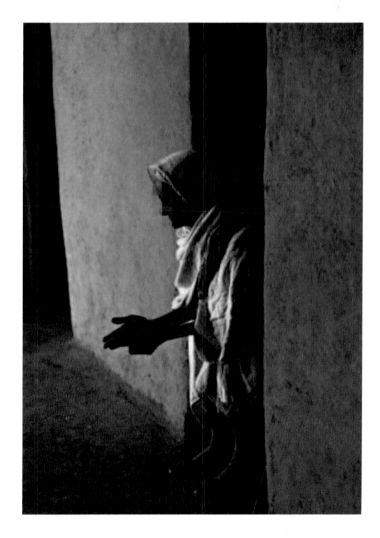

Fig. 16.8 The pubourethral ligament reconstructed with levator muscle. (Photo Credit: Andrew Browning)

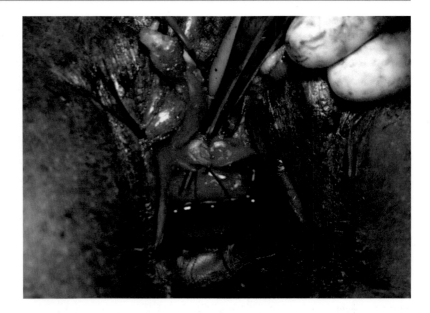

Fig. 16.9 Rectus sheath harvested. (Photo Credit: Andrew Browning)

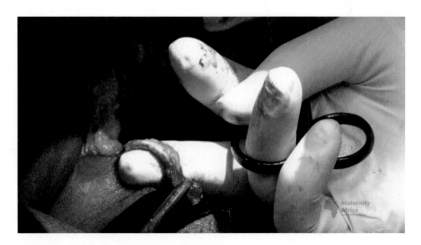

mally after a period of clean intermittent self-catheterization (CISC).[1] The remaining will have mainly stress incontinence, 3% will have detrusor overactivity and 43% will have mixed incontinence (Goh et al., 2016). Anticholinergics have been of little benefit for these women (Prof. Gordon William, Hamlin Fistula, Ethiopia, personal communication), but some still seem to gain benefit from surgery.

Several exciting and innovative techniques have been published and taught in recent years, including reconstructing the urethra, reconstructing the pubourethral ligament (Figs. 16.8, 16.9, and 16.10), and reconstructing the vagina (Figs. 16.11 and 16.12). Incontinence rates have decreased from 33–45% in the immediate post-operative period to 15–18% and these rates have largely been maintained at 6 months' follow-up (Browning, 2004, 2006; Browning et al., 2018; Browning & Menber, 2008).

---

[1] Clean Intermittent Self-Catheterization (CISC) is a method that is used to empty the bladder by the patient using a clean flexible catheter. It involves putting the catheter in and taking it out several times a day.

Fig. 16.10 Recon-
structing the puboure-
thral ligament using the
rectus sheath. (Photo
Credit: Andrew
Browning)

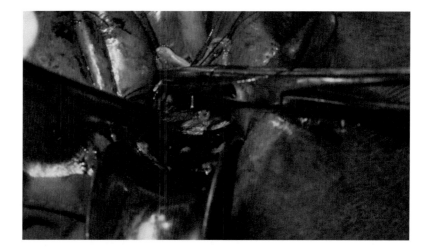

Fig. 16.11 The fistula
is closed, but there is no
remaining vaginal tissue
to cover the repair.
(Photo Credit: Andrew
Browning)

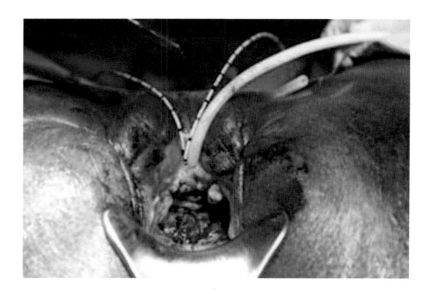

Fig. 16.12 Vagina
repaired with a
Singapore vascular flap
from the groin crease.
(Photo Credit: Andrew
Browning)

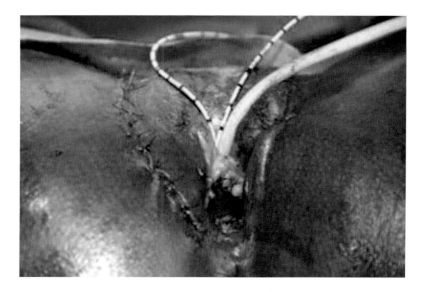

Fig. 16.13 Fourth-degree perineal tear. (Photo Credit: Andrew Browning)

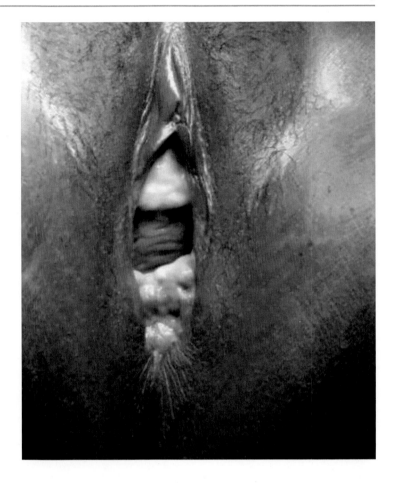

16.3   Fecal Incontinence

Perineal tears are commonly seen among patients in any fistula program (Fig. 16.13). Although they are not technically a fistula (that is, a communication between two epithelial surfaces[2]), they are a tear in the tissues, resulting in the epithelia of the anus and sometimes the rectum being in continuum with the epithelia of the vagina and perineum, and obvious fecal and flatal incontinence results. They are not caused by an obstructed labor and so are not of ischemic origin, but rather they are a traumatic tearing, usually from a precipitant labor. Being a tear, there is not the tissue loss that typifies the obstetric fistula. Perineal tears usually occur in isolation and the "field injury" of the obstructed labor injury complex does not apply.

Similarly, rectovaginal fistula can occur in isolation, usually iatrogenic, having been caused by a traumatic instrumental delivery, most commonly by a forceps delivery. They can also be caused by a direct trauma, e.g., violent intercourse, or intercourse in an undeveloped minor, or they can be the

---

[2]Epithelium refers to a thin layer of cells that line the outer surfaces of organs and blood vessels, as well as lining the inner surfaces of certain organs and body cavities. Because the epithelium does not contain blood vessels, the constituent cells receive nutrients and oxygen by diffusion.

result of a fourth-degree tear[3] being repaired incorrectly or breaking down, leaving a small fistula just proximal to the introitus.

Both the iatrogenic rectovaginal fistula (RVF) and perineal tears have a very good prognosis, both surgically; restoring normal anatomy and from a functional viewpoint. The clinical success rate for restoring fecal and flatal continence via surgery is high, approaching 100% (Goh et al., 2016).

On the other hand, an obstetric rectovaginal fistula from an ischemic origin is more severe. It almost always is associated with a vesicovaginal fistula (VVF); the labor that causes a combined VVF and RVF is almost a full day longer than the labor that causes a VVF in isolation. It is more likely to be associated with severe scarring, a more severe VVF and nerve damage resulting in foot drop (Browning & Whiteside, 2015). It is almost always possible to close an RVF, whether it is traumatic or ischemic in origin. The bladder is a more finite organ than the bowel. If much of the bladder has been destroyed, then there is nothing to repair and the prognosis is poor. However, no matter how large the RVF is there is always sigmoid colon that can be advanced to close the defect, even if the whole rectum and anus have been destroyed. There is always some anal sphincter that can be repaired and fecal continence can be restored (Browning & Whiteside, 2015).

Unfortunately, those patients with an ischemic RVF have a poor prognosis with regard to ongoing urinary incontinence, sexual and reproductive health. The more severe bladder injuries associated with an RVF can result in ongoing incontinence despite the best surgical efforts. The more extensive vaginal scaring leads to dyspareunia and in the most severe cases, apareunia. The more severe ischemic injuries that lead to the RVF can also damage the cervix and uterus, and the patient remains infertile. If there is associated foot drop,[4] it usually improves with time, but rarely it can be ongoing.

16.4   Ureteric Injuries

Fifty percent of patients will have some degree of obstructive uropathy[5] (Langundoye et al., 1976) (Fig. 16.5), and less than 5% will have a ureter involved in the fistula or an iatrogenic ureteric fistula. The obstructive uropathy leading to hydroureter,[6] hydronephrosis,[7] and even non-functioning kidneys is easy to explain if the ureter has been inadvertently tied off at the time of cesarean section or hysterectomy. In cases of obstructed labor that is not relieved by a cesarean section, it is best explained by scar formation. After the necrotic tissue comes away, scar forms within the pelvis as the remaining tissues heal. This scar is the cause of the obstruction to the ureter, either partial or complete. Surgery can relieve the obstruction by excising the scar or bypassing the obstructive scar and reimplanting the ureter on the affected side.

---

[3]A fourth-degree tear during childbirth is a tear or laceration through the perineal muscles that extends through the muscle layers that surround the anus and extends through the anal sphincter to the anal canal or rectum.

[4]Foot drop is an abnormality of gait characterized by dropping of the forefoot and inability to raise the toes or the foot from the ankle. Although there are many causes, they almost always have in common damage to the nerves.

[5]An obstructive uropathy refers to the structural or functional hindrance of the flow of urine through the ureter, bladder, or urethra. This can cause the urine to back up to the kidneys, damaging them.

[6]Hydroureter is an enlargement or dilatation of the ureter as a result of blockage of urine flow.

[7]Hydronephrosis refers to the swelling of one or both kidneys that occurs when urine cannot drain as a result of an obstruction.

16.5   Diversions

In approximately 2% of cases either the bladder fistula cannot be closed (rare), or it has been closed but the bladder capacity and/or urethra have been destroyed to such an extent that despite best efforts, continence cannot be restored. The patient might be left with what is termed a "drain pipe" urethra and/or a small non-compliant bladder, having just the same level of incontinence as she had before she was operated on. The only chance that she will have to regain continence is to have a diversion operation. The common ones are the Mainz II pouch or ileal conduit. Less commonly some continent diversion is used, for example, the Indiana Pouch. However, this is not an easy fix. If an ileal conduit is used the patient is restricted. Usually, the conduit bags are not widely available except from being imported by the hospital that did the operation. She will not be able to return to her village as she won't have access to the bags. If she was able to return to her village, she will not be accepted with her "strange condition, leaking urine from her abdomen into a bag". She will even struggle to dispose of the conduit bags for fear of them being discovered. There have been many cases of well-meaning surgeons from the West coming to "help" fistula patients and performing ileal conduits and then flying back to their own countries, not realizing these issues and leaving the patient in a worse state than when they found her.

The Mainz II pouch is an easier and perhaps more appropriate solution for the low-income countries. It is not reliant on external appliances so the woman can return to her village and even get pregnant (D'elia et al., 2004; Venn & Mundy, 1999)—but it is not for every woman. Because the prospective candidate for this procedure will need to have an intact and well-functioning anal sphincter, they must be counseled and screened appropriately. To check that the anal sphincter will hold urine, place 300 ml of blue-dyed water or saline into the rectum and get the woman to walk about for 1–2 h wearing a pad. If she leaks, she will not be suitable for the operation. If she has a weak anal sphincter and a Mainz II pouch is formed, and she will leak urine and feces mixed together after the operation. You must also carefully check if she has a rectovaginal fistula. Many patients have been diverted only to find later that she has an as yet undiscovered RVF and will leak. Despite passing the screening tests some women will still complain that they leak through the anus, usually at night when the sphincter relaxes. Still other women will refuse the operation. When they hear that they will pass urine and feces together, they exclaim "I don't want to be like a chicken"!

The operation itself is not without its morbidity and mortality (Wilkinson et al., 2016). Acidosis can result from absorption of the urine, and the woman may have to mix some bicarbonate in water and drink it each day. Patients should return for regular electrolyte checks, but in reality they don't. Several patients have been initially well but as they age, their anal sphincter will relax, again especially at night. Some surgeons have tried to plicate the anal sphincter that can give some short-term relief, but the leakage usually recurs after 1–2 years.

16.6   Cervical Injuries

During a long labor, it is not uncommon for the uterine cervix and even uterus itself to be injured. Juxtacervical or intracervical fistula invariably have the anterior cervix at least torn, if not completely necrosed and missing (Fig. 16.14) (Wilkinson et al., 2018). Care must be taken to not only repair the defect in the bladder and vagina but to also repair the cervix as well, making sure the cervical canal remains patent. If the cervical canal is closed during the surgery, amenorrhea[8] and a painful hemato-

[8]Amenorrhea is an abnormal condition in which a woman has ceased menstruation. Primary amenorrhea refers to the condition in which a young woman does not begin to menstruate by 16 years of age.

Fig. 16.14 Open cervix. It is thin anteriorly and torn on the left side. A fistula is present in the anterior cervix just proximal to the lip. (Photo Credit: Andrew Browning)

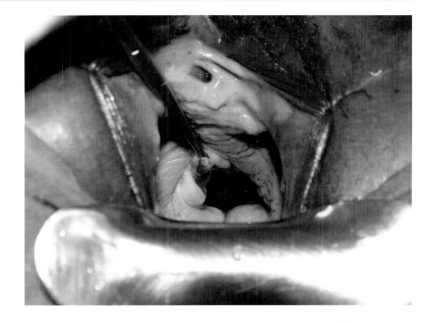

metra[9] may result if the patient is still menstruating. Despite the surgeons' best efforts, the repaired cervix might still be weak leading to an incompetent cervix and mid-trimester fetal loss if the woman gets pregnant in the future.

16.7 Infertility and Future Pregnancy

Only about 20% of women will achieve a successful, full-term delivery after a fistula repair (Delamou et al., 2016; Kopp et al., 2017; Tembely et al., 2014). There are several reasons for this. Sheehan's syndrome[10] can be caused from prolonged hypotension during the causative delivery (Naidu & Krishna, 1963). Asherman's syndrome[11] can develop presumably because of urine in the endometrial cavity affecting the endometrium and/or repeated infections whilst living with the fistula. There is very little that can be done for Sheehan's syndrome in the setting where most fistula patients occur. Asherman's syndrome can be treated with division of the adhesions in the uterine cavity, intrauterine contraceptive device (IUCD) placement to keep the cavity open, and then high-dose estrogens to try and generate an endometrium again. The success of such maneuvers for the obstetric fistula patient is unknown. Cervical injuries (above) can be repaired at the time of fistula repair with varying degrees of success, but many remain with incompetent cervices.

Other causes of amenorrhea such as severe depression and malnutrition can be managed and rectified but others, such as a cesarean hysterectomy performed for a ruptured uterus, clearly cannot.

---

[9] Hematometra refers to the abnormal accumulation of blood in the uterus, often the result of obstruction of menstrual flow at the level of the uterus, cervix, or vagina.

[10] Sheenan's syndrome is also known as postpartum pituitary gland necrosis and refers to acquired hypopituitarism that results from ischemic necrosis of the pituitary gland caused by hypovolemic shock and loss of blood during or after labor and childbirth.

[11] Asherman's syndrome is a rare condition in which scar tissue, termed adhesions, develop within the uterine cavity or cervix. In most cases, it is the result of undergoing multiple dilatation and curettage (D&C) procedures but can also result from infection.

16.8   Foot Drop and Contractures/Mobility

Up to 20% of women will have some degree of lumbosacral plexus damage or peroneal nerve damage during a long labor (Reif, 1988; Waaldjik & Elkins, 1994; Wall, 2017). Some women consider themselves immobile because of this and they can lie on the floor of their huts for weeks, months, or even years. This will eventually lead to contractures of the lower limbs, usually the ankles and knees but sometimes even the hips.

The nerve damage usually spontaneously recovers with time, but 13% of women will have some residual nerve damage at the end of 2 years (Waaldjik & Elkins, 1994). Contractures can be very difficult to treat, needing either active and often painful physiotherapy or even tendon lengthening procedures (although in practice this is rarely used).

16.9   Urine Dermatitis

The obstetric fistula patient will drink less water to pass less urine and the concentrated urine affects the skin. The resulting areas of sensitive hyperkeratosis are commonly termed urine dermatitis (Fig. 16.15). These areas can break down and become secondarily infected. The best way to treat this is to cure the incontinence. If the patient does become dry the urine dermatitis will resolve within a couple of weeks. If, however, surgical treatment has not been successful or if it is not available, urine dermatitis may be managed by encouraging the patient to drink more, diluting the urine so making it less irritating to the skin or by using a barrier lotion or cream such as Vaseline. The former is less attractive to the patient as she will then leak more, and the latter might be prohibitive because of costs.

Fig. 16.15 Urine dermatitis. (Photo Credit: Andrew Browning)

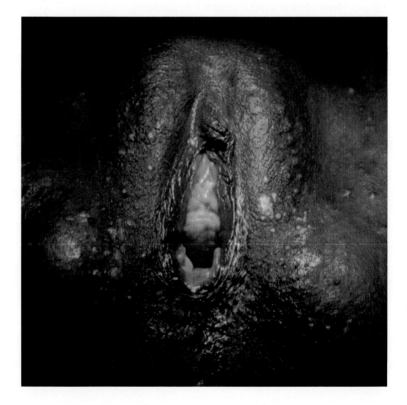

16.10   Social Issues

Patients are often left socially isolated. Social isolation may be self-inflicted or inflicted by those around her or both. The obstetric fistula sufferer will feel embarrassed about the way she smells and the state of her clothes and live with self-imposed isolation. She will avoid busy places like the market, social events, and places of worship. She will often become a recluse, staying in her small hut, being cared for by a family member (Fig. 16.7).

Isolation is often inflicted upon her. More than half of all fistula patients have been divorced because of their injuries and the rate of divorce increases if they have no live children to care for; the rate increases the longer that they suffer the fistula. She might be cared for by a parent or sibling and have very limited contact with the wider community (Kelly & Kwast, 1993; Wall, 2017)

Of course, there are remarkable exceptions to these generalizations. It is not common, but still not rare, to meet enterprising strong women who have managed despite everything working against them. Even with a fistula they will care for themselves and their hygiene, make pads from cloth and wash them regularly, attend the markets, work, run businesses, attend worship and few people know of their condition.

Curing a patient of her incontinence enables her to return to her usual social networks. If she remains with ongoing incontinence after surgery, she will remain isolated (Browning et al., 2007; Browning & Menber, 2008; Umoiyoho et al., 2011; Weston et al., 2011).

16.11   Mental Health

The mental health problems that obstetric fistula patients suffer have been well-documented in the last decade. Up to 100% of women suffering a fistula screen positive for potential psychological disorders, namely depression (Goh et al., 2005). Up to 40% of women still suffering a fistula have thought about or attempted suicide.

The surgeon's knife can go a long way in curing their mental health problems. If successfully treated and the patient becomes dry, then the number of women who screen positive with the same psychological screening tests drops back to the level of the background population (Browning et al., 2007). If, however, the fistula is not closed or the patient has severe ongoing incontinence despite a closed fistula, then she remains with depression and sometimes suicidal tendencies as well (Browning et al., 2007; Khisa & Nyamongo, 2012; Weston et al., 2011; Wilson et al., 2015).

The patients, their families and their caregivers require a great deal of support and counseling to help them cope with their condition. There has been some work in training women in various coping mechanisms, but as to whether they are effective or not is still debatable. Clearly, the best management is to get the patient fully continent, as without this the likelihood of her having a life spent free of mental health problems remains small (Wilson et al., 2015).

16.12   Iatrogenic Fistula

Perhaps one of the most disturbing facts about the etiology of obstetric fistula is that they can actually be caused by surgery. There have been great advances in the provision of obstetric care for women across the world, including the training of increased numbers of health professionals. However, in the rush to train doctors and midwives, perhaps the quality of their training has been diluted. It is not uncommon to see junior doctors not reflect and protect the bladder during cesarean section, and subsequently suture the bladder directly to the uterine repair, causing a fistula. In several recent series up to 25% of all fistula patients presenting now have the cause of their fistula as a surgical error (Barageine et al., 2014; Gele et al., 2017; Kumar et al., 2017; Raassen et al., 2017; Wright et al., 2016). This is defined as a fistula occurring in or close to the cervix after a labor of less than a day and delivering a live baby. Others have described ureteric fistula developing in isolation, usually on the left side. These only occur after a cesarean section and have not been recorded after a pure obstructed labor without a cesarean section (Raassen et al., 2017). Some cesarean sections are done after a long obstructed two to three-day labor and the fistula had already formed prior to the operation. These are not iatrogenic.

Admittedly cesarean sections are often done under difficult conditions, including urgent and even life-threatening deliveries, poor lighting, poor equipment, and poor anesthesia. This makes the surgery very difficult and it is understandable that complications can and do happen. But by simply reflecting the bladder at the time of cesarean delivery and then pushing the ureters away greatly reduces the risk for an iatrogenic fistula to occur. Vesicovaginal fistula and ureteric fistula are also being seen after routine hysterectomies. This occurs everywhere, is a known complication, and seems to be on the rise in obstetric fistula services.

If there is a good side to this, it is that iatrogenic fistulas occurring in this way are almost always small, high in the vagina or in the cervix, there is no tissue loss or broad ischemic field injury, and so their prognosis is good. The medical practitioner should aim for 100% of these women to be cured either by surgery or catheter treatment.

16.13 Conclusion: Prevention is Better Than Cure

Clearly, surgery for any condition, let alone for obstetric fistula, has its limitations. Surgical treatment for fistula incontinence, both urinary and fecal, has improved greatly over the years and clinical outcomes are better. However, some 10% of patients will remain with some degree of ongoing incontinence—most can manage well but others are left in isolation.

Surgery can do little to improve reproductive capabilities, others will remain with lifelong mobility problems due to nerve damage, and still others will have long-term renal compromise. If a diversion is needed the patient will still have lifelong risks of complications, and as they age, seepage of urine and feces via an increasingly lax anal sphincter.

However, it is ironic that where surgery has so many failings for obstetric fistula treatment, it can be used to completely prevent all of the life-long suffering that an obstructed labor might cause. Obstetric fistula was successfully eradicated in industrialized countries when women could have access to a cesarean section in labor if and when it was needed. Of course, the surgery needs to be applied carefully and skillfully, as it is of no use trying to prevent fistula by encouraging women to get to hospital for the delivery of their baby if the cesarean section itself can be the cause of a fistula. But with safe and available cesarean sections (and, at times, assisted deliveries), most if not all obstetric fistula will be prevented.

References

Arrowsmith, S., Hamlin, E. C., & Wall, L. L. (1996). Obstructed labor injury complex: Obstetric fistula formation and the multifaceted morbidity of maternal birth trauma in the developing world. *Obstetrical & Gynecological Survey, 51*, 568–574.

Barageine, J. K., Tumwesigye, N. M., Byamugisha, J. K., Almroth, L., & Faxelid, E. (2014). Risk factors for obstetric fistula in Western Uganda: A case control study. *PLoS One, 9*(11), e112299.

Browning, A. (2004). Prevention of residual urinary stress incontinence following successful repair of obstetric vesico-vaginal fistula using a fibro-muscular sling. *BJOG : An International Journal of Obstetrics and Gynaecology, 111*, 357–361.

Browning, A. (2006). Risk factors for developing residual incontinence after vesicovaginal fistula repair. *BJOG : An International Journal of Obstetrics and Gynaecology, 113*, 482–485.

Browning, A., Fentehun, W., & Goh, J. T. W. (2007). The impact of surgical treatment on the mental health of women with obstetric fistula. *BJOG: An International Journal of Obstetrics and Gynaeocology, 14*, 1439–1441.

Browning, A., & Menber, B. (2008). Obstetric fistula in Ethiopia; a six month follow up after surgical treatment. *BJOG : An International Journal of Obstetrics and Gynaecology, 115*(12), 1564–1569. https://doi.org/10.1111/j.1471-0528.2008.01900.x

Browning, A., & Whiteside, S. (2015). Characteristics, management, and outcomes of repair of rectovaginal fistula among 1100 consecutive cases of female genital tract fistula in Ethiopia. *BJOG: An International Journal Gynaecology Obstetrics, 131*(1), 70–73. https://doi.org/10.1016/j.ijgo.2015.05.012

Browning, A., Williams, G., & Petros, P. (2018). Skin flap vaginal augmentation helps prevent and cure post obstetric fistula repair urine leakage: A critical anatomical analysis. *BJOG: International Journal of Obstetrics and Gynaecology, 125*(6), 745–749. https://doi.org/10.1111/1471-0528.14953

D'elia, G., Paherhink, S., Fisch, M., Hohenfeller, R., & Thüroff, J. W. (2004). Mainz Pouch II technique: 10 years' experience. *British Journal Urology International, 93*, 1037–1042.

Delamou, A., Utz, B., Delvaux, T., Beavogui, A. H., & Shahabuddin, A. (2016). Pregnancy and childbirth after repair of obstetric fistula in sub-Saharan Africa: Scoping review. *Tropical Medicine & International Health, 21*(11), 1348–1365. https://doi.org/10.1111/tmi.12771

Gele, A. A., Salad, A. M., Jimale, L. H., Kour, P., Austveg, B., & Kumar, B. (2017). Relying on Visiting foreign doctors for fistula repair: The profile of women attending fistula repair surgery in Somalia. *Obstetrics and Gynecology International, 2017*, 6069124. https://doi.org/10.1155/2017/6069124

Goh, J. T., Tan, S. B., Natukunda, H., Singasi, I., & Krause, H. G. (2016). Outcomes following surgical repair using layered closure of unrepaired 4th degree perineal tear in rural western Uganda. *International Urogynecology Journal, 27*(11), 1661–1666. https://doi.org/10.1007/s00192-016-3024-6

Goh, J. T. W., Sloane, K. M., Krause, H. G., Browning, A., & Akhter, S. (2005). Mental health screening in women with genital tract fistulae. *BJOG: An International Journal of Obstetrics and Gynaeocology, 112*(9), 1328–1330.

Kelly, J., & Kwast, B. E. (1993). Epidemiological study of vesicovaginal fistulas in Ethiopia. *International Urogynecology Journal, 4*(5), 278–281.

Khisa, A. M., & Nyamongo, I. K. (2012). Still living with fistula: an exploratory study of the experience of women with obstetric fistula following corrective surgery in West Pokot, Kenya. *Reproductive Health Matters, 20*(40), 59–66. https://doi.org/10.1016/S0968-8080(12)40661-9

Kopp, D. M., Wilkinson, J., Bengtson, A., Chipungu, E., Pope, R. J., Moyo, M., et al. (2017). Fertility outcomes following obstetric fistula repair: A prospective cohort study. *Reproductive Health, 14*(1), 159. https://doi.org/10.1186/s12978-017-0415-1

Kumar, S., Vatsa, R., Bharti, J., Roy, K. K., Sharma, J. B., Singh, N., et al. (2017). Urinary fistula - A continuing problem with changing trends. *Journal of the Turkish German Gynecological Association, 18*(1), 15–19. https://doi.org/10.4274/jtgga.2016.0211

Langundoye, S. B., Bell, D., Gill, G., & Ogunbode, O. (1976). Urinary changes in obstetric vesico-vaginal fistulae: A report of 216 cases studied by intravenous urography. *Clinical Radiology, 27*, 531–539.

Naidu, P. M., & Krishna, S. (1963). Vesico-vaginal fistulae and certain problems arising subsequent to repair. *The Journal of Obstetrics and Gynaecology of the British Empire, 70*, 473–475.

Raassen, T., Ngongo, C. J., & Mahendeka, M. M. (2017). Diagnosis and management of 365 ureteric injuries following obstetric and gynecologic surgery in resource-limited settings. *International Urogynecology Journal, 29*(9), 1303–1309. https://doi.org/10.1007/s00192-017-3483-4

Reif, M. E. (1988). Bilateral common peroneal nerve palsy secondary to prolonged squatting in natural childbirth. *Birth, 15*, 100–102.

Tembely, A., Diarra, A., & Berthé, H. (2014). Sexuality and fertility of women operated for obstetric urogenital fistulae. *Progress in Urology, 24*(13), 876. https://doi.org/10.1016/j.purol.2014.08.202

Umoiyoho, A. J., Inyang-Etoh, E. C., Abah, G. M., Abasiattai, A. M., & Akaiso, O. E. (2011). Quality of life following successful repair of vesicovaginal fistula in Nigeria. *Rural and Remote Health, 11*(3), 1734.

Venn, S. N., & Mundy, A. R. (1999). Continent urinary diversion using the Mainz-type ureterosigmoidostomy- A valuable salvage procedure. *European Urology, 36*, 247–251.

Waaldjik, K., & Elkins, T. E. (1994). The obstetric fistula and peroneal nerve injury: An analysis of 974 consecutive patients. *International Urogynaecology Journal, 5*, 12–14.

Wall, L. (2017). *Tears for my sisters: The tragedy of obstetric fistula.* John Hopkins University Press.

Weston, K., Mutiso, S., Mwangi, J. W., Qureshi, Z., Beard, J., & Venkat, P. (2011). Depression among women with obstetric fistula in Kenya. *International Journal of Gynaecology and Obstetrics, 115*(1), 31–33. https://doi.org/10.1016/j.ijgo.2011.04.015

Wilkinson, J., Pope, R., Kammann, T. J., Scarpato, K., Raassen, T., Bishop, M. C., et al. (2016). The ethical and technical aspects of urinary diversions in low-resource settings: A commentary. *BJOG: An International Journal Gynaecology Obstetrics, 123*(8), 1273–1277. https://doi.org/10.1111/1471-0528.13934

Wilkinson, J. P., Bengtson, A. M., Chipungu, E., Pope, R. J., Makanani, B., Moyo, M., et al. (2018). Pelvic ultrasound findings in women with obstetric fistula: A cross-sectional study of cases and controls. *Obstetrics and Gynecology International, 2018*, 7409131.

Wilson, S. M., Sikkema, K. J., Watt, M. H., & Masenga, G. G. (2015). Psychological symptoms among obstetric fistula patients compared to gynecology outpatients in Tanzania. *International Journal of Behavioral Medicine, 22*(5), 605–613. https://doi.org/10.1007/s12529-015-9466-2

Wright, J., Ayenachew, F., & Ballard, K. D. (2016). The changing face of obstetric fistula surgery in Ethiopia. *International Journal of Women's Health, 8*, 243–248. https://doi.org/10.2147/IJWH.S106645

Zacharin, R. F. (1988). *Obstetric fistula*. Springer.

Obstetric Vesicovaginal Fistula: Development of a Predictive Score of Failed Surgical Repair

Joseph B. Nsambi, Olivier Mukuku,
Prosper L. Kakudji,
and Jean-Baptiste S. Z. Kakoma

Abbreviations

95% CI	95% confidence interval
AOR	Adjusted odds ratio
DHS	Demographic and Health Survey
DRC	Democratic Republic of the Congo
OF	Obstetric fistula
OR	Odds ratio
OVVF	Obstetric vesicovaginal fistula
ROC	Receiver operating characteristic
SFOVVF	Surgical failure of obstetric vesicovaginal fistula
UNFPA	United Nations Fund for Population Activities
VVF	Vesicovaginal fistula
WHO	World Health Organization

J. B. Nsambi · P. L. Kakudji
Department of Gynecology and Obstetrics,
University of Lubumbashi, Lubumbashi,
Democratic Republic of the Congo
e-mail: josephnsambi@gmail.com;
luhetekakudji@gmail.com

O. Mukuku (✉)
Department of Maternal and Child Health, High
Institute of Medical Techniques of Lubumbashi,
Lubumbashi, Democratic Republic of the Congo
e-mail: oliviermukuku@yahoo.fr

J.-B. S. Z. Kakoma
Department of Gynecology and Obstetrics,
University of Lubumbashi, Lubumbashi,
Democratic Republic of the Congo

University of Rwanda, Kigali, Republic of Rwanda
e-mail: jbszkakoma2016@gmail.com

© Springer Nature Switzerland AG 2022
L. B. Drew et al. (eds.), *A Multidisciplinary Approach to Obstetric Fistula in Africa*, Global
Maternal and Child Health, https://doi.org/10.1007/978-3-031-06314-5_17

17.1   Introduction

Obstetric fistula (OF) is an abnormal communication between the vagina and the urological or colorectal systems, caused by obstetric trauma, which causes an uncontrollable loss of urine or stool (Langkilde et al., 1999). OF is common among women living in low-income countries, where it is generally developing as a result of a prolonged/obstructed delivery and insufficient access to antenatal and intrapartum care (Wall et al., 2004).

The exact incidence of OFs remains difficult to assess because statistical data on the magnitude of this affection are difficult to determine with certainty given the absence of epidemiological surveys, case finding, and reporting. The World Health Organization (WHO) estimates that more than 2 million young women around the world live with untreated fistula and between 50,000 and 100,000 new women are affected each year. Many cases of genitourinary fistula are identified in sub-Saharan Africa and Southeast Asia (UNFPA, Engender Health, 2003; WHO, 2006). In Democratic Republic of the Congo (DRC), the 2007 Demographic and Health Survey (DHS) reports indicated that 0.3% of women report having experienced symptoms of fistula (Demographic and Health Survey, 2008).

There is no universally recognized prognostic classification for obstetric vesicovaginal fistulas (OVVF); the subject is difficult because clinical, pathological, and anatomical factors can be variable between persons with the condition. Various classifications of OFs have been developed, but none has been adopted at the international level (Kayondo et al., 2011). These classifications are based on different anatomopathological characteristics of the fistula, including distance between distal edge of the fistula and urethral meat, size of fistula, fibrotic scarring, etc. (Goh, 2004), and they are only pedagogical. Unfortunately, they are generally not useful as predictors of the outcome of surgical repair of the fistula. This deficiency of a standardized system of terminology, classification, data collection, and reports make it challenging to assess and compare surgical outcomes. In addition, there are also limited published data on characteristics of the fistula (bladder or vagina), or fistula closing techniques, that can predict the success of surgical therapy (Nardos et al., 2009). The success rate after the surgical repair varies between hospitals, and is determined by many factors such as fistula site, degree of fibrotic scarring, number of previous surgical repairs, surgical repair technique, surgeon's expertise, equipment, and post-operative nursing (Mukwege et al., 2018; Nardos et al., 2009; Rathee & Nanda, 1995; Roenneburg et al., 2006). High rates of success after surgical repair are reported by several authors ranging from 72.9% to 93% (Holme et al., 2007; Kambou et al., 2006; Muleta, 2004; Nsambi et al., 2018, 2019). However, even after the successful closure of the fistula, 15–20% of women may continue to suffer from urinary incontinence, with predictive failure factors including vaginal fibrotic scarring, prior attempts to repair, etc. (Browning, 2006; Goh et al., 2008; Nardos et al., 2009; Roenneburg et al., 2006). At present, in our environment, different factors contributing to the outcome of surgical repair of OVVF are still unknown.

This study aims to identify factors affecting surgical failure of OFVV (SFOVVF) in the southeastern part of the Province of Haut-Katanga (in DRC) and to develop a predictive score of the SFOVVF risk.

17.2   Methodology

This study is the result of several free surgical repair campaigns of OF organized by non-governmental organizations (UNFPA, *Médecins sans Frontières* and *Médecins du Désert*) in collaboration with the provincial Ministry of Public Health of Katanga Province. These organizations offer access to specialized care to the population living in the following health zones: Pweto, Kilwa, Mitwaba, Kasenga, Kashobwe, and Lubumbashi. Surgical repairs were conducted in general reference hospitals within these health zones. The hospitals were selected for their geographical accessibility and for their technical platform having made possible a large number of surgical repairs. Other patients received surgical treatment in the Benicker Center (in Lubumbashi) specializing in the management of genitourinary fistulas which is supported by the non-governmental organization "Hope Mama Africa".

This study design consisted of an analytical cross-sectional investigation identifying predictors of the SFOVVF performed from 2009 to 2018 in the Haut-Katanga province, DRC. It included women with OVVF (occurred after vaginal delivery) that had been examined after community awareness in the towns and villages of the Haut-Katanga Province. The selection was exhaustive and included all women having OVVF and fulfilling the inclusion criteria. In total, a sample size of 384 patients had been established on the basis of the inclusion criteria. To be part of the study, the inclusion criteria included those women having an OVVF that occurred after vaginal delivery, and who received an external or referred consultation, and who received surgical repair during the course of our study period. No OVVF-specific classification system had been used during the study period, but we collected the anatomopathological covariables that were included in various existing classifications.

Given the technical platform and selection criteria, 22 women having a severe OVVF (or transection) had been excluded. The collection of data was made by the medical team with a pre-established questionnaire. These data were collected from patient interrogation, external consultation records, operating room registers, and hospital registers, and thus the necessary information about each patient was available from admission to discharge. A preoperative examination was carried out in which the characteristics of the patient, fistula, bladder, and vagina were recorded. All surgical repairs were carried out in the operating room by one of the four gynecological surgeons of the campaign team assisted by general practitioners. After the establishment of a loco-regional anesthesia, the patients were placed in Trendelenburg position, the legs in "high" lithotomy position.

Variables studied were as follows:

- Socio-demographic and gynecological characteristics of the patient included age (in years) and parity at the time of surgical repair.
- Characteristics of the fistula included age of the fistula, number of fistulas, fistula size, type of fistula (vesicovaginal or rectovesicovaginal), presence of vaginal fibrotic scarring (yes or no), state of the urethra (intact, partly or completely involved), and number of previous surgical repairs of the fistula.
- Outcomes of the surgical repair (failure or closure with/without urinary incontinence) were also recorded.

The subjects constituting our population had been divided into two groups according to outcomes of the surgical repair. These results were defined as follows:

- Failed surgical repair is defined as the non-closing of the fistula. The fistula was not closed even if the urine leak has decreased considerably with retained or unpreserved urination.
- Success of the surgical repair is defined as the closure of the fistula; fistula was totally closed, with or without sphincter insufficiency (urinary incontinence). There was no urine leak where there was the fistula.

Statistical analyses were made through STATA 15 software. Women's data with SFOVVF were compared to those without SFOVVF. These analyses focused on the different independent variables one by one in order to search for any significant statistical association with SFOVVF (dependent variable). Variables with a value less than 0.02 in the bivariate analysis using Pearson's chi-squared test were included in the logistic regression model using the stepwise method. In the final model, we used variables whose significance level was less than 0.05. The logistic model thus allowed the analysis of the contribution of each independent variable to the SFOVVF in the presence of other independent variables. Score's discrimination was assessed using the ROC and C-index curves, and the score was calibrated using the Hosmer–Lemeshow test (Guessous & Durieux-Paillard, 2010; Mukuku et al., 2019; Tripepi et al., 2010). We determined the sensitivity, specificity, and percentage of correctly classified cases compared to the C-index. The robustness of the model coefficients was evaluated by bootstrap. The predictive risk score was deduced from the statistical analysis and was established by assigning points to each risk factor retained in the logistic model. To make it simple to use, the score was achieved by using rounded values of these coefficients (Mukuku et al., 2019). Risk probabilities of SFOVVF based on the values of the constructed score were calculated.

Data were collected anonymously and the authorization to conduct this study had been obtained from the Medical Ethics Committee of the University of Lubumbashi (Approval number: UNILU/CEM/101/2018).

17.3 Results

In total, 384 patients with OVVF had been the recipients of surgical repair. This repair had failed in 17.19% of the cases (66/384). Using bivariate analysis, Table 17.1 shows that there was no statistically significant association between the SFOVVF and the following covariables: age and parity of the patient, and age of the fistula ($p > 0.05$). On the other hand, a statistically significant association had been found between the SFOVVF and the following covariables: surgical approach, number of fistulas, type of fistula, state of the urethra, fibrotic scarring, and size of the fistula ($p < 0.05$). The SFOVVF was of greater significance in those cases where the surgical repair was done by trans-vesical approach (OR = 2.15; 95% CI: 1.14–3.98); in presence of two or more fistulas (OR = 9.43; 95% CI: 4.24–21.03); when the fistula had already been previously repaired (OR = 2.90; 95% CI: 1.62–5.23); when the FVV was associated with a rectovaginal fistula (OR = 4.03; 95% CI: 1.42–10.90); when the urethra was partially or completely involved (OR = 3.09; 95% CI: 1.73–5.53); in presence of the fibrotic scarring (OR = 12.37; 95% CI: 6.47–23.98); and when the fistula measured 3 cm or more in size (OR = 11.01; 95% CI: 3.14–59.78).

After logistic regression (Table 17.2), four criteria stand out as predictors of the SFOVVF: presence of the fibrotic scarring (AOR = 15.22; 95% CI: 7.34–31.58; $p < 0.0001$); presence of 2 or more fistulas (AOR = 7.41; 95% CI: 3.05–17.97; $p < 0.0001$); the trans-vesical approach (AOR = 4.26; 95% CI: 1.92–9.44; $p < 0.0001$); the urethral involvement (AOR = 3.93; 95% CI: 1.99–7.77; $p < 0.0001$).

The predictive score of the SFOVVF was constructed from the logistic model. Each risk factor was weighted by a regression coefficient representing the weight of the variable in the score calculation. The set of scores obtained is shown in Table 17.2.

The area under the ROC curve of the score was 0.8759 (Fig. 17.1). This curve shows excellent discrimination on its ability to discriminate patients who will have a SFOVVF from those who will not present it.

The presence of these four criteria corresponds to a metric score whose maximum total is 7 points. For each patient, the score varied from 0 to 7; the greater was the score, the greater the risk of SFOVVF (Table 17.2). Risk probabilities of SFOVVF based on the values of the constructed score have been calculated and are presented in Table 17.3. A score less than 4 points defines children at low risk of SFOVVF, a score between 4 and 5 points defines a moderate risk of SFOVVF, and a score beyond 5 points presents a high risk of SFOVVF. Thus, a sensitivity of 58% was obtained for a specificity of 92%. The positive predictive value was 93%. The positive predictive value was 59% and the negative predictive value was 91.25%.

Table 17.1 Bivariate analysis of risk factors associated with surgical failure of obstetric vesicovaginal fistula in Haut-Katanga Province from 2009 to 2018 in the Democratic Republic of the Congo ($n = 384$)

Variable	Failed surgical repair $n = 66$ (%)	Successful surgical repair $n = 318$ (%)	Total ($N = 384$)	Crude odds ratio [95% CI]	p-Value
Age at the time of surgical repair					
<20 years	8 (11.76)	60 (88.24)	68	1.00	0.2663
20–29 years	34 (18.70)	148 (81.30)	182	1.72 (0.75–3.94)	
≥30 years	24 (17.91)	110 (82.09)	134	1.63 (0.69–3.86)	0.3541
Parity at the time of surgical repair					
1	36 (19.25)	151 (80.75)	187	1.00	0.3632
≥2	30 (15.23)	167 (84.77)	197	1.32 (0.78–2.26)	
Age of the fistula					
≤1 year	12 (19.05)	51 (80.95)	63	1.27 (0.61–2.62)	0.6484
2–10 years	35 (15.62)	189 (84.38)	224	1.00	
>10 years	19 (19.59)	78 (80.41)	97	1.31 (0.71–2.44)	0.4782
Surgical approach					
Trans-vaginal	44 (14.57)	258 (85.43)	302	1.00	0.0091
Trans-vesical	22 (26.83)	60 (73.17)	82	2.15 (1.14–3.98)	
Number of previous surgical repairs					
None	35 (12.54)	244 (87.46)	279	1.00	<0.0001
1 or more	31 (29.52)	74 (70.48)	105	2.90 (1.62–5.23)	
Number of fistulas					
1	45 (12.93)	303 (87.07)	348	1.00	<0.0001
2 or more	21 (58.33)	15 (41.67)	36	9.43 (4.24–21.03)	
Type of the fistula					
Rectovesicovaginal	9 (42.86)	12 (57.14)	21	4.03 (1.42–10.90)	0.0013
Vesicovaginal	57 (15.70)	306 (84.30)	363	1.00	
State of the urethra					
Intact	31 (11.74)	233 (88.26)	264	1.00	<0.0001
Urethral involvement	35 (29.17)	85 (70.83)	120	3.09 (1.73–5.53)	
Fibrotic scarring					
Absent	19 (6.69)	265 (93.31)	284	1.00	<0.0001
Present	47 (47.00)	53 (53.00)	100	12.37 (6.47–23.98)	
Size of the fistula					
<1.5 cm	3 (6.12)	46 (93.88)	49	1.00	0.4404
1.5–3 cm	28 (11.11)	224 (88.89)	252	1.91 (0.55–10.24)	
>3 cm	35 (42.17)	48 (57.83)	83	11.01 (3.14–59.78)	<0.0001

Table 17.2 Logistic regression model of risk of surgical failure of obstetric vesicovaginal fistula and score of predictive factors

Variable	Adjusted odds ratio	95% Confidence interval	Coefficient	Score
Fibrotic scarring	15.22	7.34–31.58	2.72	3
Number of fistulas ≥2	7.41	3.05–17.97	2.00	2
Trans-vesical approach	4.26	1.92–9.44	1.45	1
Urethral involvement	3.93	1.99–7.77	1.37	1

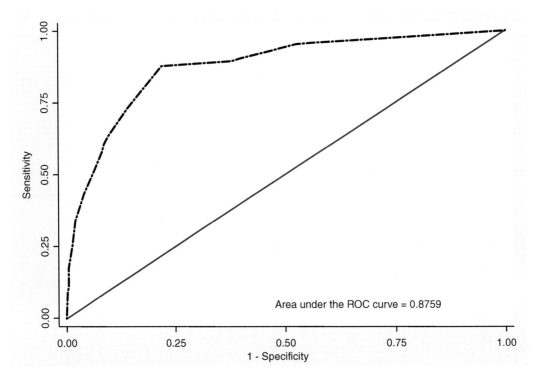

Fig. 17.1 ROC curve showing the performance of SFOVVF predictive score

Table 17.3 Probability of surgical failure of obstetric vesicovaginal fistula by score according to logistic regression model

Score	Likelihood of SFOVVF[a] (%)
0	1.82
1	4.25
2	9.64
3	20.39
4	38.07
5	59.62
6	77.99
7	89.49

[a]Obtained from the formula: $p = 1/1 + \exp (3.99 - 0.8759 \times \text{score})$

17.4 Discussion

In this study, successful obstetric fistula closure was achieved in 82.8% of patients. In a Ugandan study, the successful closure rate was 77.9% (Kayondo et al., 2011); and in a Zambian study it was 72.9% (Holme et al., 2007). However, these success rates were lower than the 90% rate reported by Hancock and Collie in Uganda (Hancock & Collie, 2004). This could be due to clinical, anatomical, and pathological differences of fistula treated in these studies. In our study, the success rate was lower than WHO requirements for a fistula treatment center with more than 85% closure. This could be due to the fact that some of our patients have not had surgery in a specialized fistula repair center; as a result, the availability of recommended suture materials, other equipment, and the quality of postoperative care may sometimes be lacking.

The study of the risk factors of SFOVVF is based on the comparison between women with and without SFOVVF. Contrary to the patient's characteristics, stronger evidence from our results corroborates the negative influence of fistula characteristics on surgical repair outcomes. In this study, SFOVVF was significantly associated with fibrotic scarring, presence of 2 or more fistulas, transvesical approach, and urethral involvement.

The present study found a significant association of SFOVVF with the fibrotic scarring that can occur around the fistula. Fibrotic scarring studies have shown an association with surgical repair outcomes, including multivariate analyses showing a negative independent effect of fibrotic scarring on closure (Barone et al., 2012; Goh et al., 2008; Kayondo et al., 2011; Kirschner et al., 2010; Lewis et al., 2009; Nardos et al., 2009; Sjøveian et al., 2011). Fistulas with fibrotic scarring are also difficult to mobilize from surrounding tissues, making them almost impossible to repair without tension; they heal on the surrounding tissues as a result of the ischemic process that led to their formation (Kayondo et al., 2011). This finding is also confirmed by Zhou et al. (2017) who point out that it is plausible that the scar tissue could lead to limited tissue mobilization for tension-free repair. In addition, viable tissue and blood intake are reduced in the presence of moderate or severe peri-fistular fibrosis.

Women with more than one fistula were seven times more likely to have a SFOVVF than those with a single fistula (AOR = 7.41; 95% CI: 3.05–17.97; $p < 0.0001$). It was confirmed that multiple fistulas (2 or more) had a significant relationship to the unsuccessful closure of VVF (Kayondo et al., 2011). This is probably due to the presence of several VVFs making it difficult to mobilize the local tissue and allowing tension-free repair due to the lack of tissue in the bladder. It is our practice to utilize a separate suture without tension on the bladder and then the vagina. This technique consists of splitting, after dissection, the bladder and the vagina, and then suturing them separately. This separation of the vaginal plane from the bladder plane around the fistula permits sufficient mobilization of the bladder plane to allow tension-free sutures after excision of the sclerotic edges of the fistula. This tissue interposition makes it possible to fill the dead spaces, to separate the vaginal and urinary sutures, and to provide a well-vascularized and flexible tissue which facilitates healing and thus prevents SFOVVF, although the results of the study by Nardos et al. (2009) did not find any difference between failure rates of fistulas repaired in one plane and those repaired in two planes.

Surgical repair of VVFs by trans-vesical approach was four times more likely to fail than transvaginal approach (AOR = 4.26; 95% CI: 1.92–9.44; $p < 0.0001$). The trans-vesical approach includes increased morbidity due to increased blood loss, long hospitalization time, and maintenance of the Foley's probe. Our preference is for the trans-vaginal approach because it offers the advantages of minimal blood loss, shorter operating time, the possibility of performing the Martius procedure, low postoperative morbidity, and short-term convalescence.

Three studies specifically described outcomes of trans-vaginal versus trans-vesical approaches, comprising a cohort of more than 500 patients (Hadzi-Djokic et al., 2009; Hilton, 2012; Ockrim et al., 2009). Of these, the overall rates of fistula closure were 90.9% and 84.0% for trans-vaginal and transvesical approaches, respectively ($p < 0.05$). Fistulas occurring in low-income countries are generally of obstetric origin and are low-located in greater than 85% of cases (Nsambi et al., 2018). As a result, VVF repairs are carried out in large proportion through trans-vaginal approach. This approach exposes places of taking of the intervening tissues between vesical and vaginal sutures, and carries less risk when aseptic conditions are rudimentary. The trans-vaginal approach of VVF repair enables higher success rates to be obtained compared with the trans-vesical approach, even if the choice of the route first depends on the complacency of the vagina, the site of the fistula, and the presence of associated lesions. In addition, even for high-located fistulas, the posterior episiotomy allows the vaginal dome to be lowered and thus the fistula to be exteriorized (Nsambi et al., 2018, 2019).

Patients with urethral involvement were 4 times more likely to have SFOVVF (AOR = 3.93; 95% CI: 1.99–7.77; $p < 0.0001$). A similar finding was observed in other studies (Delamou et al., 2016;

Goh et al., 2008; Kayondo et al., 2011; Nardos et al., 2009) where women with urethral involvement were more likely to have failed surgical repair of their fistulas than those without urethral involvement. This association could be due to the fact that the urethra is generally attached to the pubic bone and therefore difficult to mobilize. This could also be due to the difficulty of anastomosing a detached urethra that is usually shortened by the fistula (Kayondo et al., 2011).

The majority of risk factors associated with SFOVVF described in the literature are found in our study population in bivariate analysis. This is an important external validity element in defining the SFOVVF population. Some variables known to be risk factors for SFOVVF were not found in our study. Examples include the size of the fistula, the number of previous surgical repairs, and the combination of vesicovaginal and recto-vaginal fistula, which were not found in our population after multivariate analysis. This would probably be due to the fact that, by adjusting them with the other variables, they appear to be statistically less discriminating and have thus not been retained in the final predictive model. The benefit of this score is to provide the clinician with a tool to identify the patient who may have a SFOVVF in order to better manage her. To the best of our knowledge, this is the first study that links risk factors to the outcome of fistula surgical repair in our environment by scoring. This score is a simple tool that will inform clinicians in our environment about the probability of identifying patients at risk of a SFOVVF before each fistula surgical repair, and thus help guide surgical choices. All of these factors will need to be taken into account during fistula surgical repair to improve outcomes, bearing in mind that the attempt at primary surgery always carries the best chance of success. Indeed, this score requires only the rating of 4 elements. Furthermore, the good specificity of this score makes it possible to rule out the possibility of a SFOVVF. However, in order to definitively validate this score, transportability to other populations will have to be tested in advance. The prevention of SFOVVF would also allow for the prevention of repeated and traumatic surgeries for psychologically severely affected patients, with the best chance of success being in the first attempt at fistula surgical repair. Every effort must be made to succeed first, because each new intervention creates an additional sclerosis that makes future attempts more difficult. Identifying the patient at risk for SFOVVF can help prevent SFOVVF in our environment. Indeed, the risk factors reported in this study should be brought to the attention of the surgeon before any fistula surgery. Surgical practice decisions should take into account clinical parameters of the fistula.

17.5 Conclusions

Obstetric fistula is a major cause of maternal morbidity and is therefore a significant public health problem. As have been highlighted by other authors in this book, its psycho-social impact is considerable. Indeed, women carrying fistulas, pariahs because of the smell of urine that is unbearable for their surroundings, are often neglected and abandoned by their spouses, and ostracized by their communities.

Our model utilizing a predictive approach for SFOVVF is our contribution to reducing the morbidity of women with OF. This logistic model was used to develop an objective risk-based predictive score for SFOVVF in the setting of a resource-limited environment, which is where most OFs occur. We would encourage practicing physicians and other individuals involved in the management and treatment of women with OF to consider employing our model to make surgical practice decisions that can, hopefully, improve the management of OF patients.

References

Barone, M. A., Frajzyngier, V., Ruminjo, J., Asiimwe, F., Barry, T. H., Bello, A., et al. (2012). Determinants of post-operative outcomes of female genital fistula repair surgery. *Obstetrics and Gynecology, 120*(3), 524. https://doi.org/10.1097/AOG.0b013e31826579e8

Browning, A. (2006). Risk factors for developing residual urinary incontinence after obstetric fistula repair. *BJOG: An International Journal of Obstetrics & Gynaecology, 113*(4), 482–485.

Delamou, A., Delvaux, T., Beavogui, A. H., Toure, A., Kolié, D., Sidibé, S., et al. (2016). Factors associated with the failure of obstetric fistula repair in Guinea: Implications for practice. *Reproductive Health, 13*, 135. https://doi.org/10.1186/s12978-016-0248-3

Demographic and Health Survey. (2008). *Democratic Republic of Congo 2007*. Ministry of Planning and Macro International.

Goh, J. T. (2004). A new classification for female genital tract fistula. *Australian and New Zealand Journal of Obstetrics and Gynaecology, 44*(6), 502–504.

Goh, J. T., Browning, A., Berhan, B., & Chang, A. (2008). Predicting the risk of failure of closure of obstetric fistula and residual urinary incontinence using a classification system. *International Urogynecology Journal, 19*(12), 1659–1662. https://doi.org/10.1007/s00192-008-0693-9

Guessous, I., & Durieux-Paillard, S. (2010). Validation des scores cliniques: Notions théoriques et pratiques de base. *Revue Médicale Suisse, 6*(264), 1798–1802.

Hadzi-Djokic, J., Pejcic, T. P., & Acimovic, M. (2009). Vesico-vaginal fistula: Report of 220 cases. *International Urology and Nephrology, 41*(2), 299–302. https://doi.org/10.1007/s11255-008-9449-1

Hancock, B., & Collie, M. (2004). Vesico-vaginal fistula surgery in Uganda. *East and Central African Journal of Surgery, 9*(2), 32–37.

Hilton, P. (2012). Urogenital fistula in the UK: A personal case series managed over 25 years. *BJU International, 110*(1), 102–110. https://doi.org/10.1111/j.1464-410X.2011.10630.x

Holme, A., Breen, M., & MacArthur, C. (2007). Obstetric fistulae: A study of women managed at the Monze Mission Hospital, Zambia. *BJOG: An International Journal of Obstetrics & Gynaecology, 114*(8), 1010–1017.

Kambou, T., Zango, B., Outtara, T., Dao, B., & Sano, D. (2006). Point sur la prise en charge des fistules urogénitales au CHU Sourosanou de Bobo Dioulasso: Etude de 57 cas opérés en deux ans. *Médecine d'Afrique Noire, 53*(12), 665–673.

Kayondo, M., Wasswa, S., Kabakyenga, J., Mukiibi, N., Senkungu, J., Stenson, A., et al. (2011). Predictors and outcome of surgical repair of obstetric fistula at a regional referral hospital, Mbarara, western Uganda. *BMC Urology, 11*(1), 23. https://doi.org/10.1186/1471-2490-11-23

Kirschner, C. V., Yost, K. J., Du, H., Karshima, J. A., Arrowsmith, S. D., & Wall, L. L. (2010). Obstetric fistula: The ECWA Evangel VVF Center surgical experience from Jos, Nigeria. *International Urogynecology Journal, 21*(12), 1525–1533. https://doi.org/10.1007/s00192-010-1231-0

Langkilde, N. C., Pless, T. K., Lundbeck, F., & Nerstrøm, B. (1999). Surgical repair of vesicovaginal fistulae: A ten-year retrospective study. *Scandinavian Journal of Urology and Nephrology, 33*(2), 100–103. https://doi.org/10.1080/003655999750016069

Lewis, A., Kaufman, M. R., Wolter, C. E., Phillips, S. E., Maggi, D., Condry, L., et al. (2009). Genitourinary fistula experience in Sierra Leone: Review of 505 cases. *The Journal of Urology, 181*(4), 1725–1731. https://doi.org/10.1016/j.juro.2008.11.106

Mukuku, O., Mutombo, A. M., Kamona, L. K., Lubala, T. K., Mawaw, P. M., Aloni, M. N., et al. (2019). Predictive model for the risk of severe acute malnutrition in children. *Journal of Nutrition and Metabolism, 2019*, 4740825. https://doi.org/10.1155/2019/4740825

Mukwege, D., Peters, L., Amisi, C., Mukwege, A., Smith, A. R., & Miller, J. M. (2018). Panzi score as a parsimonious indicator of urogenital fistula severity derived from Goh and Waaldijk classifications. *International Journal of Gynecology & Obstetrics, 142*(2), 187–193. https://doi.org/10.1002/ijgo.12514

Muleta, M. (2004). Socio-demographic profile and obstetric experience of fistula patients managed at the Addis Ababa Fistula Hospital. *Ethiopian Medical Journal, 42*(1), 9–16.

Nardos, R., Browning, A., & Chen, C. C. G. (2009). Risk factors that predict failure after vaginal repair of obstetric vesicovaginal fistulae. *American Journal of Obstetrics and Gynecology, 200*(5), 578. https://doi.org/10.1016/j.ajog.2008.12.008

Nsambi, J. B., Mukuku, O., Kakudji, P. L., & Kakoma, J. B. S. (2019). Socio-demographic and delivery characteristics of patients with obstetric fistula in Haut-Katanga Province, Democratic Republic of Congo. *Annals of Colorectal Research, 7*(3), 1–5.

Nsambi, J. B., Mukuku, O., Yunga, J. F., Kinenkinda, X., Kakudji, P., Kizonde, J., & Kakoma, J. B. (2018). Obstetric fistulas among people living in northern Katanga province, Democratic Republic of the Congo: About 242 cases. *The Pan African Medical Journal, 29*, 34. https://doi.org/10.11604/pamj.2018.29.34.14576

Ockrim, J. L., Greenwell, T. J., Foley, C. L., Wood, D. N., & Shah, P. J. R. (2009). A tertiary experience of vesico-vaginal and urethro-vaginal fistula repair: Factors predicting success. *BJU International, 103*(8), 1122–1126. https://doi.org/10.1111/j.1464-410x.2008.08237.x

Rathee, S., & Nanda, S. (1995). Vesicovaginal fistulae: A 12-year study. *Journal of the Indian Medical Association, 93*(3), 93–94.

Roenneburg, M. L., Genadry, R., & Wheeless, C. R., Jr. (2006). Repair of obstetric vesicovaginal fistulas in Africa. *American Journal of Obstetrics and Gynecology, 195*(6), 1748–1752. https://doi.org/10.1016/j.ajog.2006.07.031

Sjøveian, S., Vangen, S., Mukwege, D., & Onsrud, M. (2011). Surgical outcome of obstetric fistula: A retrospective analysis of 595 patients. *Acta Obstetricia et Gynecologica Scandinavica, 90*(7), 753–760. https://doi.org/10.1111/j.1600-0412.2011.01162.x

Tripepi, G., Jager, K. J., Dekker, F. W., & Zoccali, C. (2010). Statistical methods for the assessment of prognostic biomarkers (Part I): Discrimination. *Nephrology, Dialysis, Transplantation, 25*(5), 1399–1401. https://doi.org/10.1093/ndt/gfq018

UNFPA, Engender Health. (2003). *Obstetric fistula needs assessment report: Findings from nine African countries.* Retrieved 9 January, 2019, from https://www.unfpa.org/sites/default/files/pub-pdf/fistula-needs-assessment.pdf

Wall, L. L., Karshima, J. A., Kirschner, C., & Arrowsmith, S. D. (2004). The obstetric vesicovaginal fistula: Characteristics of 899 patients from Jos, Nigeria. *American Journal of Obstetrics and Gynecology, 190*(4), 1011–1016. https://doi.org/10.1016/j.ajog.2004.02.007

WHO. (2006). *Obstetric fistula: Guiding principles for clinical management and programme development.* World Health Organization.

Zhou, L., Yang, T. X., Luo, D. Y., Chen, S. L., Liao, B. H., Li, H., et al. (2017). Factors influencing repair outcomes of vesicovaginal fistula: A retrospective review of 139 procedures. *Urologia Internationalis, 99*(1), 22–28. https://doi.org/10.1159/000452166

Training and Capacity Building in the Provision of Fistula Treatment Services: The FIGO Fistula Surgery Training Initiative

18

Gillian Slinger and Lilli Trautvetter

18.1 Background and Introduction

Obstetric fistula, a neglected public health and human rights issue, is a childbirth injury caused by unrelieved prolonged obstructed labour. This results in an abnormal opening between the vagina and the bladder and/or rectum, leading to uncontrollable leaking from the vagina of urine and/or faeces. The condition occurs in those countries having a high maternal mortality ratio (MMR) where women lack access to sexual and reproductive health care, notably access to safe delivery services and timely emergency caesarean section (Bangser, 2007; De Ridder et al., 2009; WHO, 2018). For women and girls, a fistula is a life-shattering condition. Prolonged and unrelieved labour not only causes 94 percent of affected women to deliver a stillborn baby (Hilton & Ward, 1998; Muleta et al., 2010; Wall et al., 2004), they also suffer severe physical trauma as well as emotional consequences because of the ordeal. The stigma attached to the condition leaves women humiliated and ashamed, often causing withdrawal from community life, and frequently leading to an ensuing downward spiral of isolation and abject poverty. Sufferers have furthermore expressed multiple losses such as the loss of body control, loss of social role as woman and wife, loss of integration in social life, loss of dignity and self-worth (Ahmed & Holtz, 2007; Mselle et al., 2011; Murphy, 1981). Obstetric fistula is also frequently associated with other health problems such as foot drop, skin ulcerations, multiple infections, renal failure, vaginal stenosis, infertility, depression and even suicide (FIGO, 2006; Hilton, 2003; Wall, 2002; Weston et al., 2011).

Safe and timely delivery services and quality obstetric care are crucial in the prevention of obstetric fistula, but economic and socio-cultural factors also play a critical role in determining where and how expectant mothers access such services. Women with obstetric fistula almost always reside in regions where gender inequality is high, and where they lack autonomy to make decisions about their sexual and reproductive health. Fistula invariably affects the most disadvantaged, marginalised and poorest of women (Akpan, 2003; Women's Dignity Project and EngenderHealth, 2006; Keri et al. 2010; Roush et al., 2012; Shen & Williamson, 1999; Wall et al., 2005). The immense physical and emotional suffering caused by the condition and the extreme socioeconomic inequalities it represents make

G. Slinger (✉) · L. Trautvetter
Fistula Surgery Training Initiative, FIGO,
London, UK
e-mail: Gillian@figo.org

© Springer Nature Switzerland AG 2022

L. B. Drew et al. (eds.), *A Multidisciplinary Approach to Obstetric Fistula in Africa*, Global Maternal and Child Health, https://doi.org/10.1007/978-3-031-06314-5_18

obstetric fistula one of the most debilitating and devastating maternal morbidities, which is rooted in gross societal and institutional neglect of women (Cook et al., 2004; Donnay & Weil, 2004; Wall, 2012) as well as a direct violation of reproductive human rights as per *The Beijing Declaration and Platform for Action* (UN, 1995) and *The Maputo Protocol* (UN, 2003).

18.2 Fistula Treatment Efforts; Old Challenges and New Achievements

Prevalence and incidence rates of obstetric fistula have always—and continue to be—topics of lively debate in the fistula community, since available datasets are largely based on estimations. The most commonly cited metrics are that fistula affects approximately two million women in more than 55 low-resource countries in Africa and Asia, with up to 100,000 additional women developing a fistula each year in some of the world's poorest and most disadvantaged communities (Browning, 2004; Cook et al., 2004; Hilton & Ward, 1998; Wall, 1998; WHO, 2018).

When left untreated, women suffering from obstetric fistula will be incontinent for the remainder of their lives. The provision of surgical treatment is, however, one of the major challenges in combating the condition. Owing to the relatively small number of skilled fistula surgeons worldwide, there is a huge unmet need to treat the backlog of women with this condition (Hancock, 2013). As a result of the long-standing global shortage of trained, skilled fistula surgeons and the absence of a harmonised training curriculum, it is further estimated that only one woman in 50 receives life-changing surgery to recover from the condition (Fistula Foundation, 2019). Although it is believed that most countries in Africa and Asia have at least one skilled fistula surgeon (Rushwan et al., 2012), these physicians are in great demand—not only to provide surgical fistula repairs, but also many other forms of health care in their home settings. This demand is also compounded by the general lack of physicians and health workers. With a few exceptions, according to WHO, in sub-Saharan Africa there are between 0.157—4 doctors per 10,000 persons, whereas in stark comparison there are 12 to 66 doctors per 10,000 in Europe (WHO, 2019). Furthermore, health professionals may be confronted with the competing demands of private health care that is available for the privileged few in their communities who can afford it. As global efforts strive to ensure universal health coverage in all countries (UN, 2015), it is exceedingly unlikely that women living with an obstetric fistula who reside in impoverished circumstances can pay into the system or even that fistula surgery is in fact covered by the system.

In the past, training in fistula surgery was normally undertaken on the physician's own initiative, who subsequently acquired his/her skills through their own efforts to observe and work alongside an experienced fistula surgeon. This, however was, and often still is conducted without a structured curriculum, a set of recognised learning objectives or infrastructure to support and facilitate progressive training in fistula surgery. Although some fistula surgeons have indeed learned the 'art of fistula surgery' in this way, this method has led to patchy, disjointed and inadequate fistula training, with a general inability to assess trainee fistula surgeons or the quality of their work, and resulting in poor outcomes for patients (Olusegun et al., 2009; Raassen et al., 2008). Meanwhile other surgeons, desperate to help their patients, familiarise themselves with available literature and then try to perform the surgery. This usually takes place without any formal training or supervision from a mentor. In most cases, the procedure fails, leaving both patient and surgeon despondent and making any subsequent curative operation all the more challenging (Hancock, 2013). There has been an increasing awareness of the 'fistula epidemic' and lack of readily accessible expert treatment. Although there are dedicated local expert fistula surgeons in many countries, unfortunately, these specialists are too few. Consequently, in recent years there has been an increase in overseas surgeons keen to 'volunteer' their services by taking part in short medical missions to perform fistula repair operations in affected countries. While most certainly motivated by a genuine desire to help, this has generated a 'tsunami' of visiting surgeons, or 'fistula tourists', rather than building the capacity and medical infrastructure of affected countries (Wall, 2007; Wall et al., 2006).

The fistula tourist approach has been recognised as problematic from both a medical and ethical perspective, as most 'volunteers' work in countries where obstetric fistula has largely been eradicated. Unless surgeons have been meticulously trained in the surgical and clinical management of women with the condition, they do not possess the necessary expertise to do this work. Consequently, despite their best intentions, they can contribute little to bridge the global treatment gap. More importantly, because they lack experience in this specialised area, they may actually do more harm than good when attempting to provide treatment for women with obstetric fistula (Arrowsmith, 2007; Gutman et al., 2007; Wall, 2014; Wall et al., 2008). This excludes foreign expert fistula surgeons, many of whom and unlike 'fistula tourists' have dedicated most of their career to the cause, and without whom much of the progress to date would not have been possible.

To initiate meaningful change, it became clear that an urgent global effort was required and in the early years of the twenty-first century, several key initiatives were established to put obstetric fistula on the global health agenda. In 2003 UNFPA and its partners launched the Campaign to End Fistula, which operates in more than 50 countries and is supported by over 80 international agencies and several hundred local organisations (UNFPA, 2003). In 2008, the International Society of Obstetric Fistula Surgeons (ISOFS) was formed; the professional body for the prevention, treatment and rehabilitation of women with obstetric fistula (ISOFS, 2019). In 2012, Direct Relief, Fistula Foundation and UNFPA developed the Global Fistula Map, to track fistula repair rates across the world each year and to identify gaps in service provision. The Global Fistula Map became the Global Fistula Hub in 2020 to provide additional benefits to the community, and is currently sharing self-reported data, collected since 2012 on 115,630 fistula repairs from 454 facilities in 39 countries (Direct Relief, 2021). Last but certainly not least, in an attempt to raise more awareness and help for women with obstetric fistula on an annual basis, in 2013 the United Nations (UN) designated May 23rd as the International Day to End Obstetric Fistula (UNFPA, 2013).

While these vital steps have undoubtedly led to an increased awareness, additional resource mobilisation, and more women treated, they have had limited impact in strengthening under-resourced, over-burdened health systems in the countries where obstetric fistula occurs. Furthermore, although governments of certain affected countries are showing much greater commitment to ending fistula, e.g. Kenya and Ethiopia, historically, the vast majority of funding for fistula treatment has come from international non-governmental organisations (NGOs), UN entities and Western philanthropic sources. This has led to an over-reliance on international support and has been labelled by some as 'running in parallel to national systems'. The delicate and precarious nature of these financing mechanisms is especially noticeable when foreign funding to countries and/or facilities for fistula treatment is reduced or even withdrawn without adequate contingency plans. Consequently, fistula treatment grinds to a halt. In addition, financial cuts are being made at the global level for crucial funds destined to support fistula work. One such case is highlighted in the 2018 Secretary General's report on 'Intensifying Efforts to End Obstetric Fistula Within a Generation' (UN, 2018) which states:

> Contributions to the Campaign to End Fistula have also declined and remain vastly insufficient to meet the current needs. Contributions to the Campaign totalled $1.58 million in 2016, but declined significantly in 2017 to $450,000

It is therefore hardly surprising that only 23 out of almost 60 fistula-affected countries have developed national strategies for obstetric fistula elimination and out of those, only 13 have implemented costed, time-bound operational plans. UNFPA's goals of eliminating obstetric fistula appear to be ambitious given the present reduction of global funding. Other prominent global actors working on fistula are experiencing similar funding cuts. With this status quo and diminishing funds across the sector, it is all the more surprising that the previous goal set by the UN to end fistula within a generation, i.e. 25 years, has recently been readjusted to 2030, in line with the United Nations' Sustainable Development Goals (UN, 2018). This presents the fistula community with an enormous challenge, and opens up a unique opportunity to mobilise more domestic resources to build national capacity for fistula prevention and treatment.

Increasing the quantity of local, competent fistula surgeons—in addition to other associated professionals like nurses, physiotherapists, counsellors, social workers, rehabilitation and social re-integration specialists—is imperative and must be included in national elimination plans so that many more women can access fistula repair surgery and a comprehensive care package in a timely manner. Resources and time also need to be allocated to share the wisdom and unique insight of expert surgeons (Waaldijk, 2016), as well as development of new surgical techniques that will give renewed hope to women with more complex injuries and so-called 'inoperable/incurable cases'. As evidence is starting to suggest, this may well require a unified approach, bringing together surgeons from different sub-specialties, including plastic surgeons. Recent publications showcase such new procedures and impressive success rates for these complex cases (Pope, Brown, Chalamanda, et al., 2018; Pope, Brown, Chipungu, et al., 2018). Yet again, the safe rollout and spread of knowledge must be ensured so that women with fistula in all countries benefit equally from innovative new techniques. This also applies to fistula publications in general, including training materials. Owing to funding limitations, such publications are often only released in English, but to extend the reach and impact of these precious resources, they should be made available in the official language of other fistula-affected countries, including French and Portuguese.

18.3 FIGO's Experience in Addressing Obstetric Fistula: History of the FIGO Fistula Surgery Training Initiative

As indicated above, a prevailing obstacle in the provision of fistula treatment has been the absence of a standardised training curriculum for fistula surgeons. This has resulted in differing training approaches and inconsistent practices, based on the personal preferences of individual expert surgeons. Efforts to systematically build the capacity of fistula surgeons on a global scale had not been considered. Due to the increasing need for a coordinated global training strategy, the International Federation of Gynecology and Obstetrics (Fédération Internationale de Gynécologie et d'Obstétrique, FIGO) decided to take concrete action by assembling leading authorities from the fistula community including expert fistula surgeons and international agencies to address the global treatment gap with a two-tiered approach; education and training.

- In 2011 after numerous stakeholder meetings, FIGO released the world's first standardised curriculum—the FIGO and partners Global Competency-Based Fistula Surgery Training Manual—to train fistula surgeons (FIGO, 2011).
- In 2012 FIGO launched the Fistula Surgery Training Initiative (Slinger et al., 2018), an ambitious multi-year programme with the aim of training more fistula surgeons—using the Global Competency-based Training Manual—in order to scale up the number of skilled fistula surgeons in affected countries so that significantly more women receive treatment.

This innovative two-tiered approach provides:

- A standardised training curriculum for fistula surgeons, using a modular competency-based approach.
- A standardised list of criteria for facilities to become FIGO Training Centres.

- A standardised process for experienced fistula surgeons to become FIGO Trainers.
- A standardised list of selection criteria for trainee fistula surgeons to join the Training Initiative.
- A standardised training approach for trainee fistula surgeons to gradually build their skills over time, assisting them to attain ascending levels of competency in fistula surgery.

Following these efforts by FIGO, between 2011 and 2014 significant advances occurred in developing this programme:

- The training manual was formally introduced to the fistula community via a series of training workshops for more than 50 fistula surgeons from Africa and Asia, to demonstrate how to implement the competency-based training system, how to appraise trainee fistula surgeons (*FIGO Fellows*), and how to facilitate their progression as fistula surgeons.
- Adhering strictly to the standardised criteria, members of the FIGO Fistula Committee visited multiple busy, well-functioning fistula treatment sites across Africa and Asia. Five of these facilities have become FIGO Training Centres in Ethiopia, Kenya, Nigeria (two centres) and Tanzania.

18.4   Organisation of the FIGO Training Programme

To ensure that the most qualified applicants enter the training programme, a list of selection criteria (Fig. 18.1) for candidates was established, including the following three essential components. These state that the applicants must: (1) have a minimum of 3 years of postgraduate surgical experience; (2) originate from and be working in a country where obstetric fistula is prevalent; and (3) have the support of their Ministry of Health for provision of fistula treatment.

This founding list of selection criteria was an invaluable guide for recruitment of Fellows in the early years, ensuring that those physicians with the 'hands and the heart' to become fistula surgeons joined the programme (Slinger et al., 2018), and would most likely continue doing fistula treatment

To be considered for a training placement, applicants:

- Must be a qualified medical doctor with a minimum of three years' surgical experience
- Must originate from and be in full-time clinical work in a fistula-affected country
- Must have a proven track record and strong commitment to caring for women with obstetric fistula
- Must be available to undergo six weeks of initial training then subsequent coaching
- Must provide assurance by Ministry of Health and hospital management that the Fellow will be able to continue providing fistula treatment after initial training placement, on return to their home country
- Must be committed to the care of women who have incurred obstetric fistula and to upholding women's basic rights to health, privacy and dignity
- Must be prepared to apply immediately and on a long-term basis the skills gained during training placements/coaching sessions upon returning to their home environment
- Must provide robust references directly to FIGO by recognised fistula surgeon(s)

Note that the FIGO Project Team and the selected FIGO Training Centre will make the selection decisions jointly.

Fig. 18.1   FIGO Fellow selection criteria as at April 2021

work long into the future. With experience, the original selection criteria have been modified and expanded over time to better convey entry requirements to interested parties and moreover, as a further measure to recruit the best candidates.

To make a meaningful contribution to building national treatment capacity in high-burden countries, the criterion *'Must originate from and be in full time clinical work in a fistula-affected country'* is particularly relevant. During the selection process, in addition to the criteria, careful consideration is also made to the situation and needs of each applicant's country, including population size, MMR, existing fistula surgeons and treatment services in that country, and the geo-political context.

As the project has expanded, two objectives have been developed, relating to both short- and long-term goals, as outlined below:

1. Short-term Objective.

    To strengthen fistula treatment capacity in each affected country, by developing an appropriate pool of trained, competent fistula surgeons, who can accelerate efforts to address the fistula treatment gap and thereby treat significantly more women in that country.

2. Long-term Objective.

    To develop a group of Fellows to trainer level, to reinforce the pool of FIGO Trainers, in order to scale up global treatment efforts by helping to train more fistula surgeons (and holistic care teams) in their own country and internationally.

The involvement of fistula surgeons on the ground is a fundamental part of the training programme, both during Fellow recruitment and at every step of a Fellow's development as a fistula surgeon. FIGO welcomes feedback from practicing fistula surgeons, recommending promising candidates with whom they have worked. In fact, some of the best performing Fellows in terms of repair numbers and success rates have been recruited in this way. Each year, many requests are sent to FIGO from physicians who are keen to join the training programme from all over the world. At any given time, however, these requests far exceed the number of available places in the training sites. While most requests come from those originating from and working in fistula-affected countries, a sizeable number are also received from those working in and originating from countries where obstetric fistula has been largely eradicated.

In line with the goals of the training programme to strengthen national fistula treatment capacity, FIGO only accepts Fellows from fistula-affected countries. Rare exceptions are occasionally made to admit Fellows from other contexts, e.g. Europe, who can show a solid track record of involvement in fistula treatment work, who are working in a high-burden fistula country, and who will almost certainly continue to provide fistula treatment long into the future.

When a candidate is deemed to meet the selection criteria, the application folder is sent to the appointed training centre, then a decision is jointly made by FIGO and the training centre, regarding acceptance (or not) of the applicant onto the programme. Where appropriate, an initial training placement is subsequently scheduled for the new Fellow. While the selection decision is jointly made by FIGO and the training centre, the whole application, training and monitoring process for all Fellows is entirely managed by FIGO in close collaboration with training centre staff, the associated Fellow(s), as well as multiple stakeholders. This includes responding to daily enquiries, coordinating the application and selection process, scheduling training placements and coaching visits, management of travel and accommodation logistics, as well as often protracted interactions with immigration and national education bodies to secure visas and medical registration in the host country.

Although applicants demonstrating ongoing commitment and experience in fistula surgery are now the preferred candidates for the training programme, professional circumstances do vary greatly between Fellows. Many hold senior clinical roles in their home facilities, with large and mixed caseloads, as well as additional management and academic responsibilities. This means that no two Fellows or their situations are identical. A flexible, continuous training approach therefore has to be adopted, which is tailored to meet the needs of each and every Fellow, to seamlessly complement their professional role without disrupting their existing work schedule or that of their hospital.

A Fellow may enter the training programme with very different amounts of experience and expertise in fistula surgery and care. While a relatively inexperienced Fellow might join having assisted 50 fistula repairs and having done 15 repairs by themselves—and hence they will contribute to goal #1 as cited earlier—others may join having already assisted 1000 repairs and having done 500 cases themselves and hence will be able to make a meaningful contribution to goal #1 and relatively quickly to goal #2 as also cited earlier. Once accepted onto the programme, using the Global Competency-based Training Manual as a standardised training tool, Fellows' skills are methodically built over time through a series of training placements in FIGO Training Centres, interspersed with coaching visits in the Fellows' home environment by an experienced fistula surgeon who is a FIGO Trainer. To accommodate the diverse circumstances and individual needs of each Fellow, no set time period has been allocated for the Fellowship training or to the attainment of the three levels of competency in fistula surgery—Standard, Advanced, and the highest level, Expert. Acquisition of competencies takes place in the form of graduated training, starting with basic principles and addressing less complex cases in Standard level, then building Fellows' skills, to allow them to perform increasingly difficult procedures such as urethral and vaginal reconstruction.

Each Fellow starts by doing an initial 4- to 6-week training placement in a FIGO Training Centre. This entails the Fellow working with the centre's expert team to build knowledge and skills in the holistic care of women with fistula, including patient recruitment, medical and surgical management, psychosocial and nutritional support, rehabilitation and post-operative follow up. During the placement, the critical development of competences in fistula surgery is achieved by the Fellow assisting the trainer, and crucially, by gaining as much hands-on experience as possible in fistula repair procedures that are at an appropriate level and performed by the Fellow under strict supervision by the trainer. While every effort is made to give as much hands-on practice as possible, building a Fellow's skills in fistula surgery is time-consuming and particularly challenging because:

- Very few fistulas are considered 'simple' or 'straightforward enough' to be repaired by a relatively inexperienced fistula surgeon.
- No two fistula cases are the same; the majority being of a complex or very complex nature (Hancock, 2009).
- The first attempt at surgical repair has the greatest chance of success, with every attempt thereafter radically reducing the patient's chance of a full recovery (Breen, 2019). This inevitably means that expert trainers may be inclined to do such repairs themselves while the Fellow observes.
- Approximately 75% of Fellows are the only fistula surgeon in the facility where they do fistula repairs, with no on site supervision by an experienced fistula surgeon to guide them or help strengthen their skills (Slinger et al., 2018).
- For patient safety, and to optimise surgical outcomes, Fellows must never attempt a repair beyond their present level of competency if unsupervised.
- Fellows are generally able to focus just part of their time on fistula treatment, which means they only have limited opportunity to build their skills and expertise.
- Each Fellow's professional circumstances and his/her opportunity to do fistula treatment work are different.

Guided by the Global Competency-based Training Manual, at the end of the first training period, Fellows are informed by the Trainer of their current level of competency in fistula surgery. Constructive

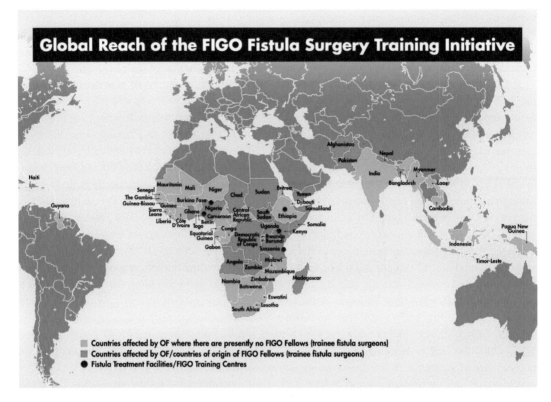

Fig. 18.2 Global reach of the FIGO fistula surgery training initiative. [Reprinted from Slinger, G., & Trautvetter, L. (2020). Addressing the Fistula Treatment Gap and Rising to the 2030 Challenge. *International Journal of Gynecology & Obstetrics*, 148(Suppl. 1):9–15, Fig. 1. https://doi.org/10.1002/ijgo.13033, licensed under the terms of the Creative Commons Attribution 4.0 International License (http://creativecommons.org/licenses/by/4.0/)]

feedback is also provided to strengthen the Fellows' surgical skills and management of fistula patients, as well as recommendations on additional training requirements. Consistent with the three levels of competency, a certification system has also been developed. As for a Fellow's initial training placement, or for any subsequent training or coaching, assessment and confirmation of a Fellow's level of competency, or progression to the next level, is the responsibility of the respective FIGO Trainer involved, whom after discussing with the Fellow, communicates the level to the FIGO Team, who then issue the appropriate certificate to the Fellow.

Of the 67 Fellows currently enrolled on the Training Programme from 22 countries (see Fig. 18.2):

- More than 50 have attained Standard level.
- 13 have attained Advanced level; and many others are working towards Advanced level
- Of the 13 who have attained Advanced level, several are approaching Expert level.

18.5 Multi-disciplinary Team Training

As the programme developed, it became evident that to ensure comprehensive care services for women with fistula, as well as training fistula surgeons, a broader training approach was required. Consequently, in recent years, multi-disciplinary health teams have been admitted to the programme

Fig. 18.3 FIGO Fellow Dr. Belquis Al-Jailani (second from the left) and team from Yemen undergoing training in Comprehensive Community-based Rehabilitation Tanzania (CCBRT)

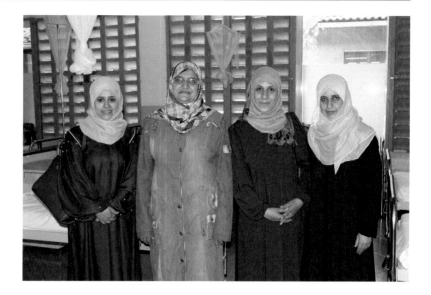

from countries like Ghana, the Democratic Republic of the Congo (DRC), Somalia, Yemen (Fig. 18.3) and Afghanistan. These teams typically consist of ward and theatre nurses from fistula departments, often with psychosocial support staff and physiotherapists, who with their Fellow, undergo team training together in a FIGO Training Centre. This inclusive training approach enables team members to learn simultaneously in a specialist centre and then apply what they have learned with their own patients and teams when they return home. A subsequent coaching visit by a trainer in their home facility provides an ideal opportunity for additional training, not only to strengthen the surgical skills of the resident Fellow, but also the quality of care provided by the entire fistula team. FIGO has received a growing number of requests for team training from high-burden countries. In collaboration with partners, this will be further expanded in the near future to incorporate other specialists responsible for patient recruitment, rehabilitation and nutrition.

18.6   Monitoring and Evaluation

Monitoring and evaluation are fundamental components of the Training Initiative to track Fellow progress and programme impact. This is achieved with the help of the password-protected *Kaizen e-Portfolio* database (Fry-It, 2019) where Fellows and trainers submit their data which is saved on each person's individual timeline. Whereas Fellows are only able to access their own information, trainers are able to access the profiles of all Fellows. Thereby Fellows can easily view their trainers' reports and their progress, as well as their fistula repair numbers and surgical outcomes. Trainers, on the other hand, can easily prepare for coaching visits and other training activities by viewing the Fellows' timelines in advance. Kaizen is also used to host new educational materials such as surgical training films and the latest fistula publications. Guided by the Global Competency-based Training Manual, the training experience and the Fellow's progress are recorded at the end of the initial training placement by the Fellow and trainer using assessment forms that are completed on Kaizen. This not only helps to assess the Fellow's level of competency, but also indicates where improvements to the training programme might be appropriate.

Upon successful completion of the initial training placement, Fellows are automatically enrolled into the programme's quarterly data collection to provide key information about their fistula repair work, including numbers, results and challenges. In response to emerging trends, the database can be swiftly adjusted to delve deeper into certain issues. Coaching visits usually take place in the Fellow's home environment, either in his/her own or a neighbouring health facility, e.g. fistula camps with partners. This gives trainers a clear impression of the services being provided and can generate discussions to improve and, where appropriate, expand holistic fistula care at the Fellow's facility. As with a placement in a training centre, the Fellow and trainer complete an assessment form on Kaizen at the end of the coaching session, describing the coaching experience, outlining progress (using the training manual), confirming current level of competency, as well as suggestions by the trainer to further strengthen the Fellow's skills and his/her corresponding fistula department. In addition to the Kaizen ePortfolio, FIGO conducts ad-hoc interviews and surveys to identify Fellow needs and major challenges in their fistula work. Highlighted in quarterly data collections, then confirmed through a specially crafted survey, the project team identified a serious fistula equipment gap, as well as multiple environmental factors hindering fistula treatment work, to which appropriate solutions were—and continue to be—found. The project team also communicates regularly with trainers and an extensive network of partners on the ground to gather and share information. These monitoring and evaluation methods create robust feedback loops, provide up-to-date information, allow the project team to monitor progress and make data-driven decisions, and consistently weave lessons-learned back into the programme.

18.7 Programme Governance

Since 2014, the Training Initiative has been managed by a very small project team with substantial experience in fistula programming and who are based at FIGO Headquarters in London. In addition to the project staff, the programme has been intermittently guided by the FIGO Committee for Fistula and Genital Trauma—a group of senior clinicians and experts in the field of obstetric fistula. In line with the project's considerable growth in both size and complexity, and to garner additional expert support, in 2017, the Training Initiative's Expert Advisory Group (EAG) was established. Composed of FIGO Trainers, the project team and a variety of the committee members, the EAG delivers expert guidance and consensus for issues central to the initiative including increasing Fellows' skills, tracking of data and surgical results, addressing problems, as well as strategic development of the broader Training Initiative.

The EAG is also the best placed body to address and agree upon previously unresolved issues together, such as setting up criteria to remove Fellows from the programme. Permanent removal can be considered in circumstances where Fellows do not meet training standards, whose professional circumstances or career path have changed, who consistently fail to submit their quarterly repair data or who are out of contact with the project team.

In order to accommodate Fellows who are undertaking a period of full-time study, either in their country of origin or abroad, the EAG has devised a system to temporarily remove them from the programme, on the condition that they resume contact with the project team once they are in a position to continue their fistula repair work, at which point they may re-enter the Initiative.

This is a win-win mechanism for all parties, including:

- *The Fellow*; who is able to confidently enhance his/her knowledge and skill set by undergoing extra study without losing his/her valuable training place on the programme.
- *The Training Initiative*; as Fellows undertaking study are not lost from the programme, nor is there any distortion in the 'reporting' of Fellow data if some are temporarily on study leave, away from clinical work.

- *The donors/sponsors*; as every precious donor dollar is used flexibly and optimally. Considering the long road required to train a fistula surgeon and the limited available funds, this is a critically important point, especially knowing how efforts by many to train fistula surgeons in the past often bore few fruits and investments were lost.
- *The women with fistula*; who are presently not able to access fistula treatment for many reasons; principally because there are not enough trained, skilled fistula surgeons.

Directly enhancing the surgical treatment and holistic management of fistula patients, the EAG works together to refine practices and protocols, develop new guidelines and training materials, identify research gaps and ensure a standardised best practice model in fistula care for the Training Initiative, as well as for the whole fistula community.

18.8 Challenges

As can be expected, setting up the first global Fistula Surgery Training Initiative has not been without its difficulties, and many valuable lessons have been learned along the way. This section highlights some of the challenges encountered and describes how they are being addressed.

18.8.1 Maintaining the Critical Yet Precarious Fistula Treatment Chain

A key challenge faced by many Fellows is practicing and developing their skills in fistula surgery. A critical factor determining how quickly they can advance their fistula repair work depends on how well the fistula treatment chain (Fig. 18.4) is working in their region (Slinger, 2018).

While some of the more fortunate surgeons work in well-equipped centres with established patient recruitment and transportation mechanisms, as well as sufficient means to pay for patients' treatment and hospital stay, the vast majority of Fellows work in facilities with meagre, often fleeting resources and irregular patient caseloads.

As mentioned earlier, while governments and local authorities endeavour to provide some funding, more often than not, the fistula treatment chain is partly or fully funded by international donor agencies. Each funder customarily supports a specific link or section of the chain, for example, patient recruitment and transportation to and from a treatment facility. However, fistula treatment services become extremely disrupted when the funding of any part of the chain is reduced or stopped. Fellows frequently report that they are '*now doing fewer or no repairs*' because a vital link of the treatment chain suddenly 'lost funding'.

Experience consistently shows that a reliably funded, functioning and coordinated fistula treatment chain, enhances collaboration and use of precious resources, thereby bringing in high patient numbers (Slinger & Trautvetter, 2020). When each crucial link of the treatment chain is fully functioning, Fellows:

- Have a regular patient caseload.
- Do a greater number of fistula repairs.
- Develop their skills at a faster pace.
- Treat a much higher number of women, to help close the fistula treatment gap in their country.

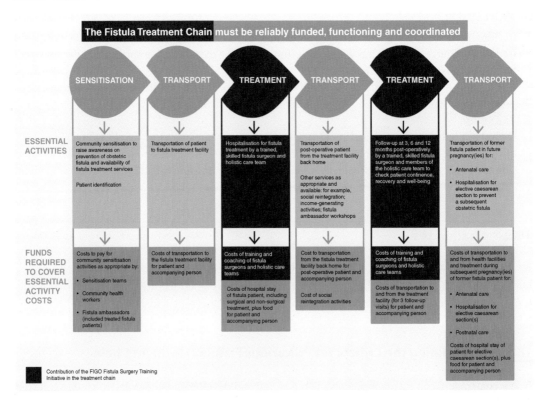

Fig. 18.4 The Fistula Treatment Chain must be reliably funded, functioning and coordinated. [Reprinted from Slinger, G., & Trautvetter, L. (2020). Addressing the Fistula Treatment Gap and Rising to the 2030 Challenge. *International Journal of Gynecology & Obstetrics*, 148(Suppl. 1):9–15, Fig. 2. https://doi.org/10.1002/ijgo.13033, licensed under the terms of the Creative Commons Attribution 4.0 International License (http://creativecommons.org/licenses/by/4.0/)]

18.8.2 Data Dilemmas and Double/Multiple Reporting

Despite a sophisticated monitoring and evaluation system, data collection has been and continues to be a challenge. Fellows are busy clinicians with multiple responsibilities and competing schedules. Submission of their fistula repair data is essential, yet timely submission is not always possible. A patient, yet persistent, approach has hence been adopted by the project team. In practice, this means sending regular reminders and follow-up telephone calls, in addition to remaining flexible with deadlines, to ensure maximum submission rates, as well as quality of content.

Another data dilemma is the double—or multiple—reporting of fistula repairs. This occurs when more than one—or numerous—donors/authorities fund the same fistula surgeon and/or his/her institution. For example, a fistula treatment facility providing routine repairs might be funded by three different donors: one funding patient recruitment and fistula treatment, the second funding patient food during hospitalisation, fistula surgery and medication, and the third funding patient transportation, fistula treatment and equipment. The surgeon is required to provide a summary of annual repairs to each funder. Unless one donor funds everything, it is difficult, if not impossible, for the surgeon to accurately report how many fistula repairs have been funded by each entity. Inevitably, the surgeon often reports total fistula repairs by the facility three times, i.e. to each funding body. In addition, it is likely that once a year the facility will report their total fistula repair number to the Global Fistula Hub, which in this scenario will result in the same repair numbers being reported four times to four different agencies. All Fellows are actively encouraged to submit their facility repair data annually to the Global Fistula Hub. Currently, FIGO only collects Fellow repair data and does not collect how many Fellows 'double or multiple report' their repair numbers. However, with relative ease this could be corrected in future reporting and quickly determined from quarterly data collections, resulting in a more accurate account of fistula repairs.

18.8.3 Competency Levels

The progression of Fellows through the different levels of competency—as outlined in the Global Competency-based Training Manual—has also been a challenge and is not as straightforward as was originally envisaged. Due to competing demands and the complexity of fistula surgery, Fellows only have limited time to do fistula repair work and in tandem, to develop these specialised skills. A further hurdle is that most Fellows provide services in resource-constrained settings, where the fistula treatment chain is particularly fragile, causing unpredictable and fluctuating patient numbers.

Presently, Fellows must be assessed by a FIGO Trainer in order to progress to the next level of competency. However, since the frequency of coaching visits directly depends on the availability of funds, as well as trainers' time, visits take place much less frequently than required. These elements, as well as other challenges, cause inevitable delays in Fellows attaining the next level of competency. To better facilitate progression as a fistula surgeon through ascending levels of competency, the training manual and certification mechanism will be re-organised in the near future so that the majority of Fellows can comfortably treat a large cadre of fistula cases, while the most complex cases will be reserved for an expert fistula surgeon.

18.8.4 Funding

Finally, and not unexpectedly, one of the biggest challenges faced by the training initiative is funding. Although the project has benefitted from ongoing funding since the start in 2012, these funds have been insufficient to meet the programme's needs, especially in more recent years. While there is presently an increased awareness about obstetric fistula, it is nonetheless a very specialised area in which to work, and remains unknown and completely 'off the radar' of many funders. Furthermore, the relatively small prevalence rate compared to other well-publicised global health issues, such as HIV, malaria and cervical cancer, puts women with obstetric fistula at the end of the priority list. The reinstatement of the global gag rule under the Trump administration in 2017 (Singh & Karim, 2017) also led to funding shifts at the time, as significant amounts from donor organisations were redirected to cover the resulting gap in safe abortion and family planning services. Funding challenges are however being experienced by the fistula community as a whole and are not just specific to the Fistula Surgery Training Initiative. Naturally, unpredictable, unreliable and inadequate funding means that the Initiative is expanding slower than desired.

18.9   Future Priorities and Key Achievements

After steady growth and notable accomplishments, the Training Initiative has clearly demonstrated the effectiveness of its two-tiered approach to train substantially more fistula surgeons and care teams in order to close the global treatment gap. As outlined below, despite various challenges, many of the original goals have been reached and even exceeded (Figs. 18.5 and 18.6).

- 67 Fellows from 22 high-burden fistula countries presently being trained
- Coaching visits provided by FIGO Trainers to more than 50 Fellows
- More than 13,000 fistula repairs collectively performed by Fellows (as at December 2020)
- Ten multidisciplinary health teams accepted for training in holistic fistula care
- Robust monitoring and evaluation mechanism developed to track Fellow progress and programme impact, allowing data-driven decisions to consistently strengthen the initiative
- High-quality customised fistula instrument sets and head torches supplied to 45 Fellows (Fig. 18.6)
- Extensive network of partners established and being coordinated to help facilitate the programme
- EAG set up to provide additional expert opinion and strategic guidance on the evolving initiative
- Considerable increase in requests to FIGO from high-profile agencies and Ministries of Health, wishing to sponsor new Fellows and fistula teams
- Growing preference by donors who are greatly reassured if the fistula surgeon they are funding has received, or is undergoing FIGO Training.

Fig. 18.5   Key achievements of FIGO's fistula surgery training initiative

Fig. 18.6   FIGO Fellow Dr. Claude Idring'i from Democratic Republic of the Congo (DRC) receiving FIGO fistula instrument sets

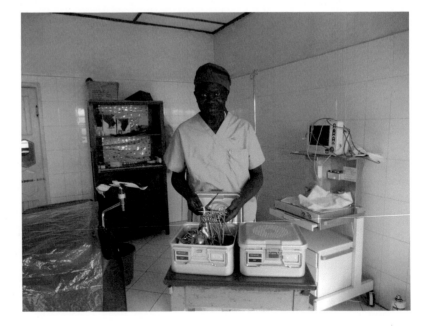

In direct collaboration with the EAG and partners at all levels, and in the continued drive to treat more women, in the next phase, the Training Initiative aims to:

- Admit more Fellows and health teams from neglected countries with high numbers of fistula cases.
- Provide ongoing training and coaching for existing Fellows to prevent delays in the development of their competencies, so more can progress to FIGO Trainer status.
- Continue to provide regular live online training sessions covering specific fistula procedures and topics, allowing a unique opportunity for Fellows to discuss directly with FIGO Trainers.
- Identify additional, well-functioning FIGO Training Centres in francophone Africa and Asia.
- Organise surgical workshops for Fellows and trainers.
- Continue upgrading and supplying specialised fistula equipment to Fellows and trainers, as well as making materials available to the broader fistula community.
- Reinforce the fistula treatment chain in close collaboration with stakeholders.
- Develop and publish more fistula educational resources, e.g. Best Practice Guidelines and an updated version of the Global Competency-based Fistula Surgery Training Manual with translations in French and Portuguese.
- Identify research gaps to reinforce the evidence base and thereby enhance clinical practices.
- In collaboration with the fistula community, accelerate efforts to raise significantly more awareness and funds in support of women with obstetric fistula.

18.10 Conclusions

With a wealth of experience, FIGO has become a cutting-edge authority on training fistula surgeons. Driven by the urgent need to address the global treatment gap, this has been achieved through establishment of the world's first standardised curriculum for fistula surgery and by launching a revolutionary training programme for fistula surgeons and their teams in affected countries. With the indispensable support of a vast network of partners across Africa and Asia, FIGO is building national capacity to provide fistula surgery, enhancing quality and providing holistic care to significantly more women.

To eliminate fistula requires ongoing prevention efforts and a substantial scaling up of fistula treatment services, including more trained, competent fistula surgeons and care teams in high-burden contexts. In parallel, more focus must be given to raising awareness and to addressing the underlying socio-economic factors giving rise to the condition in the world's most disadvantaged communities. These efforts will, of course, also require increased funding support from donors, agencies, and governments.

The recent adjustment by the UN to end fistula by 2030, in line with the United Nations Sustainable Development Goals (SDGs), presents a huge challenge, particularly with the acute shortage of domestic and international resources. Yet for affected countries and the global community, this also presents a golden opportunity to close the fistula treatment gap. The FIGO Fistula Surgery Training Initiative (Fig. 18.7) will play a major role in this noble endeavour and will continue to work tirelessly until obstetric fistula has been eradicated.

Fig. 18.7 Group photo with several FIGO Fellows, Trainers and project team attending the ISOFS conference in Kathmandu, Nepal, December 2018

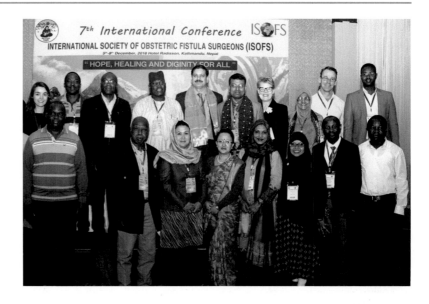

Acknowledgements Sincere thanks to the committed FIGO Fellows and Trainers of the Fistula Surgery Training Initiative as well as all supporting partners, with special mention to Fistula Foundation and Texas Children's Hospital who have contributed to the success of the project. Grateful thanks are also extended to Dr. Andrew Browning (AM) for his continued guidance and for kindly providing feedback on the initial draft of this chapter.

References

Ahmed, S., & Holtz, S. A. (2007). Social and economic consequences of obstetric fistula: Life changed forever? *International Journal of Gynecology & Obstetrics, 99*(Suppl 1), S10–S15. https://doi.org/10.1016/j.ijgo.2007.06.011

Akpan, E. (2003). Early marriage in eastern Nigeria and the health consequences of vesicovaginal fistulae (VVF) among young mothers. *Gender and Development, 11*, 70–76. https://doi.org/10.1080/741954319

Arrowsmith, S. D. (2007). Urinary diversion in the vesico-vaginal fistula patient: General considerations regarding feasibility, safety, and follow-up. *International Journal of Gynecology & Obstetrics, 99*(Suppl 1), S65–S68. https://doi.org/10.1016/j.ijgo.2007.06.028

Bangser, M. (2007). Strengthening public health priority-setting through research on fistula, maternal health, and health inequities. *International Journal of Gynecology & Obstetrics, 99*(Suppl 1), S16–S20. https://doi.org/10.1016/j.ijgo.2007.06.016

Breen, M. (2019). *Manual of obstetric fistula surgery*. The Foundation for the Global Library of Women's Medicine.

Browning, A. (2004). Obstetric fistula in Ilorin, Nigeria. *PLoS Medicine, 1*(1), e2. https://doi.org/10.1371/journal.pmed.0010002

Cook, R. J., Dickens, B. M., & Syed, S. (2004). Obstetric fistula: The challenge to human rights. *International Journal of Gynecology & Obstetrics, 87*(1), 72–77. https://doi.org/10.1016/j.ijgo.2004.07.005

De Ridder, D., Badlani, G. H., Browning, A., Singh, P., Sombie, I., & Wall, L. L. (2009). Fistulas in the developing world. In L. Cardozo, P. Abrams, S. Khoury, & A. Wein (Eds.), *Incontinence* (pp. 1419–1458). Health Publications Ltd.

Direct Relief. (2021). *Global fistula map*. Direct Relief. Retrieved April 9, 2012, from http://globalfistulahub.org/.

Donnay, F., & Weil, L. (2004). Obstetric fistula: The international response. *Lancet, 363*(9402), 71–72. https://doi.org/10.1016/S0140-6736(03)15177-X

FIGO. (2006). *Ethical guidelines*. International Federation of Obstetrics and Gynecology.

FIGO. (2011). *Global competency-based fistula surgery training manual*. International Federation of Obstetrics and Gynecology. Retrieved June 19, 2019, from https://www.figo.org/sites/default/files/uploads/wg-publications/fistula/FIGO_Global_Competency-Based_Fistula_Surgery_Training_Manual_0.pdf

Fistula Foundation. (2019). *What is fistula?* Fistula Foundation. Retrieved June 16, 2019, from https://www.fistulafoundation.org/what-is-fistula/

Fry-It. (2019). *Kaizen ePortfolio*. Fry-It. Retrieved July 5, 2019, from https://fry-it.com/kaizen/

Gutman, R. E., Dodson, J. L., & Mostwin, J. L. (2007). Complications of treatment of obstetric fistula in the developing world: Gynatresia, urinary incontinence, and urinary diversion. *International Journal of Gynecology & Obstetrics, 99*(Suppl 1), S57–S64. https://doi.org/10.1016/j.ijgo.2007.06.027

Hancock, B. (2009). *Practical obstetric fistula surgery.* The Foundation for the Global Library of Women's Medecine.

Hancock, B. (2013). *An introduction to obsetric fistula surgery.* Sapiens Publishing.

Hilton, P. (2003). Vesico-vaginal fistulas in developing countries. *International Journal of Gynecology & Obstetrics, 82*(3), 285–295. https://doi.org/10.1016/S0020-7292(03)00222-4

Hilton, P., & Ward, A. (1998). Epidemiological and surgical aspects of urogenital fistulae: A review of 25 years' experience in southeast Nigeria. *International Urogynecology Journal and Pelvic Floor Dysfunction, 9*(4), 189–194. https://doi.org/10.1007/BF01901602

ISOFS. (2019). Retrieved July 24, 2019, from https://www.isofs-global.org/

Keri L, Kaye D, Sibylle K. (2010). Referral practices and perceived barriers to timely obstetric care among Ugandan traditional birth attendants (TBA). Afr Health Sci., *10*(1):75–81.

Mselle, L. T., Moland, K. M., Evjen-Olsen, B., Mvungi, A., & Kohi, T. W. (2011). "I am nothing": Experiences of loss among women suffering from severe birth injuries in Tanzania. *BMC Womens Health, 11,* 49. https://doi.org/10.1186/1472-6874-11-49

Muleta, M., Rasmussen, S., & Kiserud, T. (2010). Obstetric fistula in 14,928 Ethiopian women. *Acta Obstetricia et Gynecologica Scandinavica, 89*(7), 945–951. https://doi.org/10.3109/00016341003801698

Murphy, M. (1981). Social consequences of vesico-vaginal fistula in northern Nigeria. *Journal of Biosocial Science, 13*(2), 139–150. https://doi.org/10.1017/S0021932000013304

Olusegun, A. K., Akinfolarin, A. C., & Olabisi, L. M. (2009). A review of clinical pattern and outcome of vesi-covaginal fistula. *Journal of the National Medical Association, 101*(6), 593–595. https://doi.org/10.1016/S0027-9684(15)30946-9

Pope, R., Brown, R. H., Chalamanda, C., Hollier, L. H., Jr., & Wilkinson, J. P. (2018). The gracilis muscle flap for irreparable, "impossible", and recurrent obstetric fistulas. *International Journal of Gynecology & Obstetrics, 143*(3), 390–392. https://doi.org/10.1002/ijgo.12643

Pope, R. J., Brown, R. H., Chipungu, E., Hollier, L. H., Jr., & Wilkinson, J. P. (2018). The use of Singapore flaps for vaginal reconstruction in women with vaginal stenosis with obstetric fistula: A surgical technique. *An International Journal of Obstetrics and Gynaecology, 125,* 751–756. https://doi.org/10.1111/1471-0528.14952

Raassen, T. J., Verdaasdonk, E. G., & Vierhout, M. E. (2008). Prospective results after first-time surgery for obstetric fistulas in East African women. *International Urogynecology Journal and Pelvic Loor Dysfunction, 19*(1), 73–79. https://doi.org/10.1007/s00192-007-0389-6

Roush, K., Kurth, A., Hutchinson, M. K., & Van Devanter, N. (2012). Obstetric fistula: What about gender power? *Health Care for Women International, 33*(9), 787–798. https://doi.org/10.1080/07399332.2011.645964

Rushwan, H., Khaddaj, S., Knight, L., & Scott, R. (2012). Need for a global obstetric fistula training strategy. *International Journal of Gynecology & Obstetrics, 119*(Suppl 1), S76–S79. https://doi.org/10.1016/j.ijgo.2012.03.022

Shen, C., & Williamson, J. B. (1999). Maternal mortality, women's status, and economic dependency in less developed countries: A cross national analysis. *Social Science & Medicine, 49,* 197–214. https://doi.org/10.1016/s0277-9536(99)00112-4

Singh, J. A., & Karim, S. S. A. (2017). Trump's "global gag rule": Implications for human rights and global health (Comment). *The Lancet, 5*(4), PE387–PE389. https://doi.org/10.1016/S2214-109X(17)30084-0

Slinger, G. (2018). *Fistula treatment chain.* ISOFS Conference.

Slinger, G., & Trautvetter, L. (2020). Addressing the fistula treatment gap and rising to the 2030 challenge. *International Journal of Gynecology and Obstetrics, 148,* 9–15. https://doi.org/10.1002/ijgo.13033

Slinger, G., Trautvetter, L., Browning, A., & Rane, A. (2018). Out of the shadows and 6000 reasons to celebrate: An update from FIGO's fistula surgery training initiative. *International Journal of Gynecology and Obstetrics, 141*(3), 280–283. https://doi.org/10.1002/ijgo.12482

UN. (1995). *Beijing declaration and Platform for Action (PFA).* UN. Retrieved July 19, 2019, from https://www.un.org/womenwatch/daw/beijing/platform/

UN (2003). Maputo protocol—Protocol to the African Charter on Human and Peoples' Rights on the Rights of Women in Africa. . Retrieved July 19, 2019, from http://www.achpr.org/files/instruments/women-protocol/achpr_instr_proto_women_eng.pdf.

UN. (2015). *Sustainable development goals.* UN. Retrieved July 2, 2019, from https://www.un.org/sustainabledevelopment/sustainable-development-goals/

UN. (2018). *Resolution adopted by the General Assembly on 17 December 2018.* UN. Retrieved June 16, 2019, from http://www.endfistula.org/sites/default/files/pub-pdf/UNGA_PUB_2018_EN_RESOLUTION_73_147.pdf

UNFPA. (2003). *Campaign to end fistula.* UNFPA. Retrieved July 24, 2019, from http://www.endfistula.org/campaign

UNFPA. (2013). *International Day to end Obstetric Fistula 23 May.* UNFPA. Retrieved July 24, 2019, from http://www.endfistula.org/campaign/international-day-end-obstetric-fistula

Waaldijk, K. (2016). *Obsetric trauma surgery—Art and science, functional female pelvis anatomy for reconstructive surgery*. Printmarkt.eu.

Wall, L. L. (1998). Dead mothers and injured wives: The social context of maternal morbidity and mortality among the Hausa of northern Nigeria. *Studies in Family Planning, 29*(4), 341–359. Retrieved from http://www.ncbi.nlm.nih.gov/pubmed/9919629

Wall, L. L. (2002). Thomas Addis Emmet, the vesicovaginal fistula, and the origins of reconstructive gynecologic surgery. *International Urogynecology Journal and Pelvic Floor Dysfunction, 13*(3), 145–155; discussion 155. Retrieved from http://www.ncbi.nlm.nih.gov/pubmed/12140707

Wall, L. L. (2007). Ethical issues in vesico-vaginal fistula care and research. *The International Journal of Gynecology and Obstetrics, 99*(Suppl 1), S32–S39. https://doi.org/10.1016/j.ijgo.2007.06.020

Wall, L. L. (2012). Obstetric fistula is a "neglected tropical disease". *PLoS Neglected Tropical Diseases, 6*(8), e1769. https://doi.org/10.1371/journal.pntd.0001769

Wall, L. L. (2014). A bill of rights for patients with obstetric fistula. *International Journal of Gynecology and Obstetrics, 127*(3), 301–304. https://doi.org/10.1016/j.ijgo.2014.06.024

Wall, L. L., Arrowsmith, S. D., Briggs, N., Browning, A., & Lassey, A. (2005). The obstetric vesicovaginal fistula in the developing world. *Obstetrical and Gynecological Survey, 60*, S3–S51. https://doi.org/10.1097/00006254-200507001-00002

Wall, L. L., Arrowsmith, S. D., & Hancock, B. D. (2008). Ethical aspects of urinary diversion for women with irreparable obstetric fistulas in developing countries. *International Urogynecology Journal and Pelvic Floor Dysfunction, 19*(7), 1027–1030. https://doi.org/10.1007/s00192-008-0559-1

Wall, L. L., Arrowsmith, S. D., Lassey, A. T., & Danso, K. (2006). Humanitarian ventures or 'fistula tourism?': The ethical perils of pelvic surgery in the developing world. *International Urogynecology Journal and Pelvic Floor Dysfunction, 17*(6), 559–562. https://doi.org/10.1007/s00192-005-0056-8

Wall, L. L., Karshima, J. A., Kirschner, C., & Arrowsmith, S. D. (2004). The obstetric vesicovaginal fistula: Characteristics of 899 patients from Jos, Nigeria. *The American Journal of Obstetrics and Gynecology, 190*(4), 1011–1019. https://doi.org/10.1016/j.ajog.2004.02.007

Weston, K., Mutiso, S., Mwangi, J. W., Qureshi, Z., Beard, J., & Venkat, P. (2011). Depression among women with obstetric fistula in Kenya. *International Journal of Gynecology and Obstetrics, 115*(1), 31–33. https://doi.org/10.1016/j.ijgo.2011.04.015

WHO. (2018). *10 facts on obstetric fistula*. WHO. Retrieved June 16, 2019, from https://www.who.int/features/factfiles/obstetric_fistula/en/

WHO. (2019). *Total density of physicians per 1000 population: Latest available year*. WHO. Retrieved June 16, 2019, from http://gamapserver.who.int/gho/interactive_charts/health_workforce/PhysiciansDensity_Total/atlas.html

Women's Dignity Project & EngenderHealth. (2006). *Risks and resilience: Obstetric fistula in Tanzania*. Women's Dignity Project & EngenderHealth. Retrieved June 16, 2019, from https://www.engenderhealth.org/files/pubs/maternal-health/risk-and-resilience-obstetric-fistula-in-tanzania.pdf

Medical and Surgical Challenges and Opportunities for Treatment at the Aberdeen Women's Centre in Sierra Leone

19

Ennet Banda Chipungu

19.1 Introduction to Aberdeen Women's Centre

Aberdeen Women's Centre (AWC) is located in Freetown, the capital city of Sierra Leone. It is the only facility in this West African country that is dedicated to providing comprehensive care for women living with obstetric fistula, which is a devastating childbirth injury that can leave women with chronic incontinence. Since its founding, AWC has provided life-restoring obstetric fistula repair to over 2000 women.

The Centre was built in 2004 in order to take over the work of obstetric fistula repair from the Mercy Ships, an international charity that provides humanitarian assistance through international hospital ships. While it initially solely provided fistula management, with the passage of years AWC expanded and now multiple services are being offered. In 2005, an out-patient paediatric clinic was built serving children from new-born infants up to 15-year-olds. The services being offered include consultations, immunizations, physiotherapy, nutritional therapy and short-stay management, including care for very ill patients. It is open on weekdays and has two outreach clinics in Kroo Bay. Sick children needing in patient management are referred to Ola During hospital for further management. Clients are seen on a first come first serve basis, after triaging, until the day's target is reached. AWC currently sees over 20,000 children a year.

There are also family planning services, which are available to everybody within the community. The family planning clinic is open on weekdays and over weekends there are outreach clinics in highly populated areas. Methods being offered are oral contraceptives, both combined and progesterone only, Depo-Provera injectable, progesterone implants, intrauterine devices, copper T and condoms. There is also management of complications and treatment of sexually transmitted infections. These family planning services were initiated in order to help in combating maternal mortality and also in helping to prevent obstetric fistula.

In 2010 a maternity unity was opened in order to serve the local community and also to help in reducing maternal deaths and preventing obstetric fistula.

E. B. Chipungu (✉)
Freedom from Fistula Foundation,
Freetown, Sierra Leone
e-mail: ennetb@yahoo.com

© Springer Nature Switzerland AG 2022
L. B. Drew et al. (eds.), *A Multidisciplinary Approach to Obstetric Fistula in Africa*, Global Maternal and Child Health, https://doi.org/10.1007/978-3-031-06314-5_19

There is also a teenage programme, Dream girls, which serves teenagers when they are pregnant and after delivery. They are taught health education, how to look after a baby, and skills in literacy, numeracy, and arts and crafts. After delivery they are encouraged to go back to school or they are given housekeeping lessons and cooking classes so that they can get jobs or start their own businesses so that they gain employment.

Additionally, the facility's laboratory is open every day and processes specimens from all of the wards. The most common investigations done are full blood count and malaria tests. It also has a blood blank that primarily serves the maternity ward.

The AWC is unique in that all of its services are offered for free. The funding for the centre is primarily from the Gloag Foundation. UNFPA contributes to the management of fistula patients and the teenage program is sponsored by the Aminata Foundation, a charity foundation from Australia.

19.2 Maternity Services

The maternal mortality ratio (MMR) in Sierra Leone is one of the highest in the world with 1165 deaths/100,000 live births. According to the maternal death surveillance and response report of 2016, the main cause of maternal deaths was postpartum haemorrhage (32%), seconded by pregnancy-induced hypertension (16%) (Directorate of Reproductive and Child Health, Ministry of Health and Sanitation [Sierra Leone] 2017). Poor quality of care was identified as the main contributor for 67% of the maternal deaths, combined with delay in seeking and accessing care. These factors are also the main contributors of obstetric fistula.

In 2010 the government of Sierra Leone introduced the free health care initiative to all pregnant women, lactating women, and under five children, in order to ease access to skilled health workers and adequate resources. This provision will also reduce maternal mortality in Sierra Leone. AWC launched its maternity unit in 2010, which offers free antenatal, intrapartum and postpartum care to the surrounding underprivileged community. This was initiated with the aim of offering a good environment for delivery, offering good quality evidence-based care, reducing maternal mortality and morbidity, and preventing obstetric fistula. AWC has five delivery beds, 10 antenatal beds in the maternity unit and 15 postnatal beds. Currently, it is the second busiest maternity facility in Freetown, next to Princess Christian Maternity Hospital, with over 3000 deliveries a year. The number of deliveries has been increasing over the years, putting constraints on the available resources. The maternity unit has about 20 government posted midwives and nurses. There are also two government posted medical officers and an international obstetrician and gynaecologist.

19.3 The Challenge of Inadequate Resources and Infrastructure

The number of deliveries that can be conducted is limited by the number of available midwives and doctors. The midwives are government posted and AWC has no control on the number of midwives or nurses posted to the unit. Due to this restriction coupled with the limited budget of drug and supplies, AWC cannot serve all the pregnant women around the centre. Therefore, AWC limits the number of deliveries by tending to only pre-booked patients. These patients are booked from the community. There are two booking days in a week and 40 patients are booked on each day. However, with a bigger space than what we have now, as well as an increase in resources, including drugs and supplies, AWC will be capable of offering quality maternity care to more mothers than the numbers at present.

AWC does not have its own neonate unit, so all neonates who need care have to be transferred to Ola During Paediatric hospital, which is quite a distance from the centre. Also, if the mother is post-

Caesarean section or still ill, the neonate is transferred without the mother, which makes early bonding and establishment of exclusive breastfeeding impossible. Most of the time, the neonates cannot be transferred without a guardian, and this takes up essential time before appropriate management can be initiated. However, this can be solved by having an extension of the paediatric unit, to have a neonatal unit with all the required equipment, so that admissions can be done within the centre with 24 h onsite paediatric doctors. However, there currently is not enough space within the compound to accommodate these extensions.

19.4 Procuring and Maintaining Medical Equipment

It is difficult to procure some of the essential equipment in the country. Therefore, we often require equipment or spare parts to be brought in from outside the country, which is expensive and time-consuming. This is mostly for sutures for caesarean sections and oxygen concentrators, which are crucial in resuscitation of neonates and management of critical maternity cases. It has been a struggle to get vacuum extractors, which are needed to expedite delivery especially when the foetus is in distress or the second stage of labour has been prolonged. Almost all the delivery sets are brought in from outside the country. Because the spare parts are being brought from outside, sometimes the part which is brought in is not right and it takes even longer for the machines to be fixed.

Additionally, there is a need for the centre to get an extra neonatal resuscitaire, in order to assist with resuscitation of hypoxic and preterm neonates. The centre also is in need of a cardiotocography machine, which will be essential in monitoring of high-risk cases in order to reduce the numbers of fresh stillbirths and hypoxic neonates. With all these struggles of getting equipment, there are often damages to the equipment within a short time. There is a dedicated biomedical engineer, who comes to do the repairs once a week, but increased staff training on the use and cleaning of new equipment could also be helpful.

19.5 Limited Interhospital Care Coordination

Another extreme challenge is it is difficult to refer patients, especially critical patients, to the tertiary hospital, Princess Christian Maternity Hospital. Having an onsite high dependency unit or intensive unit, with well-trained personnel to offer close monitoring and ventilation of very sick patients, would improve the quality of care being offered to save the lives of mothers and newborns.

19.6 Fistula Services

In Sierra Leone, AWC is the only facility which offers surgical repairs of fistula. At the moment, AWC performs about 200 surgeries a year, though it has capacity to do about 300 a year. Most of our fistulas are obstetric. The patients come from all over Sierra Leone and most of them are from the rural areas. Although a number of fistula patients are walk-ins, most patients are brought in by the screening team from AWC, which enters hard-to-reach areas to sensitize the communities about fistula and identify women with fistula who are in need of repair. AWC offers both routine surgeries and repairs during camps. There are about 45 beds dedicated to fistula patients. Currently, one of the greatest challenges is the centre primarily depends on international surgeons who are flown in to provide surgeries during the camps. Having a fistula surgeon at all times at AWC would enable the centre to provide routine surgery to women with fistulas.

19.7   Fistula Prevalence and Incidence Not Known

UNFPA estimates that about 2–4 million women live with obstetrics fistula in low-income countries and that there are about 50,000 to 100,000 new cases every year (World Health Organization, 2018). Currently, the prevalence and incidence in Sierra Leone is not known. AWC has been managing both old and new fistula cases, which means there are still clients we have not reached and that there are clients who do not have access to health facilities with skilled health workers and timely interventions.

Because the figures for fistula are not known, it is difficult to know if we are able to reach out to all women who need the centre's services. Since most patients are brought in by AWC teams who go into the rural areas, it is possible that there are areas the teams have not been able to reach, especially the areas in extremely rural parts of the country with no access roads. Therefore, there is a need to intensify sensitization of communities in these hard-to-reach areas on what fistula is, how to prevent it, and where to go if you have a fistula. Partnering with organizations who work with these communities could aid these efforts. There is also a need to sensitize health workers in rural community facilities on fistula and where they should refer women with fistula.

Currently, there is a plan to bring in midwives and nurses from as many health facilities as possible to AWC. This effort will provide an opportunity for these healthcare providers to learn more about obstetric fistula, including what it is, how it affects women, and how to screen for patients. This effort could additionally assist in identifying patients in places we cannot reach while reducing the number of screening trips and therefore the cost of the program.

Like other sites have done, a patient ambassador program was introduced at AWC. However, compared to other sites, this effort was not as successful at identifying and bringing in women who need fistula repair. This could be due to ongoing high rates of stigmatization in communities as well as financial and cultural barriers.

19.8   Poor Post-surgical Follow-up

An ongoing challenge for AWC is most of our patients do not return for follow-up, which is critical. This challenge makes it difficult for us to calculate long-term cure rates, to assess postsurgical psychological state, to assess how women have reintegrated into the community, and to determine whether they are financially independent. Follow-up via mobile phones is a possibility; however, most of our patients do not provide a phone number or they are in areas where there is no mobile network. These challenges must be addressed if we are to address the long-term outcomes and needs of women after obstetric fistula repair.

19.9   No Solution to Irreparable Fistulas and Patients with Stress Incontinence

About 80–95% of obstetric fistula can be closed after surgery (Ouedraogo et al., 2018). However, even after surgical closure, some women may still have urinary incontinence. This incontinence is more common in patients who have obstetric fistula involving the bladder neck and the urethra.

A number of procedures, including urethral plication, rectus sheath sling, pubococcygeus slings, and glacilis muscle slings have been attempted with minimal success. Many patients were benefitting from the use of urethral plugs, which were being supplied by Direct Relief. Unfortunately, the production of urethral plugs was halted and this method is no longer an option. As healthcare providers, it is frustrating to try and manage these patients because there is little to offer them to address their ongoing incontinence.

There are other fistula patients who are deemed irreparable due to multiple unsuccessful repairs, inadequate bladder tissue, or absent urethral tissue. Initially in the Malawian centre in Lilongwe, the clients were being offered urinary diversions, MAINZ II, illeal conduit or Miami pouch. However, these methods have since been put on hold due to high complication rates and need for regular follow-up, which is often difficult to achieve.

For these women, there is also a need for special counselling and support, so that they can be financially independent since they are often isolated due to ongoing incontinence. Future efforts should assess options that may be the most feasible and accessible for these women, so that their quality of life may improve despite persistent incontinence that cannot be remedied via surgery.

19.10 Challenge of Interhospital Consultation

An ongoing challenge for AWC is interhospital consultation. AWC is located in Aberdeen township, which is quite a distance from the tertiary hospital, Connaught. The distance between the two hospitals makes it difficult to have other specialists help AWC. Assistance can be coordinated for scheduled cases; however, it is extremely difficult in emergency cases.

19.11 Recurrent Fistula

Unfortunately, we have had patients return to AWC with a recurrent fistula after successful fistula repair surgery. This damage primarily presents itself following another attempted vaginal delivery. On discharge, women who have undergone fistula repair are advised to plan for delivery through Caesarean section as soon as they learn they are pregnant. However, many women do not acquire a Caesarean section, and they labour at home and develop a recurrent obstetric fistula. Other women may attempt vaginal delivery in health facilities, even though they arrive to the facility with post-op instructions from AWC outlining that Caesarean section is needed for any future deliveries following fistula repair. Unfortunately, many of these women also have a stillbirth.

To avoid developing a recurrent fistula, patients are now instructed to come to the centre once they find out they are pregnant and await delivery. They might wait at the centre for several months, so that they can have a safe delivery and a live baby. However, this method is not ideal because the women are away from their families for a long time. For the women who cannot afford to travel to AWC in Freetown, they often end up with a stillbirth and recurrent fistula. Therefore, there is a need for continued sensitization to clinicians and midwives on how to manage pregnant patients who have previously undergone fistula repair.

19.12 Conclusion

AWC is the only facility in Sierra Leone that provides surgical repair for women with obstetric fistulas. The centre continues to grow and improve the quality of care that we provide. This is accomplished via the use of evidence-based medicine, providing job training for all clinical staff, and utilising experienced staff and international mentors. Challenges persist; however, despite the challenges, AWC assists in reducing preventable maternal deaths, delivers services to vulnerable pregnant patients, provides care to children, and performs obstetric fistula repair surgeries to women whose lives have been impacted by chronic incontinence.

References

Ouedraogo, I., Payne, C., Nardos, R., Adelman, A. J., & Wall, L. L. (2018). Obstetric fistula in Niger: 6-month post-operative follow-up of 284 patients from the Danja Fistula Center. *International Urogynecology Journal, 29*(3), 345–351. https://doi.org/10.1007/s00192-017-3375-7

Sierra Leone National Reproductive, Maternal, Newborn, Child and Adolescent Health Strategy 2017–2021

World Health Organization. (2018). Obstetric fistula. https://www.who.int/news-room/facts-in-pictures/detail/10-facts-on-obstetric-fistula. Accessed Dec. 23. 2020.

Comparing Three Models of Fistula Care Among Five Facilities in Nigeria and Uganda

20

Pooja Sripad, Caroline Johnson, Vandana Tripathi, and Charlotte E. Warren

20.1 Introduction

Women living in low- and middle-income countries (LMICs), where access to quality maternal health care is often limited, are disproportionately affected by female genital fistula that is often obstetric in origin. This condition is estimated to affect one to two million women globally (Adler et al., 2013). In LMICs, health systems have mixed capacity to identify and adequately treat fistula. In sub-Saharan Africa, health systems are often perceived as or actually are unable to address the regional fistula burden because of individual and systemic economic constraints, sociocultural norms that limit women's access to care, and infrastructural barriers that make it difficult for women to reach the tertiary hospitals that conduct fistula repair.

Fistula repair demands comprehensive care and often requires surgery or physical closure, which in many LMICs, takes place under the care of a limited number of specialized surgeons (Harrison et al., 2015). In LMICs, the proportions of successful physical closure following surgery range variably from 55% to 95% (World Health Organization, 2006) as does comprehensive post-operative care. In some cases, clients continue to report fistula-like symptoms such as urinary incontinence between three months and three years' post-repair (Khisa & Nyamongo, 2012). Comprehensive fistula care requires consideration of multiple pre- and post-operative contextual factors including the severity of the fistula, the complexity of the surgery(ies), counseling quality, and the extent to which post-operative care guidelines were followed.

Global guidelines by the World Health Organization (WHO) on established treatment for fistula repair and framework for assessing quality of maternal and newborn health care increasingly encompass the need to holistically investigate care quality. Fistula treatment guidelines (2006) include principles for clinical and surgical management, nursing care, pre- and post-operative physiotherapy, and social reintegration and rehabilitation (World Health Organization, 2006). Specific WHO indicators

P. Sripad (✉) · C. E. Warren
Social Behavioral Science Research, Population Council, Washington, DC, USA
e-mail: psripad@popcouncil.org

V. Tripathi
Fistula Care Plus, EngenderHealth, New York, NY, USA

C. Johnson
Independent Contributor, Washington, DC, USA

© Springer Nature Switzerland AG 2022
L. B. Drew et al. (eds.), *A Multidisciplinary Approach to Obstetric Fistula in Africa*, Global Maternal and Child Health, https://doi.org/10.1007/978-3-031-06314-5_20

for measuring quality of fistula repair care include rates of successful first surgical repair, proportions of women who had two or more unsuccessful repairs, and proportions of women who are able to successfully return to their normal lives in their families and society (i.e., "reintegration"). Dimensions of quality fistula care related to psychological, emotional, and social normalcy warrant further attention and require integration of client insights. WHO's quality of care framework (2016) reinforces the need to assess technical quality care and respectful practices in all aspects of maternal and newborn health, emphasizing the experiential dimensions of comprehensive fistula repair; this includes understanding provider and patient perspectives of these services. Although women's experience with fistula is increasingly recognized as a measure of a health system's quality and ability to meet women's reproductive health needs, significant challenges in accurately quantifying fistula prevalence and in collating quality data remain (Harrison et al., 2015). Less evidence exists on understanding the context of fistula repair options globally and the lived experiences of both patients and providers in accessing, utilizing, and providing quality fistula repair care.

As LMICs grapple with how to address fistula in their contexts, this chapter describes multiple models of repair care in some sub-Saharan African settings based on existing health structures, policies, and human resource capacities. It explores experiences of care from individual patient, family, provider, and community perspectives through case examples within a program and research context.

20.2 Program and Research Context

In Nigeria and Uganda, the United States Agency for International Development (USAID) supported Fistula Care *Plus* project implemented by EngenderHealth, which has collaborated with the Population Council on a Research to Action partnership to identify and respond to barriers to fistula treatment. This collaboration began with a literature review on barriers affecting women's access to genital fistula treatment in low-income countries. The review identified numerous barriers that women often face, and categorized these barriers as psychosocial, cultural, awareness, social, financial, transportation, facility shortages, and quality of care factors. Building on this review, the Population Council conducted formative, qualitative research in 2015 to understand the specific barriers women face in Nigeria and Uganda and to identify enabling mechanisms that mitigate the most salient barriers. In 2016, findings from these studies informed Fistula Care *Plus* in the design of a comprehensive information, screening, and referral intervention aimed at reducing the awareness, financial, and transportation barriers that impede women's access to fistula treatment in Nigeria and Uganda. In 2016/17, Fistula Care *Plus* launched the Fistula Treatment Barrier Reduction Intervention to strengthen community-based screening and referral to the treatment facility in two sites within Nigeria and one in Uganda. The Population Council conducted implementation research to evaluate the effects of this intervention (Population Council, 2020).

20.3 Fistula Care Plus Country Contexts

It has been estimated that Nigeria has an annual obstetric fistula incidence rate of 2.11 per 1000 live births, while 1.4% of Ugandan women ages 15–49 years report experiencing fistula-like symptoms at least once in their lives (ICF, 2018; Ijaiya et al., 2010). Despite its underequipped and underfunded health system, Nigeria has the technical expertise and infrastructural support for obstetric fistula repair through accredited National Obstetric Fistula Centers (NOFIC) in each of its six geopolitical zones. Each NOFIC may serve women from up to as many as six surrounding states. Repair surgery is free of charge in many fistula treatment centers across the country and serviced by well-trained practitioners. Nonetheless, many Nigerian women still live with obstetric fistula and do not seek care, either due to lack of awareness of the existence of treatment options or sites, or simply because of economic, social, cultural, and other inhibitive factors.

Since 2002, the Federal Ministry of Health has recognized the need to comprehensively address fistula repair in Nigeria, and more than a decade ago developed the National Strategic Framework for Eradication of Fistula in Nigeria (2005–2010) whose goal was to develop and implement comprehensive interventions to fistula care including repair, rehabilitation, and reintegration. Building on this strategy, The National Framework for Elimination of Obstetric Fistula in Nigeria (2011–2015) worked to continue expanding access to fistula repair care across Nigeria with the goal of reducing the national fistula burden by 50%.

In Uganda, fistula camps are conducted a few times each year at regional referral hospitals and missions, where they provide the majority of fistula repairs. Routine fistula repair has been introduced and is gradually scaling up at a number of hospitals, but multiple social, economic, and political barriers prevent routine care from being a viable repair option for most Ugandan women. A recent study of regional fistula incidence at Kitovu hospital in Masaka, Uganda found that women traveled, on average, more than 150 km to access care and that 94% experienced successful repair (McCurdie et al., 2018). Fistula camps in Uganda boast surgical success rates of greater than 80% (The Republic of Uganda Ministry of Health, n.d.).

20.4 Methodology

This chapter draws on findings from this broader research to action collaboration, synthesizing information collected during the formative, baseline, and midline phases through patient interviews, community focus groups, and discussions with key stakeholders in five sites in Nigeria and Uganda. These five sites reflect a convenience sample that has been supported by the USAID-supported Fistula Care *Plus* Project at EngenderHealth jointly selected for formative and/or implementation research. Study locations include Katsina, Kano and Ebonyi, Nigeria and Hoima and Masaka, Uganda.

In order to assess experiences with the provision and receipt of fistula repair, researchers spoke with women currently living with fistula, their family members, providers of fistula repair care – including nurses, fistula surgeons, and health center managers – and women who underwent previous fistula repair surgery. In-depth interviews with 139 stakeholders as well as 18 focus group discussions took place in Nigeria and Uganda between 2015 and 2017. Details of data collection activities are outlined in Table 20.1.

Following transcription and translation, data was inductively coded using Nvivo 12 software alongside memos written during data collection and analysis phases. A grounded theory principle-driven approach enabled groupings of barriers and enablers of care across numerous dimensions, as well as the organic groupings of typologies of fistula care provision environments across our sample sites. Among other barriers to care, health systems factors—the focus of this chapter, particularly facility shortages and political and structural aspects of fistula repair centers—distinguished three models of care: basic routine, pooled/camp-based, and holistic-routine. The following section draws inductively from the qualitative data collected across study sites and highlights the experiences of women, providers, community, and family members with each model of care.

Table 20.1 Data collection

	Nigeria			Uganda		
	Kano	Ebonyi	Katsina	Hoima	Masaka	Total
In-depth interviews						
Women affected by fistula	8	9	30	20	15	**82**
Spouses & other family members	4	2	0	6	5	**17**
Providers at camps, facility & district managers	4	7	2	14	13	**40**
Total	16	18	32	40	33	**139**
Focus group discussions						
Post-repair clients	1	1	0	2	2	**6**
Community stakeholders—women	1	1	2	1	1	**6**
Community stakeholders—men	1	1	2	1	1	**6**
Total	3	3	4	4	4	**18**

20.5 Models of Fistula Care

Three models of fistula care were identified across the five settings in Nigeria and Uganda examined through this study. While the models of care described here are not a comprehensive report of the fistula care approaches extant in LMICs, they do illustrate the varied strategies and approaches that our study sites' health systems have taken to address the fistula burden.

- **Basic routine care model**: fistula repair surgeries are performed throughout the year in specialized fistula centers at designated hospitals. (Relevant study sites: Kano and Ebonyi, Nigeria).
- **Pooled/camp-based model**: fistula repair surgeries are performed 3–4 scheduled times throughout the year at designated tertiary hospitals; sometimes heavily donor-supported, these models mobilize extensive outreach resources (through radio ads and village health teams) to bring women to their facilities during "camps"; often involve holistic rehabilitative and re-integration services, but few routine care options. (Relevant study sites: Hoima and Masaka, Uganda).
- **Holistic-routine care model**: fistula repair surgeries are performed throughout the year in specialized, fistula centers at designated hospitals where women also receive up to six months of rehabilitation and re-integration services. (Relevant study site: Katsina, Nigeria).

Each model below describes the structure and process of repairs and post-operative care—including funding and external support—and awareness and access barriers described as experienced by women and perceived by health providers in these settings.

20.5.1 Model 1: Basic Routine Care

20.5.1.1 Structure and Process

In Nigeria, fistula treatment has often been provided through both routine care and the "pooled" or camp model described below. However, at many government National Obstetric Fistula Centers (NOFIC), routine care has become a predominant service delivery approach. In the most recent project fiscal year (September 2017–2018), of the surgical fistula repairs supported by Fistula Care *Plus*, 64% were provided through routine care and 36% were provided as "pooled" efforts. At NOFICs, women can seek year-round repair care at no cost and return home within 2 weeks of surgery (Keya et al., 2018). Two of the five sites assessed through the Fistula Care *Plus*/Population Council collaboration in Nigeria provide fistula treatment predominantly through this basic routine care model.

The Laure Fistula Center at Murtala Muhammed Specialist Hospital in Kano State was accredited in 2015 as an official fistula training site by the International Federation of Gynecology and Obstetrics (FIGO). With support from the Kano state government and non-governmental organizations, the Laure Vesicovaginal Fistula (VVF) Center provides routine fistula care during which women undergo surgical repair and are discharged home shortly following their procedure. In the past project fiscal year, ninety-one percent of the surgical fistula repairs supported by Fistula Care *Plus* at the Laure VVF Center were through routine care, with the remainder delivered through "pooled efforts".

At the center, the surgical procedure to repair fistula is free, but women are obliged to pay for food, water, medication, toiletries, and any treatment needed for co-morbidities. Nurse matrons in the Post-operative Ward offer health education and counseling to women during their brief stay with the goal of maintaining the fistula's closure through appropriate hygiene.

"My husband brings food... everyone brings food. When [drugs] are prescribed, we go and buy them." Post-repair client, Kano

"It is truly free; you don't pay for anything when it comes to surgical management. But then if the patient comes down with malaria, she has to pay for that, and she has to feed herself." Fistula surgeon, Kano

Despite accreditation to provide routine fistula repair, a shortage of full-time trained fistula surgeons often means that surgeries can only be conducted at Laure VVF when volunteer or visiting surgeons are present. This leads to extended wait times for women seeking care or requiring women to return home without surgical repair and travel back to the hospital later when a surgeon is available. Long wait times are often due to provider insufficiencies at fistula centers, including surgeon engagement in dual practice.

"This is four weeks now. We were called and given the admission card, but I was told to go home, that if it was time for the operation I would be admitted. I was reporting here every day, and then I was admitted on Sunday... Wednesday I was operated." Post-Repair Client, Kano

Physicians in Kano corroborate women's experiences as most trained fistula surgeons are employed at larger, university-affiliated hospitals and act as consultants to fistula repair centers, often conducting surgeries once per week at most.

"I look at this patient holistically; I am not just about closing the hole. If I operate, how will this patient cope post-op? Because I know there are not enough capable hands that will see this patient when I am away, that limits the number of cases I take." Fistula surgeon, Kano

"This is a serious challenge at this facility in Kano – currently, there is no doctor dedicated to the facility by the state government. The state coordinator on VVF is supposed to be the one that oversees the facility activities, but he is not based at the hospital, he is a medical officer somewhere." Fistula Surgeon, Kano

The NOFIC in Ebonyi state is staffed by four trained fistula surgeons and regularly supported by obstetrics/gynecological specialists from the neighboring Federal Teaching Hospital in Abakiliki, less than 3 km away. Surgeons at the Ebonyi NOFIC conduct daily fistula repair surgeries and one senior advisor describes the routine fistula surgeries as opportunities for training resident and student surgeons in fistula repair. During the past project fiscal year, eighty-five percent of the surgical fistula repairs supported by Fistula Care *Plus* at the Ebonyi NOFIC were provided through routine care, with 15% delivered through "pooled" efforts.

Women from beyond Ebonyi often seek repair care at the NOFIC including women from as far away as Imo, Enugu, and other parts of southeast Nigeria, likely because, with substantial funding from the federal government, the Ebonyi NOFIC offers free surgery, food, water, sheets, and medications.

"Nobody has collected a penny from me except the day I was asked to buy a small drip which was little or nothing, it was NGN 100 (USD $0.28). They also put blood for me; I expected they would collect money but until now, nobody has asked me about money." Post-Repair Client, Ebonyi

In addition to a full team of fistula surgeons, the NOFIC in Ebonyi offers short-term psychological services to facilitate women's holistic care and to support social reintegration. Following surgery, women are discharged home after a maximum of 14 days in the NOFIC. Completely free treatment in Ebonyi does not dispel the perceived financial barriers of women unaware of their medical options or availability of free services available. Consequently, families often seek surgery at private facilities, incurring high medical costs and resulting in varying levels of surgical success.

"The support is this feeding and the rest too. Yesterday they told me some kind words [psychological/ emotional support] that made me calm down." Post-Repair Client, Ebonyi

"When I came for a checkup at that other hospital, they discharged me after 7 days, but the doctor told me before the operation that I would stay there 14 days. But as the thing started leaking again, I lost hope and told him to discharge me, that I can come and lose the stitches later… before the surgery we agreed on NGN 100,000 (USD $276), but as he went to that place [operating theater] what he saw is not [what he expected] so he increased. Finally, when they discharged us, they give us NGN 180,000 (USD $497) bill." Post-Repair Client on Previous Repair Attempts at Private Hospital, Ebonyi

Despite government support at federally funded centers, fistula surgeons increasingly face challenges with commodity shortages because government funding is often only sufficient to pay for personnel salaries. There is a gap between what is necessary for routine care and what government funding can cover. Consequently, providers often use personal salaries to ensure that critical surgical equipment functions effectively and consistently.

"Finance is a very big problem because the money we get from the federal government is a far cry from what we need to run the center. I myself spend 20%-30% of my salary to make sure things work." Fistula Surgeon, Ebonyi

20.5.1.2   Awareness and Access Barriers

Limited knowledge about affordable and available fistula care options among communities and providers poses challenges to effective surgical care. Women living with fistula are largely unaware that their condition is treatable, and are even less aware that facilities are available to conduct repairs; this lack of awareness dominates in Ebonyi where the government-sponsored NOFIC is newer than in Kano. Women who do hear about repair care options most often learn from friends or family members while a limited number learn about it on the radio. In some contexts, NOFIC nurses have the capacity and financial support to conduct outreach visits in surrounding areas, strengthening community awareness. In both settings, outreach activities by community partners and programs like Fistula Care *Plus* are ongoing, though at times these have limited reach.

"We were always asking, nobody said they know. My colleagues that live here [say] that it is always announced on the radio." Post-Repair Client, Kano

"My own community didn't know about this repair. I went to the [community] meeting the last three years, and I gave them the health talk. Afterwards, many of my community women started coming here for repair – I didn't even know they were having the problem." Post-Operative Nurse Matron, Kano

Primary healthcare providers throughout Nigeria have similarly limited knowledge of centers that repair fistula, causing many women to undergo surgery at the hands of unskilled providers or endure years of an open fistula before learning from knowledgeable community neighbors or other providers about appropriate repair care options. One fistula surgeon practicing in Ebonyi since 2008 reported that ongoing lack of awareness of treatment options leads to long-term damage from fistula, ultimately requiring more complex medical care.

"In the north there is awareness but not in the south. This is the first fistula center owned by the government for the south-east region, but the awareness isn't really there despite the campaign. Most patients move from hospital to hospital and from state to state seeking treatment and most of the time fall into the hands of the untrained, and a lot of harm is done. When they come here it becomes very tough. You find a woman here maybe 30- or 50-years history of leakage, and that is a difference compared to the north." Fistula Surgeon, Ebonyi

20.5.2   Model 2: Pooled/Camp-Based

20.5.2.1   Structure and Process

While government support for routine care in Uganda has increased in recent years, the camp-based care model continues to support a majority of repairs, including the two sites assessed through the Fistula Care *Plus*/Population Council collaboration. In the past project fiscal year, seventy-eight percent of the surgical fistula repairs supported by Fistula Care *Plus* in Uganda were delivered through camps, with 22% provided through routine care. At Kitovu Hospital, the primary repair site engaged with the Fistula Care *Plus*/Population Council intervention to reduce fistula treatment barriers, eighty-nine percent of surgical fistula repairs were provided through camps, compared to 11% provided through routine care.

Camps align repair opportunities at fistula camps with influxes of external financial support or availability of skilled providers. In practice, as support dissipates between camps, hospitals lack human and material resources to sustain fistula repair.

"The availability is always there when we have a camp around and when the announcements have been made. I do not know whether our doctors have finished training as fistula surgeons... if our doctors are done training then we shall have a surgeon all the time in the hospital to repair the fistula." Policymaker, Hoima

At most fistula camps, in addition to free surgical treatment, women receive an array of rehabilitation and social re-integration services (Keya et al., 2018). Nurse counselors offer advice on a range of pragmatic post-operative strategies for women to maintain their repairs, physiologically heal, and maximize their opportunities for successful socioeconomic re-integration.

"For those that have been repaired, we tell them about abstinence of three months; that they should improve on their diet; and they should join community groups for income-generating activities." Nurse Counselor, Hoima

Fistula camps are organized by the government in collaboration with implementing partners including, but not limited to, UNFPA, USAID Fistula Care *Plus* project, Amref Health Africa, and Terrewode. Implementing partners support the cost of surgery, media and community awareness campaigns and in some cases, patients' transport to and from the camp as well surgeons' costs of living while the camp is ongoing. Some women, however, pay out of pocket for transportation and must cover the costs of any companions who travel and stay with them at the fistula camps; this is often in addition to prior expenses of seeking care at centers ill-equipped to manage fistula.

"At every camp, according to [the resources budgeted by] USAID, we are supposed to do sixty patients. Now if we do seventy, eighty, these extra ones are not covered by USAID, and our director has to look for extra funds from somewhere. There is not a line in the budget dedicated for fistula, but we have the Fistula Foundation and these doctors from the Royal College in the UK who are also supporting where there is need. The ministry of health sometimes offers sundries." Health manager, Masaka

"It cost me NGN 25,000 (USD $69) for transport from home to here, but I had enough money which we also used to eat for the first time once we came here. Now we have a problem of money to buy soap and salt." Mother of post-repair client, Masaka

Once a date has been selected for a fistula camp, community awareness campaigns utilize government agencies such as District Health Management Teams and Village Health Teams, as well as television and radio advertisements, to inform community women about the upcoming repair availability. Fistula camps require a large team of dedicated personnel including a minimum of three fistula surgeons, two nurse/midwife obstetric counselors, and one anesthetist supported by one to two anesthetic assistants. Despite efforts at counseling and re-integration advice, some policymakers view long-term follow-up for women's successful reintegration into their communities as an ongoing challenge.

"Prior to the [camps] we usually do sensitization that helps to reduce barriers. For example, when I am talking on the radio, I give a health education talk and about the management we are going to do. That we are going to do the operations free, that the meals are going to be free, that they are going to be with their attendant, and that the transport to and from is going to be refunded." Fistula surgeon, Masaka

"What we lack is reinforcing the continuum of care. If a mother is discharged from the hospital to the community, is there a mechanism to follow up with this woman to ensure she has healed very well or is doing very well in her community?" Policy maker, Hoima

Kitovu and Mulago hospitals retain at least three trained surgeons, the minimum number required to facilitate an obstetric fistula camp. Other regional hospitals employ at least one trained fistula surgeon, but re-assignment to other facilities, professional pursuits, and other career factors limit the number of available surgeons, inhibiting fistula repairs. Structural and sociocultural factors, including shortages of trained surgeons and low prioritization of repair care in potential routine repair facilities, require most women to wait to be treated in fistula camps by visiting fistula surgeons. Persistent delays to women's repair lead to over-filling at fistula camps and cause providers, often equipped or funded to repair sixty women at a time, to see up to 100 patients. While providers consistently report that all women are seen who arrive to fistula camps, women often wait multiple days to be seen for surgery and frequently are not ever seen and must return at the next camp.

"The unit is opened four times a year for camps, for about two months each time. But we do not have permanent staff. We have four permanent staff." Fistula surgeon, Masaka

"This is my third time coming here, the first time was October 7, 2014. I came back on March 10, 2015 and spent like a month, and this time I have so far spent four days here. They provide us with food and tea free of charge, so we are taken care of. Treatment is also free." Woman awaiting surgical repair, Masaka

20.5.2.2 Awareness and Access Barriers

While women and communities in Uganda are somewhat aware of the symptoms of fistula (ICF, 2018), our data shows that less is understood about its causes, prevention strategies, treatability, and where and when to seek care. Varying beliefs that fistula is caused by witchcraft, negligent providers, the stature and age of the mother, and who can and cannot seek care (i.e., women of different faiths being able to access care at faith-based hospitals) suggests limited, basic understanding of fistula as an abnormal medical condition. Moreover, the shame associated with the condition remains a deterrent to care-seeking. Insufficient primary healthcare provider awareness of and knowledge about screening for and treating fistula often further prevents women from accessing timely and appropriate linkages to repair care. In pooled/camp-based settings, this gap in awareness at primary health center level modifies knowledge and other care-seeking barriers in the community. Given the non-routine nature of repairs, this added layer of delay may explain, in part, high prevalence of fistula (Maheu-Giroux et al., 2015).

"We went to a doctor in Masindi and they gave me drugs and I took it—they gave me three weeks and it did not work and we went to another doctor. Then he told us to come to a gynecologist here in Hoima, so I came here—they gave me more medicine and she told me to come to the hospital here." Post-repair client, Hoima

"Women with such a disease—we don't know them because we have not seen them. For us men, we don't know what brings this disease, so we are requesting you bring a health education talk to us here for both men and women to know what causes it, how it can be treated, and how they can be brought to the hospital." Male community member, Hoima

"It's embarrassment that is killing us—how will I go and talk about it, now the whole village will know that I am the one who has been leaking, no!" Female community member, Hoima

20.5.3 Model 3: Holistic-Routine Care

20.5.3.1   Structure and Process

A third, "holistic" model of care was identified in Katsina State in northwest Nigeria, where women receive free surgical treatment and up to six months of housing and job training in a chosen trade to help facilitate their successful reintegration into society once they return home (Keya et al., 2018). The FIGO-accredited Babbar Ruga NOFIC is located in urban Katsina and, in addition to providing fistula surgical training, offers workers' housing as an impetus to maintain a full-time trained surgical staff. The 200-bed NOFIC boasts two operating theaters dedicated specifically to fistula repair and two wards for up to 80 post-operative clients. The NOFIC is primarily funded by the federal Ministry of Health (MOH) with added support from the state MOH, implementing partners, and donors. The provision of reintegration services in the Post-operative Ward frequently depends on added support from the state and implementing partners. During the past fiscal year 90% of the surgical fistula repair supported by Fistula Care *Plus* at the Babbar Ruga NOFIC were provided through routine care, with 10% provided through "pooled efforts".

The Babbar Ruga NOFIC is a key fistula repair center in the region staffing three fistula surgeons and two medical officers who, together, perform free, routine fistula repair. Limitations in the number of available fistula surgeons result in fewer surgical repairs conducted than the NOFIC has capacity for. Although the NOFIC has a high physical capacity to attend to women, increasing patient volume due to increasing awareness of repair center availability conflicts with low numbers of fistula surgeons available, resulting in some women being admitted to the hospital and prepared for surgery but facing delays in receiving repairs.

"Sometimes, we prepare seven patients for surgery – they will end up doing five. If we had enough staff, enough doctors, I think they could even do up to ten in a day." NOFIC nurse, Katsina

20.5.3.2   Awareness and Access Barriers

Community members in Katsina describe additional socio-cultural barriers that delay women's care, including an inadequate number of female hospital providers that prevent women from being able to seek care in this cultural context. Women's husbands, particularly those living in rural areas, often do not allow them to seek care from or be treated by male providers. Community women discuss the need for more female providers as a solution not only to barriers to fistula care but as a preventive measure to avoid fistula development by enabling women to attend antenatal care—many women continue to face barriers to care throughout their pregnancies, increasing their risk of labor complications that can lead to fistula development.

"No matter how much you try to go to hospital for ANC, if the husband says no, there is nothing you can do. In my own case, my husband did not allow me to go for ANC. I later had a miscarriage; he was informed, and I tried to go to the hospital, but he refused." Female community member, Katsina

"It is improper for men to look at or to repair women, this is one reason why the husband will not allow his wife to go for ANC [antenatal care]. It is good to have female health workers, so the husband will allow his wife to attend hospital services." Female community member, Katsina

In comparison to other fistula care centers, the Babbar Ruga NOFIC maximizes its Post-operative Ward capacity by offering fistula repair clients up to six months of rehabilitation and reintegration services. Women who stay in the "transit camp" at Babbar Ruga learn a trade of their choosing ranging from sewing and hair dressing to detergent and soap making. Women are provided two to three meals per day in addition to follow-up medical care and classes on the Quran and personal health. A culminating graduation ceremony attended by the women's relatives is intended to facilitate full reintegration into society and foster family reconnection in instances where women may have experienced social or familial isolation because of their previous fistula condition.

"They said if anybody wants to go to school, they should indicate interest. Now that we are discharged and have shown interest, they said once they graduate this set, they will enroll us next." Post-repair client, Katsina

Providers at the Katsina NOFIC describe women becoming increasingly comfortable and relaxed during their stay in the Fistula Ward and attribute women's emotional improvement to the interaction with and recognition of other women living with fistula.

20.6   Discussion

The routine, pooled/camp-based, and holistic-routine care models observed across these specific Nigerian and Ugandan contexts illustrate varying responses to the needs of women living with fistula. Across all three model settings, supply shortages at the fistula center and lacking awareness of communities and primary health providers of options for fistula repair comprise barriers; quality post-repair counseling and social services supporting reintegration enable more holistic fistula care. This points to a challenge of fistula surgical and rehabilitative services requiring improved supply-side financing of care provision and demand-enhancing efforts at the community level.

The effectiveness of different models in addressing the needs of women with fistula are also moderated by the socio-cultural, structural, and disease burden contexts of the communities in which they are located. Some barriers reflect socio-cultural norms such as the preference of women and men for female surgeons and counselors in Katsina (holistic-routine) model. In this context, the gender norms favoring husbands' decisions around their wives' care-seeking fistula prevention (e.g., antenatal, delivery and postnatal care services) translates into a reluctance to facilitate access to fistula repair which is often provided by male surgeons. Additionally, while women in Katsina face similar awareness barriers as women in other parts of Nigeria, gender normative constraints that restrict women's agency in seeking health care generally affect access to care. Structurally, under-resourced health systems, mixed funding sources, and perceived fears around quality of care notably affect long wait times in pooled/camp-based and holistic-routine care models. In both contexts, it is important to note that not only are backlogs of fistula patients higher than those of routine fistula care settings, but the enhanced positive effects of reintegration services often respond to funding shifts. For example, the potential positive effects of the holistic-routine care model's long-term rehabilitation services are jeopardized when external funding decreases unless a federal, state, or regional government assumes the costs. Across all three models, delays in women's receipt of care can be attributed to these compounding structural aspects alongside complexity of the repair procedure, low prevalence of fistula compared to other health focal areas, the high cost of surgical repair and ancillary costs, and complexity and variability of post-repair prognoses that may render fistula surgeries a lesser priority in hospitals (Baker et al., 2017).

Experiences of providers and patients across the three models reflect shared and diverging views in terms of quality and effectiveness of repair access and reintegration opportunities. In the routine care context, despite remaining community awareness gaps, once women are linked to care, free medical care is viewed favorably. Contrastingly, routine fistula care providers are challenged by free care provision as governments may be financially limited in supporting material supplies and sufficient human resources (e.g., qualified surgeons and post-operative nurse-counselors) to treat the number of women requiring services. In pooled/camp-based contexts, challenges of non-routine care are paramount, though providers and policymakers express more positive experiences than patients. Providers describe the influx of resources and attention to repair options and post-operative social reintegration support that arrives with donor-supported camps as enablers of women's access and provider ability to treat; they also recognize the unanticipated consequences of increased attention, including excess patient referral which donor resources and provider capacity are under-equipped to manage. In pooled/camp-based contexts, women face long wait times, often make multiple trips, and bear the financial burden of ancillary needs of companions during their extended post-operative stay. Finite financial donor resources and out-of-pocket patient expenditures persist as challenges to the model's sustainability. In the context of the holistic-routine care model in Katsina, while providers are available to conduct surgeries and reintegration services are comprehensive, human resource capacities remain insufficient to adequately address the fistula burden in the area.

It is important to consider the structure, process, awareness, and access barriers to fistula care in the context of the overall impact that fistula has on women's well-being and livelihood in physical, psychological, social, and economic ways (Barageine et al., 2015). These factors correlate with the first and third delays to service use (delay in women's decisions to seek care and in their receipt of care upon arrival to a health facility) as suggested in a systematic literature review of barriers to fistula repair for women in Sub-Saharan Africa (Baker et al., 2017). As seen elsewhere, in making the decision whether to seek fistula repair care, women consider the relative burden of actual costs, including treatment, transportation, and ancillary needs, the opportunity costs of leaving their work and family for an extended time, and any previous experiences they may have had with the health system, either positive or negative (Keya et al., 2018). Women also often face stigmatization, ostracism from their friends and families, and gradual depreciation of their senses of esteem and personal value. Social isolation, loss of joy in their marriages and other relationships, and feelings of shame associated with constant odor and wetness can relegate women to the fringes of their societies and their families (Barageine et al., 2015; McCurdie et al., 2018). These social barriers, compounded by limited postnatal care, cause women in LMIC to hide their fistula for extended periods, resulting in added delay to early fistula identification and treatment (Baker et al., 2017). These multi-dimensional challenges complicate many women's access to and receipt of quality repair care.

We recognize this study's limitation in presenting a sample of service models across our study sites within a program and research context, rather than the comprehensive description of the full range of fistula repair models in these countries and globally. Limitations of the comparisons made across the three models in this chapter stem from our inability to triangulate experience with accurate quantitative data on fistula prevalence and incidence level. While few studies have been able to estimate fistula repair success rates, fewer still have explored women's experiences living with fistula or their experiences accessing and receiving repair care (Baker et al., 2017; Barageine et al., 2015; Maheu-Giroux et al., 2015). Deficiencies in national and subnational data on fistula prevalence are partly due to the hidden nature of the populations who suffer the condition and in part, but also because questions about fistula experience are not routinely collected in all contexts (Hardee et al., 2012; Harrison et al., 2015; Keya et al., 2018). Demographic health surveys (DHS) in some countries do ask women about their experience with fistula-like symptoms in their lifetime, but not whether they have been treated; these data are less likely to be captured at the level of the routine health information system. Until women's frequent concerns about privacy and stigma at the community level and experience of reintegration services are captured within the DHS, underreporting of obstetric fistula is likely to continue. Linking basic-routine, pooled/camp-based, holistic-routine, and other care models to population outcomes will require integrating multi-level data sources and modeling estimation techniques (Tunçalp et al., 2015).

20.7 Conclusions

The three models of care for fistula repair identified through the five sites included in the Fistula Care *Plus*/Population Council research collaboration reveal both prevailing barriers as well as promise in the sub-Saharan African contexts of study as recounted by patients and providers. Mixed awareness of repair options, insufficient human resources, and limited financing remain significant structural factors to effective and quality fistula repair. Further research and reproductive and maternal health programs in LMICs would benefit from recognizing the multi-layered needs of complex and stigmatizing conditions like obstetric fistula, as well as the bottlenecks induced by intermittent financing that affect the lived experiences of women, communities and medical practitioners. Eliciting voices of those providing and receiving fistula repair, as described in this chapter, is a critical starting point to not only appreciate the positive and negative features of the current models of fistula care, but to consider how each can be improved, integrated with routine systems, and leveraged to better address women's needs in fistula prevention, treatment, and rehabilitation.

Acknowledgements We would like to acknowledge Charity Ndwiga (Population Council-Kenya, Emmanuel Nwala (Population Council-Nigeria), and Hassan Kanakulya (EngenderHealth-Uganda) for their provision of contextual insights and thank Erin Mielke and Mary Ellen Stanton of the U.S. Agency for International Development for their review of this chapter.

References

Adler, A. J., Ronsmans, C., Calvert, C., & Filippi, V. (2013). Estimating the prevalence of obstetric fistula: A systematic review and meta-analysis. *BMC Pregnancy and Childbirth, 13*(1), 246. https://doi.org/10.1186/1471-2393-13-246

Baker, Z., Bellows, B., Bach, R., & Warren, C. (2017). Barriers to obstetric fistula treatment in low-income countries: A systematic review. *Tropical Medicine & International Health, 22*(8), 938–959. https://doi.org/10.1111/tmi.12893

Barageine, J. K., Beyeza-Kashesya, J., Byamugisha, J. K., Tumwesigye, N. M., Almroth, L., & Faxelid, E. (2015). "I am alone and isolated": A qualitative study of experiences of women living with genital fistula in Uganda. *BMC Women's Health, 15*(1), 73. https://doi.org/10.1186/s12905-015-0232-z

Hardee, K., Gay, J., & Blanc, A. K. (2012). Maternal morbidity: Neglected dimension of safe motherhood in the developing world. *Global Public Health, 7*(6), 603–617. https://doi.org/10.1080/17441692.2012.668919

Harrison, M. S., Mabeya, H., Goldenberg, R. L., & McClure, E. M. (2015). Urogenital fistula reviewed: A marker of severe maternal morbidity and an indicator of the quality of maternal healthcare delivery. *Maternal Health, Neonatology and Perinatology, 1*(1), 20. https://doi.org/10.1186/s40748-015-0020-7

ICF. (2018). *Uganda demographic and health survey 2016*. UBOS and ICF. http://dhsprogram.com/pubs/pdf/FR333/FR333.pdf

Ijaiya, M., Rahman, A., Aboyehi, A., Olatinwo, A., Esuga, S., Ogah, O., et al. (2010). Vesicovaginal fistula: A review of Nigerian experience. *West African Journal of Medicine, 29*(5), 293–298. https://www.ajol.info/index.php/wajm/article/view/68247

Keya, K. T., Sripad, P., Nwala, E., & Warren, C. E. (2018). "Poverty is the big thing": Exploring financial, transportation, and opportunity costs associated with fistula management and repair in Nigeria and Uganda. *International Journal for Equity in Health, 17*(1), 70. https://doi.org/10.1186/s12939-018-0777-1

Khisa, A. M., & Nyamongo, I. K. (2012). Still living with fistula: An exploratory study of the experience of women with obstetric fistula following corrective surgery in west Pokot, Kenya. *Reproductive Health Matters, 20*(40), 59–66. https://doi.org/10.1016/S0968-8080(12)40661-9

Maheu-Giroux, M., Filippi, V., Samadoulougou, S., Castro, M. C., Maulet, N., Meda, N., & Kirakoya-Samadoulougou, F. (2015). Prevalence of symptoms of vaginal fistula in 19 sub-Saharan Africa countries: A meta-analysis of national household survey data. *The Lancet Global Health, 3*(5), e271–e278. https://doi.org/10.1016/S2214-109X(14)70348-1

McCurdie, F. K., Moffatt, J., & Jones, K. (2018). Vesicovaginal fistula in Uganda. *Journal of obstetrics and gynaecology: the journal of the Institute of Obstetrics and Gynaecology, 38*(6), 822–827. https://doi.org/10.1080/01443615.2017.1407301

Population Council. (2020). Reducing barriers to accessing fistula repair in nigeria and uganda: an implementation research study. *Washington, D.C.*

The Republic of Uganda Ministry of Health. (n.d.). National Obstetric Fistula Strategy, 2011/12–2015/16 (Draft).

Tunçalp, Ö., Tripathi, V., Landry, E., Stanton, C. K., & Ahmed, S. (2015). Measuring the incidence and prevalence of obstetric fistula: Approaches, needs and recommendations. *Bull World Health Organ, 93*(1), 60–62.

World Health Organization. (2006). Obstetric fistula: Guiding principles for clinical management and programme development. Geneva. http://apps.who.int/iris/bitstream/handle/10665/43343/9241593679_eng.pdf;jsessionid=6B8A47E77CA69E6E6352048A5B98ED6C?sequence=1.

Obstetric Fistula in the Democratic Republic of the Congo: Neglected Care of Young Women in Rural Areas

21

Joseph B. Nsambi, Olivier Mukuku, and Jean-Baptiste S. Z. Kakoma

21.1 Introduction

Every day, about 830 women die worldwide from complications of pregnancy or childbirth with about 99% of deaths occurring in developing countries (Alkema et al., 2016; WHO, 2018). Current estimates indicate that for every woman who dies from pregnancy-related complications, 15–30 suffer from serious co-morbidities (Schwartz, 2015)—these include urogenital fistula, and all of these conditions are preventable and treatable (UNFPA, 2009). Urogenital fistulas are defined as abnormal communication, congenital or acquired, between the urinary tract and the female genital tract. This communication may appear between the bladder and the uterus or urethra and vagina. There are various varieties of urogenital fistulas: urethro-vaginal fistulas, vesico-uterine fistulas, and vesico-vaginal fistulas (Langkilde et al., 1999; Tafesse, 2008).

Urogenital fistulas can occur congenitally, but are most often acquired from obstetrical, surgical, radiological, malignant, and various causes. In developing countries, including most of those in Africa, more than 90% of fistulas are of obstetric etiology, while in resource-rich countries such as the United Kingdom and the United States more than 70% occur after pelvic surgery (Hilton, 2003, 2016). In this chapter, we will discuss obstetric fistulas (OF) occurring as a complication of pregnancy.

Obstetric fistula is a condition that results from prolonged obstructed labor, most commonly affecting women living in resource-poor countries where access to Emergency Obstetric and Newborn Care (EmONC) including obtaining an operative delivery is difficult for a variety of reasons. Those women living in rural areas and those in households with low socioeconomic status have fewer opportunities to benefit from such EmONC, and especially cesarean delivery, and therefore are more likely to be at

J. B. Nsambi
Department of Gynecology and Obstetrics, University of Lubumbashi,
Lubumbashi, Democratic Republic of the Congo

O. Mukuku (✉)
Department of Maternal and Child Health, High Institute of Medical Techniques of Lubumbashi,
Lubumbashi, Democratic Republic of the Congo
e-mail: oliviermukuku@yahoo.fr

J.-B. S. Z. Kakoma
Department of Gynecology and Obstetrics, University of Lubumbashi,
Lubumbashi, Democratic Republic of the Congo

University of Rwanda, Kigali, Republic of Rwanda

© Springer Nature Switzerland AG 2022
L. B. Drew et al. (eds.), *A Multidisciplinary Approach to Obstetric Fistula in Africa*, Global Maternal and Child Health, https://doi.org/10.1007/978-3-031-06314-5_21

risk of having an obstetric fistula. The prevention and management of obstetric fistula is included in the Sustainable Development Goal 3 (SDG3) of improving maternal health by the United Nations (United Nations, 2018).

Obstetric fistula is rarely seen in developed countries, but it continues to cause pervasive physical, emotional, and social suffering for many women in developing countries (Donnay & Weil, 2004). Despite its devastating impact, it is one of the most neglected diseases of maternal health in low-income countries (Wall, 2012). Among its serious repercussions on the patient's life are urogenital discomfort, psychosocial morbidity, and disruption of conjugal life.

Obstetric fistula is a major global health challenge, although it is difficult to determine its global, national, or even regional prevalence for a number of reasons: (1) it is not a reportable condition; (2) there is no routine surveillance for this condition in countries where it is prevalent; (3) women with OF may not be forthcoming about having the condition; (4) it mainly affects women living in the most remote areas; and (5) women with OF are often stigmatized.

The World Health Organization (WHO) estimates that between 2 and 3.5 million women world-wide live with untreated fistula and that between 50,000 and 100,000 women are newly affected with it each year (WHO, 2006). The vast majority of cases are in sub-Saharan Africa and South-East Asia (Creanga et al., 2007; UNFPA & EngenderHealth, 2003). The exact prevalence in the Democratic Republic of the Congo (DRC) is not well-known, but the United Nations Population Fund (UNFPA) estimates that about 40,000 women suffer from obstetric fistula in this country (UNFPA, 2009; UNFPA & EngenderHealth, 2003). The 2007 DRC Demographic and Health Survey reports indicated that 0.3% of women report having already experienced fistula symptoms (Ministère du Plan et Macro International, 2008). Due to the hidden nature and the complex veil of misperceptions that surround this condition, many researchers consider these figures largely underestimated, mainly because many fistula women do not seek care or are unaware of the possibilities of surgical repair (Creanga et al., 2007; Nsambi et al., 2018).

The Democratic Republic of the Congo is a developing country where a large part of the population lives in rural areas. The urbanization rate, the urban population in relation to the total population of the Democratic Republic of the Congo, was estimated at 32% in 2007 (Flouriot, 2008).

This chapter focuses on obstetric fistulas as they are observed in the Democratic Republic of the Congo and more specifically in the province of Haut-Katanga which is located in the south-east of the country.

21.2   Haut-Katanga and Its People

21.2.1   Geography

Since 2015, Haut-Katanga has been a province in the Democratic Republic of the Congo following the break-up of the province of Katanga. This new province's territory corresponds to that of the historic Katanga-Oriental that existed during the early period of post-colonial Democratic Republic of the Congo between 1963 and 1966. It is located in the south-east of the country, on the border with Zambia (INS, 2016). Haut-Katanga has an area of 128,264 km^2 and shares its borders:

- in the North with the provinces of Haut-Lomami and Tanganyika,
- in the West with the province of Lualaba,
- in the East and South with the Republic of Zambia.

Haut-Katanga comprises six territories (Kipushi, Mitwaba, Pweto, Sakania, Kasenga, and Kambove) and two major cities (the capital city of Lubumbashi and Likasi). Its climate is temperate in the South, and warm in the North. The average temperature varies between 10 °C and 40 °C. It is marked by two seasons: dry season from April to September and rainy which goes from October to April (INS, 2016). The soil is sandy in the north and sandy clay in the south with the dominant vegetation being the "savanna". There are mountain ranges and two main lakes (Moëro and Tshangalele) as well as large rivers (Luapula, Lufira, Luvua). The Luvua River connects Lake Moëro with the Congo River (INS, 2016).

21.2.2 Population and Activities

In 2015, its population was 4,391,146 (50.4% male and 49.6% female), which represents approximately 4.4% of the population of the country as a whole. Its density is 34 inhabitants/km². The dominant ethnicities and tribes are: Lamba, Sanga, Bemba, Bakunda, Balomotwa, and Kaonde (INS, 2016).

The main activities are fishing, trade, mining, and agriculture. Lubumbashi, the second largest city in DRC, is the mining capital of the country and is a base for many of the country's biggest mining companies. The various resources of this province constitute a major asset for its economic development. All the territories of this province are rich in wealth. Its subsoil is rich in copper, zinc, manganese, cobalt, gold, etc., and attracts large mining companies to set up on its territory. These create jobs and generate considerable resources for the State (INS, 2016).

The province of Haut-Katanga is becoming more and more a crossroads of large mining companies as a consequence of the considerable increase of the population. The soil of Haut-Katanga is rich and thus constitutes an important source of income for its inhabitants. Food crops are cultivated in a traditional manner and without the use of chemical fertilizers (INS, 2016). Livestock, including cattle, is practiced in the Kundelungu plateaus and in many other areas. Fishing occurs in the Luapula and Moëro lakes, as well as in rivers such as the Lufira and Luvua. The territory is also rich in tourist reserves. These tourist sites constitute one of the main sources of income for the State. Among these are the waterfalls such as those of Lofoï (the highest waterfall in Africa, sheltered by the Haut-Katanga, which falls from a slope of 384 m in height) and those of the Luapula River called the "Falls of Johnson", close to Kasenga on the Luapula, which forms a natural border between Katanga and Zambia, between the Moëro and Bangwelo lakes. Another natural resource is the Kundelungu National Park that was created in 1970, which covers 7600 km² and contains many animal species including monkeys, lions, leopards, antelopes, and zebras (INS, 2016).

Although French is the official language, the main spoken lingua franca in the province is Kiswahili.[1] In addition, the influx of many people from rural areas for employment has resulted in a variety of imported languages including Kiluba,[2] Chokwe,[3] Bemba,[4] and Kisanga,[5] among others.

---

[1]Kiswahili, or Swahili, is a widely spoken Bantu language that is the lingua franca of the African Great Lakes region. A member of the Southern Bantoid branch of the Benue-Congo subdivision of the Niger-Congo language family, it is spoken by many millions of persons. Much of its vocabulary is derived from Arabic, and it was originally written in Arabic script.

[2]The Kiluba language, also termed Luba-Katanga and Luba-Shaba, is a member of the Niger-Congo language family and is one of the two major Bantu languages spoken in the DR Congo called "Luba". It is spoken in the Southeast region of the DR Congo by the Luba people.

[3]Chokwe is a Bantu language which is the national language of Angola. It is also spoken by the Chokwe people of DR Congo and Zambia.

[4]Bemba, or Kibemba, is a major Bantu language spoken in DRC (Haut-Katanga) and Zambia (North East and North Provinces). It has approximately 4.1 million speakers.

[5]Kisanga is known by other names—Sanga, Southern Luba and Luba-Sanga. It is a Bantu language of the Democratic Republic of the Congo.

306   J. B. Nsambi et al.

21.3 Environmental and Cultural Context of Childbirth

Obstetric fistula is associated with certain socio-economic and cultural factors (Holme et al., 2007; Kasamba et al., 2013; Muleta, 2004). Obstetric fistula (called "*kasusu*" or "*kinswi*" in the Bemba language) is more the preserve of rural than urban women because of the qualitative disparity of the health structures concerning in particular the qualification of its personnel. The rural setting is characterized by under-qualification of antenatal clinic staff and lack of access to surgical interventions, while most qualified physicians live in urban areas and most rural hospitals have inadequate facilities for surgical emergency care (Cavallaro et al., 2013; Hsia et al., 2012; Kinenkinda et al., 2017). In addition, the reference health structures in which a cesarean section can be performed are too remote from environments where most rural populations live (sometimes beyond 100 km). Added to this are the geographical inaccessibility and the lack of roads to access hospitals. The rural population resides for the most part in remote and isolated areas with a mediocre road network making emergency evacuation for dystocia difficult or late. It often takes hundreds of kilometers to reach a health center with a hypothetical functional surgical unit (Meyer et al., 2007; Nsambi et al., 2018), and the bicycle is most of the time used as an ambulance (called "*kitebo*" in the Bemba language) (Fig. 21.1).

In addition, there are ethnocultural beliefs that regard as sacred early marriages, home deliveries, and delivery by vaginal birth, the latter praised as the method of delivery whatever the cost. This pronatalist ethnocultural attitude characterizing sub-Saharan Africa makes cesarean births highly unpopular, and operative deliveries can be stigmatizing to a mother. In some villages where we have recruited patients with obstetric fistula, cesarean section is seen as a curse and in addition, a woman who undergoes a cesarean section is considered unfit for marriage and can even be divorced.

The combination of these environmental and socio-cultural factors explains the fact that most women (70.7%) deliver their infants at home (Table 21.1) (Nsambi et al., 2018), mainly under the supervision of a traditional birth attendant (called "*nakimbela*" in the Bemba language). Other authors have also reported high rates of home-based delivery ranging from 91.1% to 97.1% (Hilton & Ward,

Fig. 21.1 Bicycle being used as an ambulance. (Photo Credit: Olivier Mukuku)

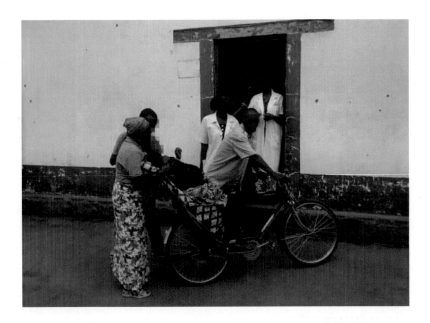

Table 21.1 Distribution of patients by location of delivery. [Source: Adapted from Joseph Bulanda Nsambi, Olivier Mukuku, Jean-de-Dieu Foma Yunga, et al. (2018) Obstetric fistulas in Haut-Katanga province, Democratic Republic of Congo: report of 242 cases. *Pan African Medical Journal.* 29(34). Some modifications were made. https://doi.org/10.11604/pamj.2018.29.34.14576, licensed under the terms of the Creative Commons Attribution License (https://creativecommons.org/licenses/by/4.0/)]

Location of delivery	N = 242	Percent
Home	171	70.7
Health center	48	21.6
Reference general hospital	23	10.4

Fig. 21.2 Hut used as a delivery room—*musakuta*. (Photo Credit: Olivier Mukuku)

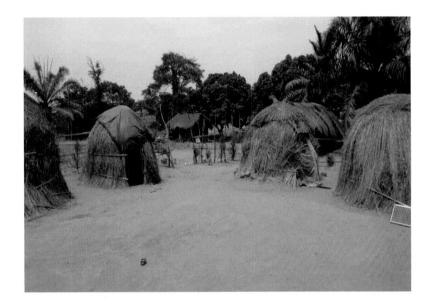

1998; Ijaiya & Aboyeji, 2004; Meyer et al., 2007). The duration of labor leading to the development of obstetric fistula was, on average, 2.25 days with 99.6% of mothers having a labor duration of 24 h or more (Nsambi et al., 2018). In the literature, this average duration varied from 2.5 to 4 days (Harouna et al., 2001; Hilton & Ward, 1998; Melah et al., 2007; Meyer et al., 2007; Nafiou et al., 2007), while 72.5% to 95.7% of obstetric fistula patients had labored for 24 h or more (Ahmad et al., 2005; Holme et al., 2007; Melah et al., 2007; Nafiou et al., 2007; Wall et al., 2004).

The major risk factors associated with the development of obstetric fistula include neglected obstructed labor, accidental injury during cesarean section, forceps delivery, craniotomy, symphysiotomy, and traditional obstetric practices. In rural areas, deliveries are conducted at home in the huts (Fig. 21.2) used as delivery rooms (called "*Musakuta*" in Bemba) by traditional birth attendants, who are in most cases untrained. They have no knowledge of dystocia and are unaware of the normal duration of parturition. For them, all pregnant women must give birth vaginally at all costs; this helps to explain the long duration of labor until childbirth (average: more than 2 days). Sometimes, the *nakimbela* make use of prohibited maneuvers (e.g., use of mortar and pestle pressure on the belly of the parturient) to force the expulsion of the fetus, thus leading to obstetric morbidities such as uterine rupture or obstetric fistula.

Obstetric fistula leads to serious social and economic impacts on the lives of these affected women (Mselle & Kohi, 2015). The majority of women are abandoned by their spouses or partners who cannot bear the stain originating from the permanent flow of urine and stool with foul-smelling odors. In the series of 242 women with obstetric fistula recruited in rural areas of the province of Haut-Katanga

(Nsambi et al., 2018), we reported that 71.5% of them were abandoned by their spouses. The divorce rate due to fistula is about 50% in Nigeria (Wall, 2006) and 87% in Niger (Harouna et al., 2001). Socially, these patients (called "*bakinswi*" in Bemba) fear stigma and discrimination end up evading the community to avoid the gaze of others and live in a state of ostracism without sharing their state. This is a factor aggravating the social experience of the patient who is subjected to physical and moral suffering (total loss of status and dignity) (Mselle & Kohi, 2015; Ndiaye et al., 2009).

21.4   Characteristics of Women with Obstetric Fistula

21.4.1 Sociodemographic Characteristics

Obstetric fistula occurs preferentially in young parturients: the very young age of the woman with obstetric fistula has been noted by several authors (Falandry, 1992; Harouna et al., 2001; Holme et al., 2007). Among 242 women with obstetric fistula (Table 21.2), we noted that the mean age at onset was 23.20 ± 7.72 years (range: 13–51 years); 65.3% of them (158/242) were under 25 years of age and 40.1% (97/242) were teenagers (age under 20) (Nsambi et al., 2018). The increased obstetrical risk in adolescent girls may be partially explained by anatomical immaturity. In adolescents, the pelvis grows more slowly and gradually until old age. In addition, the acquisition of the adult size does not imply an equivalent growth of the pelvis because "*the pelvis does not definitively finish its configuration until the 25th year, although the adult forms are reached around the age of 16*" (Maryam & Ali, 2008). This immaturity of the pelvis is responsible for the anomalies of the basin (limited basin, basin usually shrunk) in the teenager, who is prone to more frequent obstetric complications (Faucher et al., 2002).

In our study, the majority of women (90.9%) were primiparous at the time of fistula onset (Table 21.2) (Nsambi et al., 2018). Studies in Uganda and Zambia reported that one in two women with obstetric fistula was primiparous at the time of fistula development (Hancock & Collie, 2004; Holme et al., 2007). This shows that obstetric fistula usually affects primiparous adolescents probably because of pelvic insufficiency leading to obstructed labor (for cephalopelvic disproportion and prolonged labor) (Jokhio & Kelly, 2006; Munan et al., 2017; Nafiou et al., 2007; Rosenfield et al., 2007).

Table 21.2 Distribution of patients by age and parity at the onset of obstetric fistula. [Source: Adapted from Joseph Bulanda Nsambi, Olivier Mukuku, Jean-de-Dieu Foma Yunga, et al. (2018) Obstetric fistulas in Haut-Katanga province, Democratic Republic of Congo: report of 242 cases. *Pan African Medical Journal*. 29(34). Some modifications were made. https://doi.org/10.11604/pamj.2018.29.34.14576, licensed under the terms of the Creative Commons Attribution License (https://creativecommons.org/licenses/by/4.0/)]

Variable	$N = 242$	Percent
Age		
<20 years	97	40.1
20–24 years	61	25.2
25–29 years	42	17.4
30–34 years	18	7.4
35–39 years	11	4.5
≥40 years	13	5.4
Parity		
1	220	90.9
2	14	5.8
≥3	8	3.3

In the villages where we conducted our study (Nsambi et al., 2018), marriage takes place traditionally at an early age. The girl, as soon as she has her menarche, is directly considered ready for marriage (early marriage), and this results in school abandonment. The vast majority of our patients (94.7%) were out of school, and this is in line with the findings of most African authors who have observed that girls and women with obstetric fistula have rates of out-of-school attendance ranging from 90.5% to 94.7% (Jokhio & Kelly, 2006; Kaboré et al., 2014; Kambou et al., 2006; Nielsen et al., 2009). Studies by Holme et al. (2007) in Zambia and Roka et al. (2013) in Kenya reported that the level of education in girls and women was statistically very low compared to those without fistula. Uneducated or poorly educated women are often deprived of the necessary information on the importance of antenatal care and hospital delivery; they also do not often have access to quality care, as the low level of education is an indirect reflection of the low socioeconomic level.

21.4.2 Anthropometric Characteristics

Women with obstetric fistula are usually small. In our study (Nsambi et al., 2018), 68.2% of the patients had a weight of less than 50 kg and 73.2% of the patients were less than 150 cm in size (average: height of 145.1 ± 7.1 cm). In a study by Wall et al. (2004), 55% of fistula patients weighed less than 50 kg and 79.4% of them were less than 150 cm in height. Holme et al. (2007) and Ahmad et al. (2005) reported average heights of 148 and 145 cm respectively. The small size and weight deficit in obstetric fistula patients have been confirmed in most published series (Ahmad et al., 2005; Holme et al., 2007; Melah et al., 2007; Wall et al., 2004). This deficit of stature and weight reported by various studies is due to several factors: anemia, malnutrition, early pregnancies occurring before the end of puberty, and early cessation of growth. Previous studies found that girls and women with obstetric fistula were thin and short, two independent risk factors for obstructed labor (Malonga et al., 2018; Sokal et al., 1991). According to Lansac et al. (2006), small stature is a classically known risk factor for dystocia. Since growth in height typically stops shortly after menarche, as pelvic growth continues (Moerman, 1982), women who are married at a young age (as are most cases in our series) may become pregnant before they reach full adult pelvic status. The combination of early marriage with short stature, incomplete pelvic growth, and generally contracted pelvis predisposes this female population to cephalopelvic disproportion during labor.

21.5   Characteristics of Obstetric Fistula

In our environment, the delay between the development of obstetric fistula and its repair (age or duration of obstetric fistula) is often very long. The average duration of obstetric fistula was 4.76 years with extremes of 6 months and 34 years; more than one in three patients had fistula for 5 years or more (Nsambi et al., 2018). In Pakistan, Jokhio and Kelly (2006) reported that 40% of patients had fistula for more than 5 years. In Tanzania, Cichowitz et al. (2018) reported that 48.3% of patients had lived more than 10 years with obstetric fistula. This advanced age of fistula in our patients was multifactorial, encompassing social, technical, financial, and environmental issues:

- The stigmatizing nature of the pathology that leads patients to isolation.
- The long clinical tolerance of the disease which is not immediately life-threatening, with many women who do not seek medical attention preferring to live alone with their illness.

- Lack of information about the possibilities of surgical management of the condition that results in women resorting to traditional treatment.
- Lack of financial resources to cope with healthcare expenses, which is also a contributing factor to the delay in medical consultation.
- Lack of integrated prevention and management policy of obstetric fistulas in our health system.

The duration of obstetric fistulas is an important factor in preventing socioeconomic and psychological consequences. The long delay in the development of the disease is a source of stigma, discrimination, and abandonment, and is among potential factors influencing the separation of married couples (Ndiaye et al., 2009).

Regarding the anatomical variety of obstetric fistulas, vesico-vaginal fistulas are the most frequent with proportions ranging from 70.6% to 96.3% (Fig. 21.3) (Harouna et al., 2001; Holme et al., 2007; Kaboré et al., 2014; Kayondo et al., 2011; Washington et al., 2015). In some of our patients in Haut-Katanga, we found vesico-vaginal fistulas associated with a rectovaginal fistula. This high frequency of vesico-vaginal fistula compared with other types of fistulas is probably due to the greater likelihood of compression of the anterior vaginal wall by the fetal head against the pelvis causing more frequent ischemia of the bladder than that of the rectum.

Fig. 21.3 An obstetric fistula. (Photo Credit: Olivier Mukuku)

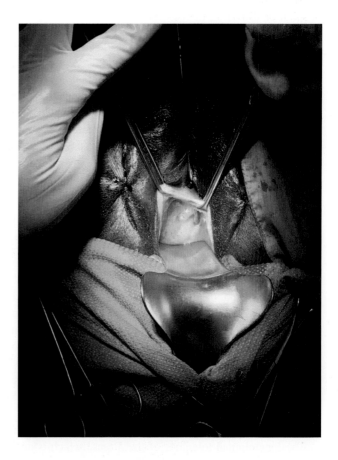

21.6   Management of Obstetric Fistula

21.6.1   Status of Organized Surveillance and Planning

At the national level, no strengthened plan for the eradication of obstetric fistula has been developed (i.e., subsidizing deliveries, making delivery kits available in rural maternity hospitals, giving priority to doctors working in rural areas, etc.). Up to the present time, obstetric fistula is not listed as a notifiable disease in the DRC's health information system.

Obstetric fistula appears to be a silent morbidity among Congolese women that has attracted the interest of donors, non-governmental organizations, local partners, and United Nations' reproductive health organizations who have joined forces for the elimination of obstetric fistula. Technically, there is a lack of infrastructure, staff, and healthcare workers specialized in the repair of obstetric fistulas. As in other African countries where fistula is prevalent, patients who are poor are not able to afford the cost of medical care and transportation to consult in a specialized medical center.

Not long ago, there were no public facilities specialized in the management of fistulas throughout the province of Haut-Katanga. Nevertheless, in our country, there were only two public centers that were created with the support of international organizations. These centers are located in the capital city of Kinshasa (Saint Joseph Medical Center) and in the province of South Kivu (Reference General Hospital of Panzi). In the province of Haut-Katanga, there was no specialized center, and obstetric fistula care was performed in the form of campaigns in rural areas by *Médecins sans Frontières* (Doctors without Borders) and *Médecins du Désert*.

Beginning in 2013, a private structure has emerged in the city of Lubumbashi. This structure works in collaboration with a non-governmental organization of Congolese rights called "*Hope Mama Africa*". It provides specialized care in the field of repair of urogenital fistula permanently and thus covers the entire province of Haut-Katanga. It is composed of four doctors trained in vaginal surgery (specifically in the repair of fistulas) including a gynecologist-obstetrician, eight nurses, and two anesthesiologists (Figs. 21.4 and 21.5). This structure, although private, is in close collaboration with the rural health zones for the search for and selection of patients with obstetric fistula.

Fig. 21.4 Dr. Nsambi (middle) and his assistants in the operative theatre repairing an obstetric fistula. (Photo Credit: Olivier Mukuku)

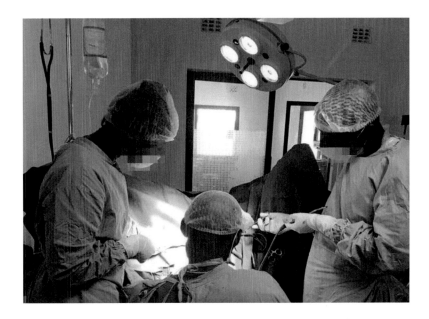

Fig. 21.5 Dr. Nsambi
(second from left) and
his fistula repair team in
the operating room in
Lubumbashi. (Photo
Credit: Olivier Mukuku)

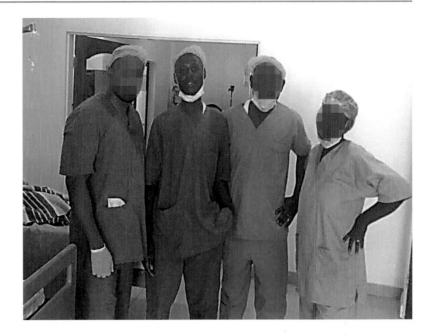

21.6.2 Recruitment of Patients

Recruitment of affected women is implemented through awareness messages distributed via community relays and non-governmental organizations working in rural areas. These non-governmental organizations are reaching out to more remote areas of the province for patients with obstetric fistula. Some patients are referred by public health facilities such as health centers and general referral hospitals.

Given the technical plateau and the short period for campaigns, women in care were those carrying a simple urogenital fistula (or type 1) or a type 2 or 3 complex urogenital fistula according to the Goh classification (Goh, 2004). No woman with a complex type 4 urogenital fistula or severe urogenital fistula (transection) was treated.

21.7   Results

Surgical repair is the mainstay of treatment for fistula management (Figs. 21.6 and 21.7). Recall that abnormal communication between the viscera tends to close spontaneously before the end of epithelialization, provided that the natural flow pathways are not obstructed.

To promote an early closure, especially in cases where the fistula is small, it is necessary to circumvent the mechanisms of the urethral sphincter by catheterization. Continuous drainage of the bladder, combined with antibiotics to limit tissue damage caused by infection, is an initial treatment for obstetric fistulas that develop after a dystocic delivery. Indeed, spontaneous closure of obstetric fistula has been reported in up to 28% of cases when catheterization was used (Waaldijk, 1997).

The success rate after surgical repair of obstetric fistula—defined by complete closure of the fistula—varies from one center to another and is determined by many factors such as fistula site, degree of healing, previous attempts at repair, repair technique, surgeon's expertise, equipment, and post-operative nursing. The success rate in our study was 86% (Nsambi et al., 2018). Such high rates of success after repair are reported by other authors ranging from 71.7% to 93.4% (Gessessew & Mesfin,

Fig. 21.6 An obstetric fistula undergoing surgical repair. (Photo Credit: Olivier Mukuku)

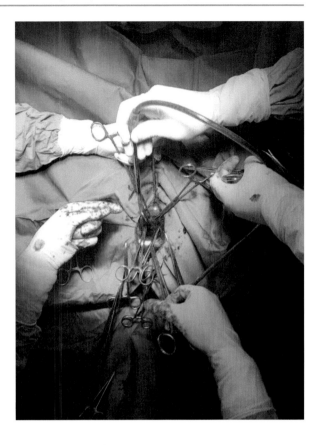

Fig. 21.7 An obstetric fistula before undergoing surgical repair. (Photo Credit: Olivier Mukuku)

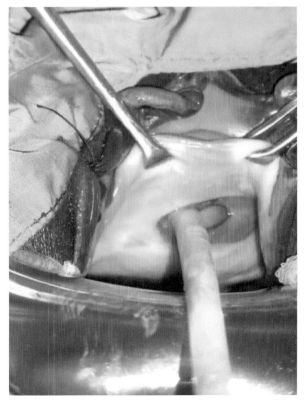

2003; Holme et al., 2007; Kambou et al., 2006; Kayondo et al., 2011; Loposso et al., 2016; Moudouni et al., 2001; Muleta, 1997; Paluku & Carter, 2015; Sori et al., 2016). However, even after successful closure, 15–20% of cases may continue to suffer from urinary incontinence. Predictors of failure include vaginal scarring, circumferential fistula, and previous attempts at repair (Browning, 2006; Goh et al., 2008; Nardos et al., 2009; Roenneburg et al., 2006). The most important factor in successful fistula repair is adherence to basic surgical principles, including careful preoperative evaluation, exposure of the fistula and surrounding tissue scale, tension-free closure, excision of all fibrotic tissue, and maintenance of a suture line that is kept uninfected and dry (Kayondo et al., 2011). Closing the bladder is much more important in achieving a successful repair than vaginal closure. As long as these principles are followed, the surgical approach often concludes successfully. In most cases, the choice is essentially dictated by the procedure which the surgeon is more comfortable and familiar with.

The same is true about the method of approach when repairing the fistula. The arguments differ as to whether the abdominal or vaginal approach is the most appropriate for fistula repair. But we must recognize the need for individualized care based on anatomical relationships, extent of injury, and co-morbidities. In our series from Lubumbashi, 69.4% of fistulas were repaired vaginally (Nsambi et al., 2018). The vaginal way represents for us the best path, because it is the most anatomically simple and offers an optimal surgical exposure, thanks to the traction on the balloon of a Foley probe. We have favored the vaginal approach when vesico-vaginal fistula was near the neck of the bladder. The benefits include a low rate of complications, less bleeding, rapid postoperative recovery, and short hospital stay (Kayondo et al., 2011). Almost all types of vesico-vaginal fistula can be repaired vaginally. There are technical devices to widen the vaginal way (Dupont & Raz, 1996). These include:

- Schuckhar lateral episiotomy (used to repair a rectovaginal fistula associated with a vesico-vaginal fistula).
- Posterior episiotomy of Picot-Couvelaire (considered dilapidated, but which lowers the vaginal dome and makes it possible to externalize a high-situated fistula).
- Disinsertion of the anterior face of the bladder to the pubis.

We reserve the abdominal surgical approach for those cases that had a fistula that could not be properly visualized and exposed vaginally behind the orifices of the ureter, either because of vaginal stenosis, or in rare cases where an intra-abdominal pathological condition required simultaneous care, or in cases of vesico-uterine fistulas.

21.8 Conclusion and Perspectives

In summary, obstetric fistula remains an important obstetric problem in low-resource countries. It is strongly associated with stillbirth because both are related to obstructed labor in the absence of EmONC. Reliable epidemiological and demographic data on obstetric fistula in low-resource countries are lacking.

Safe delivery is a basic human right; the real challenge is to make it a practical reality for everyone. National strategies for prevention are much more important for the ultimate eradication of this devastating disease. These strategies include government's recognition of fistula as a major public health concern, improving the status of women in society, expanding primary education especially for girls; development of supportive infrastructure and trained specialists; and affordable, accessible, and acceptable services for all pregnant women.

Emphasis should also be placed on the involvement of religious and traditional leaders in circumventing certain socio-cultural barriers.

The government, as the ultimate guarantor of the country's health policy, should:

- Implement a coherent health coverage plan and ensure equilibrium in terms of equipment and human resources between urban and rural areas (in particular, motivation of the nursing staff).
- Give women access to a health center, skilled medical care, and cesarean section in those cases of obstructed delivery.
- Train nurses in these facilities to perform antenatal referral consultations and EmONC.
- Implement legal instruments that condemn early marriage and increase the number of doctors repairing fistulas (training and encouragement of sustainable care projects).

The community should help and support the government's efforts in this area by relaying information through community health workers who would be in charge of sensitizing the community on the use of health services.

References

Ahmad, S., Nishtar, A., Hafeez, G. A., & Khan, Z. (2005). Management of vesico-vaginal fistulas in women. *International Journal of Gynecology & Obstetrics, 88*, 71–75.

Alkema, L., Chou, D., Hogan, D., Zhang, S., Moller, A. B., Gemmill, A., et al. (2016). Global, regional, and national levels and trends in maternal mortality between 1990 and 2015, with scenario-based projections to 2030: A systematic analysis by the UN Maternal Mortality Estimation Inter-Agency Group. *The Lancet, 387*(10017), P462–P474. Retrieved January 15, 2019, from https://www.thelancet.com/journals/lancet/article/PIIS0140-6736(15)00838-7/fulltext.

Browning, A. (2006). Risk factors for developing residual urinary incontinence after obstetric fistula repair. *BJOG: An International Journal of Obstetrics & Gynaecology, 113*(4), 482–485. Retrieved January 16, 2019, from https://obgyn.onlinelibrary.wiley.com/doi/full/10.1111/j.1471-0528.2006.00875.x

Cavallaro, F. L., Cresswell, J. A., França, G. V., Victora, C. G., Barros, A. J., & Ronsmans, C. (2013). Trends in caesarean delivery by country and wealth quintile: Cross-sectional surveys in southern Asia and sub-Saharan Africa. *Bulletin of the World Health Organization, 91*, 914–922D. Retrieved January 16, 2019, from: https://www.who.int/bulletin/volumes/91/12/13-117598/en/

Cichowitz, C., Watt, M. H., Mchome, B., & Masenga, G. G. (2018). Delays contributing to the development and repair of obstetric fistula in northern Tanzania. *International Urogynecology Journal, 29*(3), 397–405.

Creanga, A. A., Ahmed, S., Genadry, R. R., & Stanton, C. (2007). Prevention and treatment of obstetric fistula: Identifying research needs and public health priorities. *International Journal of Gynecology & Obstetrics, 99*(Suppl 1), S151–S154.

Donnay, F., & Weil, L. (2004). Obstetric fistula: The international response. *The Lancet, 363*(9402), 71–72. https://doi.org/10.1016/S0140-6736(03)15177-X

Dupont, M. C., & Raz, S. (1996). Vaginal approach to vesicovaginal fistula repair. *Urology, 48*(1), 7–9.

Falandry, L. (1992). Vesicovaginal fistula in Africa. 230 cases. *Presse Médicale, 21*(6), 241–245.

Faucher, P., Dappe, S., & Madelenat, P. (2002). Maternité à l'adolescence: Analyse obstétricale et revue de l'influence des facteurs culturels, socio-économiques et psychologiques à partir d'une étude rétrospective de 62 dossiers. *Gynécologie Obstétrique & Fertilité, 30*(12), 944–952.

Flouriot, J. (2008). Congo RDC: Population et aménagement d'un immense pays. *Population and Avenir, 2*, 4–8. https://doi.org/10.3917/popav.687.0004

Gessessew, A., & Mesfin, M. (2003). Genitourinary and rectovaginal fistulae in Adigrat zonal hospital, Tigray, North Ethiopia. *Ethiopian Medical Journal, 41*(2), 123–130.

Goh, J. T. (2004). A new classification for female genital tract fistula. *Australian and New Zealand Journal of Obstetrics and Gynaecology, 44*(6), 502–504.

Goh, J. T., Browning, A., Berhan, B., & Chang, A. (2008). Predicting the risk of failure of closure of obstetric fistula and residual urinary incontinence using a classification system. *International Urogynecology Journal, 19*(12), 1659–1662. https://doi.org/10.1007/s00192-008-0693-9

Hancock, B., & Collie, M. (2004). Vesico-vaginal fistula surgery in Uganda. *East and Central African Journal of Surgery, 9*(2), 32–37.

Harouna, Y. D., Seibou, A., Maikano, S., Djambeidou, J., Sangare, A., Bilane, S., et al. (2001). La fistule vesico-vaginale de cause obstetricale: Enqueteaupres de 52 femmes admises au village des fistuleuses. *Médecine d'Afrique Noire, 48*(2), 55–59.

Hilton, P. (2003). Vesico-vaginal fistulas in developing countries. *International Journal of Gynecology & Obstetrics, 82*(3), 285–295.

Hilton, P. (2016). Trends in the aetiology of urogenital fistula: A case of 'retrogressive evolution'? *International Urogynecology Journal, 27*(6), 831–837. Retrieved February 7, 2019 from https://www.ncbi.nlm.nih.gov/pmc/articles/PMC4879169/

Hilton, P., & Ward, A. (1998). Epidemiological and surgical aspects of urogenital fistulae: A review of 25 years' experience in Southeast Nigeria. *International Urogynecology Journal, 9*(4), 189–194.

Holme, A., Breen, M., & MacArthur, C. (2007). Obstetric fistulae: A study of women managed at the Monze Mission hospital, Zambia. *BJOG: An International Journal of Obstetrics & Gynaecology, 114*(8), 1010–1017. Retrieved February 7, 2019, from https://obgyn.onlinelibrary.wiley.com/doi/full/10.1111/j.1471-0528.2007.01353.x

Hsia, R. Y., Mbembati, N. A., Macfarlane, S., & Kruk, M. E. (2012). Access to emergency and surgical care in sub-Saharan Africa: The infrastructure gap. *Health Policy and Planning, 27*(3), 234–244.

Ijaiya, M. A., & Aboyeji, P. A. (2004). Obstetric urogenital fistula: The Ilorin experience, Nigeria. *West African Journal of Medicine, 23*(1), 7–9.

INS (Institut National de la Statistique). (2016). *La province du Haut-Katanga*. INS. Retrieved December 16, 2018, from http://www.inskatanga.com/hautkatanga.html.

Jokhio, A. H., & Kelly, J. (2006). Obstetric fistulas in rural Pakistan. *International Journal of Gynecology & Obstetrics, 95*(3), 288–289. https://doi.org/10.1016/j.ijgo.2006.08.008

Kaboré, F. A., Kambou, T., Ouattara, A., Zango, B., Yaméogo, C., Kirakoya, B., et al. (2014). Aspects épidémiologiques, étiologiques et impact psychosocial des fistules urogénitales dans une cohorte de 170 patientes consécutives, prises en charge dans trois centres du Burkina Faso de 2010 à 2012. *Progrès en Urologie, 24*(8), 526–532.

Kambou, T., Zango, B., Outtara, T., Dao, B., & Sano, D. (2006). Point sur la prise en charge des fistules urogénitales au CHU Sourosanou de Bobo Dioulasso: Etude de 57 cas opérés en deux ans. *Médecine d'Afrique Noire, 53*(12), 665–673.

Kasamba, N., Kaye, D. K., & Mbalinda, S. N. (2013). Community awareness about risk factors, presentation and prevention and obstetric fistula in Nabitovu village, Iganga district, Uganda. *BMC Pregnancy and Childbirth, 13*(1), 229. Retrieved February 7, 2019, from https://www.ncbi.nlm.nih.gov/pmc/articles/PMC4028862/

Kayondo, M., Wasswa, S., Kabakyenga, J., Mukiibi, N., Senkungu, J., Stenson, A., et al. (2011). Predictors and outcome of surgical repair of obstetric fistula at a regional referral hospital, Mbarara, western Uganda. *BMC Urology, 11*(1), 23. Retrieved February 7, 2019, from https://www.ncbi.nlm.nih.gov/pmc/articles/PMC3252285/

Kinenkinda, X., Mukuku, O., Chenge, F., Kakudji, P., Banzulu, P., Kakoma, J. B., et al. (2017). Cesarean section in Lubumbashi, Democratic Republic of the Congo I: Frequency, indications and maternal and perinatal mortality. *The Pan African Medical Journal, 27*, 72. https://doi.org/10.11604/pamj.2017.27.72.12147

Langkilde, N. C., Pless, T. K., Lundbeck, F., & Nerstrøm, B. (1999). Surgical repair of vesicovaginal fistulae: A ten-year retrospective study. *Scandinavian Journal of Urology and Nephrology, 33*(2), 100–103. https://doi.org/10.1080/003655999750016069

Lansac, J., Marret, H., & Oury, J.-F. (2006). *Pratique de l'accouchement* (4th ed.). Elsevier Masson.

Loposso, M., Hakim, L., Ndundu, J., Lufuma, S., Punga, A., & De Ridder, D. (2016). Predictors of recurrence and successful treatment following obstetric fistula surgery. *Urology, 97*, 80–85. https://doi.org/10.1016/j.urology.2016.03.079

Malonga, F. K., Mukuku, O., Ngalula, M. T., Luhete, P. K., & Kakoma, J. B. (2018). Anthropometric and pelvic external measurements in nulliparas of Lubumbashi: Risk factors and predictive score of mechanical dystocia. *Pan African Medical Journal, 31*, 69. https://doi.org/10.11604/pamj.2018.31.69.16014. Retrieved November 13, 2018, from http://www.panafrican-med-journal.com/content/article/31/69/full/

Maryam, K., & Ali, S. (2008). Pregnancy outcome in teenagers in east sauterne of Iran. *The Journal of the Pakistan Medical Association, 58*(10), 541–544.

Melah, G. S., Massa, A. A., Yahaya, U. R., Bukar, M., Kizaya, D. D., & El-Nafaty, A. U. (2007). Risk factors for obstetric fistulae in North-Eastern Nigeria. *Journal of Obstetrics and Gynaecology, 27*(8), 819–823. https://doi.org/10.1080/01443610701709825

Meyer, L., Ascher-Walsh, C. J., Norman, R., Idrissa, A., Herbert, H., Kimso, O., et al. (2007). Commonalities among women who experienced vesicovaginal fistulae as a result of obstetric trauma in Niger: Results from a survey given at the National Hospital Fistula Center, Niamey, Niger. *American Journal of Obstetrics & Gynecology, 197*(1), 90.e1–90.e4. https://doi.org/10.1016/j.ajog.2007.03.071

Ministère du Plan et Macro International. (2008). *Enquête Démographique et de Santé, République Démocratique du Congo 2007*. Ministère du Plan et Macro International. Retrieved from https://dhsprogram.com/pubs/pdf/FR208/FR208.pdf

Moerman, M. L. (1982). Growth of the birth canal in adolescent girls. *American Journal of Obstetrics & Gynecology, 143*(5), 528–532.

Moudouni, S., Nouri, M., Koutani, A., Ibn Attya, A., Hachimi, M., & Lakrissa, A. (2001). Les fistules vésico-vaginales obstétricales. À propos de 114 cas. *Progrès en Urologie, 11*, 103–108.

Mselle, L. T., & Kohi, T. W. (2015). Living with constant leaking of urine and odour: Thematic analysis of socio-cultural experiences of women affected by obstetric fistula in rural Tanzania. *BMC Women's Health, 15*(1), 107. https://doi.org/10.1186/s12905-015-0267-1. Retrieved November 13, 2018, from https://bmcwomenshealth.biomedcentral.com/articles/10.1186/s12905-015-0267-1/

Muleta, M. (1997). Obstetric fistulae: A retrospective study of 1210 cases at the Addis Ababa fistula hospital. *Journal of Obstetrics and Gynaecology, 17*(1), 68–70.

Muleta, M. (2004). Socio-demographic profile and obstetric experience of fistula patients managed at the Addis Ababa fistula hospital. *Ethiopian Medical Journal, 42*(1), 9–16.

Munan, R., Kakudji, Y., Nsambi, J., Mukuku, O., Maleya, A., Kinenkinda, X., & Kakudji, P. (2017). Childbirth among primiparous women in Lubumbashi: Maternal and perinatal prognosis. *The Pan African Medical Journal, 28*, 77. https://doi.org/10.11604/pamj.2017.28.77.13712

Nafiou, I., Idrissa, A., Ghaichatou, A. K., Roenneburg, M. L., Wheeless, C. R., & Genadry, R. R. (2007). Obstetric vesico-vaginal fistulas at the National Hospital of Niamey, Niger. *International Journal of Gynecology & Obstetrics, 99*(S1), 71–74.

Nardos, R., Browning, A., & Chen, C. C. (2009). Risk factors that predict failure after vaginal repair of obstetric vesicovaginal fistulae. *American Journal of Obstetrics and Gynecology, 200*(5), 578, e1–4. https://doi.org/10.1016/j.ajog.2008.12.008

Ndiaye, P., Amoul Kini, G., Idrissa, A., Camara, D. M., & Tal-Dia, A. (2009). Parcours de la femme souffrant de fistule obstétricale au Niger. *Médecine Tropicale, 69*, 61–65.

Nielsen, H. S., Lindberg, L., Nygaard, U., Aytenfisu, H., Johnston, O. L., Sørensen, B., et al. (2009). A community-based long-term follow up of women undergoing obstetric fistula repair in rural Ethiopia. *BJOG: An International Journal of Obstetrics & Gynaecology, 116*(9), 1258–1264.

Nsambi, J. B., Mukuku, O., FomaYunga, J. D., Kinenkinda, X., Kakudji, P., Kizonde, J., et al. (2018). Obstetric fistula in the province of Haut-Katanga, Democratic Republic of Congo: About 242 cases. *The Pan African Medical Journal, 29*, 34. https://doi.org/10.11604/pamj.2018.29.34.14576. Retrieved December 13, 2018, from http://www.panafrican-med-journal.com/content/article/29/34/full/

Paluku, J. L., & Carter, T. E. (2015). Obstetric vesico-vaginal fistulae seen in the northern Democratic Republic of Congo: A descriptive study. *African Health Sciences, 15*(4), 1104–1111.

Roenneburg, M. L., Genadry, R., & Wheeless, C. R., Jr. (2006). Repair of obstetric vesicovaginal fistulas in Africa. *American Journal of Obstetrics and Gynecology, 195*(6), 1748–1752.

Roka, Z. G., Akech, M., Wanzala, P., Omolo, J., Gitta, S., & Waiswa, P. (2013). Factors associated with obstetric fistulae occurrence among patients attending selected hospitals in Kenya, 2010: A case control study. *BMC Pregnancy and Childbirth, 13*(1), 56. https://doi.org/10.1186/1471-2393-13-56. Retrieved November 13, 2018, from https://bmcpregnancychildbirth.biomedcentral.com/articles/10.1186/1471-2393-13-56/

Rosenfield, A., Min, C. J., & Freedman, L. P. (2007). Making motherhood safe in developing countries. *New England Journal of Medicine, 356*(14), 1395–1397. Retrieved February 7, 2019, from: https://www.nejm.org/doi/full/10.1056/nejmp078026

Schwartz, D. A. (2015). Pathology of maternal death – The importance of accurate autopsy diagnosis for epidemiologic surveillance and prevention of maternal mortality in developing countries. In D. A. Schwartz (Ed.), *Maternal mortality: Risk factors, anthropological perspectives, prevalence in developing countries and preventative strategies for pregnancy- related death* (pp. 215–253). Nova Scientific Publishing.

Sokal, D., Sawadogo, L., Adjibade, A., & Operations Research Team. (1991). Short stature and cephalopelvic disproportion in Burkina Faso, West Africa. *International Journal of Gynecology & Obstetrics, 35*(4), 347–350.

Sori, D. A., Azale, A. W., & Gemeda, D. H. (2016). Characteristics and repair outcome of patients with Vesicovaginal fistula managed in Jimma University teaching hospital, Ethiopia. *BMC Urology, 16*(1), 41. Retrieved January 13, 2019, from https://bmcurol.biomedcentral.com/articles/10.1186/s12894-016-0152-8

Tafesse, B. (2008). A new classification of female genital fistula. *Journal of Obstetrics and Gynaecology Canada, 30*, 394–395. Retrieved December 14, 2018 from: https://www.jogc.com/article/S1701-2163(16)32823-7/pdf

UNFPA. (2009). *Campaign to end fistula. The year in review. Annual report 2008.* UNFPA. Retrieved January 8, 2019, from https://www.unfpa.org/publications/campaign-end-fistula-year-review

UNFPA, EngenderHealth. (2003). *Obstetric fistula needs assessment report: Findings from nine African countries.* UNFPA, EngenderHealth. Retrieved January 9, 2019, from https://www.unfpa.org/sites/default/files/pub-pdf/fistula-needs-assessment.pdf

United Nations. (2018). *Sustainable development goals.* UN. Retrieved January 6, 2019, from https://www.un.org/sustainabledevelopment/sustainable-development-goals/

Waaldijk, K. (1997). Immediate indwelling bladder catheterization at postpartum urine leakage—Personal experience of 1200 patients. *Tropical Doctor, 27*(4), 227–228. https://doi.org/10.1177/004947559702700414

Wall, L. L. (2006). Obstetric vesicovaginal fistula as an international public-health problem. *The Lancet, 368*(9542), 1201–1209. Retrieved February 7, 2019, from https://www.thelancet.com/journals/lancet/article/PIIS0140-6736(06)69476-2/fulltext

Wall, L. L. (2012). Obstetric fistula is a "neglected tropical disease". *PLoS Neglected Tropical Diseases, 6*(8), e1769. Retrieved December 10, 2018, from https://journals.plos.org/plosntds/article?id=10.1371/journal.pntd.0001769

Wall, L. L., Karshima, J. A., Kirschner, C., & Arrowsmith, S. D. (2004). The obstetric vesicovaginal fistula: Characteristics of 899 patients from Jos, Nigeria. *American Journal of Obstetrics and Gynecology, 190*(4), 1011–1016. https://doi.org/10.1016/j.ajog.2004.02.007

Washington, B. B., Raker, C. A., Kabeja, G. A., Kay, A., & Hampton, B. S. (2015). *International Journal of Gynecology & Obstetrics, 129*(1), 34–37. https://doi.org/10.1016/j.ijgo.2014.09.033

WHO. (2006). *Obstetric fistula: Guiding principles for clinical management and programme development.* World Health Organization.

WHO. (2018). *Maternal mortality.* World Health Organization. 16 February 2018. Retrieved January 10, 2019, from: https://www.who.int/news-room/fact-sheets/detail/maternal-mortality

Therapeutic Management of Obstetric Fistula: Learning from Implementation of Insertable Devices to Improve the Health and Well-being of Women and Girls in Low- and Middle-Income Countries

Nessa Ryan and Ann E. Kurth

22.1 Introduction

Obstetric fistula is a preventable birth injury that results from pelvic tissue damage during a prolonged, obstructed labor when a connection forms between a woman's bladder and vagina.[1] Women and girls who are already socially, geographically, or economically marginalized are at increased risk, including those who have low social status, low educational attainment, living rurally, or living in contexts where early coitarche and child marriage are normalized; development of obstetric fistula further exacerbates their marginalization (Wall, 2012). An affected woman will experience chronic incontinence, pain, and discomfort. Women's observable chronic urinary leakage and related odor make them vulnerable to stigma, including external stigma (i.e., overt discrimination, verbal abuse, relationship dissolution, social isolation) and internal stigma (i.e., internalization of negative stereotypes), causing poor mental health consequences and reduced opportunity for income-generating activities (Ahmed & Holtz, 2007; Alio et al., 2011; Bangser, 2006; Changole

---

[1] Vesico-vaginal fistula (VVF) occurs when an abnormal connection forms between the genital and urinary tracts, while recto-vaginal fistula (RVF) occurs between the genital tract and rectum. Although VVF and RVF are both possible complications of prolonged, obstructed labor, this work will exclusively focus on self-management of the more common VVF.

N. Ryan (✉)
New York University School of Global Public Health, New York, NY, USA

Susan and Henry Samueli College of Health Sciences, Irvine, CA, USA
e-mail: ryann01@nyu.edu

A. E. Kurth
Yale University School of Nursing, New Haven, CT, USA

Epidemiology of Microbial Diseases, Yale School of Public Health, New Haven, CT, USA
e-mail: ann.kurth@yale.edu

© Springer Nature Switzerland AG 2022
L. B. Drew et al. (eds.), *A Multidisciplinary Approach to Obstetric Fistula in Africa*, Global Maternal and Child Health, https://doi.org/10.1007/978-3-031-06314-5_22

et al., 2017). This significantly reduces quality of life and delays treatment seeking (Adefris et al., 2017; Khisa et al., 2017; Ruder et al., 2018). Family and friends are also vulnerable to stigma and the associated negative outcomes due to association with an affected woman (Jarvis et al., 2017; Jarvis, Richter, Vallianatos, & Thornton, 2017). As many as two million women are living with the stigmatizing birth injury globally, primarily in low- and middle-income countries (LMICs) in sub-Saharan Africa and South Asia (Adler et al., 2013).

Obstetric fistula persists due to various multi-level barriers (i.e., individual, social, and structural) to successful fistula prevention and management (Baker et al., 2017; Banke-Thomas et al., 2014), like failure to provide timely emergency obstetric care to prevent prolonged, obstructed labor, lack of adequate services for surgical fistula repair, and low status of women and girls that may lead to low educational attainment and normalization of child marriage thus increasing risk of labor complications. Surgical capacity to repair the injury is increasing; however, current global capacity is low and many women with this 'neglected tropical disease' (Wall, 2012) are left behind. From 2003 to 2018, the Population Fund (UNFPA), the UN agency tasked with addressing obstetric fistula, reports directly supporting over 100,000 fistula repair surgeries globally (UNFPA, 2018); however, as many as 100,000 new cases develop each year (Adler et al., 2013).

Scale-up of surgical fistula repair services is ongoing and must overcome various barriers to implementation (UN, 2014), including factors at the individual level (i.e., depression, shame), social level (i.e., stigma, gender power imbalances), and structural level (i.e., lack of community-based referral mechanisms, financial cost of the procedure, transportation difficulties, the availability of facilities that offer fistula repair, community reintegration, and the competing priorities of political leadership) (Baker et al., 2017). In the meantime, women who have not accessed successful repair attempt to creatively manage their incontinence and related odor with available low-cost materials, however, with limited perceived effectiveness and appropriateness (Barageine et al., 2015; Gebresilase, 2014; Heller, 2018; Kabayambi et al., 2014). In settings where adult diapers or sanitary pads are prohibitively expensive or unavailable, women use absorptive fabrics that hold urine against the skin, causing severe irritation; moreover, these fabrics require continuous washing for reuse (Ryan, 2019). Clinically effective options for incontinence self-management are inaccessible for most, and durable low-cost innovations to implement within the context of current fistula programming are urgently needed to support the unmet needs of women living with fistula.

Evidence to support use of one such innovation for self-management of fistula-related incontinence, an insertable vaginal cup, is growing (Ganyaglo et al., 2018; Goldberg et al., 2016; New Vision Reporter, 2012; Russell et al., 2016; Ryan, 2019). This flexible reservoir cup is acceptable, safe, and effective for managing menstrual blood among women and girls in LMICs where fistula is prevalent (Beksinska et al., 2015; Juma et al., 2017; van Eijk et al., 2019). Within a feasibility study on the use of the cup among women with fistula at a health facility in Ghana, the insertable cup was found to be feasible, acceptable, and appropriate (Ganyaglo et al., 2018). Initial discussions with fistula stakeholders (i.e., clinicians, policymakers, and researchers) suggest this device could be compatible with ongoing fistula programming (Ryan, 2019); however, fistula care services are delivered in various different ways and implementation will need to be contextualized for local settings.

Previous research on insertables can highlight valuable lessons for implementation of this novel device. This work is informed by the lessons learned from implementation challenges when large-scale clinical trials of multipurpose preventive technologies (MPTs) were carried out without appreciation of the context in which the intervention would be used and delivered in sub-Saharan Africa, leading to a critical misunderstanding of the vaginal practices and cultural taboos represented within the target population that potentially confounded a positive treatment effect.

This chapter will provide a review of the evidence on the use of insertable devices for the health and well-being of women and girls in LMICs, including for the purposes of contraception and/or prevention of sexually transmitted infection (STI), menstrual hygiene management, pelvic organ prolapse, and urinary incontinence. Although a strong evidence base exists to support the use of insertable devices in LMICs, there exists a "know-do" gap between these proven interventions and their reliable implementation at scale. As many factors can influence the successful implementation of an evidence-based intervention, here we focus on identifying potential challenges in implementation among last mile populations (Chao et al., 2014), or those who are poorest, in greatest need, and furthest from health services. In understanding these challenges, we can apply lessons learned to the planning and implementation of a therapeutic insertable device to address obstetric fistula-related incontinence for women and girls in LMICs. Analysis of the successes and challenges of intervention and implementation will be guided by various intervention and implementation frameworks, including the Social Ecological Model (SEM) (Bronfenbrenner, 1989), acceptability and adherence of MPTs (Tolley et al., 2013), and implementation research outcomes (Proctor et al., 2011). Findings will be used to discuss with policymakers and donors to encourage their engagement and investment in implementation, as well as to inform future research. Ultimately, such an innovation could reduce the stigma burden and significantly improve the quality of life of affected women and their families (Mwini-Nyaledzigbor et al., 2013; Sullivan et al., 2016).

22.2   Conceptual Framework

22.2.1   Social Ecological Model

This work is predominantly informed by the Social Ecological Model (SEM) (Bronfenbrenner, 1989) to examine factors from the intrapersonal and interpersonal levels to the broader community and systems levels. The SEM, originally developed by Urie Bronfenbrenner in 1979 (Bronfenbrenner, 1989) to encourage a more ecological focus on contextual factors influencing human development, has frequently informed the development of various effective multi-level, multi-component global public health strategies. The insertable cup for non-surgical management of fistula, if implemented as a component of comprehensive fistula programming, could be associated with successful therapeutic management of this chronic condition that could allow for improved health and well-being among women and girls in LMICs. The underlying logic of the model suggests that behavior affects and is affected by multiple levels of influence and that interventions should be informed by reciprocal causation, or the concept that individual behaviors shape and are shaped by the social environment. A key strength of the SEM that encourages its application to multiple topics of public health concern is its ability to illustrate the interactive relationship between individuals and their environment while nesting various influencing factors within the hierarchical levels of individual (intrapersonal), interpersonal, community, organizational, and policy/enabling environment.

Implementation should be examined from the individual level to the policy level, by exploring attributes of the product itself, through to the skills and preferences of the intended user, to the perceived perspectives of partners and family members, to community attitudes to cultural norms (Tolley et al., 2013). In their model, Tolley et al. (2013) map onto the SEM the continuum of relevant factors that influence acceptability of, as well as adherence to, multipurpose prevention technologies (MPTs), including insertable devices that target prevention of unintended pregnancy and STIs, like HIV (Tolley et al., 2013). This is a helpful approach that encourages an ecological framing to factors that might influence the implementation of such products; however, this framework can be strengthened by supplementing with additional factors, beyond acceptability and adherence that are known to influence implementation.

22.2.2 Implementation Science Framework

Various factors contribute to the successful implementation of an evidence-based intervention, and implementation research, the scientific study of methods to promote the systematic uptake of proven interventions into routine practice (and thus to improve health), provides us with an approach to integrating implementation concerns into interventional research. Research on an insertable device to manage fistula-related incontinence should be guided by an implementation science framework. Proctor et al. (2011) developed a taxonomy for implementation research outcomes, which, in addition to acceptability and fidelity, includes appropriateness, feasibility, adoption, cost, user penetration, and sustainability (defined in Box 22.1 in expanding hierarchical level of analysis—i.e., from level of the user to provider to organization). This taxonomy, which has been utilized in various settings and disciplines, enables global assessment of implementation effectiveness and provides a means to expand the focus of the conceptual framework developed by Tolley and colleagues regarding acceptability and fidelity of MPTs (Tolley et al., 2013).

Box 22.1 Implementation Research Outcomes Defined and Level of Analysis (Proctor et al., 2011)
- *Acceptability*: the perception among implementation stakeholders (beneficiaries and implementers) that the innovation is agreeable, palatable, or satisfactory (level of analysis: user, provider).
- *Appropriateness*: the perceived fit, relevance, or compatibility of the innovation for a given practice setting, provider, or beneficiary; and/or perceived fit of the innovation to address a particular issue or problem (level of analysis: user, provider, organization).
- *Fidelity*: degree to which the innovation can be implemented as it was prescribed in the original protocol or as it was intended by the program developer (level of analysis: provider).
- *Adoption*: the intention, initial decision, or action to try or employ the innovation (i.e., uptake) (level of analysis: provider, organization).
- *Feasibility*: the extent to which the innovation can be successfully used or carried out within a given agency or setting (level of analysis: provider, organization).
- *Cost*: (incremental or implementation cost) is defined as the cost impact of an implementation effort (level of analysis: provider, organization).
- *Penetration*: the integration of a practice within a service setting and its subsystems (level of analysis: organization).
- *Sustainability*: the extent to which a newly implemented innovation is maintained or institutionalized within a service setting's ongoing, stable operations (level of analysis: organization).

Ultimately the integration of Tolley et al.'s ecological framing of factors contributing to acceptability and adherence and Proctor's et al.'s implementation outcomes provides a broad but specific conceptual framework to guide the assessment of implementation of various insertable devices for women's health in LMICs.

22.3 Types of Insertable Devices for Women's Health in LMICs

Insertables are technologies that reside within the body. When we talk about insertable devices (IDs) for women's health, we are focused on technologies predominantly for sexual, reproductive, menstrual, or gynecological health and well-being. More often than not, this term refers to products or devices that are inserted intravaginally and can be removed and replaced by the user. Insertables have long been valued by global health practitioners and policymakers as products with the potential to improve women's health and quality of life but are potentially under-used by intended populations in low-resources settings. Because they are user-controlled technologies, IDs are more likely to be accessible and acceptable to women and girls within the last mile, or those who are poorest, in greatest need, and furthest from health services.

In low-resource settings, women face unique barriers to obtaining effective methods for prevention of unintended pregnancy and STI, as well as methods for menstrual hygiene management, pelvic organ prolapse, and incontinence management. Various insertables provide discreet female-controlled methods that allow women to protect and care for themselves, even in a context where there are other threats to their sexual, reproductive, menstrual, and gynecological health and well-being beyond their control, such as negotiation of sexual activity and taboo surrounding the female body and natural processes like menstruation.

22.3.1 Insertable Devices for Contraception and Sexually Transmissible Infection Prevention

IDs for prevention of unintended pregnancy range from barrier methods to hormonal methods, while IDs for prevention of STI solely include barrier methods (see Box 22.2). Barrier methods block sperm from entering the uterus and can be used with spermicidal foam or film. Hormonal methods contain either estrogen and progestin, or progestin only and prevent pregnancy by preventing ovulation (release of egg from the ovaries), by thickening the mucus in the cervix to make the uterus impenetrable to sperm, and by thinning the lining of the uterus to prevent implantation.[2]

Box 22.2 Insertable Devices Listed Here by Their Intended Health Target Are Described in Further Detail Below
- Contraception.
  - Barrier method (i.e., internal condom, diaphragm, cervical cap, contraceptive sponge).
  - Hormonal method (i.e., intravaginal ring).
- Sexually transmitted infection (STI) prevention.
  - Barrier method (i.e., internal condom).
- Multipurpose prevention (of STI, unintended pregnancy, and/or HIV).
  - Intravaginal ring.
- Pelvic organ prolapse.
  - Pessary.
- Menstrual hygiene management.
  - Tampon.
  - Vaginal menstrual cup.
  - Cervical menstrual cup.
- Urinary incontinence management.
  - Urethral plug.
  - Modified vaginal menstrual cup.

---

[2]Although the intrauterine device (IUD) and the sub-dermal contraceptive implant are also insertable devices for prevention of unintended pregnancy, they are not included here as they have limited perceived relevance to research on an insertable device for management of fistula-related urinary incontinence.

22.3.2 Barrier Contraceptive Methods

22.3.2.1   Internal Condom

The internal condom, also known as the universal or female condom, is a small nitrile (soft plastic) disposable pouch that is inserted within the vagina or anus and provides a safe, effective non-hormonal option for dual protection against unintended pregnancy (females) and STIs (females and males). It offers a similar effectiveness at pregnancy prevention (79% effective) as the external condom (85% effective) but is inserted intravaginally for STI and pregnancy protection or into the anus for STI prevention.

22.3.2.2   Diaphragm

The diaphragm is a shallow, dome-shaped, reusable silicone cup that is inserted in the vagina with spermicide to cover the cervix, the opening of the uterus, during sex to prevent unintended pregnancy, with 88% effectiveness (Mauck et al., 2017). This device was reportedly less commonly used at the turn of the twenty-first century than in decades before (Ramjee et al., 2008).

Traditional diaphragms have come in various sizes; therefore, a woman needed to receive a pelvic exam from a provider and be fitted for an appropriate size to initiate use. New designs, such as the contoured diaphragm, are one size fits most, thus eliminating the need to access a provider. As a diaphragm can serve as a delivery platform for spermicidal or microbicidal gel, studies of a combined cervical barrier and gel delivery system informed the development and evaluation of the MPTs (mentioned next).

22.3.2.3   Cervical Cap

The cervical cap is a soft, silicone cup that is inserted vaginally, covers the cervix, and, when used with spermicide, is 71–86% effective. The cervical cap is slightly smaller than the diaphragm and shaped like a sailor's hat. With proper care, the reusable cup can last for 1 year before needing to be replaced.

22.3.2.4   Contraceptive Sponge

The contraceptive sponge, or the birth control sponge is a small, disk-shaped sponge made from soft, plastic foam that contains spermicide and is 76–88% effective. Like the cervical cap, it is inserted vaginally and fits against the cervix. The spermicide slows sperm so it cannot reach an egg.

22.3.3 Hormonal Methods

22.3.3.1   Intravaginal Ring

The intravaginal ring is a small, flexible ring that can be easily inserted and removed to prevent unintended pregnancy through the delivery of contraceptive hormones. It is 91% effective at preventing pregnancy. The traditional intravaginal ring is inserted for 3 weeks then removed for 1 week to allow for menstruation; the user then disposes of it. The device can be worn undetected during sexual activity (Huang et al., 2015).

A recent vaginal ring innovation is a progestin vaginal system that provides a full year of protection against unintended pregnancy. It does not require refrigeration, which is particularly important for distribution and use in low-resource settings, where challenges exist to maintaining the cold chain while accessing populations in the last mile. Another innovation, the progesterone contraceptive vaginal ring, is a three-month ring designed specifically for spacing while breastfeeding. This takes into account that women's contraceptive needs are dynamic throughout the life span.

22.3.4 Insertable Devices for Multipurpose Prevention

Technologies that best address the multiple sexual and reproductive health risks of women and girls in many LMICs are the multipurpose prevention technologies (MPTs). These methods include gels, intravaginal rings, or barrier devices that serve as an STI preventative (particularly HIV) and contraceptive product to reduce or prevent multiple and overlapping sexual and reproductive health risks (Brady & Manning, 2013). The conceptual approach assumes that the device could be more acceptable and easier to adhere to if it served more than one function.

22.3.4.1   Multipurpose Prevention Intravaginal Ring (IVR)

The multipurpose prevention intravaginal ring, similar to the traditional intravaginal ring described in Sect. 22.3.3.1, is a polyurethane reservoir technology that is inserted vaginally and provides a controlled release of a diverse range of drugs for 3 months or longer. The ring can deliver drug combinations from either a single or dual reservoir design, which allows for delivery of multiple active agents from independently controlled segments of the ring.

22.3.5 Insertable Devices for Pelvic Organ Prolapse

22.3.5.1   Pessary

The pessary is a soft device that is fitted into the vagina and provides support to vaginal tissues displaced by pelvic organ prolapse (when the bladder, rectum, or uterus drops or bulges down toward the vagina). This intravaginal support device can also help with managing stress incontinence, or urinary incontinence occurring with coughing, straining, or exercising (Barber & Maher, 2013), and with preventing preterm birth. This device is rarely studied in LMICs (Jarde et al., 2019).

The pessary comes in various shapes: ring (circle-shaped and can be inserted and removed without physician fitting), Gehrung (U-shaped and requires physician fitting), Gellhorn (disk-shaped, with a small knob in the center), and cube (uses suction to provide support).

22.3.6 Insertable Devices for Menstrual Hygiene Management

22.3.6.1   Tampon

The tampon, cylindrical in shape and made of cotton, rayon, or a blend of the two, is a disposable insertable device for managing menstruation. Tampons are designed either to be inserted with the use of a plastic or cardboard applicator or to be directly inserted manually without an applicator.

The invention of the applicator tampon dates back to the late nineteenth century (The British Medical Journal, 1879), although multiple examples predating this publication observe women in various cultural settings had developed tools for self-managing their menstrual flow using absorptive materials to which they had access, including wool, vegetable fibers, paper, and grasses (Fetters, 2015).

22.3.6.2   Vaginal Menstrual Cup

The vaginal menstrual cup is a bell-shaped device that is inserted in the vagina, typically made of medical-grade silicone (or alternatively of rubber, latex, or elastomer), that is used to collect menstrual flow and eliminate odor. It is washed after being emptied, and boiled after each period, and, with proper care, can be reused up to 10 years. Disposable single-use menstrual cups also exist. Results from a recent systematic review and meta-analysis suggest reported leakage is similar or lower for menstrual cups than for disposable pads or tampon (van Eijk et al., 2019).

22.3.6.3 Cervical Menstrual Cup

The cervical menstrual cup, like the contraceptive diaphragm, is placed around the cervix high in the vagina. In one study in Zimbabwe of the hypothetical acceptability of a one-size-fits-all, polyurethane insertable MPT which could also be used as a cervical menstrual cup, results suggest the product was feasible and devices for multiple purposes (i.e., menstrual hygiene management, contraception, prevention from STI) have a perceived benefit among users and should be further studied (Averbach et al., 2009). The cup's effectiveness for menstrual hygiene management in an LMIC has not been reported (van Eijk et al., 2019).

22.3.7 Insertable Devices for Urinary Incontinence

22.3.7.1 Urethral Plug

The internal urethral device, also referred to as intraurethral device, is a small silicone cylinder that is temporarily inserted into the urethra using an applicator or insertion probe. A small balloon is inflated after insertion which is also designed to secure the device in the urethra. Urethral plugs have been used among women with urethral incontinence as an alternative therapy to additional surgery to address urinary incontinence. Urethral plugs have been found to help 75.7% of women leaking urine from the urethra after successful fistula repair in Ethiopia, although risks include plug rupture, migration into the bladder, and infection (Brook & Tessema, 2013). The only version currently available on the market is made from a soft, compressible, mineral oil-filled silicone material and comes in one size only.

22.3.7.2 Modified Vaginal Menstrual Cup for Vesico-Vaginal Fistula Management

This flexible reservoir cup is acceptable, safe, and effective in preventing leakage of menstrual blood among women and girls in LMICs where fistula is prevalent (Beksinska et al., 2015; Juma et al., 2017; van Eijk et al., 2019). Programmatic and clinical case reports suggest the utility of the menstrual cup, when used appropriately, for collection or control of urinary leakage in women with vesicovaginal fistula (VVF), the anatomical classification of the injury which could benefit from such a novel use (Goldberg et al., 2016; New Vision Reporter, 2012; Russell et al., 2016). Within a feasibility study on the use of the cup among women with fistula (who had or had not previously attempted surgical repair) at a health facility in Ghana, researchers observed via a pad test a 46 mL (95% CI: 11.4–81.4) or 61.0% (95% CI: 35.9–86.2) mean reduction in volume of urine leakage over 2 h (Ganyaglo et al., 2018). Most participants perceived a reduction in leakage and reported this prototype was acceptable based on ease of insertion and removal and comfort while wearing. No adverse events attributed to the cup were reported by participants or observed on clinical exam. Because this was a small sample, subgroup analyses were not possible. Research on longer use and follow-up is warranted, including for design modifications, or the addition of tubing and a leg bag that could be attached and allow for urine storage of a greater capacity (i.e., 500 mL with a leg bag vs 30 mL with cup alone). Additionally, it will be necessary to identify which type of woman could most benefit from the use of this insertable device, based on preferences, anatomical characteristics, leakage severity, socio-demographics, and contextual factors.

It is clear that IDs have multiple applications for women's health and well-being across the lifespan—from adolescence through the reproductive years to older age—and for multiple purposes, including menstrual hygiene management, contraception and/or prevention of sexually transmitted infection, pelvic organ prolapse, and urinary incontinence. Although these devices may be clinically effective, respective to their targets for women's health and well-being, various shared challenges to their implementation in LMICs exist and may inform development and implementation of future insertable devices, including for the purpose of therapeutic management of fistula-related urinary incontinence.

22.4 Barriers and Facilitators to Development and Implementation of Insertable Devices for Women's Health in LMICs

Just as lessons learned from the development of hormonal and barrier methods of insertable devices for reproductive health went on to inform the later development of insertable devices, such as MPTs (Brady & Manning, 2013; Fernandez-Romero et al., 2015; Friend et al., 2013), and various global health interventions, such as PrEP and HIV prevention technologies, so too can previous challenges and successes of insertable devices for women's health in LMICs inform research on a therapeutic insertable device to manage fistula-related incontinence. The multi-level factors contributing as barriers or facilitators to development and implementation are indicated below.

22.4.1 Challenges and Barriers to Development and Implementation

Although there are various challenges to the development and implementation of insertable devices for women's health in LMICs, some barriers identified earlier on during introduction were addressed in later research and implementation. As indicated in the aforementioned conceptual framework, challenges to development and implementation are presented from the micro to the meso to the macro level, respectively, including product characteristics, user and provider attributes, social and environmental issues, health system influences, and cultural factors.

At the level of the individual, user attributes can significantly influence implementation, attributes which may be directly related to the characteristics of the device itself, such as its design, duration of action, and type and severity of related side effects. For example, internal condoms initially suffered from a lack of design varieties that affected ease of insertion and removal, comfort, and sensation while using, thus reducing acceptability (Brady & Manning, 2013). Additionally, some global health programs focused their efforts for internal condom distribution on reaching female sex workers, a highly stigmatized group at high risk of HIV infection; this resulted in the unintended consequence of lasting stigma associated with the use of internal condoms and reduced acceptability in other populations. Reduced user acceptability of other MPTs also proved a challenge within early, large clinical trials in LMICs (Ramjee et al., 2008). Trials were planned without understanding product-user interaction, including misunderstanding normative vaginal washing or douching practices and insertion of substances, which may have confounded treatment effect (Atujuna et al., 2018; Sivapalasingam et al., 2014). The menstrual cup, an innovation highlighted more recently as the topic of menstruation gains priority within the global health agenda, is an acceptable innovation for women and girls in LMICs; however, the cup is not as readily available as existing menstrual products on the market (Tellier et al., 2012; Tellier & Hyttel, 2018).

In addition to user influences, the implementer (i.e., clinical provider) and their interaction with and perceptions of the insertable device are also an individual-level factor that can influence implementation. Indeed, adoption of the internal condom in LMICs has been negatively affected by provider bias (i.e., low provider acceptability), as well as comparatively high cost, even though there is generally interest among many women, along with global health advocates, for a user-controlled device for dual protection from STIs and prevention of unintended pregnancy (Brady & Manning, 2013). Moreover, healthcare providers may not be trained on IDs or available to provide the counseling and services that women require in order to address their reproductive health, incontinence, or gynecological needs with the use of an insertable device (Abdool, 2011). There is a marked lack of standardized guidelines for devices like the pessary, which reduces implementation fidelity.

Challenges to the uptake of insertable devices based on social relationships and environmental considerations persist in LMICs. Socio-behavioral issues, such as social costs, risk perception, and self-efficacy, contribute to demand and use of insertable devices. Adoption of insertable devices for menstrual hygiene management, for example, reminds us of the importance of encouraging and shaping a supportive social environment when introducing technocratic solutions. Persistent cultural taboos regarding menstruation may reduce or prevent adoption of menstrual cups by girls in LMICs, just as resistance from a sexual partner prevents adoption of insertables for contraception and STI prevention (Hyttel et al., 2017; Tolley et al., 2013). Challenges to uptake of menstrual cups further touch on environmental barriers, including lack of running water as well as appropriate water and sanitation facilities in schools that would allow girls to appropriately use menstrual cups. Hygiene concerns, including hand hygiene when using these devices, play an important role for safety and effectiveness with all insertable devices.

Today there are additional structural factors at the level of the health system which challenge uptake and sustainability of insertable devices in LMICs, including limited funding, lack of donor commitment, and competing budget priorities (Abdool, 2011; Brady & Manning, 2013; Tellier & Hyttel, 2018). Indeed, the main source of contraception in most LMICs comes from the public sector, which typically offers limited options, thus insertable devices are not always available. Stock outs and procurement issues challenge the feasible implementation of IDs in these contexts (Abdool, 2011). Additionally, the requirement for interaction with a provider in a clinical setting prior to initiation may also serve as a barrier. For example, earlier designs, such as for the contraceptive diaphragm, required a clinical assessment and fitting by a physician before initiation; this reduced accessibility and thus feasible implementation, particularly among women and girls in lowest resource settings. Additionally, comparatively high cost led to an imbalance in supply and demand, which ultimately reduced user acceptability and uptake (Brady, 2011; Pratt, 2008). Reduced market competition can leave women with limited options for acceptable, appropriate devices. For example, the manufacturer of the most commonly used urethral plug has ceased production, resulting in many women being left without options to self-manage their urethral urinary incontinence.

22.4.2 Successes and Facilitators to Development and Implementation

Various successes for the development and implementation of insertable devices for the health and well-being of women and girls in LMICs have been informed by incorporation of design thinking; utilization of mixed methodological approaches to understand needs, impact, and processes; and recent integration of implementation research methods.

Regarding the individual level facilitators, there have been notable successes regarding increased acceptability, appropriateness, and adoption. New iterations of insertable devices (i.e., for the internal condom and MPTs) developed through human-centered design processes (Bazzano et al., 2017), allow for greater user acceptability. In fact, the human-centered design presents a design paradigm, as described by Giacomin (2014), that places user acceptability at the focal point, examining human behaviors and meanings through "techniques which communicate, interact, empathize and stimulate the people involved, obtaining an understanding of their needs, desires, and experiences which often transcends that which the people themselves actually realized" (p. 610). Research efforts regarding the effectiveness of MPTs, like the IVR (Ugaonkar et al., 2015), have begun to embed acceptability studies and qualitative examination early on in clinical studies (Guthrie et al., 2018) and prioritize user perspectives (Rosen et al., 2015) in LMICs (Minnis et al., 2018). Studies have shown that acceptability increases over time as the user becomes more comfortable with insertion and removal and builds comfort with touching one's vagina (Brady & Manning, 2013; Tellier & Hyttel, 2018; van Eijk et al., 2019). This has been recently observed with the menstrual cup, but also with the diaphragm and internal condom. Recent interventions with IDs in LMICs that moderately improved knowledge, attitudes, and practices for menstrual hygiene management in particular prioritized user acceptability (Tellier & Hyttel, 2018). This turn toward acceptability research was informed by earlier studies of IDs for dual and multipurpose prevention in which lack of understanding of context confounded impact. Successful insertable device implementation is now coupled with targeted marketing and education regarding the product (i.e., product effectiveness, side effects, etc.).

Successes have also been noted by encouraging facilitators at the interpersonal and community levels. Research and programs have evolved to recognize that women have different needs for contraception based on individual and family characteristics and those needs may change throughout the reproductive lifespan. For example, a hormonal method used prior to childbirth may not be appropriate once a woman has a child and is breastfeeding. The MPTs consider women's preference for discreet use without knowledge of sexual partner, for use in a context where women may have reduced capacity to negotiate sexual activity (Fernandez-Romero et al., 2015). The progestin IVR, one MPT which provides a full year of protection against unintended pregnancy and does not require refrigeration, seems increasingly appropriate for general use in LMICs; whereas the progesterone IVR is designed specifically for spacing while breastfeeding. Contraceptive prevalence increases if the contraceptive mix increases, or additional methods are made available in a given location. Increased choice might increase user acceptability and encourage new users.

However, individual decision making should not be prioritized without consideration of a supportive environment in which to use these devices. Building support for use by girls and women from peers, partners, and other influential community members can provide an enabling environment (Tellier & Hyttel, 2018). Research in LMICs suggests programmers have to include the product with supplies which make it possible to wash the cup, including soap, washbasins, drying facilities, and possibilities for boiling, if required. (Hyttel et al., 2017; Tellier et al., 2012; Tellier & Hyttel, 2018) The usability, acceptability, and adherence of insertables provide examples of how it is necessary to understand the cultural, social, and institutional context of how gender practices influence the use of a device.

22.5   Application of Lessons Learned with Insertable Devices for Health and Well-being of Women and Girls in LMICs to Inform Development and Implementation of an Insertable Device for Therapeutic Management of Obstetric Fistula

Research and implementation of a therapeutic tool for self-management of fistula-related urinary incontinence are informed by various challenges and successes of the development and implementation of existing insertable devices for women's health in LMICs, including those for the purposes of management of urinary incontinence, contraception and/or pregnancy prevention, or menstrual hygiene management. Learning from lessons past, previous challenges to avoid or mitigate include: non-optimal design that limits user acceptability; provider bias due to limited training or lack of clinical guidelines for the provision of IDs; a misunderstanding of user-device interaction and context for use; lack of enabling social and physical environment, including limited support from peers, partner, and other community members and appropriate supportive supplies and facilities for use; concerns regarding individual cost and low donor commitment; and difficulties with procurement reducing availability and provider acceptability. Previous successes addressed some of these earlier challenges and should be modeled in the development and implementation of this novel device (see Box 22.3). These include the utilization of design thinking and human-centered design approaches to prioritize user's dynamic needs and increase acceptability and appropriateness; increasing user-controlled device options to improve penetration within a population; increasing accessibility to safe, appropriate ID options by reducing the need for travel to a clinical facility prior to initiation; and delivering products with supportive materials (i.e., relevant education, soap and washbasin to clean and maintain device) and within enabling environments (i.e., encouraging social support for use).

Box 22.3 Lessons Learned to Apply to Development and Implementation of IDs for Obstetric Fistula Management

- Prioritize acceptability early on in research process.
  - Improved user acceptability, improved appropriateness.
- Introduce user-controlled therapeutic ID options.
  - Increased penetration.
- Anticipate provider training needs and provide clinical guidelines.
  - Improved provider acceptability, increased adoption, increased fidelity.
- Integrate a community-based approach with a facility-based approach based on context.
  - Improved accessibility, increased penetration.
- Deliver product with supportive materials (i.e., user education, soap and wash basin to clean and maintain device).
  - Improved appropriateness, improved user acceptability, increased feasibility.
- Implement within an enabling environment (i.e., encouraging social support for use).
  - Improved appropriateness, increased feasibility.

Applying this knowledge, future research should utilize various intervention and implementation strategies accordingly (see Box 22.4). Research will use human-centered design processes to prioritize user acceptability and input through qualitative assessment nested in clinical trials. Women with a lived experience of repaired or existing obstetric fistula should be involved in the design and implementation of this product, much as post-repair fistula patients have gone on to provide a critical role as survivor advocates to assist with various activities, including supporting anti-stigma campaigns and recruitment for repair. Although comprehensive fistula programming already focuses on prevention, repair, and reintegration, therapeutic management could also be prioritized. If therapeutic devices are found to be effective in such trials, they should be integrated into comprehensive fistula programming to reach all women and girls in need. This could be achieved by developing research and implementation partnerships with important fistula stakeholders, identifying champions to support implementation, and creating educational materials to increase acceptability among clinical providers. It will be critical to develop buy in among frontline health workers, who are the gatekeepers for fistula patients and who regularly go above and beyond provision of fistula care—many times serving dual roles as care provider and patient advocate. Use of the cup, as with other insertables, requires repeated behaviors (i.e., insertion, removal, cleaning, maintenance) and there may be a learning curve for appropriate use; users may need women-centered, supportive counseling to initiate and continue use.

Multi-sectoral partnerships have already been successfully prioritized by the Population Fund (UNFPA), the UN agency tasked with fistula prevention, treatment, and reintegration, and sustainable, scalable intervention for therapeutic management of obstetric fistula should also be incorporated. Implementation of effective therapeutic tools will need lasting donor and government commitment for a sustainable intervention and reliable product supply, as end users cannot be expected to purchase cups themselves. This could be encouraged through integration into existing programs and structures. As with the provision of insertables for other purposes, fistula care is delivered through multiple sectors within a healthcare system (i.e., public, non-profit, and faith-based sectors). The best mix of program entry points and distribution channels for therapeutic self-management of fistula-related urinary incontinence will depend on regional and national context and should be integrated into ongoing programming. Researchers will need to study implementation in different contexts to balance the tension between implementation fidelity and appropriateness for the local context. This research should be guided by health behavior and implementation science theory.

Although some fistula care settings provide support for therapeutic self-management for residual incontinence (Castille et al., 2015), less attention has been paid to therapeutic self-management for fistula-related incontinence. This has ethical implications for women who are receiving multiple surgical attempts that are likely to be unsuccessful. As integration of therapeutic self-management into fistula management options introduces a change in approach from surgical management alone, this poses a somewhat radical departure from existing clinical practices which may suggest that the speed of uptake will be slow. Significant marketing efforts may be necessary, including market development which may manifest as educating health care professionals, forming partnerships with advocacy organizations, and conducting public awareness campaigns (Brady & Manning, 2013). Although this vaginal cup is innovative in its application to a new target population and ongoing design modifications, this chapter shows that the use of insertable devices for women's health is widespread for various functions. We should also remind ourselves that women have always utilized materials from their environment to address their gynecological needs, such as using plant material for menstrual hygiene management or fabrics for incontinence management, but this is less likely to be recognized as "an innovation". The provision of an insertable cup for management of fistula-related urinary incontinence merely provides a safer and more effective tool. Indeed, research of women living with fistula in LMICs has already suggested the transformative power of concealing leakage so that one may "pass" (Goffman, 1963) as a non-stigmatized, non-discredited individual (Heller, 2018). If the cup allows women to effectively manage leaking and conceal their stigmatized identity, they may gain self-efficacy to overcome stigma and will seek available fistula treatment; therefore, integration of therapeutic self-management tools into comprehensive fistula programs could improve access to surgical repair.

Existing research has focused on the surgical approaches in the management of fistula; (Arrowsmith et al., 2010; Tebeu et al., 2012; Waaldijk, 1995); however, comparatively less focus has been applied to understanding women's options for self-management of this chronic condition for women who cannot or will not get timely, effective surgical repair. As the mean length of time a woman lives with fistula before obtaining repair is 4–10 years (Delamou et al., 2015; Maulet et al., 2013; Sori et al., 2016), due to various individual, social, and structural barriers to repair, and successful surgical repair is not guaranteed for all who undergo surgery, user-controlled tools for therapeutic self-management have the potential to improve the quality of life of many women living with this chronic condition. An assets-based approach to understanding women's lived experience with fistula, which focuses on the actual or potential strengths within the capacity of affected women to improve their quality of life, highlights that women who have not accessed successful repair attempt to creatively manage their incontinence and related odor with available low-cost materials, however, with limited perceived effectiveness and appropriateness (Ryan, 2019) Future research on an insertable device to manage fistula-related urinary incontinence is necessary to truly address the needs of women and girls in LMICs suffering with this highly stigmatized condition.

Box 22.4 Potential Strategies for Implementation of IDs for Obstetric Fistula Management
- Utilize design thinking and human-centered design approaches.
- Develop research and implementation partnerships with fistula stakeholders.
- Identify and include champions to support implementation.
- Create educational materials to increase acceptability among clinical providers.
- Develop guidelines to guide clinical practice of frontline health workers.
- Market development (i.e., conducting public awareness campaigns).

22.6   Conclusions

In this chapter, we survey the widespread use of insertable devices for various purposes related to women's health. To our knowledge, this is the first review to gather evidence on these tools to support health and well-being among women and girls in LMICs, in part due to the fact that research has been previously siloed by target health condition. Examining the successes and challenges of implementing these insertable devices across the literature highlights lessons learned for development and implementation of an insertable vaginal cup for non-surgical management of obstetric fistula. This cup may allow users to self-manage leaking, conceal their stigmatized identity, gain self-efficacy to overcome stigma, and thus seek surgical repair. Therapeutic use of this product would not replace surgical repair of fistula, rather it could improve quality of life for those identified with vesico-vaginal fistula and waiting for surgery (or who are not ready for surgery for whatever personal reasons). Simultaneously, systems-level interventions to scale-up surgery to prevent and repair fistula should be ongoing—but these structural initiatives require major investment, political will, prolonged engagement, and time.

The cup, which may provide a temporary solution to prevent vulnerability to stigma that in many cases can be quite severe, could be implemented with various strategies. These range from prioritizing user acceptability via human-centered design approaches to improving provider adoption, fidelity, and acceptability via provider training and provision of clinical guidelines to developing research and implementation partnerships with fistula stakeholders. While trials to assess clinical effectiveness of this cup are ongoing, ultimately, successful implementation will in part be based on women's needs and fistula care services already in place. Future research will need to assess context-specific factors that shape intervention and implementation success, in hopes of building an appropriate implementation strategy.

References

Abdool, Z. (2011). Evaluation of vaginal pessary use by south African gynaecologists. *South African Journal of Obstetrics and Gynaecology, 17*(3), 64–67. https://doi.org/10.7196/sajog.386

Adefris, M., Abebe, S. M., Terefe, K., Gelagay, A. A., Adigo, A., Amare, S., et al. (2017). Reasons for delay in decision making and reaching health facility among obstetric fistula and pelvic organ prolapse patients in Gondar University hospital, Northwest Ethiopia. *BMC Womens Health, 17*(1), 64. https://doi.org/10.1186/s12905-017-0416-9. Retrieved February 1, 2020, from https://www.ncbi.nlm.nih.gov/pmc/articles/PMC5567648/

Adler, A. J., Ronsmans, C., Calvert, C., & Filippi, V. (2013). Estimating the prevalence of obstetric fistula: A systematic review and meta-analysis. *BMC Pregnancy and Childbirth, 13*, 246. https://doi.org/10.1186/1471-2393-13-246. Retrieved February 1, 2020, from https://www.ncbi.nlm.nih.gov/pmc/articles/PMC3937166/

Ahmed, S., & Holtz, S. A. (2007). Social and economic consequences of obstetric fistula: Life changed forever? *International Journal of Gynaecology and Obstetrics, 99*(Suppl 1), S10–S15. https://doi.org/10.1016/j.ijgo.2007.06.011

Alio, A. P., Merrell, L., Roxburgh, K., Clayton, H. B., Marty, P. J., Bomboka, L., et al. (2011). The psychosocial impact of vesico-vaginal fistula in Niger. *Archives of Gynecology and Obstetrics, 284*(2), 371–378. https://doi.org/10.1007/s00404-010-1652-5

Arrowsmith, S. D., Ruminjo, J., & Landry, E. G. (2010). Current practices in treatment of female genital fistula: A cross sectional study. *BMC Pregnancy and Childbirth, 10*, 73. https://doi.org/10.1186/1471-2393-10-73. Retrieved February 3, 2020, from https://www.ncbi.nlm.nih.gov/pmc/articles/PMC2995487/

Atujuna, M., Newman, P. A., Wallace, M., Eluhu, M., Rubincam, C., Brown, B., et al. (2018). Contexts of vulnerability and the acceptability of new biomedical HIV prevention technologies among key populations in South Africa: A qualitative study. *PLoS One, 13*(2), e0191251. https://doi.org/10.1371/journal.pone.0191251

Averbach, S., Sahin-Hodoglugil, N., Musara, P., Chipato, T., & van der Staten, A. (2009). Duet for menstrual protection: A feasibility study in Zimbabwe. *Contraception, 79*(6), 463–468. https://doi.org/10.1016/j.contraception.2008.12.002

Baker, Z., Bellows, B., Bach, R., & Warren, C. (2017). Barriers to obstetric fistula treatment in low-income countries: A systematic review. *Tropical Medicine & Interntional Health, 22*(8), 938–959. https://doi.org/10.1111/tmi.12893. Retrieved February 3, 2020, from https://onlinelibrary.wiley.com/doi/full/10.1111/tmi.12893

Bangser, M. (2006). Obstetric fistula and stigma. *Lancet, 367*(9509), 535–536. https://doi.org/10.1016/s0140-6736(06)68188-9

Banke-Thomas, A. O., Wilton-Waddell, O. E., Kouraogo, S. F., & Mueller, J. E. (2014). Current evidence supporting obstetric fistula prevention strategies in sub-Saharan Africa: A systematic review of the literature. *African Journal of Reproductive Health, 18*(3), 118. Retrieved February 3, 2020, from http://www.bioline.org.br/pdf?rh14049

Barageine, J. K., Beyeza-Kashesya, J., Byamugisha, J. K., Tumwesigye, N. M., Almroth, L., & Faxelid, E. (2015). "I am alone and isolated": A qualitative study of experiences of women living with genital fistula in Uganda. *BMC Womens Health, 15*, 73. https://doi.org/10.1186/s12905-015-0232-z. Retrieved February 3, 2020, from https://www.ncbi.nlm.nih.gov/pmc/articles/PMC4566494/

Barber, M. D., & Maher, C. (2013). Epidemiology and outcome assessment of pelvic organ prolapse. *International Urogynecology Journal, 24*(11), 1783–1790.

Bazzano, A., Martin, J., Hicks, E., Faughnan, M., & Murphy, L. (2017). Human-centred design in global health: A scoping review of applications and contexts. *PLoS One, 12*(11), e0186744. https://doi.org/10.1371/journal.pone.0186744. eCollection 2017. Retrieved February 1, 2020, from https://www.ncbi.nlm.nih.gov/pmc/articles/PMC5665524/

Beksinska, M. E., Smit, J., Greener, R., Todd, C. S., Lee, M. L., Maphumulo, V., et al. (2015). Acceptability and performance of the menstrual cup in South Africa: A randomized crossover trial comparing the menstrual cup to tampons or sanitary pads. *Journal of Womens Health (Larchmt), 24*(2), 151–158. https://doi.org/10.1089/jwh.2014.5021

Brady, M. (2011). *Constructing a critical path for product development, commercialization and access*. Population Council. https://doi.org/10.31899/hiv1.1006. Retrieved June 2018.

Brady, M., & Manning, J. (2013). Lessons from reproductive health to inform multipurpose prevention technologies: Don't reinvent the wheel. *Antiviral Research, 100*(Suppl), S25–S31. https://doi.org/10.1016/j.antiviral.2013.09.019

Bronfenbrenner, U. (1989). Ecological systems theory. *Annals of Child Development, 6*, 187–249.

Brook, G., & Tessema, A. B. (2013). Obstetric fistula: The use of urethral plugs for the management of persistent urinary incontinence following successful repair. *International Urogynecology Journal, 24*(3), 479–484. https://doi.org/10.1007/s00192-012-1887-8

Castille, Y. J., Avocetien, C., Zaongo, D., Colas, J. M., Peabody, J. O., & Rochat, C. H. (2015). One-year follow-up of women who participated in a physiotherapy and health education program before and after obstetric fistula surgery. *International Journal of Gynaecology and Obstetrics, 128*(3), 264–266. https://doi.org/10.1016/j.ijgo.2014.09.028

Changole, J., Thorsen, V. C., & Kafulafula, U. (2017). "I am a person but I am not a person": Experiences of women living with obstetric fistula in the central region of Malawi. *BMC Pregnancy and Childbirth, 17*(1), 433. https://doi.org/10.1186/s12884-017-1604-1. Retrieved February 1, 2020, from https://www.ncbi.nlm.nih.gov/pmc/articles/PMC5740704/

Chao, T., Lo, N., Mody, G., & Sinha, S. (2014). Strategies for last mile implementation of global health technologies. *The Lancet Global Health, 2*(9), e497–e498. Retrieved February 1, 2020, from https://www.thelancet.com/journals/langlo/article/PIIS2214-109X(14)70253-0/fulltext

Delamou, A., Delvaux, T., Utz, B., Camara, B. S., Beavoqui, A. H., Cole, B., et al. (2015). Factors associated with loss to follow-up in women undergoing repair for obstetric fistula in Guinea. *Tropical Medicine & International Health, 20*, 1454–1461. Retrieved February 1, 2020, from https://onlinelibrary.wiley.com/doi/full/10.1111/tmi.12584

Fernandez-Romero, J. A., Deal, C., Herold, B. C., Schiller, J., Patton, D., Zydowsky, T., et al. (2015). Multipurpose prevention technologies: The future of HIV and STI protection. *Trends in Microbiology, 23*(7), 429–436. https://doi.org/10.1016/j.tim.2015.02.006

Fetters, A. (2015, June 1). The tampon: A history, the cultural, political, and technological roots of a fraught piece of cotton. *The Atlantic.* https://www.theatlantic.com/health/archive/2015/06/history-of-the-tampon/394334/

Friend, D. R., Clark, J. T., Kiser, P. F., & Clark, M. R. (2013). Multipurpose prevention technologies: Products in development. *Antiviral Research, 100*(Suppl), S39–S47. https://doi.org/10.1016/j.antiviral.2013.09.030

Ganyaglo, G. Y. K., Ryan, N., Park, J., & Lassey, A. T. (2018). Feasibility and acceptability of the menstrual cup for non-surgical management of vesicovaginal fistula among women at a health facility in Ghana. *PLoS One, 13*(11), e0207925. https://doi.org/10.1371/journal.pone.0207925. Retrieved February 1, 2020, from https://www.ncbi.nlm.nih.gov/pmc/articles/PMC6261596/

Gebresilase, Y. T. (2014). A qualitative study of the experience of obstetric fistula survivors in Addis Ababa, Ethiopia. *International Journal of Women's Health, 6,* 1033–1043. Retrieved February 3, 2020, from https://www.ncbi.nlm.nih.gov/pmc/articles/PMC4266262/

Giacomin, J. (2014). What is human centred design? *Design, 17*(4), 606–623.

Goffman, E. (1963). *Stigma: Notes on the management of spoiled identity.* Prentice-Hall.

Goldberg, L., Elsamra, S., Hutchinson-Colas, J., & Segal, S. (2016). Delayed diagnosis of vesicouterine fistula after treatment for mixed urinary incontinence: Menstrual cup management and diagnosis. *Female Pelvic Medicine & Reconstructive Surgery, 22*(5), e29–e31. https://doi.org/10.1097/SPV.0000000000000301

Guthrie, K. M., Rosen, R. K., Vargas, S. E., Getz, M. L., Dawson, L., Guillen, M., et al. (2018). User evaluations offer promise for pod-intravaginal ring as a drug delivery platform: A mixed methods study of acceptability and use experiences. *PLoS One, 13*(5), 1–18. https://doi.org/10.1371/journal.pone.0197269. Retrieved February 2, 2020, from https://www.ncbi.nlm.nih.gov/pmc/articles/PMC5951541/

Heller, A. (2018). Transforming obstetric fistula through concealment in Niger. *Human Organization, 77*(3), 239–248. https://doi.org/10.17730/0018-7259.77.3.239

Huang, Y., Merkatz, R. B., Hillier, S. L., Roberts, K., Blithe, D. L., Sitruk-Ware, R., et al. (2015). Effects of a one year reusable contraceptive vaginal ring on vaginal microflora and the risk of vaginal infection: An open-label prospective evaluation. *PLoS One, 10*(8), e0134460. https://doi.org/10.1371/journal.pone.0134460. Retrieved February 3, 2020, from https://www.ncbi.nlm.nih.gov/pmc/articles/PMC4534458/

Hyttel, M., Thomsen, C. F., Luff, B., Tellier, M., Storrusten, H., & Nyakato, V. N. (2017). Drivers and challenges to use of menstrual cups among schoolgirls in rural Uganda: A qualitative study. *Waterlines, 36*(2), 109–124. https://doi.org/10.3362/1756-3488.16-00013

Jarde, A., Lutsiv, O., Beyene, J., & McDonald, S. D. (2019). Vaginal progesterone, oral progesterone, 17-OHPC, cerclage, and pessary for preventing preterm birth in at-risk singleton pregnancies: An updated systematic review and network meta-analysis. *BJOG: An International Journal of Obstetrics & Gynaecology, 126*(5), 556–567. https://doi.org/10.1111/1471-0528.15566

Jarvis, K., Richter, S., & Vallianatos, H. (2017). Exploring the needs and challenges of women reintegrating after obstetric fistula repair in northern Ghana. *Midwifery, 50,* 55–61. https://doi.org/10.1016/j.midw.2017.03.013

Jarvis, K., Richter, S., Vallianatos, H., & Thornton, L. (2017). Reintegration of women post obstetric fistula repair: Experience of family caregivers. *Global Qualitative Nursing Research, 4,* 2333393617714927. https://doi.org/10.1177/2333393617714927. Retrieved February 3, 2020, from https://www.ncbi.nlm.nih.gov/pmc/articles/PMC5528919/

Juma, J., Nyothach, E., Laserson, K. F., Oduor, C., Arita, L., Ouma, C., et al. (2017). Examining the safety of menstrual cups among rural primary school girls in western Kenya: Observational studies nested in a randomised controlled feasibility study. *BMJ Open, 7*(4), e015429. https://doi.org/10.1136/bmjopen-2016-015429. Retrieved February 3, 2020, from https://www.ncbi.nlm.nih.gov/pmc/articles/PMC5566618/

Kabayambi, J., Barageine, J. K., Matovu, J. K. B., Beyeza, J., & Ekirapa, E. (2014). Living with obstetric fistula: Perceived causes, challenges and coping strategies among women attending the fistula clinic at Mulago hospital, Uganda. *International Journal of Tropical Disease and Health, 4*(3), 352–361. https://doi.org/10.9734/ijtdh/2014/7505

Khisa, A. M., Omoni, G. M., Nyamongo, I. K., & Spitzer, R. F. (2017). 'I stayed with my illness': A grounded theory study of health seeking behaviour and treatment pathways of patients with obstetric fistula in Kenya. *BMC Womens Health, 17*(1), 92. https://doi.org/10.1186/s12905-017-0451-6. February 3, 2020, from https://www.ncbi.nlm.nih.gov/pmc/articles/PMC5622500/

Mauck, C. K., Brache, V., Kimble, T., Thurman, A., Cochon, L., Littlefield, S., et al. (2017). A phase I randomized postcoital testing and safety study of the Caya diaphragm used with 3% Nonoxynol-9 gel, ContraGel or no gel. *Contraception, 96*(2), 124–130. https://doi.org/10.1016/j.contraception.2017.05.016. Epub 2017 Jun 9.

Maulet, N., Keita, M., & Macq, J. (2013). Medico-social pathways of obstetric fistula patients in Mali and Niger: An 18-month cohort follow-up. *Tropical Medicine & International Health, 18*(5), 524–533. https://doi.org/10.1111/tmi.12086. Retrieved February 2, 2020, from https://onlinelibrary.wiley.com/doi/full/10.1111/tmi.12086

Minnis, A. M., Roberts, S. T., Agot, K., Weinrib, R., Ahmed, K., Manenzhe, K., et al. (2018). Young women's ratings of three placebo multipurpose prevention technologies for HIV and pregnancy prevention in a randomized, cross-over study in Kenya and South Africa. *AIDS & Behavior, 22*(8), 2662–2673. https://doi.org/10.1007/s10461-018-2078-5. Retrieved February 3, 2020, from https://www.ncbi.nlm.nih.gov/pmc/articles/PMC6097726/

Mwini-Nyaledzigbor, P. P., Agana, A. A., & Pilkington, F. B. (2013). Lived experiences of Ghanaian women with obstetric fistula. *Health Care for Women International, 34*(6), 440–460. https://doi.org/10.1080/07399332.2012.755981

New Vision Reporter. (2012). *Menstrual cup: Temporary relief for fistula patients*. New Vision. Retrieved from https://www.newvision.co.ug/new_vision/news/1307335/menstrual-cup-temporary-relief-fistula-patients

Pratt, B. (2008). Female condoms: Access to dual protection technologies. In L. Frost & M. Reich (Eds.), *Access: How do good health technologies get to poor people in poor countries?* Harvard Center for Population and Development Studies.

Proctor, E., Silmere, H., Raghavan, R., Hovmand, P., Aarons, G., Bunger, A., et al. (2011). Outcomes for implementation research: Conceptual distinctions, measurement challenges, and research agenda. *Administration and Policy in Mental Health, 38*, 65–76. Retrieved February 3, 2020, from https://www.ncbi.nlm.nih.gov/pmc/articles/PMC3068522/

Ramjee, G., van der Straten, A., Chipato, T., de Bruyn, G., Blanchard, K., Shiboski, S., et al. (2008). The diaphragm and lubricant gel for prevention of cervical sexually transmitted infections: Results of a randomized controlled trial. *PLoS One, 3*(10), e3488. https://doi.org/10.1371/journal.pone.0003488

Reports and Analyses and Descriptions of New Inventions in Medicine, Surgery, Dietetics, and the Allied Sciences. (1879). *British Medical Journal, 1*(947), 273.

Rosen, R. K., van den Berg, J. J., Vargas, S. E., Senocak, N., Shaw, J. G., Buckheit, J. R. W., et al. (2015). Meaning-making matters in product design: Users' sensory perceptions and experience evaluations of long-acting vaginal gels and intravaginal rings. *Contraception, 92*(6), 596–601. https://doi.org/10.1016/j.contraception.2015.08.007

Ruder, B., Cheyney, M., & Emasu, A. A. (2018). Too long to wait: Obstetric fistula and the sociopolitical dynamics of the fourth delay in Soroti, Uganda. *Qualitative Health Research, 28*(5), 721–732. https://doi.org/10.1177/1049732317754084

Russell, K. W., Robinson, R. E., Mone, M. C., & Scaife, C. L. (2016). Enterovaginal or vesicovaginal fistula control using a silicone cup. *Obstetrics and Gynecology, 128*(6), 1365–1368. https://doi.org/10.1097/AOG.0000000000001745

Ryan, N. (2019). *Stigma and coping among women living with obstetric fistula in Ghana: A mixed methods study*. New York University College of Global Public Health. (PhD).

Sivapalasingam, S., McClelland, R. S., Ravel, J., Ahmed, A., Cleland, C. M., Gajer, P., et al. (2014). An effective intervention to reduce intravaginal practices among HIV-1 uninfected Kenyan women. *AIDS Research and Human Retroviruses, 30*(11), 1046–1054. https://doi.org/10.1089/aid.2013.0251

Sori, D. A., Azale, A. W., & Gemeda, D. H. (2016). Characteristics and repair outcome of patients with vesicovaginal fistula managed in Jimma University teaching Hospital, Ethiopia. *BMC Urology, 16*, 41.

Sullivan, G., O'Brien, B., & Mwini-Nyaledzigbor, P. (2016). Sources of support for women experiencing obstetric fistula in northern Ghana: A focused ethnography. *Midwifery, 40*, 162–168. https://doi.org/10.1016/j.midw.2016.07.005

Tebeu, P. M., Fomulu, J. N., Khaddaj, S., de Bernis, L., Delvaux, T., & Rochat, C. H. (2012). Risk factors for obstetric fistula: A clinical review. *International Urogynecology Journal, 23*(4), 387–394. https://doi.org/10.1007/s00192-011-1622-x. Retrieved February 3, 2020, from https://link.springer.com/article/10.1007/s00192-011-1622-x

Tellier, M., Hyttel, M., & Gad, M. (2012). *Assessing acceptability and hygienic safety of menstrual cups as a menstrual management method for vulnerable young women in Uganda red cross Society's life planning skills project: Pilot study report*. WoMena, Uganda Red Cross Society. Retrieved from https://www.changemakers.com/sites/default/files/red_cross_and_womena_ltd_-_uganda_pilot_study_report_dec_2012_.pdf

Tellier, S., & Hyttel, M. (2018). *Menstrual health management in east and southern Africa: A review paper*. United Nations Population Fund, WoMena.

Tolley, E. E., Morrow, K. M., & Owen, D. H. (2013). Designing a multipurpose technology for acceptability and adherence. *Antiviral Research, 100*(Suppl), S54–S59. https://doi.org/10.1016/j.antiviral.2013.09.029

Ugaonkar, S. R., Wesenberg, A., Wilk, J., Seidor, S., Mizenina, O., Kizima, L., et al. (2015). A novel intravaginal ring to prevent HIV-1, HSV-2, HPV, and unintended pregnancy. *Journal of Controlled Release, 213*, 57–68. https://doi.org/10.1016/j.jconrel.2015.06.018

UN. (2014). *UN Secretary General Report: Supporting efforts to end obstetric fistula*. UN. Retrieved from https://www.unfpa.org/resources/supporting-efforts-end-obstetric-fistula-report-secretary-general

UNFPA. (2018). *Intensifying efforts to end obstetric fistula within a generation: Report of the Secretary-General*. UNFPA. Retrieved from http://www.unfpa.org/obstetric-fistula

van Eijk, A. M., Zulaika, G., Lenchner, M., Mason, L., Sivakami, M., Nyothach, E., et al. (2019). Menstrual cup use, leakage, acceptability, safety, and availability: A systematic review and meta-analysis. *The Lancet Public Health, 4*(8), e376–e393. https://doi.org/10.1016/S2468-2667(19)30111-2

Waaldijk, K. (1995). Surgical classification of obstetric fistulas. *International Journal of Gynecology & Obstetrics, 49*(2), 161–163. https://doi.org/10.1016/0020-7292(95)02350-L

Wall, L. L. (2012). Obstetric fistula is a "neglected tropical disease". *PLoS Neglected Tropical Diseases, 6*(8), e1769. https://doi.org/10.1371/journal.pntd.0001769

The Aberdeen Women's Centre: Providing Care for Girls and Women with Fistula and Other Conditions in Sierra Leone

23

Ivy Kalama

23.1 Introduction: The Aberdeen Women's Centre

The Aberdeen Women's Centre in Freetown is the sole point of care for women and girls who are suffering from obstetric fistula throughout the country. The Republic of Sierra Leone is a country on the West African coast with an estimated population of 7813, 000 in 2019 (United Nations, 2019) (Fig. 23.1). Freetown is the capital and largest city in Sierra Leone, which is recognized as one of the poorest countries in the world. For this reason, many Sierra Leoneans, particularly women, face a unique set of health challenges that are influenced by many factors.

The United Nations Population Fund's most recent report estimates that two million women in sub-Saharan Africa, the Arab States, and Latin America and the Caribbean regions currently live with obstetric fistula, with approximately 50,000 to 100,000 new cases every year (UNFPA, 2018). In 2019, 87% of deliveries were attended by skilled personnel, and the most recent national-level maternal mortality estimates found Sierra Leone has one of the highest maternal mortality rates in the world with 1,120 maternal deaths per 100,000 live births in 2017 (UNICEF, 2019). In Sierra Leone, maternal deaths account for more than a third of all deaths of women aged 15 to 49 (UNFPA, 2018). A myriad of factors contribute to the high maternal and neonatal mortality rates in Sierra Leone. In 2014, Lancet produced a new journal series "Every Newborn" which identified that the majority of maternal deaths occur within a 24-hour time frame from labour. This report also identified that the most compounding factor attributing to this was poor quality of care (The Lancet, 2014).

The Freedom from Fistula Foundation's Aberdeen Women's Centre has become the second busiest maternity hospital in Sierra Leone. It is also the safest, with 0.17% maternal death rate in 2018 (FFF 2019). It is also the only dedicated fistula treatment centre in the country. AWC provides expert surgical care to women and girls who have experienced prolonged, obstructed labour and consequently suffer from obstetric fistula. The Centre's focus has been to treat fistula by providing high-quality, holistic and free care to patients and prevent fistula through the provision of safe maternal health care.

I. Kalama (✉)
Freedom from Fistula Foundation, Freetown, Sierra Leone
e-mail: Ivy.Kalama@gloagfoundation.com

© Springer Nature Switzerland AG 2022
L. B. Drew et al. (eds.), *A Multidisciplinary Approach to Obstetric Fistula in Africa*, Global
Maternal and Child Health, https://doi.org/10.1007/978-3-031-06314-5_23

Fig. 23.1 Map of Sierra Leone, highlighting Freetown where the Aberdeen Women's Centre is situated. (Source: Sierra Leone map showing major population centres as well as parts of surrounding countries and the North Atlantic Ocean. The World Factbook, 2021. Washington, DC: Central Intelligence Agency, 2021. https://www.cia.gov/the-world-factbook/)

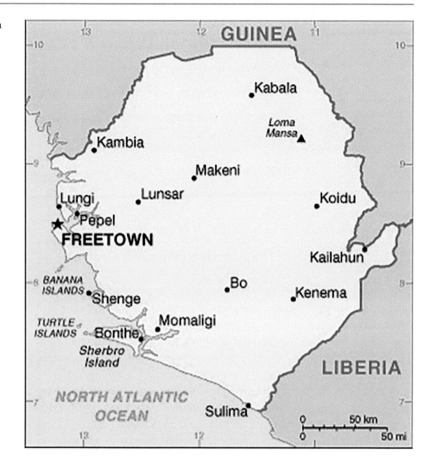

Additionally, AWC provides a free outpatient children's clinic for children up to 15 years of age who were either born in our maternity unit or live in the surrounding communities.

Since its inception in 2008, AWC has safely delivered more than 14,000 babies, performed 6700 fistula surgeries and provided primary care to more than 110,000 children (FFF, , 2019). The Scottish-based Gloag Foundation provides the management oversight of AWC and has financial responsibility for the project, through its Freedom from Fistula Foundation charity. Additional donors to AWC include the Aminata Maternal Foundation, UNFPA, Mercy Ships and others. This generous support assists the Centre's three main functions: the fistula clinic, the maternity clinic and the outpatient children's clinic.

23.2   Fistula Programme at AWC

Obstetric fistula is a child birth injury caused by prolonged, obstructed labour without access to timely medical intervention. Obstetric fistula leaves women and girls with chronic incontinence of urine and/or faeces. Women and girls who have fistulas are often outcast by their families and communities due to the smell of their incontinence. This leads to lives of isolation, poverty and shame. As devastating as fistula is, there is hope. Obstetric fistula is both preventable and treatable. The prevention and treatment of obstetric fistula are central efforts at AWC.

AWC is the only comprehensive fistula repair service in Sierra Leone, and AWC has the capacity to perform up to 300 surgeries per year. Obstetric fistula patients at AWC come from across the country and are identified and mobilised to come to the Centre through a variety of activities, including screening trips into remote areas, radio advertising, referrals from other health facilities, and our former patient Ambassador programme. The majority of our patients come from the provinces through screening trips. The transport infrastructure in Sierra Leone is limited and financially unavailable to many women and girls with fistula. Therefore, screening trips take place most months and involve visiting communities and health centres to find women and girls who have fistula and are living in isolation. We advertise the visits in advance through radio announcements in the local dialects, as well as church and community networks. During these trips, the driver and nurses travel for up to two weeks, identifying and collecting fistula patients who would otherwise have no means of accessing our services.

We also run fistula jingles in nine Sierra Leonean local languages, which have been developed into episodes across several local radio stations. The messages are centred on fistula awareness and reproductive health information as we continue to address the need for increased awareness within the target population across the country. This work is supplemented by road shows on fistula awareness and treatment, which are carried out on market days in key locations throughout the country.

Our Fistula Ambassador Programme trains and utilizes former fistula patients to be advocates within the communities and identify fellow women and girls suffering from obstetric fistula. Outreach and identifying women in need of repair are crucial components of our work, as women often do not know their condition can be treatable and they therefore do not seek care. Because of the shame and stigma that is associated with fistula, most of our patients live in the outskirts of their communities and have been shunned by others. AWC trains former patients, nurses and community health workers to identify women and girls with fistula within their communities while promoting education about the prevention and treatment for obstetric fistula. They are also supported financially with funds to cover transportation and airtime costs so they can refer women for treatment at AWC. Patient ambassador training began in 2019. Since then, thirteen patients have been referred to us by patient ambassadors. Our mission is to reach the last woman in the last village so she can regain her life after suffering from obstetric fistula. The ambassador program is essential in educating and providing information to women and girls within various communities and hospitals. These efforts ensure progress towards the eradication of fistula.

Fistula patients stay at Aberdeen Women's Centre for approximately 3–4 weeks, but they may stay for as long as 12 months depending on the severity of their condition and general health. During this time, we have the opportunity to extend care beyond fistula treatment alone. Most women and girls who endured obstetric fistula were ostracized by their families and communities due to the smell of their incontinence. They are often left to live as outcasts and suffer from a number of negative physical, social and psychological consequences due to fistula (Drew et al., 2016). Therefore, the need for a holistic approach, which addresses the many consequences of obstetric fistula, is vital to rebuild their confidence and reintegrate them back into society. At AWC, our in-house counsellor offers support to all our patients over their duration of stay. The counselling service session serves as a platform that provides psychosocial care for patients. These services are provided in efforts to assist and support patients in handling anxiety, anger management, depression, mood disorders, stress and family dynamics.

The fistula surgery is supplemented by our Patient Rehabilitation and Empowerment Programme where we uplift and engage patients with the aim of providing them with a better future. We offer classes in literacy and numeracy, income-generating skills, health education and counselling services. The literacy and numeracy class are aimed at providing and equipping our fistula patients with education that may aid them on their journeys to restore their dignity and self-worth. The education and skills training components work to remove two of the key socioeconomic barriers that make women more at risk of fistula injury—education and financial security. Educational classes are conducted three times a week by a trained teacher. We also conduct group sessions where the fistula patients and teenagers are given the tools to be creative and develop new skills. These skills empower women so they may earn their own incomes when they leave the centre and return to their communities. We additionally offer classes on creating goods and crafts that can be sold in local markets. For many women, art can also be used as a form of therapy and self-expression.

Upon discharge, we have a *"gladi gladi ceremony"* where we celebrate the healing of the women. Gladi means "glad" in Krio, the official language spoken in Sierra Leone. This celebration demonstrates that we are glad they are dry after fistula repair. As part of this celebration, we give the women a new dress signifying the start of a "new" life that is free from obstetric fistula. Additionally, should a former fistula patient have a subsequent pregnancy, we offer free caesarean sections to all former fistula patients as well as quality antenatal and postnatal care.

23.3 Conclusion

Over the last 10 years of working in Sierra Leone, Aberdeen Women's Centre has collaborated with the Ministry of Health and Sanitation, the local communities in the Aberdeen district of Freetown, local clinics and hospitals around the country, and our patients and staff to adapt our services to address the needs of the women and girls we treat. For example, we opened our maternity unit in 2010 after two years of treating fistula patients, in response to the dire need for free, quality maternal health care for the poorest women and girls and to prevent other women from experiencing obstetric fistula. In 2017, we also opened a children's clinic in the Kroo Bay slum of Freetown at the request of the local community in order to provide desperately needed free health care to children under five years of age in that community.

Through our work in Sierra Leone, Malawi, Kenya and Madagascar over the last 10 years, Freedom from Fistula Foundation has developed core programmes to compliment and strengthen the maternal healthcare systems in Africa and our work is in response to each country's specific needs for their women and girls. All of our projects have been designed in consultation with the respective Ministries of Health in each country, the target population and local communities. Additionally, we have developed programmes beyond the provision of health care in response to the needs of our patients. We have also implemented programmes that are designed to improve the quantity and quality of services that are provided and contribute to the sustainability of the countries in which we serve.

Aberdeen Women's Centre takes pride in providing a holistic model of care for the women and girls who visit our centre. Our aim is to ensure that women leave with better care and knowledge about their health than when they arrived at the centre. This includes repairing women of obstetric fistula, ensuring the safe delivery of a child and providing social worker and counsellor support to women and girls. Through these efforts, we can work towards our mission to ensure that women and girls are empowered to live better, healthier and happier lives.

References

Drew, L. B., Wilkinson, J. P., Nundwe, W., Moyo, M., Mataya, R., Mwale, M., & Tang, J. H. (2016). Long-term outcomes for women after obstetric fistula repair in Lilongwe, Malawi: A qualitative study. *BMC Pregnancy Childbirth, 16*, 2. https://doi.org/10.1186/s12884-015-0755-1

Freedom from Fistula. (2019). The power of 10: A decade of freedom. https://freedomfromfistula.org/FFFUS/mobile/index.html - p=1. Accessed 18 Jan. 2021.

UNICEF. (2019). Sierra Leone – Key Demographic Indicators. https://data.unicef.org/country/sle/. Accessed 20 July 2022.

United Nations. (2019). Country profile. Sierra Leone. http://data.un.org/en/iso/sl.html. Accessed 18 Jan 2021.

United Nations Population Fund – Sierra Leone (UNFPA). (2018). Situational analysis of quality improvement in maternal and neonatal health care, Sierra Leone. https://sierraleone.unfpa.org/en/publications/situational-analysis-quality-improvement-maternal-and-neonatal-health-care-sierra-leone. Accessed 18 Jan. 2021.

The Lancet (2014). Every Newborn Series. https://www.thelancet.com/series/everynewborn. Accessed 18 Jan. 2021.

The World Factbook 2021. Washington, DC: Central Intelligence Agency, 2021. https://www.cia.gov/the-world-factbook/

Part IV

Beyond Surgery—Preventing Obstetric Fistula and Addressing Its Many Consequences

Height and External Measurement
of Pelvic Diameters to Predict
Obstetric Fistula in Congolese
Women: A Case–Control Study

24

Joseph B. Nsambi, Olivier Mukuku,
Xavier K. Kinenkinda, Prosper L. Kakudji,
Robert Andrianne,
and Jean-Baptiste S. Z. Kakoma

24.1 Introduction

Maternal morbidity and mortality remain a major health problem in many low-resource regions of the world, particularly in sub-Saharan Africa and South Asia where access to high-quality obstetric care is limited. An estimated 20–30% of these complications are due to cephalopelvic disproportion (CPD), a condition in which the fetal head is too large to fit through the maternal pelvis during delivery (Benjamin et al., 2012). Among these, obstetric fistulas (OF) are considered the most debilitating—during the prolonged, obstructed labor the fetal head is lodged in the mother's pelvis thereby cutting off the blood flow to surrounding tissues. The prolonged obstruction causes tissue necrosis leading to fistula formation between the woman's bladder and/or rectum and vagina, causing uncontrollable incontinence (Nsambi et al., 2018; Wall et al., 2004). Obstetric fistulas are widely recognized as a public health indicator of the availability and quality of health services provided to women. In

J. B. Nsambi · X. K. Kinenkinda · P. L. Kakudji
Department of Gynecology and Obstetrics, University of Lubumbashi,
Lubumbashi, Democratic Republic of the Congo
e-mail: josephnsambi@gmail.com; kinenkindaxavier@yahoo.fr; luhetekakudji@gmail.com

O. Mukuku (✉)
Department of Maternal and Child Health, High Institute of Medical Techniques of Lubumbashi,
Lubumbashi, Democratic Republic of the Congo
e-mail: oliviermukuku@yahoo.fr

R. Andrianne
Department of Urology, University Hospital, University of Liège, Liège, Belgium
e-mail: robert.andrianne@gmail.com

J.-B. S. Z. Kakoma
Department of Gynecology and Obstetrics, University of Lubumbashi,
Lubumbashi, Democratic Republic of the Congo

University of Rwanda, Kigali, Republic of Rwanda
e-mail: jbszkakoma2016@gmail.com

© Springer Nature Switzerland AG 2022
L. B. Drew et al. (eds.), *A Multidisciplinary Approach to Obstetric Fistula in Africa*, Global
Maternal and Child Health, https://doi.org/10.1007/978-3-031-06314-5_24

low-resource countries, women with OF are literally the embodiment of the health system's inability to provide quality maternal health care and appropriate delivery services (Harrison et al., 2015).

The Democratic Republic of the Congo (DRC), similar to many other low-resource countries in sub-Saharan Africa, faces several challenges in delivering quality maternal health care, including the lack of essential equipment, poor training and underqualification of personnel working in peripheral maternity hospitals, inadequate or poor distribution of health services, difficulties in accessing timely referrals, and the increase in informal and unviable maternity units (Kinenkinda et al., 2017). As a result, many women in the DRC are unable to access and benefit from high-quality maternity care. It is therefore essential to define simple and reliable screening parameters that can be used by all health personnel, including midwives and trained nurses.

Pelvimetry refers to the evaluation of the diameters of the bony pelvis to assess the pelvic cavity for the passage of a fetus. The maternal pelvis morphological feature is important predictive factor of vaginal delivery. For successful vaginal delivery, proper shape and size of the pelvis are necessary (Mirgalobayat et al., 2019). For centuries, the different methods of antenatal assessment of the pelvis have produced varying results. These methods include manual pelvimetry, instrumental pelvimetry, radiological pelvimetry, magnetic resonance imaging, and computed tomodensitometry (CT) (Hamm & Forstner, 2007; Lenhard et al., 2010; Molina & Nicolaides, 2010). Previous studies have shown that CT is convenient and accurate technique to measure the obstetrical external pelvic diameters (Kolesova et al., 2017; Siccardi et al., 2019), yet this technique is not available in rural areas in DRC (Nsambi et al., 2018). External pelvimetry is a manual examination, using a simple instrument, and is available for routine obstetrics practice in clinical settings (Siccardi et al., 2021).

Contracted pelvis and mechanical dystocia are more likely to be implicated in obstructed labor. CPD occurs in 2–15% of births; antenatal prediction of this condition and its rapid management are essential to reduce its share in obstetric accidents (Bansal et al., 2011). External pelvimetry helps estimate the pelvis size and thus draw attention to the possibility of CPD. Previous studies have demonstrated the efficiency of external pelvimetry as a screening tool for CPD prevention (Kakoma, 2016; Kakoma et al., 2010; Liselele, Boulvain, et al., 2000; Liselele, Tshibangu, & Meuris, 2000; Malonga et al., 2018; Rozenholc et al., 2007).

No study in DRC has thus far examined the relationship between the occurrence of OF and anthropometric measurements (height and external pelvimetry). The objective of this study was to see whether height and external measurement of pelvic diameters could be a useful tool for preventing OF in women from the Haut-Katanga Province, in DRC.

24.2 Methods

A case-control study was conducted from July 2018 to June 2019 in Haut-Katanga Province (DRC). Women with OF had been previously identified during the community outreach in the towns and villages of the Haut-Katanga Province. Oral information about the survey and its objectives was provided to all study participants after obtaining their free and informed consent to participate.

Cases (n = 54) were women with OF admitted to the Benicker Medical Center in Lubumbashi for surgical repair of OF. In this group of 54 cases, there were no women from Twa, or Pygmy, ancestry. Controls (n = 108) were randomly recruited from women who consulted the Mzee Medical Center in Lubumbashi during the study period. They were free from OF and any other abnormalities in the pelvis and had already vaginally delivered a newborn weighing 2500 g or more. Case-control matching was done on an age basis with one case for two controls. The same reviewer took measurements of all subjects included in the study.

As study variables, we collected the following anthropometric measurements: height (cm), weight (kg), body mass index (BMI) (kg/m^2), and external pelvic measurements (cm). These pelvic measurements included the bi-crestal diameter (between the iliac crests), the iliac bi-spines diameter (between the outer edges of the anterior superior iliac spines), the bi-trochanteric diameter (between the two femoral trochanters), the inter-tuberosities diameter (between the ischial tuberosities), the external obstetric conjugate or the anteroposterior diameter (the Baudelocque's diameter: between the first sacral segment and the upper border of the pubic symphysis), and the base of the Trillat's triangle (on the upper edge of the pubis, between the inguinal ligaments' fold). To perform these measurements, we used a stadiometer, a scale, and a Breisky pelvimeter (an instrument used in obstetrics to assess the size of the female pelvis to determine the necessity of performing a cesarean section) (Malonga et al., 2018; Siccardi et al., 2019, 2021). Anthropometric measurements used as threshold values were defined as values below the tenth percentile of the Malonga et al.'s study population (2018).

STATA® software (version 15) has been used for the statistical analyses. The Student t-test was used to compare means. A linear regression with a meaning threshold set at $p < 0.05$ was used.

Ethics approval was obtained from the Medical Ethics Committee of the University of Lubumbashi (approval number: UNILU/CEM/101/2018). Free and informed oral consent from all participants in the study was obtained verbally. Confidentiality and anonymity have been respected.

24.3 Results

Comparison of anthropometric measurements' means shows that the targeted measurements are significantly smaller in women with OF than in women without OF (Table 24.1 and Fig. 24.1).

Using the tenth percentiles of different anthropometric measurements of the Malonga et al.'s study population (2018), compared with women without OF, we find that women with OF were in high proportions below tenth percentiles for all anthropometric measurements (Table 24.2).

By looking for the relationship between fistula occurrence and anthropometric measurements, the linear regression model shows a strongly significant linear relationship between fistula occurrence and the following measurements: height, inter-tuberosities diameter, external obstetric conjugate, bi-trochanteric diameter, bi-crest diameter, and base of the Trillat's triangle (Table 24.3).

Table 24.1 Comparison of means (Standard Deviations) of age and anthropometric measurements

Variable	Women with obstetric fistula ($n = 54$) *Mean* (SD)	Women without obstetric fistula ($n = 108$) *Mean* (SD)	t-value	p-value
Age (years)	25.96 (8.10)	24.62 (5.68)	−1.22	0.2229
Height (cm)	147.57 (3.96)	160.00 (7.04)	12.04	<0.0001
Weight (kg)	46.38 (7.23)	67.04 (11.73)	11.85	<0.0001
Body mass index (kg/m²)	21.25 (2.85)	26.14 (3.97)	8.05	<0.0001
Inter-tuberosities diameter (cm)	8.26 (0.64)	9.89 (1.23)	9.12	<0.0001
Base of Trillat's triangle (cm)	11.55 (1.62)	15.26 (0.70)	20.34	<0.0001
External obstetric conjugate (cm)	16.64 (1.81)	20.94 (1.56)	15.69	<0.0001
Iliac bi-spinous diameter (cm)	21.04 (1.80)	23.54 (2.21)	7.19	<0.0001
Iliac bi-crestal diameter (cm)	23.30 (2.52)	25.15 (2.63)	4.28	<0.0001
Bi-trochanteric diameter (cm)	27.37 (2.59)	30.64 (2.93)	6.94	<0.0001

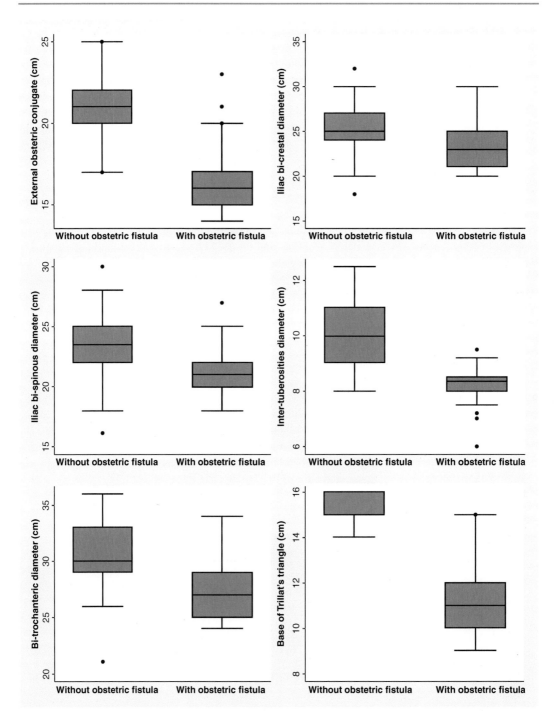

Fig. 24.1 Box plot showing anthropometric measurements of women with and without obstetric fistula

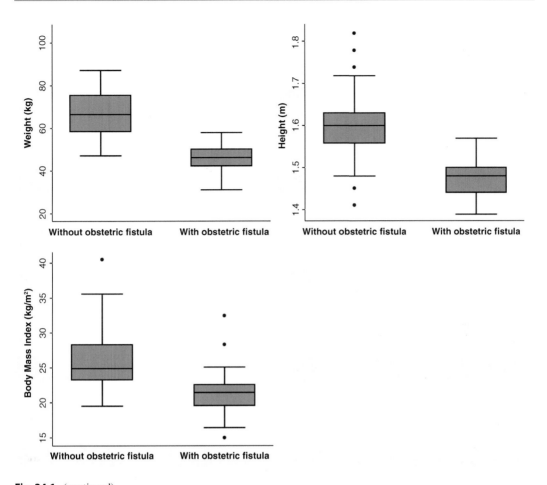

Fig. 24.1 (continued)

Table 24.2 Relationship between anthropometric measurements and obstetric fistula

Variable	Women with obstetric fistula (*n* = 54)		Women without obstetric fistula (*n* = 108)		Crude odds ratio [95% Confidence interval]	*p*-value
	n	(%)	*n*	(%)		
Height						
<150 cm	35	(64.81)	7	(6.48)	26.57 [10.30–68.59]	<0.00001
≥150 cm	19	(35.19)	101	(93.52)	1.00	
Iliac bi-crestal diameter						
<22 cm	16	(29.63)	12	(11.11)	3.37 [1.45–7.78]	0.0065
≥22 cm	38	(70.37)	96	(88.89)	1.00	
Iliac bi-spinous diameter						
<20 cm	8	(14.81)	2	(1.85)	9.08 [2.01–64.71]	0.0025
≥20 cm	46	(85.19)	106	(98.15)	1.00	
Bi-trochanteric diameter						
<26 cm	16	(29.63)	1	(0.93)	44.02 [7.53–961.60]	<0.00001

(continued)

Table 24.2 (continued)

Variable	Women with obstetric fistula (*n* = 54)		Women without obstetric fistula (*n* = 108)		Crude odds ratio [95% Confidence interval]	*p*-value
	n	(%)	*n*	(%)		
≥26 cm	38	(70.37)	107	(99.07)	1.00	
Inter-tuberosities diameter						
<8 cm	24	(44.44)	15	(13.89)	4.96 [2.31–10.66]	<0.0001
≥8 cm	30	(55.56)	93	(86.11)	1.00	
External obstetric conjugate						
<18.1 cm	41	(75.93)	1	(0.93)	315.46 [46.30–3763.96]	<0.0001
≥18.1 cm	13	(24.07)	107	(99.07)	1.00	
Base of Trillat's triangle						
<11 cm	17	(31.48)	0	(0)	Undefined	<0.0001
≥11 cm	37	(68.52)	108	(100)	1.00	
Weight						
<52 kg	47	(87.04)	7	(6.48)	90.89 [28.97–341.43]	<0.0001
≥52 kg	7	(12.96)	101	(93.52)	1.00	

Table 24.3 Linear regression of anthropometric measurements associated with obstetric fistula

Variable	Coefficient	Standard error	*t*-value	*p*-value	95% Confidence interval		Sig
Iliac bi-crestal diameter	0.037	0.007	4.97	0.000	0.022	0.052	***
Iliac bi-spinous diameter	−0.009	0.010	−0.95	0.342	−0.029	0.010	*
Base of Trillat's triangle	−0.145	0.012	−11.97	0.000	−0.169	−0.121	***
Bi-trochanteric diameter	0.026	0.007	3.53	0.001	0.011	0.040	***
External obstetric conjugate	−0.031	0.010	−3.04	0.003	−0.052	−0.011	***
Inter-tuberosities diameter	−0.073	0.015	−4.84	0.000	−0.102	−0.043	***
Weight	−0.003	0.002	−1.73	0.085	−0.007	0.000	*
Height	−0.978	0.271	−3.61	0.000	−1.513	−0.443	***
Constante	3.918	0.366	10.72	0.000	3.196	4.641	***

$***p < 0.01, **p < 0.05, *p > 0.05$

24.4   Discussion

If there are anthropometric measurements that reflect a severely contracted pelvis that can lead to obstructed labor and formation of OFs, these measurements could potentially be used as a screening tool. Anthropometric measurements (height, weight, BMI, and external pelvimetry) are simple, not technology-dependent, easy to learn, less intrusive than an internal pelvic evaluation, and can be performed in rural areas with poorly resourced health facilities. Thus, this simple screening tool could potentially help identify women who are at risk of developing OF.

In this study, patients with OF were considered to have had a CPD in the delivery that led to fistula. Fetal physiopathology is attributed to the stagnation of the fetus being expelled, and the prolonged compression of tissues in the back of pubic symphysis (prolonged obstruction of labor in the absence of emergency obstetric care) (Zheng & Anderson, 2009). It follows a perforation between the vagina and the bladder and/or the rectum. Several studies have shown a close link between anthropometric characteristics and the occurrence of CPD (Kakoma, 2016; Kakoma et al., 2010; Liselele, Boulvain, et al., 2000; Liselele, Tshibangu, & Meuris, 2000; Malonga et al., 2018; Rozenholc et al., 2007). In addition, it is well established that the height of the mother is correlated with the size of the pelvis; several studies have shown that mothers with CPD are shorter than mothers who have normal vaginal births (Merchant et al., 2001; Rozenholc et al., 2007; Sheiner et al., 2005; Shittu et al., 2007). In this study, women with OF had significantly smaller anthropometric measurements compared to women without OF. The trend may also be explained by the fact that small size is likely associated with a high risk of contracted pelvis and CPD. Similar results have been found in other studies in Africa comparing anthropometric measurements of women who presented with CPD compared to those who did not (Kakoma, 2016; Kakoma et al., 2010; Liselele, Boulvain, et al., 2000; Liselele, Tshibangu, & Meuris, 2000; Malonga et al., 2018; Wall et al., 2004). However, there is no consensus on the height below which CPD is likely to occur. Several studies used a threshold value of 150 cm for height to predict CPD. However, this height cut-off is not be appropriate for all ethnic populations due to cultural height variation; additionally, the nutritional status of the mother and genetic factors both impact the size fetus (Alijahan et al., 2014; Lee et al., 2009). A method of determining a threshold limit for anthropometric measurement to predict the CPD is to identify and use the tenth percentile of the measurement for the study population (Liselele, Boulvain, et al., 2000; Liselele, Tshibangu, & Meuris, 2000; Malonga et al., 2018; Rozenholc et al., 2007). Again, this is an arbitrary value that does not take into account the size fetus, which confers a low sensitivity to the CPD prediction (Liselele, Boulvain, et al., 2000; Liselele, Tshibangu, & Meuris, 2000). Although CPD may also depend on several maternal and fetal factors other than maternal pelvis size and fetal size (Ferguson & Sistrom, 2000), the results of this study are very important and demonstrate the relevance of anthropometric measurements (height and external pelvimetry) in predicting OF in women. However, it is also possible to recognize CPD in the absence of a disproportional diagnosis (narrow pelvis) (Benjamin et al., 2012).

This study points to the importance of external pelvic diameters in predicting CPD and thus preventing OF. The results of this study are of paramount importance to midwives and obstetricians working in this field, especially in low-resource settings with high rates of OF. In these settings, the simple anthropometric measurements utilized in this study could be evaluated with small statured women in labor for close monitoring and timely referral to a facility capable of cesarean delivery.

24.5 Limitations

This study has several limitations. First, this study has a very small sample size of women with OF, which needs to be acknowledged. Second, we use the tenth percentile of the Malonga et al.'s study population (2018) as a method of determining a threshold limit for anthropometric measurement for predicting OF. This limits the application of this method in other populations. Our study was performed in the population of one province of the DRC. Anthropometric measurements and body features differ across different regions and people groups. More research is needed in other regions and populations with a larger sample size in order to evaluate the effectiveness of these anthropometric measurements on a larger number of women. If anthropometric measurements are to be used to identify women at risk of CPD, the general reproducibility of these measurements must be confirmed.

24.6 Conclusion

This study shows that anthropometric measurements in Congolese women with OF in this sample are significantly smaller compared to women without OF. The findings demonstrate the potential of using the combination of the maternal height with external pelvimetry to assess the risk of CPD in Congolese women. Taking these measurements is a simple and inexpensive screening method to identify women who will require supervised delivery in a facility capable of providing cesarean sections. Furthermore, this simple antenatal screening tool could be implemented in health centers without operative capability for timely referral of women at risk of CPD to higher level facilities, thus preventing maternal death and injury.

References

Alijahan, R., Kordi, M., Poorjavad, M., & Ebrahimzadeh, S. (2014). Diagnostic accuracy of maternal anthropometric measurements as predictors for dystocia in nulliparous women. *Iranian Journal of Nursing and Midwifery Research, 19*(1), 11.

Bansal, S., Guleria, K., & Agarwal, N. (2011). Evaluation of Sacral Rhomboid Dimensions to Predict Contracted Pelvis: A Pilot Study of Indian Primigravidae. *J Obstet Gynecol India, 61*(5), 523–527. https://doi.org/10.1007/s13224-011-0078-8

Benjamin, S. J., Daniel, A. B., Kamath, A., & Ramkumar, V. (2012). Anthropometric measurements as predictors of cephalopelvic disproportion: Can the diagnostic accuracy be improved? *Acta Obstetricia et Gynecologica Scandinavica, 91*(1), 122–127. https://doi.org/10.1111/j.1600-0412.2011.01267.x

Ferguson, J. E., 2nd, & Sistrom, C. L. (2000). Can fetal–pelvic disproportion be predicted. *Clinical Obstetrics and Gynecology, 43*(2), 247–264.

Hamm, B., & Forstner, R. (Eds.). (2007). *MRI and CT of the female pelvis*. Springer Science & Business Media.

Harrison, M. S., Mabeya, H., Goldenberg, R. L., & McClure, E. M. (2015). Urogenital fistula reviewed: A marker of severe maternal morbidity and an indicator of the quality of maternal healthcare delivery. *Maternal Health, Neonatology and Perinatology, 1*(1), 1–8. https://doi.org/10.1186/s40748-015-0020-7

Kakoma, J. B. (2016). Cesarean section indications and anthropometric parameters in Rwandan nulliparae: Preliminary results from a longitudinal survey. *The Pan African Medical Journal, 24*, 310. https://doi.org/10.11604/pamj.2016.24.310.9603

Kakoma, J. B., Karibushi, J., & Ramazani, K. R. (2010). Height, weight, external pelvic diameters and cesarean section: A cohort study in Southern Province of Rwanda (Huye District). *Rwanda Medical Journal, 68*(3), 21–24.

Kinenkinda, X., Mukuku, O., Chenge, F., Kakudji, P., Banzulu, P., Kakoma, J. B., & Kizonde, J. (2017). Césarienne à Lubumbashi, République Démocratique du Congo II: Facteurs de risque de mortalité maternelle et périnatale. *The Pan African Medical Journal, 26*, 208. https://doi.org/10.11604/pamj.2017.26.208.12148

Kolesova, O., Kolesovs, A., & Vetra, J. (2017). Age-related trends of lesser pelvic architecture in females and males: A computed tomography pelvimetry study. *Anatomy & Cell Biology, 50*(4), 265–274.

Lee, A. C., Darmstadt, G. L., Khatry, S. K., LeClerq, S. C., Shrestha, S. R., & Christian, P. (2009). Maternal-fetal disproportion and birth asphyxia in rural Sarlahi, Nepal. *Archives of Pediatrics & Adolescent Medicine, 163*(7), 616–623. https://doi.org/10.1001/archpediatrics.2009.75

Lenhard, M. S., Johnson, T. R., Weckbach, S., Nikolaou, K., Friese, K., & Hasbargen, U. (2010). Pelvimetry revisited: Analyzing cephalopelvic disproportion. *European Journal of Radiology, 74*(3), e107–e111. https://doi.org/10.1016/j.ejrad.2009.04.042

Liselele, H. B., Boulvain, M., Tshibangu, K. C., & Meuris, S. (2000). Maternal height and external pelvimetry to predict cephalopelvic disproportion in nulliparous African women: A cohort study. *BJOG: An International Journal of Obstetrics & Gynaecology, 107*(8), 947–952.

Liselele, H. B., Tshibangu, C. K., & Meuris, S. (2000). Association between external pelvimetry and vertex delivery complications in African women. *Acta Obstetricia et Gynecologica Scandinavica, 79*(8), 673–678.

Malonga, F. K., Mukuku, O., Ngalula, M. T., Luhete, P. K., & Kakoma, J. B. (2018). Étude anthropométrique et pelvimétrique externe chez les nullipares de Lubumbashi: Facteurs de risque et score prédictif de la dystocie mécanique. *The Pan African Medical Journal, 31*, 69. https://doi.org/10.11604/pamj.2018.31.69.16014

Merchant, K. M., Villar, J., & Kestler, E. (2001). Maternal height and newborn size relative to risk of intrapartum caesarean delivery and perinatal distress. *BJOG: An International Journal of Obstetrics & Gynaecology, 108*(7), 689–696. https://doi.org/10.1111/j.1471-0528.2000.tb10394.x

Mirgalobayat, S., Ghahari, L., Allahqoli, L., Mostafavi, S. R. S., Safari, K., Rikhtehgar, M., et al. (2019). Evaluation of the link between pelvimetry based on computed tomography and predicting status' delivery. *Journal of Contemporary Medical Sciences, 5*(6), 313–316.

Molina, F. S., & Nicolaides, K. H. (2010). Ultrasound in labor and delivery. *Fetal Diagnosis and Therapy, 27*(2), 61–67. https://doi.org/10.1159/000287588

Nsambi, J. B., Mukuku, O., Kinenkinda, X., Kakudji, P., Kizonde, J., & Kakoma, J. B. (2018). Fistules obstétricales dans la province du Haut-Katanga, République Démocratique du Congo: à propos de 242 cas. *Pan African Medical Journal, 29*(1), 1–14. https://doi.org/10.11604/pamj.2018.29.34.14576

Rozenholc, A. T., Ako, S. N., Leke, R. J., & Boulvain, M. (2007). The diagnostic accuracy of external pelvimetry and maternal height to predict dystocia in nulliparous women: A study in Cameroon. *BJOG: An International Journal of Obstetrics & Gynaecology, 114*(5), 630–635. https://doi.org/10.1111/j.1471-0528.2007.01294.x

Sheiner, E., Levy, A., Katz, M., & Mazor, M. (2005). Short stature—An independent risk factor for Cesarean delivery. *European Journal of Obstetrics & Gynecology and Reproductive Biology, 120*(2), 175–178. https://doi.org/10.1016/j.ejogrb.2004.09.013

Shittu, A. S., Kuti, O., Orji, E. O., Makinde, N. O., Ogunniyi, S. O., Ayoola, O. O., & Sule, S. S. (2007). Clinical versus sonographic estimation of foetal weight in southwest Nigeria. *Journal of Health, Population, and Nutrition, 25*(1), 14.

Siccardi, M., Valle, C., & Di Matteo, F. (2021). Dynamic external pelvimetry test in third trimester pregnant women: Shifting positions affect pelvic biomechanics and create more room in obstetric diameters. *Cureus, 13*(3), e13631. https://doi.org/10.7759/cureus.13631

Siccardi, M., Valle, C., Di Matteo, F., & Angius, V. (2019). A postural approach to the pelvic diameters of obstetrics: The dynamic external pelvimetry test. *Cureus, 11*(11), e6111. https://doi.org/10.7759/cureus.6111

Wall, L. L., Karshima, J. A., Kirschner, C., & Arrowsmith, S. D. (2004). The obstetric vesicovaginal fistula: Characteristics of 899 patients from Jos, Nigeria. *American Journal of Obstetrics and Gynecology, 190*(4), 1011–1016. https://doi.org/10.1016/j.ajog.2004.02.007

Zheng, A. X., & Anderson, F. W. (2009). Obstetric fistula in low-income countries. *International Journal of Gynecology & Obstetrics, 104*(2), 85–89. https://doi.org/10.1016/j.ijgo.2008.09.011

Designing Preventive Strategies for Obstetric Fistula: Evidence from a Survey Conducted Among Rural and Urban Women in Burkina Faso

25

Aduragbemi Banke-Thomas

25.1 Introduction

Most cases of obstetric fistula are confined within an area of the globe known as the "fistula belt." This belt comprises the northern half of sub-Saharan Africa—from Mauritania to Eritrea—and the developing countries of Middle East Asia (Tebeu et al., 2012). While obstetric fistula is known to be prevalent in these regions, measurement of its incidence and prevalence can at best be described as challenging, especially as many women with obstetric fistula do not present at health facilities, and are mostly poor, young women who are often illiterate and live in rural areas (Cowgill et al., 2015; WHEC, 2013). However, efforts to estimate incidence and prevalence of the condition have shown that approximately 2 of every 1000 women of reproductive age within the sub-Saharan Africa region live with untreated fistula (Adler et al., 2013). It is estimated that the incidence of new cases of obstetric fistula varies between 1 and 3 per 1000 births in West Africa (Kalembo & Zgambo, 2012), with higher rates of 5–10 new cases per 1000 births reported in rural areas of sub-Saharan Africa (Vangeenderhuysen et al., 2001).

The results of a needs assessment conducted by Engender Health in sub-Saharan African countries revealed that poverty, lack of skilled birth care, lack of emergency obstetric care (EmOC), lack of transportation, limited knowledge and the shortage of qualified providers for fistula repair, poor integration of services and marginalization of women with fistula are some of the factors contributing to the high prevalence of obstetric fistula among women in the region (Cook et al., 2004). In addition, the high prevalence of early marriage and teenage pregnancy, which in turn means that girls do not have pelvises which have sufficiently developed to allow for procreation, has been linked to

---

This chapter presents findings from a postgraduate dissertation of the corresponding author and an updated version of a paper first published as: Banke-Thomas, A. O., Kouraogo, S. F., Siribie, A., Taddese, H. B., & Mueller, J. E. (2013). Knowledge of obstetric fistula prevention amongst young women in urban and rural Burkina Faso: A cross-sectional study. *PLoS ONE*, 8(12), e85921. https://doi.org/10.1371/journal.pone.0085921.

A. Banke-Thomas (✉)
School of Human Sciences, University of Greenwich, London, UK
e-mail: a.bankethomas@gre.ac.uk

© Springer Nature Switzerland AG 2022
L. B. Drew et al. (eds.), *A Multidisciplinary Approach to Obstetric Fistula in Africa*, Global Maternal and Child Health, https://doi.org/10.1007/978-3-031-06314-5_25

the high occurrence of obstetric fistula in these areas (Tebeu et al., 2012). This is further compounded by the poor nutritional status of most of the girls who live in these highly deprived settings (Konje & Ladipo, 2000).

Similar to many other sub-Saharan African countries, obstetric fistula remains a huge problem in Burkina Faso (Maheu-Giroux et al., 2015; Tebeu et al., 2012). Of 1000 consultations in surgery across the various levels of care, from 5 to 17 are fistula repair cases (UNFPA, 2004). In a 2015 study that assessed the prevalence of the symptoms of vaginal fistula in sub-Saharan Africa countries including Burkina Faso, lifetime prevalence of vaginal fistula symptoms was estimated as 0.4 (0.0–1.1) per 1000 women of reproductive age (Maheu-Giroux et al., 2015). However, since the early 2000s, obstetric fistula has been recognized as a significant public health problem that has required concerted efforts to address in Burkina Faso, mostly due to the global campaign to end fistula launched by the United Nations Population Funds (UNFPA) in nine sub-Saharan African countries (UNFPA, 2004).

Burkina Faso is a francophone West African country with an economy that is mainly based on agriculture and livestock. It has an estimated population of over 14 million inhabitants and an annual population growth rate of 3.1%. Women represent 51.8% of the population, including 24% being women of childbearing age (15–49 years). Burkina Faso has a predominantly young population with 47.9% of the entire population within the 0- to 14-year-old age bracket. About 80% of the population lives in rural areas. There is also a relatively high early fertility rate (130‰ at 15–19 years), which increases rapidly to a peak at 25–29 years (269‰) (INSD, 2007, 2017; INSD & ICF International, 2012). According to the World Bank classification, Burkina Faso is a low-income country, whereby about 45.3% of the population lives below the poverty line and the income per capita is estimated at just 72,690 FCFA (US$146) per person per year (INSD, 2007; World Bank, 2018).

As it relates to maternal health indices in Burkina Faso, the adjusted maternal mortality ratio (MMR) is estimated at 560 per 100,000 live-births, with a ratio of children under-five mortality of 176 per 1000. Forty-eight per cent of women are married by 18 years of age and women will typically go on to have an average of six children with a median of 34.8 months between each pregnancy. As of 2010, the rate of female genital mutilation was 73% (INSD, 2007; UNICEF, 2013). In a survey conducted by the Burkina Faso Family Health Directorate, it was found that the majority of fistulas seen in health facilities were uro-genital (89.1%), followed by recto-vaginal (6.7%) and uro-recto-vaginal (4.2%) (UNFPA & DSF, 2004). The duration of the disease was less than 1 year in 48.5% of cases and 5 years or more in 21% of cases. The median age of women with fistula was 25 years old; 96.3% were housewives and had no income of their own (UNFPA & DSF, 2004).

Previously, there was a 4-year programme, covering the period, 2011–2015, to eradicate obstetric fistula from Burkina Faso (UNFPA & Ministère de la Santé—Burkina Faso, 2012). However, the task of eradicating this condition remains daunting. This chapter reports a survey conducted in Boromo health district, in the Boucle du Mouhoun region of Burkina Faso. The region has one of the highest fertility rates in Burkina Faso and harmful practices such as female genital mutilation, early marriage and wife inheritance persist throughout the region despite repeated campaigns (DRS Boucle du Mouhoun, 2012). The women residing in the health district are mostly served by a Medical Centre with Surgical Services [Centre Médical avec une Antenne Chirurgicale (CMA)] (Fig. 25.1). In the survey, prevalence of knowledge on obstetric fistula prevention among young women was assessed in both rural and urban communities of Boromo. This was done as a means to gather critical evidence to aid design of preventative programmes aimed at reducing incidence of obstetric fistula.

Fig. 25.1 Maternity unit of the Medical Centre with Surgical Services [Centre Médical avec une Antenne Chirurgicale (CMA)] that serves most women in Boromo health district. (Photo Credit: Aduragbemi Banke-Thomas)

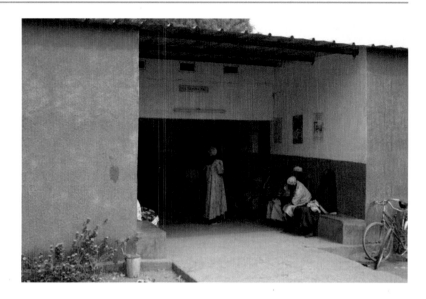

25.2 Methods and Statistical Analysis

A descriptive cross-sectional study was conducted to assess and compare knowledge of young women (ages 18–20 years) and their sources of information on obstetric fistula in urban and rural areas of the Boromo health district. We employed a cluster sampling method, which included two groups: the only urban area and three of the nine rural areas in Boromo. The sample size was estimated, selecting a statistical power of 80% and an α-error of 0.05 for the comparison of population-level knowledge in both groups (rural Boromo and urban Boromo). Ideally, the knowledge should be 100% widespread, but in this study, we assumed that 80% knowledge prevalence was "sufficient" to effectively propagate any piece of information that needs to be disseminated. The sample size was calculated with the intention of being able to describe a 20% significant difference in knowledge, that is, an observed prevalence of 60% or lower. These two proportions were used to generate the sample size, with a design effect (D_{eff}) of 2. The assumption made to estimate "ρ" clusters was similar within each sample, to bring the value to "1." The computation under these assumptions prescribed a sample size of 24 for each group (urban and rural), which adds to 48 for the whole study. Subsequently, factoring in the design effect led to an estimation of a sample size of 96. The method used in populating the groups had been utilized previously in studies of prevalence of meningococcal carriage in rural and urban communities of Bobo-Dioulasso, Burkina Faso (Mueller et al., 2011). The multi-stage sampling entailed that streets or departments would be selected purposely while compounds or villages would be identified by systematic random sampling method. This sampling technique was preferred as it was found to be more feasible and as it allowed enumerators to work more efficiently (Barnett, 2002).

For urban Boromo, the first stage involved selecting three streets beginning with a randomly identified starting point. This was done after reviewing all streets on the cadastral plans. For the second stage, identification of compounds to be included in the survey was done by spinning a pen on a notebook and progressing in the direction indicated by the tip and entering every second compound that was encountered during the walk. If no eligible young woman met the inclusion criteria within the compound, the investigators continued to the next compound. In each compound, the investigators included only one person, who was in turn identified randomly.

For rural Boromo, the first stage involved randomly selecting three of the nine administrative departments. For the second stage, 50 hamlets were identified from the selected departments, through systematic random sampling. The villages to be included in the survey were identified by spinning a pen on a notebook and moving in the direction indicated by the tip of the pen, entering every second village encountered. One eligible woman was included per hamlets. A hamlet in this setting typically represents small settlements of around seven to ten households.

In each compound (urban Boromo) and hamlet (rural Boromo), a resident young woman of Burkinabé origin, between 18 and 20 years of age and who had not suffered or was not currently suffering from obstetric fistula, was randomly selected and recruited into the study. The eligible age range was set between 18 and 20 years following the rationale that assessing the prevalence of knowledge in a young group would have important ramifications, as they constitute the most affected age group and as they present with opportunities for early intervention with prevention messages. However, we limited the lower age bracket to 18 years as going below that would entail including children in this sensitive subject area, which would in turn led to quite strenuous and time-consuming processes in terms of obtaining ethics approval from the ethics approval boards of the different institutions involved in the research and the host country. Female interviewers administered the designed semi-structured questionnaires to assess the knowledge of participants on obstetric fistula.

A pretesting of the questionnaire used for the survey was conducted prior to the main study using five respondents, who were excluded from the main study. Following the pilot study, the necessary modifications were made to the instrument to simplify the language and facilitate comprehension on the part of participants. The questionnaire was written in French, and the most common local languages Mossi[1] and Dioula.[2] All versions were tested as part of the pretesting. Female research assistants who were trained to conduct the instrument and who had experience in previous research were involved in administering the questionnaire.

For design of the questionnaire, we consulted previous attempts at assessing knowledge in the area (Hassan & Ekele, 2009), albeit for patients rather than the general population. We also drew upon our understanding of the critical etiological and programmatic considerations in the area. Accordingly, the first section of the questionnaire collected information on the socio-demographic background of the respondents including age, level of education, marital status, age at first marriage, number of previous pregnancies and age of first pregnancy (for those who reported being pregnant previously). The second section of the questionnaire inquired about the awareness of respondents about obstetric fistula. "Awareness" in this study simply referred to whether the respondent had previously heard about obstetric fistula. For those respondents who answered, "Yes," they were classified as being "aware," while those who responded "No" were classified as "unaware."

The third section of the questionnaire was used to assess participants' knowledge. "Knowledge" in this study was defined as "the knowledge of risk factors and symptoms of obstetric fistula, normal duration of labour and possible sources of emergency obstetric care." An assumption was made in this study that knowledge of these four critically important aspects would contribute towards the reduction of the incidence and prevalence of obstetric fistula. All aspects were given equal weight. To test for knowledge of risk factors, we put forth a range of inaccurate propositions (evil spirits, bad luck, prohibited act committed by a woman) and a set of accurate ones (female genital mutilation, home delivery, prolonged labour and malnutrition). We applied the same multiple-choice format to inquire about

---

[1]The Mossi language is a Gur language belonging to the Oti–Volta branch. It is one of two official regional languages of Burkina Faso and is closely related to the Frafra language which is spoken in the northern half of neighboring Ghana. It is the language of the Mossi people and is spoken by approximately five million people.

[2]The Dioula, or Jula, language is a Mande language that is one of the Manding languages, closely related to Bambara, and is spoken by many millions of persons in West Africa as either a first or second language.

respondents' knowledge on symptoms of obstetric fistula. Inaccurate propositions that were put forward in this regard included continuous sleeping and stomach ache, while urinary incontinence, faecal incontinence and vulvar irritation constituted the accurate ones. On the other hand, we adopted a "Yes" or "No" response format to assess knowledge on duration of labour and possible sources of emergency obstetric care. Participants who scored 50% or more (providing correct answers to two or more of the questions) were classified as "sufficiently informed" while those with a score of less than 50% were classified as "insufficiently informed." The percentage of "informed participants" was the "prevalence of knowledge." Based on their responses, adolescents were classified into one of these two categories.

We used standard statistical methods for the analyses, including accounting for design effect. Participant characteristics were compared between the rural and urban group using Fisher's exact test for categorical and Wilcoxon rank-sum test for continuous variables. Odds ratios for the association between rural residency and awareness or knowledge about obstetrical fistula were calculated using logistic regression. To evaluate whether characteristics differing between rural and urban participants (educational status, previous pregnancy and marital status) could explain or had masked an association between rural residency and the outcomes, we calculated adjusted odds ratios. To evaluate whether educational status or previous pregnancy influenced the association between rural residency and outcomes, we also calculated stratified odds ratios.

Ethics approval for this study was obtained from the ethics committee of the School of Health and Related Research (ScHARR), University of Sheffield, in the United Kingdom, as well as Ecole des Hautes Études en Santé Publique (EHESP), in France, and the National Centre for Scientific and Technological Research (CNRST), and the National Health Research Ethics Committee (CERS), in Burkina Faso. Written informed consent was obtained from participants using a predesigned form, which had been reviewed and approved by all four ethics committees. For those participants who could not read and write, the enumerators read out the research information sheet and the informed consent form, and their thumbprint was taken as proof of consent. All investigators were trained on data collection to ensure data quality and ethical integrity of the research. Female research assistants were employed for data collection due to the sensitivity of the research subject. All information collected on personal data during the search was strictly confidential. Participant names were coded, and anonymity maintained.

25.3 Findings from the Survey

In total, 126 contacts were made, five declined to participate, making the total number of respondents to be 121. Of the five who declined to participate, three were from the urban group and two from the rural group. The median age of participants was 19 years old. Approximately one-half of participants (50.4%) in the total sample had not received school education, 45.5% were married and 45.5% had been pregnant in the past (regardless of outcome) (Table 25.1). Maternal age at first pregnancy varied between 15 and 20 years. Participants residing in rural areas (62.0% of total) were significantly less educated, had more frequently experienced pregnancy and were a larger proportion of married women, than their urban counterparts (Table 25.1). There was no divorced or widowed participant.

Only one-third of participants were aware of obstetric fistula, with a marginal difference between rural (37.9%) and urban residents (34.9%), which was not biased by educational status, experience of pregnancy (Table 25.2) or marital status (data not shown). Regarding sources of information, most of the women who were aware of obstetric fistula got the information through the media (45.5%) or word of mouth from family and friends (41.0%), with predominance of word of mouth among rural women (68.2%). Compared to urban women, and irrespective of education status, previous pregnancy or

Table 25.1 Characteristics of participants included in the survey. Women ages 18–20 years in Boromo district, Burkina Faso, 2013

		Total (N = 121)	Rural Boromo (N = 58)	Urban Boromo (N = 63)	P value for difference between rural and urban[a]
Age	Mean (SD)	19.0 (0.9)	19.1 (0.9)	18.9 (0.9)	0.352
Level of education	Non-educated	61 (50.4%)	36 (62.0%)	25 (39.7%)	0.004
	Primary	21 (17.4%)	12 (20.7%)	9 (14.3%)	
	Secondary	39 (32.2%)	10 (17.2%)	29 (46.0%)	
Marital status	Married	55 (45.5%)	38 (65.5%)	17 (27.0%)	0.000
	Single	66 (54.5%)	20 (34.5%)	46 (73.0%)	
Previous pregnancy	Yes	55 (45.5%)	34 (58.6%)	21 (33.3%)	0.006
Age at first pregnancy (years)	Median (min, max)	18.0 (15, 20)	17.5 (15, 20)	18.0 (15, 20)	0.894
Number of pregnancies	Median (min, max)	1 (1, 3)	1 (1, 3)	(1, 3)	0.479

[Source: Reprinted from Banke-Thomas AO, Kouraogo SF, Siribie A, Taddese HB, Mueller JE. (2013) Knowledge of Obstetric Fistula Prevention amongst Young Women in Urban and Rural Burkina Faso: A Cross-Sectional Study. *PLOS ONE.* 8(12):e85921. https://doi.org/10.1371/journal.pone.0085921, licensed under the terms of the Creative Commons Attribution License (https://creativecommons.org/licenses/by/4.0/)]

[a] Fisher exact or Wilcoxon rank-sum test

Table 25.2 Awareness and knowledge on obstetric fistula and effect of rural residency to these outcomes. Women ages 18–20 years in Boromo district, Burkina Faso, 2013

		Total (N = 121)	Rural Boromo (N = 58)	Urban Boromo (N = 63)	Crude OR (95%-CI)	OR (95%-CI) adjusted for education	OR (95%-CI) adjusted for previous pregnancy
Awareness of obstetric fistula	Yes	44 (36.4%)	22 (37.9%)	22 (34.9%)	1.14 (0.47, 2.76)	1.69 (0.61, 4.70)	1.06 (0.43, 2.62)
Source of awareness	Word of mouth	18 (40.9)	15 (68.2)	3 (13.6)			
	School	6 (13.6)	2 (9.1)	4 (18.2)			
	Media	20 (45.5)	5 (22.7)	15 (68.2)	0.14 (0.04, 0.46)[a]	0.12 (0.02, 0.81)	0.13 (0.03, 0.61)
Knowledge of obstetric fistula	Informed	44 (36.4%)	14 (24.1%)	30 (47.6%)	0.35 (0.16, 0.79)	0.41 (0.18, 0.93)	0.27 (0.09, 0.79)
Awareness of risk of complications during delivery	Yes	13 (10.7%)	10 (17.2%)	3 (4.8%)	4.17 (1.63, 10.66)	3.95 (1.41, 11.07)	4.11 (1.18, 14.31)
Knowledge of transport means in case of emergency	Ambulance	19 (15.7%)	7 (12.1%)	12 (19.0%)	0.58 (0.24, 1.44)[b]	0.74 (0.31, 1.72)	0.87 (0.32, 1.41)
	Motorcycle	87 (71.9%)	41 (71.7%)	46 (73.0%)			
	Donkey	1 (0.82%)	1 (1.7%)	0 (0.0%)			
	Foot	14 (11.6%)	9 (15.5%)	5 (7.9%)			

Figures present N (%); *OR* odds ratio

[Source: Reprinted from Banke-Thomas AO, Kouraogo SF, Siribie A, Taddese HB, Mueller JE. (2013) Knowledge of Obstetric Fistula Prevention amongst Young Women in Urban and Rural Burkina Faso: A Cross-Sectional Study. *PLOS ONE.* 8(12): e85921. https://doi.org/10.1371/journal.pone.0085921, licensed under the terms of the Creative Commons Attribution License (https://creativecommons.org/licenses/by/4.0/)]

[a] OR for having had information on obstetric fistula by media, vs. word of mouth or school

[b] OR for mentioning ambulance as the means of transport in case of emergency, vs. other means

Table 25.3 Association between of rural residency and knowledge on obstetric fistula by group, by level of education. Women ages 18–20 years in Boromo district, Burkina Faso, 2013

	Crude odds ratio (95%-CI)	Odds ratio (95%-CI) adjusted for education and/or previous pregnancy
Overall (N = 121)	0.35 (0.16, 0.79)	0.31 (0.10, 0.92)
Non-educated (N = 61)	0.26 (0.11, 0.64)	0.17 (0.05, 0.55)
Primary education (N = 21)	0.67 (0.15, 2.89)	0.69 (0.20, 2.43)
Secondary education (N = 39)	0.62 (0.08, 4.94)	0.57 (0.05, 5.96)
Previous pregnancy (N = 55)	0.18 (0.05, 0.67)	0.20 (0.05, 0.71)
No previous pregnancy (N = 66)	0.43 (0.11, 1.68)	0.51 (0.13, 2.06)

marital status, rural women were about eight times less likely to have received information through the media. More participants from urban Boromo were classified as "sufficiently informed" on obstetric fistula (47.6% vs. 24.1%) (Table 25.2). Women in rural areas were three times less likely (OR 0.35, CI-95%, 0.16, 0.79) to demonstrate sufficient knowledge, and this effect was only slightly explained by lack of education and only slightly underestimated by previous pregnancy (see adjusted odds ratios in Table 25.2).

All 121 participants identified the hospital as a site where they could access emergency obstetric care, but only 11.0% of women thought they could have pregnancy complications that would require emergency treatment (Table 25.2). Rural residents were four times more likely to exhibit this understanding (OR 4.17, 95% CI, 1.63, 10.66), irrespective of education or previous pregnancy. Most women (71.9%) identified the motorcycle, and only 15.7% the ambulance, as the means for transport in case of emergency, with no significant association with rural residency (Table 25.2).

In stratified analyses using the adjusted model (Table 25.3), the negative association between rural residence and knowledge of obstetric fistula was particularly strong among women without school education (OR 0.17; 95% CI, 0.05, 0.55), but was attenuated and no longer significant among women with any schooling (OR 0.45; 95% CI, 0.13, 1.56). Among women with previous experience of pregnancy, rural residency was even more strongly associated with lack of knowledge than among women without. Sufficient knowledge on obstetric fistula tended to be more common among women with previous pregnancy than without: 66.7% vs. 38.1% among urban residents, and 26.5% vs. 20.8% among rural residents (differences not statistically significant). Inclusion of marital status as a covariate did not impact any of the effect estimates but weakened the model due to limited sample size (data not shown).

25.4   Discussion

The results of this survey among young women in Burkina Faso suggest that the prevalence of awareness of obstetric fistula and knowledge on its prevention are low in both urban and rural areas. From the results in the study reported in this chapter, women in rural areas were almost three times less likely to have preventive knowledge on obstetric fistula compared to urban women, and these differences could not be explained by differences in education, experience of previous pregnancy or marital status. A qualitative study conducted among males and females ages 18–49 years in Nabitovu village, Iganga district, Eastern Uganda, showed that preventive knowledge on obstetric fistula was generally low (Kasamba et al., 2013), in keeping with our data. A similar cross-sectional study on knowledge of women on antenatal care conducted in Alexandria, Egypt, also showed that urban women had a higher mean total score for antenatal care knowledge than their rural counterparts, with a statistically significant difference (11.23 ± 2.91 and 6.59 ± 4.14, respectively, and $Z = 9.73$, $P < 0.001$) (Kishk, 2002). This urban–rural knowledge gap signifies the need for focusing on rural women with targeted messages on maternal health generally and on the risks and consequences of fistula and ways of preventing it, specifically.

Higher levels of education among urban young girls could explain their higher health literacy, as more young urban women speak and understand the French language, even though there are other factors that could contribute to this rural–urban health literacy gap (Zhang, 2006). This could have a massive impact on the amount of information that rural young women can access, as French is the lingua franca and the most spoken language for health media programmes, in contrast to the local dialects. Our results from stratifying for education suggest that schooling, even basic primary education, can reduce the rural–urban gap in knowledge related to obstetric fistula and ultimately contribute to prevention of its occurrence. In a study conducted in Shanghai, education was found to be the most important determinant of maternal health knowledge among rural-to-urban migrant women (Zhao et al., 2009). Furthermore, it has been shown that schools provide an important medium for propagating health education, especially sexual health education. A programme implemented in 62 primary schools in rural Mwanza, Tanzania, based on a curriculum which was teacher-led and peer-assisted, showed improved knowledge of risks and benefits of behaviours (Plummer et al., 2007).

It is now widely accepted that keeping girls in school, especially, and ensuring that they complete at least a primary education, contributes to women empowerment, curtails harmful traditional practices such as child marriage, promotes gender equality and reduces incidences of maternal morbidity and mortality, including obstetric fistula (Barageine et al., 2014; Capes et al., 2011; Shefren, 2009). Based upon these facts, there are strong calls for strengthening inter-sectoral collaboration between the ministries of health and education. A working World Health Organization (WHO) document emphasizes this need to promote multi-sectoral linkages between ministries of health, education and social protection, if improvements are to be made on the state of global maternal health (Lule et al., 2003). Specifically, there is need to further develop sex education as a whole in the school curriculum. A qualitative study conducted in Burkina Faso in 1993 recommended that sex education should be introduced earlier than the beginning of high school and that the programme should include discussions on social norms and beliefs about contraception and their modes of action, their advantages and disadvantages, fear of infertility and the choice of partner (Diesfeld, 1993). In addition to these suggestions, based on findings from the research reported in this chapter, there is a need to include discussions on risk associated with unsupervised childbirth, complications of early marriage and early pregnancy, and especially, obstetric fistula. This would ensure that young women are already empowered with critical information to aid their decision-making when they get pregnant, as it has been reported as a barrier to preventive interventions against obstetric fistula in sub-Saharan Africa (Banke-Thomas et al., 2014; Lufumpa et al., 2018).

Web platforms such as the "Comité National de Lutte contre la Pratique de l'Excision" (National Committee Against the Practice of Excision) (http://www.sp-cnlpe.gov.bf/) and the "SOS excision" phone line (80-00-1112) provide some relevant information to individuals in communities. However, findings from the study presented in this chapter show that there are several young women who may not be able to access information on prevention of obstetric fistula from such platforms. Young women who were "aware" of obstetric fistula in rural areas mostly attributed their awareness to their family and friends, that is, through word of mouth. In this regard, it is difficult to ascertain the authenticity and quality of the information they receive, in contrast to structured and targeted messages from health professionals, counsellors or through the media. A systematic review and meta-analysis demonstrated the positive effects of face-to-face tailored messages from health workers on health behaviours of participants (Wanyonyi et al., 2011). Similar to the study reported in this chapter, another study carried out in Tanzania showed that young rural women have limited access to mass media when compared to their urban counterparts and that even though word of mouth communication between family and friends plays a large role in the spread of news and information, its role in spreading family planning, and other maternal and child health information is low (Montez, 2011). Therefore, there is a need to employ innovative approaches in order to ensure distribution of targeted, structured and accurate information about obstetric fistula among rural young women. These methods should utilize one of the most common means of information distribution in these settings, that is, word of mouth communication. These could include adoption of peer-education health clubs that has been proven to be effective in similar settings in other countries, such as the five-year social marketing adolescent sexual health project implemented in Cameroon, South Africa, Botswana and Guinea, that has had positive effects on contraceptive use (Agha, 2002). Approaches that leverage design of what works in specific context also guarantee value for money (Banke-Thomas et al., 2017; Eborieme et al., 2020).

There has been a rise in the annual rate of institutional deliveries in Burkina Faso, with the most significant incremental increase of 27.3% occurring a year after the introduction of the subsidy for emergency care in 2007 (Ridde et al., 2011). However, this level of coverage has not translated into ensuring the dissemination of critical maternal health information, especially in the case of rural residents, as evidenced by the observation that there was only a marginal difference in obstetric fistula prevention knowledge between those who had been pregnant in the past and those that had never been pregnant. This could be due to the persistent popularity of traditional birth attendants in such settings or due to missed opportunities to disseminate health messages during hospital consultations. Indeed, most of the participants of this study stated that they believed that they would not have complications during childbirth (approximately 90% of the study population). Opportunities to engage young women should be optimally utilized to enable mainstreaming of obstetric fistula messages into routine services such as antenatal and postnatal care services. Successful integration of family planning messages have been implemented with community-based maternal health services such as antenatal and postnatal counselling services in Bangladesh, whereby a mid-term evaluation of the programme showed that women in the intervention areas were more likely to use modern family planning methods within 12 months of childbirth, compared to the control area (42% vs. 27%) (Ahmed et al., 2013).

In the study presented in this chapter, almost one-half of the females were already married, which is very similar to figures cited by UNFPA (2012). The demographic characteristics of our study are similar to data available from the 2010 national health survey for Burkina Faso. Specifically, our result corroborates the higher levels of teenage marriage and teenage pregnancy in rural areas reported in that study (INSD & ICF International, 2012). This finding is also corroborated by the Population Council, which reported that nearly two thirds (62% of girls ages 20–24 years), living in rural areas, were married before the age of 18 (Brady et al., 2007). This is a finding that also exposes the contradiction between situations on the ground and what the law prescribes, whereby the legal age for marriage is set at 17 years for girls in Burkina Faso (Ministère de la Justice, 1989). In the study reported in this chapter, 9% of young women reported that they got married by the age of 15 years, a finding that is supported by another study conducted in Burkina Faso which showed that 6% of rural girls were married under the age of 15 years (Brady et al., 2007). This effectively signifies the importance of reaching out to girls before this age with reproductive health messages. Findings in this study show the need to understand the unique challenges and needs of rural areas in Burkina Faso and other developing countries, as young women living in rural areas have a higher risk of obstetric fistula and as they are at marked disadvantage when it comes to health literacy.

While it was evident that the motorcycle was the most frequently used mode of transportation in the district, as it was relatively cheaper than a vehicle and faster than a donkey. The concern was for the women who believed an ambulance was the best mode of transport in an emergency. Only the district hospital provides ambulance services (DRS Boucle du Mouhoun, 2012). As of the conclusion of this survey, there was only one functional ambulance in the hospital. It was key to highlight this finding, as ultimately, structural improvements geared at health system strengthening need to accompany health promotion strategies to be successful.

One of the limitations of our study includes the relatively small sample size. Also, due to cluster sampling, participants in our study may be more homogeneous than the population as a whole (Barnett, 2002). In addition, there is potential for inter-observer bias, due to the use of more than one interviewer; a standard and intensive training was conducted for all data enumerators with a view of minimising this bias. The standard operating procedure utilized in this study also helps to reduce the risk of this form of bias.

25.5 Conclusions

Findings from this study show clearly that planning programmes focused on prevention cannot simply be a case of "one size fits all." This study has provided essential information for framing policies and designing programmes to prevent obstetric fistula. Strategies must be adapted to local settings, whether urban or rural, in order to be more effective. Efforts geared towards tackling obstetric fistula should be made explicit and strengthened within the context of wider developmental objectives and global targets such as the Sustainable Development Goals whereby multi-sectoral approaches (including education, health and gender) are deployed, while harnessing the respective contributions of all stakeholders, to ensure that "no one (including disadvantaged young girls) is left behind." It is also crucial to strengthen local research efforts that focus on identifying information gaps and that explore the most effective methods for disseminating information for behaviour change in health.

Although the study reported in this chapter has focused on the preventative aspects of obstetric fistula programmes, it is essential to note the importance of the other two components that make up an effective fistula response, that is, treatment and reinsertion (social and economic). Slinger describes the importance of a holistic approach in her commentary, where she compared obstetric fistula interventions to a tub that is filling with water; while one tries to remove the water from the bath with a cup, there is also the need to work towards closing the tap (Slinger, 2011). Hence, it follows this analogy that approaches to tackling public health ills such as obstetric fistula, which have major societal ramifications, require concerted, multi-sectoral efforts that span the whole prevention–care continuum. Indeed, the eradication of obstetric fistula fundamentally constitutes a human rights issue; a societal ill that has inequality written all over it. It embodies gender inequality as well as geographic inequality within the same feminine gender, as women in rural communities are more disadvantaged compared to those in urban areas. Indeed, *"in an unequal world, these women are the most unequal among unequals"* (de Bernis, 2007).

References

Adler, A. J., Ronsmans, C., Calvert, C., & Filippi, V. (2013). Estimating the prevalence of obstetric fistula: A systematic review and meta-analysis. *BMC Pregnancy and Childbirth, 13*, 246. Retrieved December 23, 2018, from https://www.ncbi.nlm.nih.gov/pmc/articles/PMC3937166/

Agha, S. (2002). A quasi-experimental study to assess the impact of four adolescent sexual health interventions in sub-Saharan Africa. *International Family Planning Perspectives, 28*(2), 67–70. & 113–118. Retrieved December 21, 2018, from https://www.guttmacher.org/sites/default/files/pdfs/pubs/journals/2806702.pdf

Ahmed, S., Norton, M., Williams, E., Ahmed, S., Shah, R., Begum, N., Mungai, J., Lefevre, A., Al-Kabir, A., Winch, P. J., McKaig, C., & Baqui, A. H. (2013). Operations research to add postpartum family planning to maternal and neonatal health to improve birth spacing in Sylhet District, Bangladesh. *Global Health, Science and Practice, 1*(2), 262–276. Retrieved December 21, 2018, from https://www.ncbi.nlm.nih.gov/pmc/articles/PMC4168577/

Banke-Thomas, A. O., Kouraogo, S. F., Siribie, A., Taddese, H. B., & Mueller, J. E. (2013). Knowledge of obstetric fistula prevention amongst young women in urban and rural Burkina Faso: A cross-sectional study. *PLoS One, 8*(12), e85921.

Banke-Thomas, A. O., Wilton-Waddell, O. E., Kouraogo, S. F., & Mueller, E. (2014). Current evidence supporting obstetric fistula prevention strategies in sub Saharan Africa: A systematic review of the literature. *African Journal of Reproductive Health, 18*(3), 118–127. Retrieved December 30, 2018, from https://www.ajol.info/index.php/ajrh/article/viewFile/109210/99004

Banke-Thomas, A., Madaj, B., Kumar, S., Ameh, C., & van den Broek, N. (2017). Assessing Value-for-Money in Maternal and Newborn Health. *BMJ Global Health, 2*, e000310. https://doi.org/10.1136/bmjgh-2017-000310.

Barageine, J. K., Tumwesigye, N. M., Byamugisha, J. K., Almroth, L., & Faxelid, E. (2014). Risk factors for obstetric fistula in Western Uganda: A case control study. *PLoS One, 9*(11), e112299. Retrieved December 30, 2018, from https://www.ncbi.nlm.nih.gov/pmc/articles/PMC4234404/

Barnett, V. (2002). *Sample survey: Principles and methods* (3rd ed.). Arnold.

Brady, M., Saloucou, L., & Chong, E. (2007). *L'adolescence des filles au Burkina Faso: Une clé de voûte pour le changement social.* Population Council. Retrieved December 30, 2018, from https://www.popcouncil.org/uploads/pdfs/2010PGY_AdolGirlsBurkinaFaso_fr.pdf

Capes, T., Ascher-Walsh, C., Abdoulaye, I., & Brodman, M. (2011). Obstetric fistula in low and middle income countries. *The Mount Sinai Journal of Medicine, 78*(3), 352–361. https://doi.org/10.1002/msj.20265

Cook, R., Dickens, M., & Syed, S. (2004). Obstetric fistula: The challenge to human rights. *International Journal of Gynecology & Obstetrics, 87*, 72–77. https://doi.org/10.1016/j.ijgo.2004.07.005

Cowgill, K. D., Bishop, J., Norgaard, A. K., Rubens, C. E., & Gravett, M. G. (2015). Obstetric fistula in low-resource countries: An under-valued and under-studied problem—systematic review of its incidence, prevalence, and association with stillbirth. *BMC Pregnancy and Childbirth, 15*, 193. Retrieved December 30, 2018, from https://www.ncbi.nlm.nih.gov/pmc/articles/PMC4550077/

de Bernis, L. (2007). Obstetric fistula: Guiding principles for clinical management and programme development, a new WHO guideline. *International Journal of Gynaecology and Obstetrics, 99*(Suppl 1), S117–S121. https://doi.org/10.1016/j.ijgo.2007.06.032

Diesfeld, R. G. (1993). Problems related to schoolgirl pregnancies in Burkina Faso. *Studies in Family Planning, 24*(5), 283–294.

DRS Boucle du Mouhoun. (2012). *Presentation Generale de la Region Sanitaire.* DRS Boucle du Mouhoun.

Eboreime, E. A., Olawepo, J. O., Banke-Thomas, A., Abejirinde, I.-O. O., & Abimbola, S. (2020). Appraising and addressing design and implementation failure in global health: A pragmatic framework. *Global Public Health*, 1–9. https://doi.org/10.1080/17441692.2020.1814379.

Hassan, M., & Ekele, B. (2009). Vesicovaginal fistula: Do the patients know the cause? *Annals of African Medicine, 8*(2), 122–126. Retrieved December 20, 2018, from http://www.annalsafrmed.org/article.asp?issn=1596-3519;year=2009;volume=8;issue=2;spage=122;epage=126;aulast=Hassan

INSD. (2007). *Resultats Preliminaires du recensement general de la population et de l'habitation de 2006.* INSD.

INSD. (2017). *Annuaire statistique 2016.* INSD. Retrieved December 20, 2018, from http://www.insd.bf/n/contenu/pub_periodiques/annuaires_stat/Annuaires_stat_nationaux_BF/Annuaire_stat_2016.pdf

INSD, & ICF International. (2012). *Enquête démographique et de santé et à indicateurs multiples (EDSBF-MICS IV) 2010.* INSD et ICF International. Retrieved December 30, 2018, from http://www.insd.bf/n/contenu/actualites/edsbf_mics_rapport.pdf

Kalembo, F., & Zgambo, M. (2012). Obstetric fistula: A hidden public health problem in sub-Saharan Africa. *Arts and Social Sciences Journal, 2012*(ASSJ-41), 1–8. Retrieved December 30, 2018, from https://www.omicsonline.org/open-access/obstetric-fistula-a-hidden-public-health-problem-in-subsaharan-africa-2151-6200-1000041.php?aid=13420

Kasamba, N., Kaye, D. K., & Mbalinda, S. N. (2013). Community awareness about risk factors, presentation and prevention and obstetric fistula in Nabitovu village, Iganga district, Uganda. *BMC Pregnancy and Childbirth, 13*, 229. Retrieved December 30, 2018, from https://www.ncbi.nlm.nih.gov/pmc/articles/PMC4028862/

Kishk, N. A. (2002). Knowledge, attitudes and practices of women towards antenatal care: Rural-urban comparison. *The Journal of the Egyptian Public Health Association, 77*(5–6), 479–498.

Konje, J. C., & Ladipo, O. A. (2000). Nutrition and obstructed labor. *The American Journal of Clinical Nutrition, 72*(1), 291S–297S.

Lufumpa, E., Doos, L., & Lindenmeyer, A. (2018). Barriers and facilitators to preventive interventions for the development of obstetric fistulas among women in sub-Saharan Africa: A systematic review. *BMC Pregnancy and Childbirth, 18*(1), 155. Retrieved December 30, 2018, from https://www.ncbi.nlm.nih.gov/pmc/articles/PMC5946543/

Lule, E., Oomman, N., Epp, J., & Ramana, G. N. V. (2003). *Achieving the millennium development goal of improving maternal health: Determinants, interventions and challenges.* World Bank. Retrieved December 30, 2018, from http://documents.worldbank.org/curated/en/551751468330300620/pdf/320370LuleAchievingtheMDGFinal.pdf

Maheu-Giroux, M., Filippi, V., Samadoulougou, S., Castro, M. C., Maulet, N., Meda, N., & Kirakoya-Samadoulougou, F. (2015). Prevalence of symptoms of vaginal fistula in 19 sub-Saharan Africa countries: A meta-analysis of national household survey data. *Lancet Global Health, 3*(5), e271–e278. Retrieved December 30, 2018, from https://www.thelancet.com/action/showPdf?pii=S2214-109X%2814%2970348-1

Ministère de la justice. (1989). *Code des personnes et de la famille.* Ministère de la justice. Retrieved December 30, 2018, from https://www.refworld.org/docid/3ae6b4da27.html

Montez, D. (2011). *Family planning and maternal health in Tanzania: Women demand for more information.* Africa Development Research Brief. Retrieved December 30, 2018, from https://pdfs.semanticscholar.org/1d51/9ba18eabc1141c4cf60676244595fc497e5b.pdf?_ga=2.7588214.552392036.1546171338-1752513074.1545923383

Mueller, J. E., Yaro, S., Njanpop-Lafourcade, B.-M., Drabo, A., Idohou, R. S., Kroman, S. S., Sanou, O., Diagbouga, S., Troaré, Y., Sangaré, L., Borrow, R., & Gessner, B. D. (2011). Study of a localized meningococcal meningitis epidemic in Burkina Faso: Incidence, carriage, and immunity. *The Journal of Infectious Diseases, 204*(11), 1787–1795. Retrieved December 30, 2018, from https://www.ncbi.nlm.nih.gov/pmc/articles/PMC3247801/

Plummer, M. L., Wight, D., Obasi, A. I. N., Wamoyi, J., Mshana, G., Todd, J., Mazige, B. C., Makokha, M., Hayes, R. J., & Ross, D. A. (2007). A process evaluation of a school-based adolescent sexual health intervention in rural Tanzania: The MEMA kwa Vijana programme. *Health Education Research, 22*(4), 500–512. Retrieved December 30, 2018, from https://academic.oup.com/her/article/22/4/500/632618

Ridde, V., Richard, F., Bicaba, A., Queuille, L., & Conombo, G. (2011). The national subsidy for deliveries and emergency obstetric care in Burkina Faso. *Health Policy and Planning, 26*(Suppl 2), ii30–ii40. Retrieved December 30, 2018, from https://academic.oup.com/heapol/article/26/suppl_2/ii30/640606

Shefren, J. M. (2009). The tragedy of obstetric fistula and strategies for prevention. *American Journal of Obstetrics and Gynecology, 200*(6), 668–671. https://doi.org/10.1016/j.ajog.2009.03.008

Slinger, G. (2011). *Preventing obstetric fistula: A public health priority.* Rewire. Retrieved November 28, 2018, from https://rewire.news/article/2011/03/04/preventing-obstetric-fistulapublic-health-priority/

Tebeu, P. M., Fomulu, J. N., Khaddaj, S., de Bernis, L., Delvaux, T., & Rochat, C. H. (2012). Risk factors for obstetric fistula: a clinical review. *International Urogynecology Journal, 23*(4), 387–394. Retrieved February 4, 2019, from https://www.ncbi.nlm.nih.gov/pmc/articles/PMC3305871/

UNFPA. (2004). *Etude Socioanthropologique des Fistules Obstetricales dans la Zone d'Intervention du Projet «Appui a la Lutte contre la Mortalite Maternelle» (Projet BKF No. 05/01/13).* UNFPA. Retrieved December 30, 2018, from https://burkinafaso.unfpa.org/fr/publications/etude-sur-les-fistules-obstétricales

UNFPA. (2012). *Marrying too young: End child marriage.* UNFPA. Retrieved December 30, 2018, from https://www.unfpa.org/sites/default/files/pub-pdf/MarryingTooYoung.pdf

UNFPA & DSF. (2004). *Analyse de la Prise en charge des Fistules Urogenitales au Niveau des Services de Santé de Référence du Burkina* (pp. 2001–2003). UNFPA & DSF.

UNFPA & Ministère de la Santé—Burkina Faso. (2012). Programme national de lutte contre les fistules obstétricales 2011–2015. Retrieved December 30, 2018, from https://burkinafaso.unfpa.org/fr/publications/programme-national-de-lutte-contre-les-fistules-obst%C3%A9tricales-2011-2015

UNICEF. (2013). *Burkina Faso.* UNICEF. Retrieved November 26, 2018, from https://www.unicef.org/french/infoby-country/burkinafaso_statistics.html

Vangeenderhuysen, C., Prual, A., & Ould el Joud, D. (2001). Obstetric fistulae: Incidence estimates for sub-Saharan Africa. *International Journal of Gynecology & Obstetrics, 73*(1), 65–66.

Wanyonyi, K. L., Themessl-Huber, M., Humphris, G., & Freeman, R. (2011). A systematic review and meta-analysis of face-to-face communication of tailored health messages: Implications for practice. *Patient Education and Counseling, 85*(3), 348–355.

WHEC. (2013). *Global efforts to end obstetric fistula (part 1).* WHEC. Retrieved December 30, 2018, from http://www.womenshealthsection.com/content/print.php3?title=urogvvf011&cat=78&lng=english

World Bank. (2018). *World Bank country and lending groups.* World Bank. Retrieved December 30, 2018, from https://datahelpdesk.worldbank.org/knowledgebase/articles/906519

Zhang, Y. (2006). Urban-rural literacy gaps in sub-Saharan Africa: The roles of socioeconomic status and school quality. *Comparative Education Review, 50*(4), 581–602.

Zhao, Q., Kulane, A., Gao, Y., & Xu, B. (2009). Knowledge and attitude on maternal health care among rural-to-urban migrant women in Shanghai, China. *BMC Women's Health, 9*, 5. Retrieved October 31, 2018, from https://www.ncbi.nlm.nih.gov/pmc/articles/PMC2674037/

Sexual Function in Women with Obstetric Fistulas

26

Rachel Pope

26.1 Introduction

After months to years of urinary incontinence, women with obstetric fistulas often experience a disturbance of their emotional and physical relationships for a variety of reasons. Patients have cited incontinence and odor as a barrier to relationships with romantic partners. This also affects sexual behavior. Although it is culturally taboo to discuss sexual practices in many places where obstetric fistula exists, the medical nature of the fistula allows space for the discussion of sexual health from a medical perspective. This is especially true as women with fistulas often discover their sexual dysfunction only after they have undergone fistula repair as they may not have had intercourse while the fistula was present, or they were inadvertently having intercourse into the base of the bladder while the fistula was present. As a result, they only experience dyspareunia or dysfunction once the bladder is closed as part of the vesicovaginal fistula repair (Wilkinson et al., 2011).

Sexual wellbeing is part of the holistic care of a woman with obstetric fistula. A report from a meeting held on meeting the needs of women with "fistula deemed incurable" in Boston, Massachusetts noted that women who are unable to resume sexual function may not consider their condition cured (Harvard, 2011). Few studies have looked into the sexual effects of an obstetric fistula as well as repair, but those that have will be reviewed here. It is noted, however, that culturally in most places where obstetric fistula exists, heterosexuality is the only acceptable type of relationship to query. Therefore, this review uses language reflective of a heteronormative perspective. Finally, ways to prevent sexual dysfunction and innovative treatment for sexual dysfunction among women with obstetric fistulas are discussed.

26.2 Sexual Dysfunction Among Women with Obstetric Fistulas

Sexual dysfunction consists of female sexual interest/arousal disorder and genito-pelvic/penetration disorder by the DSM-V. The symptoms must last a minimum duration of 6 months and occur 75–100% of the time. In addition, the disorder should not be better explained by a "nonsexual mental disorder,

R. Pope (✉)
University Hospital, Cleveland Medical Center, Urology Institute, Cleveland, OH, USA
e-mail: rachel.pope@uhhospitals.org

© Springer Nature Switzerland AG 2022
L. B. Drew et al. (eds.), *A Multidisciplinary Approach to Obstetric Fistula in Africa*, Global Maternal and Child Health, https://doi.org/10.1007/978-3-031-06314-5_26

a consequence of severe relationship distress (e.g., partner violence) or other significant stressors" (American Psychiatric Association, 2013). Although a fistula could be a significant stressor, this would fall under the category of medical factors attributing to sexual dysfunction. For many reasons, having an obstetric fistula causes significant dysfunction. Although sexuality is a taboo topic in many parts of the world where obstetric fistula exists, the relevance to vaginal surgery creates the cultural space for understanding many facets that women experience.

Of a study of 115 women with fistulas in Malawi, 40% of participants experienced sexual dysfunction after developing a vesicovaginal fistula (Pope et al., 2018). Many described pain inside of the vagina when they attempted intercourse and many described frustration with incontinence. Similarly, a study in Nigeria found 22.5% of women experience difficulty with intercourse at the time they have a fistula due to vaginal narrowness, pain, and/or lack of sexual desire themselves or their partner (Anzaku et al., 2017).

Many women with obstetric fistulas spend much of their time hiding and/or managing their incontinence. Due to the involuntary leakage of urine, they often wear and change cumbersome cloths or pads and find themselves bathing multiple times a day. Many women relate using lotions and powders to mask the smell. In clinical centers, we see evidence of women limiting their fluid intake as an effort to reduce leakage of urine. This unfortunately only causes the urine to become more concentrated and therefore caustic, leading to urinary dermatitis (Arrowsmith et al., 1996), which is a condition in which the skin reacts to the components of the urine by producing lesions. This can be mild or extensive (see Fig. 26.1). Many clinicians mistake urinary dermatitis for signs of syphilis, herpes or other skin conditions. Fortunately, zinc oxide and other skin barriers rapidly improve the dermatitis.

Socially, women find that their communities often ostracize them; if not for the odor, then for the belief that they have been cursed or bewitched. This belief of the fistula being a result of a curse is widespread in West, East, and South Africa, although it has not been mentioned where fistula exists in Asia. This belief and stigmatization translates to anyone who associates with the woman. Therefore, for a woman with obstetric fistula, her romantic relationships are usually in jeopardy. Studies from various regions have demonstrated that women with fistulas commonly experience divorce and physical separation from their spouses (Khisa et al., 2017; Mselle et al., 2011). Reasons for divorce include

Fig. 26.1 Example of urine dermatitis. (Photo credit: Rachel Pope)

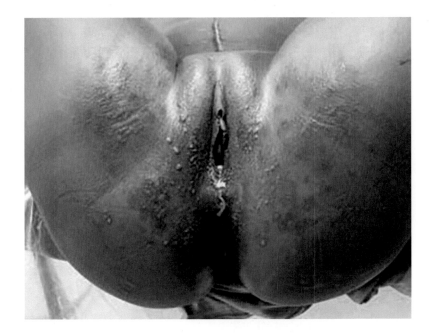

the incontinence, the belief that she is now infertile, etc. If she has no other children and the delivery that caused the fistula resulted in a stillbirth, divorce is especially common (Stokes et al., 2018). One woman in Malawi stated that her husband remained married to her but abstained from intercourse for fear that he might "catch" fistula from her (Pope et al., 2018). Others have stated they similarly worried that the curse would extend to them if they were to have intercourse.

As many communities strongly link intercourse to reproduction, some women state that they do not believe they can conceive while they have a fistula and therefore, they were likely to lose their spouse (Pope et al., 2011). However, as seen in communities throughout Madagascar, partners tend to remain with their spouses despite having an obstetric fistula and remain sexually active (personal account, 2016). Therefore, in this setting, many women continue to reproduce while they have a fistula and before they undergo surgical repair. In Malawi, 64% of total participants interviewed in the study mentioned earlier remained sexually active while having a fistula (Pope et al., 2018). Fifty-four percent engaged in nonvaginal sexual intimacy and 36% of them were coerced to engage in vaginal penetration; 15.6% of this cohort mentions their husbands taking a co-wife due to the problems with her sexuality and 3.5% states this was due to believed infertility. In Nigeria, Anzaku et al. (2017) found 77.5% of those interviewed were sexually active while they had a fistula; however, 12% were not sexually active due to what they described as physical inability with a "narrow" vagina.

Emotionally, women have stated that they are not interested in intercourse while they leak urine. There is a sense of a loss of control over one's body that likely negatively affects libido (Mselle et al., 2011; Pope et al., 2011). Mselle et al. (2011) found that women living with a fistula experience a "deep sense of loss that has negative impact on their identity and quality of life". Wilson et al. (2015) describe women who have developed a fistula as suffering from a post-traumatic stress disorder which effects emotions and social relationships. Many women are also occupied with seeking a cure, which may divert interest in physical intimacy.

In the Malawian study, roughly half of interviewees believed their husbands were having extramarital relationships and many participants blamed themselves for this. Additionally, this also caused them to fear contracting HIV or other sexually transmitted infections (Pope et al., 2018). Therefore, the compounding of loss of self-worth and the belief that one's partner is seeking out other relationships due to her physical condition, likely negatively affects sexuality and overall quality of life for a woman living with a fistula.

26.3   Sexual Function After Surgery

Coetzee (Coetzee & Lithgow, 1966) states that "optimal fistula repair should allow for complete continence with adequate bladder capacity, normal coitus without dyspareunia, and a normal reproductive capacity". Therefore, when providing vesicovaginal fistula repair services, it is imperative to address factors associated with sexual function and this discussion should be considered part of comprehensive fistula care. Although several articles on vesicovaginal fistula repair mention sexual function as a concern for patients as a residual problem, only one study has focused on the objective changes after surgery or the factors that contribute to new onset dysfunction (Anzaku et al., 2017; Gutman et al., 2007; Pope et al., 2018; Tembely et al., 2014; Wall et al., 2005).

It is hopeful that repair of the fistula would result in a return to sexual activity as previously experienced; however, this is not always the case. Urogenital disorders with and without surgical intervention have been found to be closely linked to sexual dysfunction (Wehbe et al., 2010). We see this in women with obstetric fistulas as well. Although continence may have been restored, the soft tissue of the pelvic floor may be contracted and scarred. The lack of compliance of the pelvic tissue could be from the initial obstructed labor and pelvic trauma, and chronic dermal irritation from urine can result in profound dermatitis and fibrosis. Fistula surgeons have cited that patients sometimes return after successful surgical closure of a fistula and request to have the surgery reversed (Wilkinson et al., 2011). Before repair, many of these patients were having sexual intercourse with their bladder as a replacement for the vagina. The closure of the fistula in the setting of marked vaginal stenosis or complete obliteration resulted in a subsequent inability for them to continue sexual intercourse. Two studies published on the subject found worsening sexual function after surgery, but did not note any physical characteristics or factors associated with dysfunction (Anzaku et al., 2017; Tembely et al., 2014). Evoh and Akinla (1978) describe 17% of the 162 women included in their study to have gynatresia, or a vaginal narrowing before fistula repair and 10% with a worsening condition after surgery. In one small series, half of 16 women who had large fistulas (diameter 4 cm or larger) developed vaginal narrowing with surgery (Elkins et al., 1990). Anzaku and colleagues found that about half of the women they interviewed report reduced or no sexual satisfaction after surgical repair compared to their experiences prior to a fistula (Anzaku et al., 2017). In this study, 47% report occasional or frequent pain with intercourse since surgery as compared to previously.

Sexual function and risks for dysfunction have only been explored in one study (Pope et al., 2018). This study interviewed and collected physical measurements before surgery and 6 months after surgery. The majority of women (90%, $n = 104$) expected surgery to make intercourse the same as it was prior to surgery. All women (100%, $n = 115$) stated they could wait 6 months to have intercourse after surgery and most (95.6%, $n = 110$) thought their partners could also wait. At the time of the postoperative visit, 6–12 months after fistula surgery, 20% ($n = 17$) experienced marital status changes since prior to surgery. Seven married new partners or resumed a relationship with their previous partner, three were engaged to be married, and two were divorced (one participant's husband said he could not wait 6 months, and another left while she was in the hospital). Five women mentioned new co-wives since surgery.

In our study in Malawi, vaginal length and caliber were evaluated before and after surgery using paired t-tests (Table 26.1). Vaginal length was found to decrease by 5 mm after surgery, while vaginal caliber was found to increase by 3 mm after surgery, though this was not enough difference to affect dysfunction. Both were statistically significant changes. Surprisingly, fibrosis did not statistically significantly change and was not found to be associated with sexual function. Of the variables examined, the factors statistically significantly associated with dysfunction included a larger the size of the fistula as determined by the Goh classification (>3 cm) and decreased vaginal caliber.

About one-third of the women interviewed for this study (35.6%, $n = 41$) reported trying to have intercourse since returning from surgery. Others had no partner or their partner had left town or the country for work or were concerned about developing another fistula (20.9%, $n = 24$). Many women stated they were waiting for their doctor's permission or for additional healing (31.3%, $n = 36$) to have intercourse despite already passing the 6-month waiting period. One woman avoided intercourse due to fears of becoming pregnant again. All women were interviewed using the validated revised female sexual distress scale (FSDS-R) both before and after surgery (Derogatis et al., 2001). Only 12.2% ($n = 14$) stated that they experienced problems with intercourse since surgery, though 16.5% ($n = 19$) of the participants scored in the range of dysfunction as assessed by the FSDS-R tool. Seven were still leaking with intercourse and seven were still experiencing pain. Some women find that although they are generally continent, they experience incontinence with sexual intercourse. This leakage causes embarrassment for them and becomes a reason to avoid intimate relationships.

About one-third (35.6%, $n = 41$) stated that intercourse has returned to the way it was before a fistula. Mean FSDS-R scores from before surgery were 27.1 (s.d. = 13.1) and decreased to 4.9 (s.d. = 11.0) after surgery (the higher the score, the more indicative of distress). The reason for problems with intercourse changed from leaking urine before surgery to lack of partner and concern for HIV infection (Table 26.1). Of the women who were sexually active within 30 days of the interview

Table 26.1 Change in characteristics before and after surgery

	Before surgery Mean (s.d.) (95% CI)	After surgery Mean (s.d.) (95% CI)	P value
Vaginal length (cm)	7.8 (1.9) (7.4–8.2)	7.3 (1.6) (7.0–7.6)	Paired t-test 0.0018
Vaginal caliber	5.2 (1.7) (4.9–5.5)	5.5 (1.6) (5.2–5.8)	0.0092
Fibrosis			Fishers
Yes	44 (40.9)	36 (31.6)	p = 0.1462
No	65 (59.1)	78 (68.4)	
Pain with exam			Chi
None	63 (57.8)	70 (61.4)	p = 0.111
Mild	35 (32.1)	41 (36.0)	
Moderate	8 (7.3)	3 (2.6)	
Severe	3 (2.8)	0 (0.0)	
Vaginal atrophy			Fishers
Yes	10 (9.2)	10 (8.8)	p = 0.901
No	99 (90.8)	104 (91.2)	
Pelvic floor strength			Chi
No strength (0)	1 (0.9)	1 (0.9)	p = 0.091
(1)	2 (1.9)	2 (1.8)	
(2)	5 (4.7)	3 (2.7)	
(3)	34 (31.8)	23 (20.4)	
(4)	24 (22.4)	46 (40.7)	
Full strength (5)	41 (38.3)	38 (33.6)	
Ability to relax pelvic floor			Chi
Not able to relax (0)	4 (3.7)	1 (0.9)	p = 0.113
(1)	2 (1.9)	1 (0.9)	
(2)	1 (0.9)	2 (1.8)	
(3)	9 (8.3)	11 (9.7)	
(4)	22 (20.4)	40 (35.4)	
Fully relaxed (5)	70 (64.8)	58 (51.3)	
FSDS	27.1 (13.1) (24.6–29.6)	4.9 (11.0) (2.9–7.0)	Paired t-test 0.000
Problem with sex			Chi
No partner	4 (3.5)	14 (17.1)	0.000
Partner not interested	10 (8.9)	1 (1.2)	
Do not want pregnancy	12 (10.6)	5 (6.1)	
Dryness	1 (0.9)	8 (9.8)	
Pain	4 (3.5)	0	
Vagina too small	2 (1.8)	0	
Leaking urine	59 (52.2)	11 (13.4)	
Concern for HIV	4 (3.5)	14 (17.1)	
Concern for witchcraft	5 (4.4)	6 (7.3)	
Presence of incontinence			Fishers
Yes (1)	115 (100.0)	26 (22.8)	p = 0.000
No (0)	0 (0.0)	88 (77.2)	

postsurgery, proportionally more of the participants with sexual dysfunction described vaginal ($n = 3$, 60%) and labial pain ($n = 2$, 40%) and less satisfaction with their sex lives.

Some women fear another pregnancy and delivery leading to ongoing physical problems or the recurrence of a fistula (Pope et al., 2011). Unfortunately, the women usually return to the same setting that resulted in the fistula in the first place. This means that they will probably still experience a lack of access to medical care due to infrastructure, physical distance, or poor medical facilities. Therefore, in order to avoid incurring another fistula, they must prepare for a delivery differently from their previous experiences. A scheduled cesarean delivery is recommended. Due to this stress, women may desire to avoid pregnancy altogether. In Tanzania, many women stated that after all of the trauma they had been through, they were no longer interested in a relationship. Others describe never wanting to engage in intercourse or pregnancy again for fear of developing another fistula (Donnelly et al., 2015; Pope et al., 2011). Additionally, women in Malawi expressed fear of contracting sexually transmitted infections and HIV due to the suspicion and sometimes knowledge that their partners had engaged in intercourse with other women either while they had the fistula or while they were away having their fistula repaired (Pope et al., 2018). In Madagascar, one father requested that the surgeons perform a tubal ligation for his daughter who had developed a fistula. His explanation was that their family would not be able to afford a cesarean delivery and he did not want her to develop another fistula if she were to become pregnant again (personal account, 2015). This request for tubal ligation was not performed after thorough counseling and discussion with the family; however, it illustrates the difficulty in changing one's circumstances with subsequent pregnancies after a fistula repair.

In many other sub-Saharan African countries, sexual relations are associated with marital, social, and economic stability and therefore are paramount concerns for patients who have been divorced or otherwise shunned by their communities because of a fistula. Studies have shown that future childbearing and economic security are matters of concern to women after repair (Désalliers et al., 2017). Due to the complexity of the issue, counseling services would be helpful in health facilities providing care to women with obstetric fistulas.

However, encouraging women to abstain from sexual activity so the tissues can adequately heal after fistula repair is challenging. "Pelvic rest" or abstinence is recommended after surgery for 6 weeks to 6 months; however, the optimal time required for adequate healing before sexual relations is unknown. Some patients describe difficulty in abstaining from sexual intercourse due to their husbands' demands and some women experience rape (Khisa et al., 2017). Understanding the precise amount of time required for healing from a fistula would be helpful, although would likely differ based on the extent of the injury, repair, and individual factors. In general, including partners in the counseling and expectations prior to fistula surgery could potentially help avoid women being coerced into sexual activity too soon. In some settings where fistula exists, intercourse is seen as a "right" to husbands. If women with fistulas do not possess the agency to overcome these cultural pressures, the health facilities providing repairs could assist in the safety of the woman through involving partners in appropriate discussions and counseling.

Due to the taboo associated with sexuality, it is likely that women in many settings will not divulge their issues unless asked specifically. This reluctance has been cited in Nigeria (Anzaku et al., 2017). Whereas in Malawi, it seems the individual who complained of the problem with vaginal stenosis had undergone multiple interventions already with the healthcare providers and was experiencing a problem severe enough that it threatened her marriage (Pope et al., 2017a). This severity may exist for many other women who may be less willing to advocate for themselves due to cultural inhibition.

26.4 Prevention and Treatment of Sexual Dysfunction

Some authors estimate that approximately 30% of patients require some type of vaginal reconstruction or vaginoplasty at the time of obstetric fistula repair (Wall et al., 2005). Gutman et al. (2007) explains that in acquired vaginal narrowness or "gynatresia," such as seen in women with obstetric fistulas, the devitalized vaginal tissue is similar to that in women who have undergone radiation treatment for pelvic malignancy. Therefore, a new paradigm is required for treatment of women with obstetric fistulas in order to enhance functionality.

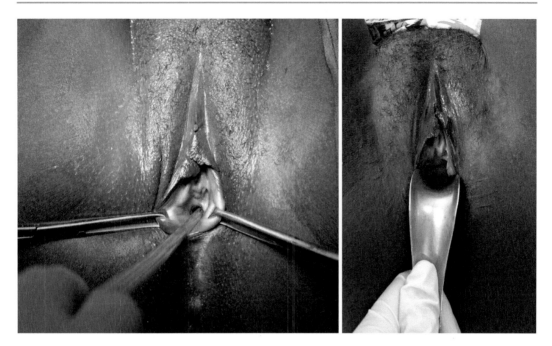

Fig. 26.2 Before and after vaginal reconstruction with bilateral Singapore flaps and use of silicone dilators for 6 months. (Photo credit: Rachel Pope) (Pope et al., 2017a; Reprinted with permission of John Wiley and Sons)

At our facility in Malawi, we have started using the combination of a pedicled pudendal fasciocutaneous flap (Singapore flap) and silicone dilators 1 month after surgical healing for women with vaginal stenosis (Pope, 2017a). This paradigm shift is the result of collaboration with plastic surgeons due to the perceived need of new techniques required to improve a patient's quality of life (Pope, 2017b). For the series of women who received a Singapore flap for vaginal reconstruction, few operative and postoperative complications were noted and overall outcomes are promising (Pope et al., 2017a). Six months after repair, the average FSDS-R score was low, indicating little to no sexual dysfunction. Initially, all participants in the study had no functional vagina due to small caliber. Six months after surgery, which includes use of silicone dilators, they were all progressing toward functional use of the vagina (see Fig. 26.2).

The surgeries to include Singapore flaps are longer and more labor intensive than a standard vesicovaginal fistula repair; however, if it prevents the need for subsequent surgeries to correct vaginal stenosis, it is worth the effort. Similarly, in the cases of women who have already undergone repair for an obstetric fistula but are experiencing vaginal stenosis complicating their sexual function, it is possible that a Singapore flap could be used to reconstruct the vagina. Dilators would still be recommended after the surgical site has healed. While dilators may help other women with vaginal stenosis, the scar tissue and fibrosis seen in patients with obstetric fistulas often cause the tissue to be hardened, contracted, and not amenable to dilation. The Singapore flap introduces healthy tissue that maintains its vascular supply and therefore, should remain pliable indefinitely. This is certainly the reason that dilators are useful as adjunct therapy for reconstruction. Once the woman has reached a dilator size that is comfortable to attempt intercourse, then intercourse alone will maintain the vaginal caliber.

In general, maintaining a heightened awareness during surgery that anatomically affects sexual function should theoretically result in fewer patients experiencing sexual dysfunction. As we have been using flaps and shifted our paradigm during the time of our study on sexual function, this could be why we found a small proportion of women with sexual dysfunction after surgery compared to other studies (Elkins et al., 1990; Evoh & Akinla, 1978; Tembely et al., 2014). It is likely that even more patients require a flap than we think as we still found that a fistula with a diameter > 3 cm is a risk factor for dysfunction. This potential criterion could be used to decide if the use of a Singapore flap is appropriate during vesicovaginal fistula surgery. However, more criteria are needed to create an objective guide for surgeons.

One unexpected finding from the study in Malawi is that many women avoid intercourse after surgery even beyond 6 months, primarily due to fear of interfering with the fistula healing or due to the lack of a partner for several reasons. The fear of another fistula or interrupting the healing process of the repair as a reason for abstaining from intercourse has been cited by other authors (Donnelly et al., 2015; Tembely et al., 2014). Like in the case of vaginal reconstruction, it is important to properly counsel women on the when they can resume intercourse and to educate them on the healing process, but also how to reinitiate intercourse when they are ready and the time is appropriate. With the "wound" of the fistula being internal, it could be difficult for an individual to feel safe and comfortable enough to initiate intercourse, despite instructions that she can resume sexual activities after a given amount of time.

26.5 Cultural Taboo and Research

Only three papers in total have been published specifically on sexuality among women with obstetric fistulas; one in Malawi, one in Mali, and one in Nigeria (Anzaku et al., 2017; Pope et al., 2017a; Tembely et al., 2014). Other papers have included sexuality as part of their inquiry (Evoh & Akinla, 1978; Gutman et al., 2007; Khisa et al., 2017). More information from other settings is needed, yet challenges in this area persist. Cultural issues may keep some aspects of research in the dark, as Anzaku et al. (2017) describe only married women were included in their study as sexual relationships outside of marriage are seen as taboo, therefore, not asked about their sexuality. In addition, in many countries where women have fistulas, homosexuality is illegal and therefore asking questions in this area of sexuality could present ethical challenges.

Additional clinical information is also needed. The difference for women with a vesicovaginal fistula and rectovaginal fistula or both types of fistula also has not been explored. Additionally, long-term sexual function of those undergoing vaginal reconstruction has not been explored.

26.6 Conclusion

Although many women with an obstetric fistula experience sexual dysfunction, most recover after surgery. During the time of living with a fistula, sexuality seems to be negatively affected to the same degree that other psychosocial aspects of life are affected. While some women maintain their relationships, many lose their partners directly due to their incontinence during intercourse or the belief that they are not fertile while leaking urine. In addition, many women find their partners engaging in intercourse with other women during this time, causing a different set of stressors to the woman living with a fistula. Connecting women with fistulas to surgery as soon as possible could also help to reduce some of these relationship quandaries.

Of those who do not recover or experience de novo dysfunction, further assistance is needed. Women who experience ongoing or de novo dysfunction are likely to have a larger fistula and decreased vaginal caliber. This change to the vaginal structure is likely due to the anterior tissue loss and subsequent vaginal shortening with the closure of the bladder and vaginal tissue, which could potentially be prevented with improved surgical technique and the use of plastic surgery techniques at the time of fistula repair.

Employing surgical techniques such as vaginal reconstruction at the time of repair with a Singapore flap, could correct the anatomical defect that leads to this dysfunction and merits further study. Additionally, including partners in counseling prior to surgery could assist in the postoperative recovery and help women avoid coercion. Discussing safe sexual practices could also assist in preventing sexually transmitted infections, including HIV in endemic areas.

Sexual education and counseling is a necessary part of surgical consent and discharge counseling as many women indicate expecting surgery to fix their sexual dysfunction as well as their incontinence. Empowering women to discuss difficulties or concerns regarding sexual function may represent a cultural challenge but is worth pursuing with appropriate cultural tactics. The high number of women who express fear of intercourse after the 6 months of healing is an obstacle for social reintegration. Attention to a woman's reproductive and sexual needs after obstetric fistula surgery is an important component to obstetric fistula care. Such efforts help to ensure the sexual and reproductive health and rights of women, particularly women who have endured meaningful impacts to their sexual and reproductive lives due to obstetric fistula.

References

American Psychiatric Association. (2013). *DSM-5: Diagnostic and statistical manual for mental disorders* (5th ed.). American Psychiatric Press.

Anzaku, S. A., Lengman, S. J., Mikah, S., Shephard, S. N., & Edem, B. E. (2017). Sexual activity among Nigerian women following successful obstetric fistula repair. *International Journal of Gynecology & Obstetrics, 137*(1), 67–71.

Arrowsmith, S., Hamlin, C., & Wall, L. L. (1996). Obstructed labor injury complex: Obstetric fistula formation and the multifaceted morbidity of maternal birth trauma in the developing world. *Obstetrical & Gynecological Survey, 51*(9), 568–574.

Coetzee, T., & Lithgow, D. M. (1966). Obstetric fistulae of the urinary tract. *Journal of Obstetrics and Gynaecology British Commonwealth, 73*, 837–844.

Derogatis, L. R., Burnett, A., Heiman, J., Leiblum, S., & Rosen, R. (2001). *Development and continuing validation of the Female Sexual Distress Scale (FSDS)*. Annual Female Sexual Function Forum. October 29.

Désalliers, J., Pare, M. E., Kouraogo, S., & Corcos, J. (2017). Impact of surgery on quality of life of women with obstetrical fistula: A qualitative study in Burkina Faso. *International Urogynecology Journal, 28*(7), 1091–1100.

Donnelly, K., Oliveras, E., Tilahun, Y., Belachew, M., & Asnake, M. (2015). Quality of life of Ethiopian women after fistula repair: Implications on rehabilitation and social reintegration policy and programming. *Culture, Health, and Sexuality, 17*(2), 150–164.

Elkins, T. E., DeLancey, J. O., & McGuire, E. J. (1990). The use of modified Martius graft as an adjunctive technique in vesicovaginal and rectovaginal fistula repair. *Obstetrics & Gynecology, 75*, 727–733.

Evoh, N. J., & Akinla, O. (1978). Reproductive performance after obstetric vesico-vaginal fistulae. *Annals of Clinical Research, 10*(6), 303–306.

Gutman, R., Dodson, J., & Mostwin, J. (2007). Complications of treatment of obstetric fistula in the developing world: Gynatresia, urinary incontinence, and urinary diversion. *International Journal of Gynecology & Obstetrics, 99*, S57–S64.

Harvard. (2011). *Fistula care; Meeting the needs of women with fistula deemed incurable: Creating a culture of possibility. Report of a consultative meeting*. Harvard Club. September 19–20, 2011.

Khisa, W., Wakasiaka, S., McGowan, L., Campbell, M., & Lavender, T. (2017). Understanding the lived experience of women before and after fistula repair: A qualitative study in Kenya. *BJOG: An International Journal of Obstetrics & Gynaecology, 124*(3), 503–510.

Mselle, L. T., Moland, K. M., Evjen-Olsen, B., Mvungi, A., & Kohi, T. W. (2011). "I am nothing": Experiences of loss among women suffering from severe birth injuries in Tanzania. *BMC Women's Health, 11*, 49.

Pope, R., Bangser, M., & Harris-Requejo, J. (2011). Restoring dignity social reintegration after obstetric fistula repair in Ukerewe, Tanzania. *Global Public Health, 6*(8), 859–873.

Pope, R., Brown, R. H., Chipungu, E., Hollier, L. H., Jr., & Wilkinson, J. P. (2017a). The use of Singapore flaps for vaginal reconstruction in women with vaginal stenosis with obstetric fistula: A surgical technique. *BJOG: An International Journal of Obstetrics and Gynaecology, 125*(6), 751–756.

Pope, R., & Wilkinson, J. (2017b). Surgical innovation for obstetric fistula patients. *BJOG: An International Journal of Obstetrics and Gynaecology, 125*(6), 750.

Pope, R., Ganesh, P., Chalamanda, C., Nundwe, W., & Wilkinson, J. P. (2018). Sexual function before and after vesicovaginal fistula repair. *Journal of Sexual Medicine, 15*, 1125–1132.

Stokes, M., Ganesh, P., Nundwe, W., Wilkinson, J., & Pope, R. (2018). *Persistent depression in women with obstetric fistula*. International Society of Fistula Surgeons. Oral Presentation.

Tembely, A., Diarra, A., & Berthé, H. (2014). Sexuality and fertility of women operated for obstetric urogenital fistulae. *Progrès en Urologie, 24*(13), 876.

Wall, L. L., Arrowsmith, S. D., Briggs, N. D., Browning, A., & Lassey, A. (2005). The obstetric vesicovaginal fistula in the developing world. *Obstetrical and Gynecological Survey, 60*, S3–S51.

Wehbe, S. A., Kellogg, S., & Whitmore, K. (2010). Urogenital complaints and female sexual dysfunction, part 2. *Journal of Sexual Medicine, 7*, 2304–2317.

Wilkinson, J. P., Lyerly, A. D., Masenga, G., Hayat, S. K., & Prabhu, M. (2011). Ethical dilemmas in women's health in under-resourced settings. *International Journal of Gynecology & Obstetrics, 113*(1), 25–27.

Wilson, S. M., Sikkema, K. J., Watt, M. H., & Masenga, G. G. (2015). Psychological symptoms among obstetric fistula patients compared to gynecology outpatients in Tanzania. *International Journal of Behavioral Medicine, 22*(5), 605–613.

Social and Reproductive Health of Women After Obstetric Fistula Repair: Insights from Guinea

27

Alexandre Delamou

27.1 Introduction

Obstetric fistula remains a health and human rights tragedy due to its devastating consequences and debilitating sequela. It is often referred to as a neglected tropical disease due to its higher prevalence among vulnerable populations in lower-resource countries (Osotimehin, 2013; Wall, 2012a). In addition to incontinence, its primary presenting symptom, common physical and psychosocial comorbidities of fistula include stillbirth, foot-drop, vaginal stenosis, secondary infertility, chronic urinary tract infection, depression, and stigmatization (Ahmed et al., 2016; Arrowsmith et al., 1996; Wall, 2012a). Obstetric fistula persists in sub-Saharan African countries where the quality of maternal health services is poor, particularly emergency obstetric care (Lozano et al., 2011; World Health Organization, 2014).

Over the past two decades, global efforts have improved women's access to fistula care, including prevention, treatment, and reintegration services (Osotimehin, 2015). From 2005 to 2013, more than 30,000 fistula repairs have been supported across 15 sub-Saharan African countries through EngenderHealth's USAID-funded Fistula Care Project, (USAID and EngenderHealth, 2014) and more than 57,000 repairs through UNFPA (Osotimehin, 2015). Surgical closure rates are usually high, particularly at first repair attempt (up to 90%), but vary based on repair site and fistula characteristics (Arrowsmith et al., 2013). Subsequent repair attempts are technically difficult and typically have lower success rates (Gupta et al., 2012; Maulet et al., 2013).

Less is known about the reproductive and social lives of women after fistula repair; although a variety of key services may be required to prevent adverse outcomes and achieve gains in quality of life. Preventing fistula recurrence relies on avoiding heavy work, waiting to resume sexual intercourse until 6 months after surgery, and carefully managing any postrepair pregnancies and deliveries in alignment with recommendations for elective cesarean section (Browning, 2009). In addition, successful social and economic reintegrations are key to helping women resume regular social lives, overcome the isolation and psychological trauma they experienced, and prevent the occurrence of

A. Delamou (✉)
Department of Public Health & Africa Center of Excellence (CEA-PCMT),
University Gamal Abdel Nasser of Conakry, Conakry, Guinea
e-mail: adelamou@gmail.com

© Springer Nature Switzerland AG 2022
L. B. Drew et al. (eds.), *A Multidisciplinary Approach to Obstetric Fistula in Africa*, Global Maternal and Child Health, https://doi.org/10.1007/978-3-031-06314-5_27

adverse health outcomes, such as stillbirth, recurrence of the fistula or maternal death (Drew et al., 2016; Lombard et al., 2015). However, the extent to which recommendations are followed and needed services are implemented is not known due to lack of longitudinal follow-up following fistula repair.

Little data are available on any aspects of the postfistula repair period. Very few studies have estimated fistula recurrence after successful repair, using various study designs and case definitions along with different lengths of follow-up (Browning & Menber, 2008; Kopp et al., 2017; Nielsen et al., 2009; Wilson et al., 2011). Similarly, there is a paucity of data on fertility, pregnancy, and childbirth after successful fistula repair, especially employing robust study designs able to provide precise estimates and risk factors of pregnancy and delivery outcomes (Browning, 2009; Mafo Degge et al., 2017).

Although available data are limited, many women are relatively young at the time their fistula is repaired, and most return to their community after surgery with the desire to resume a normal social life and fertility desires including becoming sexually active and having children (Browning & Menber, 2008; Drew et al., 2016; Landry et al., 2013; Nielsen et al., 2009; Wilson et al., 2011). Pregnancy and childbirth increase the risk of recurrence of a previously repaired fistula or the formation of a second, new fistula, especially if the woman does not undergo elective cesarean section as recommended (Browning & Menber, 2008; Nielsen et al., 2009). Fistula recurrence is stressful for women and burdensome for fistula care programs and the communities (Donnelly et al., 2015; Maulet et al., 2013), especially given the relative high cost of fistula care (Epiu et al., 2018).

This chapter seeks to contribute to the nascent evidence base on the reproductive and social lives of women after successful obstetric fistula closure through quantitative and qualitative inquiry from a series of studies conducted in Guinea between 2014 and 2018. I conducted a situational analysis of fistula care programs in Guinean context and studied the key factors that influence pregnancy and childbirth after repair of the fistula. I also sought to understand the factors associated with fistula recurrence, and the process and outcomes of social reintegration after repair along with the expectation of stakeholders on the health and social life of women treated for fistula in Guinea.

27.2   Framework for Analyzing the Reproductive Health of Women After Fistula Repair

A holistic model of fistula care should include prevention of fistula reoccurrence, case management, and reintegration after repair and should address both women with and without successful repair (Wall, 2012b). My framework for approaching this research series is oriented by a holistic model and continuum of care approach (Kerber et al., 2007; Mattison & Fiorentino, 2011) and influenced by the "Framework for analyzing the determinants of obstetric fistula formation" (Wall, 2012b) and the framework for analyzing maternal mortality (McCarthy & Maine, 1992).

Each sequence in the continuum of care is influenced by a set of distal and proximate determinants. For example, fistula occurrence is the result of remote, intermediate, and acute determinants described by Wall (2012b), while surgical repair outcomes are influenced by the clinical characteristics of the fistula, the skill level of the surgeon, and the quality of the local health facility (Arrowsmith et al., 2010; Barone et al., 2012). Postrepair outcomes depend on fistula clinical characteristics (Barone et al., 2012; Frajzyngier et al., 2012) and reintegration context including social and economic support, place of residence (rural vs. urban), access and use of health services, knowledge and use of family planning methods (Lombard et al., 2015; Mafo Degge et al., 2017). Finally, engagement in the continuum of care for women who develop fistula depends on the availability of information on fistula care services, availability and affordability of services provided along with access, and use of these services along with community perspectives on women and the disease (Wegner et al., 2007).

Table 27.1 Overview of the methods of the study included in this chapter

Study and setting	Population, period, and sample	Design, data source, and collection tools	Analysis and outcome
1. Physical and reproductive health after fistula repair; Guinea (Delamou et al., 2017).	Women discharged with a closed fistula between 1 January 2012 and 30 June 2015. (N = 481)	Longitudinal cohort study. Individual medical records of repaired patients and face to face interviews; Standardized questionnaires.	Cumulative incidence, incidence proportion, and incidence ratio using Kaplan-Meier methods. Assessment of fistula recurrence, residual incontinence, pregnancy, and childbirth.
2. Stakeholders perceptions on women after fistula repair; Guinea.	Women having experienced fistula, health providers, health managers, community, December 2016 to January 2017. (N = 83)	Descriptive qualitative study. In-depth interviews. Focus group discussions.	Emerging themes Similarities and differences Women's vulnerability, coping strategies, strategies to improve health after repair.
3. Reintegration after fistula repair through social immersion; Guinea.	Women having experienced fistula, health providers, health managers, community, 2017. (N = 55)	Descriptive qualitative study. In-depth interviews; Focus group discussions	Emerging themes Similarities and differences. Process and experience with social immersion and social reintegration up 3 months postrepair.

27.3   Methods

A mixed methods approach was used in this analysis. First, I used a longitudinal study conducted in Guinea in 2016 that analyzed the physical and reproductive health of women after repair (Delamou et al., 2017). I then triangulated these findings with a qualitative study conducted in Guinea on stakeholder perceptions of women's health after obstetric fistula repair (unpublished) and a second qualitative study on social reintegration after repair of obstetric fistula in Guinea (unpublished). The process included reviewing both the quantitative and qualitative findings and employing the qualitative findings to explain and contrast with the quantitative data. An overview of the methods by study included is provided in Table 27.1.

27.4   Results

27.4.1 Profiles of Women After Fistula Repair

Among 481 women out of 682 who underwent fistula repair in Guinea from 2012 to 2015 [and were followed postrepair], most were married or in union (72%), had no education (94%), delivered vaginally (66%), and had a stillbirth at the delivery resulting in fistula (93%) (Delamou et al., 2017). The majority were of reproductive age (85%), of whom 75% (305 women) reported being sexually active after surgery.

After repair, some sociodemographic characteristics of women benefiting from fistula surgery were found to evolve. For instance, the proportion of women reporting urban residence doubled and that of women reporting an occupation other than housewife had increased (Table 27.2).

Table 27.2 Comparison between selected socio-demographic characteristics of study participants at surgery and at follow-up, 2012 to 2016 in Guinea ($n = 481$)

Characteristic	At hospital at surgery ($N = 481$); Number (%)	At follow-up visit ($N = 481$); Number (%)	P-value[a]
Residence			<0.001
Rural	449 (93.4)	419 (87.1)	
Urban	30 (6.2)	62 (12.9)	
Unknown	2 (0.4)	0	
Marital status			0.370
Married/union	339 (70.5)	360 (74.8)	
Other[b]	133 (27.6)	121 (25.2)	
Unknown	9 (1.9)	0	
Occupation			<0.001
Housewife	445 (92.5)	311 (64.7)	
Other occupation[c]	29 (6.0)	170 (35.3)	
Unknown	7 (1.5)	0	

[Reprinted from Delamou, A., Delvaux, T., El Ayadi, A.M., Tripathi, V., Camara, B.S., et al. (2017). Fistula recurrence, pregnancy, and childbirth following successful closure of female genital fistula in Guinea: a longitudinal study. *The Lancet Global Health*. 5(11):e1152–e1160, Table 2. https://doi.org/10.1016/S2214-109X(17)30366-2, licensed under the terms of the Creative Commons Attribution 4.0 International License (http://creativecommons.org/licenses/by/4.0/).]
[a] P-value was derived after excluding "Unknown" values
[b] Single, widow or divorced/separated
[c] Office worker, farming, market vendor or student

27.4.2 Stakeholders' Perceptions on Health of Women Who Underwent Obstetric Fistula Repair

My research on fistula exploring the perceptions of stakeholders on women who underwent fistula repair aimed to understand their perspectives on the health of women postrepair of obstetric fistula in Guinea. Stakeholders included a variety of key informants (representatives from the Ministry of Health, regional, district, and hospital managers, representatives of NGOs and funding bodies, local leaders), women who underwent fistula surgery and their relatives (husbands, family members), health providers, and community health workers. Based on the findings and review of the existing literature, I developed a model to describe general perceptions of women's health after repair of obstetric fistula in sub-Saharan Africa (Fig. 27.1). Findings from the study indicate that women who underwent fistula surgery and were discharged with a closed fistula were generally perceived to carry higher health risks compared to women who have not experienced fistula. Many stakeholders, including women themselves and their relatives, health providers, and program managers, believed such women are more likely to experience maternal and neonatal complications during pregnancy and childbirth than women who have not experienced fistula. As a female community member from Kissigdougou explains:

> You know that someone who already has undergone fistula surgery is no longer as before. If they have operated on you, you have a disability while the others do not; they have never undergone surgery. So, the one who underwent the operation has more risks, especially when she carries early pregnancy. [Focus group discussion (FGD)]

The core theme that emerged from this research describing women treated for fistula was "vulnerability". Women treated for fistula are considered "vulnerable" as compared to "normal" women who have never experienced fistula. This concept of "vulnerability" includes physical, social-emotional, and economic dimensions (Fig. 27.2).

Women treated for fistula were described by stakeholders as physically diminished by the disease and the surgery.

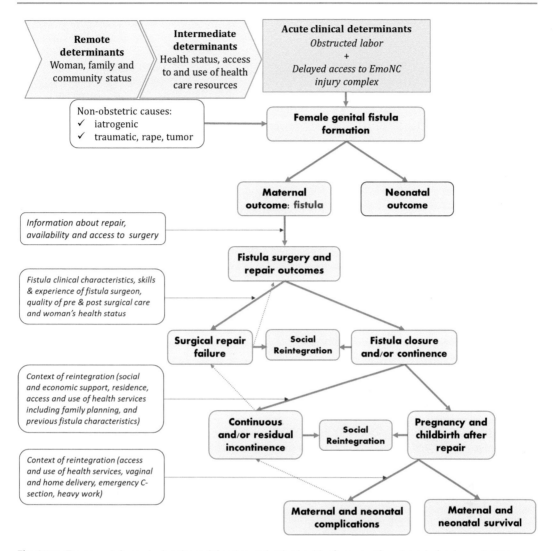

Fig. 27.1 Framework for analyzing the social and reproductive health of women after obstetric fistula repair (Delamou, 2018)

She must know that she is no longer as the others; she now is a 'half-woman', so I would tell her to be careful [during physical and sexual activities] for she already is disabled. If she now behaves like the others, it can't work. (Female, Community member, FGD, Kissidougou)

Physical vulnerability encompasses the sequela of obstructed labor complex injury, pain, fatigue or infertility.

When we are having sex, [my partner] is satisfied while I am suffering from backache… all my body aches after sexual intercourse…. Since [sex] is an obligation in the household, I buy medicines to take [beforehand] so that before the pain comes, the medicine is [already] circulating in my body. [Woman treated for fistula, In-depth interview (IDI), Labé]

The risk of maternal and neonatal complications such as fistula recurrence, abortion or stillbirth is perceived to be high, especially for those who do not follow the advice provided by healthcare workers about safe delivery at a health facility by elective C-section. Women who experienced fistula were themselves aware of this risk:

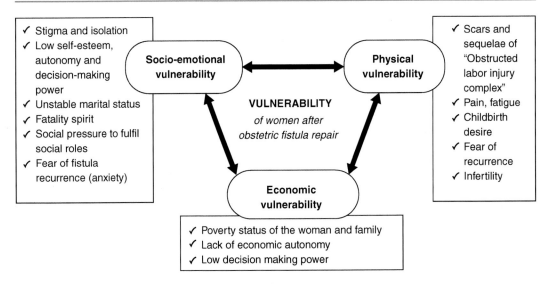

Fig. 27.2 Concepts of vulnerability in women who have undergone obstetric fistula repair

An operated and healed woman should not give birth by herself. Once at term, she should go to hospital to be operated; she should not dare to push; if she pushes, she may suffer back from the disease. (Female, Community member, IDI, Labé)

Healthcare providers corroborated these findings, emphasizing the fact that the risk of complications is high if the woman begins labor with subsequent deliveries before seeking care in a health facility.

Most participants thought that early resumption of sexual intercourse (i.e., before prescribed 3 months postsurgery) and home delivery or late (after labor has started) hospital delivery were the key risk factors of adverse health outcomes after women return to the community. Women complained that some husbands/partners are not supportive when it comes to recommended abstinence to allow for complete healing.

The problem is that if for instance you undergo [fistula surgery], you recover, you get back home, your husband refuses to abstain until the required deadline, and you have nowhere to take refuge. (Woman treated for fistula, FDG, Labé)

Socio-emotional vulnerability that includes mental vulnerability was characterized by reliance on others, stigmatization of women who lack support from their relatives (spouses, parents), and social pressure to fulfill marital duties such as resuming farm activities or sexual intercourse, becoming pregnant again or cooking. Added to that was the anxiety of fistula recurrence that keeps some women isolated from usually normal activities (sexual intercourse, dance, expression of joy, etc.).

Heavy work can re-open the disease. If your husband does not keep you far from that, what can you do? (Woman treated for fistula, FGD, Labé)

Economically, stakeholders were concerned that returning to their communities will again expose women to the same determinants that led to the formation of the previously repaired fistula given the level of household poverty. This poverty results in continuing financial barriers to accessing health care and lack of autonomy and decision-making.

Our parents and husbands are the one who are supposed to help us, but we are aware that they can't because of poverty. There are many hospitals but if they are paying and we do not have what must be paid, here is the suffering. (Woman treated for fistula, IDI, Labé)

27.4.3 Suggestions for Improving Women's Health After Repair

Improving the reproductive and social lives of women following fistula repair has to be holistic and oriented using a human rights framework. Key Guinean stakeholders agreed with this perspective, with most respondents sharing that this represents a multifaceted problem requiring a multidisciplinary approach involving a broad variety of stakeholders, e.g., providers, managers, women and their families, policy makers, local health insurance, and microcredit companies.

> *If there is good coordination, each stakeholder can take care of a given component of fistula care. This brings synergy and complementarity instead of duplication and competition.* (NGO Representative, IDI, Conakry)

Overall, stakeholders emphasized the need for interventions that can reduce women's "vulnerability" after fistula repair. These interventions should focus on restoring women's physical, socio-emotional, and economic strengths to make them "normal" women again (see Box 27.1). Policymakers suggested that these interventions be integrated into existing fistula prevention and management programs.

Box 27.1 Content of Interventions to Improve the Health of Women After Obstetric Fistula Repair Proposed by Stakeholders

1. *Social support*
   (a) Social immersion in a host family (e.g., 3 weeks).
   (b) Home visit to woman and her family.
   (c) Hosting of woman around delivery or for treatment of specific health issue.
2. *Economic empowerment*
   (a) Training of woman on income-generating activity.
   (b) Support and follow-up of woman over time to ensure she starts an income-generating activity.
3. *Medical follow-up*
   (a) Training of health providers and facilities managers.
   (b) Health insurance subscription for woman (e.g., 1 year).
   (c) Regular home visit to woman.
   (d) Awareness raising with family during home visits.

One community member suggested the implementation of community-based medical follow-up, whereby healthcare workers (HCWs) or community health workers (CHWs) working near by the woman's residence would schedule regular home visits as part of their usual outreach activities. Some managers advised subscribing women to local health insurance scheme.

> *It is important to enroll women in a health assurance scheme because most often, we have problems with referrals. Here, the delay in seeking care is the root cause of maternal and neonatal mortality and obstetric fistula. If the health insurances are strengthened, referrals and transportation of women will be done timely.* (Health Manager, IDI, Kissidougou)

Providers cited the social immersion program (a program that assigns the repaired woman for 3 weeks to a trained volunteer host family to help her gradually resume social roles before her return home) as a means to mitigate socio-emotional vulnerability and restore self-confidence and self-esteem.

After the intervention, once the woman is cured, it is good to send her to a family for a few days before she returns home. (Midwife, FGD, Labé)

Stakeholders also mentioned the need to involve women's families, including parents and partners.

In some families, it is the parents or the husband who decides, so they must be involved to keep the woman in good health. Most of the time, they must accept for the woman to do anything, including seeking health. (Manager, IDI, NZerekore)

To complement this, women treated for fistula and their families suggested home visits or even phone calls to maintain contact with the repair hospitals and be able to seek advice when it is needed.

Healthcare providers should maintain phone contact with women to encourage them to present themselves or to call the hospital if they have health concerns. (Manager, IDI, Kankan)

To address the economic vulnerability, most respondents suggested economic empowerment activities to improve women's contribution to healthcare decision-making, increase their value in the home, and address any medical or other social issues. To this end, facility managers and representatives of fistula management NGOs suggested training on income-generating activities to make them autonomous and reinforce their decision-making power.

These women are often deprived. That is why, after the operation, it is necessary to help them economically by teaching them to set up income-generating activities such as saponification, either individually or in groups. (NGO Representative, IDI, Kankan)

Providers requested that economic empowerment activities be conducted by local microfinance organizations that already are active in rural Guinea. However, most stakeholders recommended support given over time rather than one direct payment to the women. The reason given was that with one payment women tend to give the money to their families in an effort to gain their esteem and break the pity paradigm built around them rather than use it for the economic empowerment activities it was intended.

27.4.4 Reproductive Health After Obstetric Fistula Repair

I sought to estimate the magnitude of these postrepair reproductive health outcomes through a longitudinal study of 481 Guinean women (Delamou et al., 2017). After a median follow-up of 28.0 months (Interquartile range 14.6–36.6), 73 recurrent fistulas were recorded, corresponding to 18.4% (95% Confidence interval: 14.8–22.8). In the 447 women who were continent at hospital discharge, 24 cases of postrepair residual urinary incontinence were recorded, corresponding to 10.3% (95% CI: 5.2–19.6).

The study recorded 67 first pregnancies among 305 women at risk of pregnancy (aged between 15 and 49 years, with no history of hysterectomy and not using family planning) for a pregnancy rate of 28.4% (95% CI: 22.8–35.0) through 28 months postdischarge. Most of these first pregnancies (72%) occurred within the first 18 months, and 85% within the first 24 months following surgery. A total of 50 women had delivered by the time of study follow-up. Despite clinical guidance for women to deliver by elective C-section in postrepair pregnancies, 82% of women did not. Deliveries resulted in 12 stillbirths (24%), seven delivery-related fistula recurrences (14%), and one maternal death (Fig. 27.3). Among the nine women who delivered by elective C-section, no adverse maternal or neonatal outcomes were recorded.

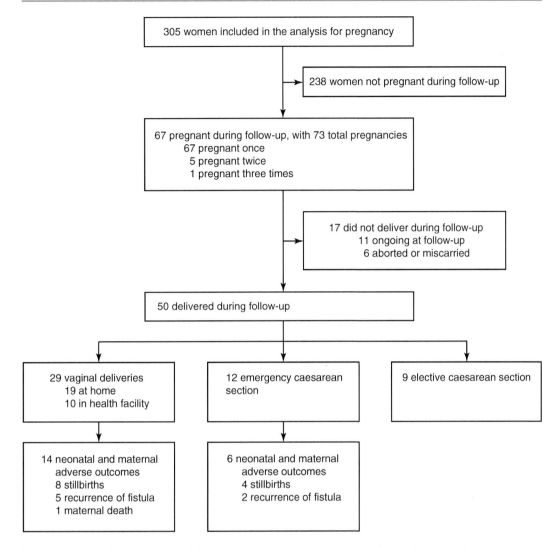

Fig. 27.3 Postrepair pregnancy and delivery outcomes among sexually active study participants of reproductive age. [Reprinted from Delamou, A., Delvaux, T., El Ayadi, A.M., Tripathi, V., Camara, B.S., et al. (2017). Fistula recurrence, pregnancy, and childbirth following successful closure of female genital fistula in Guinea: a longitudinal study. *The Lancet Global Health.* 5(11):e1152–e1160, Fig. 4. https://doi.org/10.1016/S2214-109X(17)30366-2, licensed under the terms of the Creative Commons Attribution 4.0 International License (http://creativecommons.org/licenses/by/4.0/)]

Reasons that elective C-section was not achieved by the majority of women are unknown; however, antenatal care receipt was low among this population, with 76% achieving the first antenatal visit but less than half (46%) completing the recommended four antenatal care visits. In addition, women who became pregnant within the first 6 months postdischarge were more likely to experience stillbirth at delivery compared to women who became pregnant at least 6 months after their fistula repair ($p = 0.0470$). Yet women are usually advised to delay the next pregnancy for at least 6 months so their body can recover well after surgery.

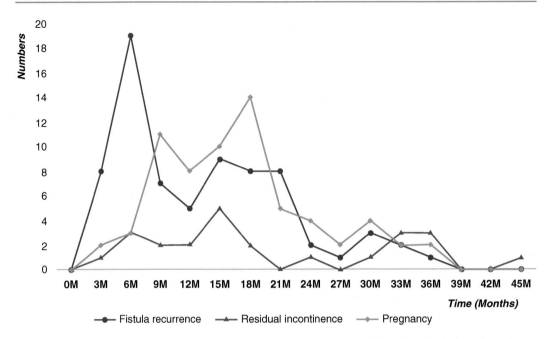

Fig. 27.4 Incidence of fistula recurrence ($n = 73$), first postrepair pregnancy ($n = 67$), and residual urinary incontinence ($n = 24$) over time in study participants. [Adapted from Delamou, A., Delvaux, T., El Ayadi, A.M., Tripathi, V., Camara, B.S., et al. (2017). Fistula recurrence, pregnancy, and childbirth following successful closure of female genital fistula in Guinea: a longitudinal study. *The Lancet Global Health*. 5(11):e1152–e1160, Fig. 3. Some modifications were made. https://doi.org/10.1016/S2214-109X(17)30366-2, licensed under the terms of the Creative Commons Attribution 4.0 International License (http://creativecommons.org/licenses/by/4.0/)]

27.4.5 Physical Health After Obstetric Fistula Repair

In the longitudinal study (Delamou et al., 2017), I found that more than half of the fistula recurrences occurred during the first 12 months after discharge and 37% were during the first 6 months (Fig. 27.4). As for residual urinary incontinence, eight (33%) occurred during the first 12 months after discharge.

I also identified factors that were associated with fistula recurrence, meaning the factors that would play a role in the breakdown of the fistula after successful repair. These factors included sexual activity, status of the urethra, bladder neck at fistula surgery, and vaginal scarring. Women who were not sexually active were three times as likely to resume leaking after surgery compared to women who were sexually active. It appeared that these women were less socially reintegrated (i.e., not living with a partner) and, therefore, had to engage in physical activities themselves. Women with urethral involvement in the fistula at the time of surgery were about three times as likely to resume leaking after surgery compared to women who had no urethral involvement. Those women who had a damaged bladder neck or vaginal scarring were about two times as likely to resume leaking after surgery compared to women who had a normal bladder neck or had no vaginal scarring. For some women, the incontinence occurred after the vaginal delivery ($n = 5$) or emergency C-section ($n = 2$) of their first postrepair pregnancy.

27.4.6 Social Reintegration After Fistula Repair

Social reintegration of women after fistula repair remains a challenge because of the variety of contexts and needs for women. To explore this issue, I conducted a study on social immersion using an innovative approach developed in Guinea by EngenderHealth, a US-based NGO. My aim was to assess the importance of "social immersion" in successful social reintegration of women receiving fistula repair. Understanding the reintegration pathway and how women's disease experience plays a role seemed critical to improving their living conditions (see Box 27.2).

The study was conducted with fistula women (pre and postsurgery, postsocial immersion, and 3 months postdischarge) and with stakeholders involved in the program (care providers, host families, and community leaders) in Labé and Kissidougou health districts in Guinea.

Box 27.2 Social immersion program

The goal of the social immersion program is to help women receiving fistula services reintegrate into family life and society after receiving clinical care.

- The program assigns each woman discharged from hospital after fistula repair who accepts, to a volunteer host family for 2–3 weeks.
- During this convalescence period, the women make a gradual and smooth return to normal life with the support of the host family.
- The role of the host family is to gradually involve the visiting woman into family activities such as cooking, eating meals together, washing, shopping, and participating in social occasions such as weddings and baptisms.
- During the stay, host families are honored through several special visits from the Mayors or their representatives along with rural radio stations.
- Host families are interviewed about their experiences with women and their messages are broadcasted to sensitize communities on fistula.

Members of the host families reported that overall women had a positive experience with the social immersion program.

It was a pleasant stay. She gradually integrated with my family; she participated in the preparation of food for the family. (Male, Host family, Kissidougou)

Host families added that the social immersion program constitutes a means of giving them back hope and self-esteem by providing women with family warmth, which they have been cut off during their lives with fistula. However, the success of this program is dependent on the success of surgery—women with a failed repair were unable to enjoy their stay with their host families due to the ongoing incontinence.

Some families encouraged women to get involved in daily activities, starting with simple activities like housework, so the women can adjust gradually to life in the host family.

We brought the woman to feel as part of our family, involving her in any activity of her choice within the family and paying respect to her. (Girl, host family, Labé)

However, some families asked women not to work hard for them, to rest well, and above all promote their full recovery.

The program had a positive impact on women's lives according to health providers, ranging from hope to social well-being, as shown in the following quote:

This program has allowed women to learn to live with families and begin their social reintegration. (Anesthetist, Kissidougou)

According to host families, the program provided women with happiness, health, joy, new knowledge, autonomy, relief, and peace.

She was very worried when I saw her in the hospital, but after this stay here, she now has the smile. This is important for her return to the village. (Female, Host family, Kissidougou)

Host families also testified that they received benefits in hosting the women, including joy, new knowledge, new relationships, and honor.

Today, when I go to the municipality for an administrative document, I do not suffer because I am recognized. The Mayor has come to visit me and my name was said on the rural radio. (Male, host family, Kissidougou)

They also cited the strengthening of the relationship and blessing as another advantage gained through the program.

Three months after discharge and after the social immersion program, most women had resumed social activities they had before fistula.

I have blended in well and I am able to do anything a woman can do. (35-years old, Labé)

Their return home was joyful.

When I returned to my family, everybody was happy and I managed to adjust back to my daily life. (34-years old, Kissidougou)

Their social reintegration was underway. Family life and relationship with relatives were described as a source of happiness and relief by women.

I am back in touch with my social acquaintances, my female friends now visit me and I visit them. (35-years old, Kissidougou)

Some couples were even re-united following the success of the repair.

When my husband found out that I was cured, he came to visit my family and asked that I go home with him. (30-years old, Labé)

In contrast, women whose repair was not successful (discharged incontinent) reported that they could not resume their social activities due to urine leakage and smell. They continued to undergo stigmatization, which was worsened by the failure of the repair, as people attributed this failure to a curse.

Given that I could not be cured, I cannot approach people. They say that it is a curse and that I cannot do anything about it. I keep looking for a cure but I prefer to stay isolated so I do not get humiliated when I go to other people's homes. (38-years old, Kissidougou)

Women who were discharged continent seemed to be better integrated socially than those who did not, the latter having chosen social isolation to mitigate the effects of stigmatization.

To improve social reintegration of women after fistula repair, health providers suggested providing career training and psychosocial support for these women. They also recommended raising women's awareness to help them recognize that they no longer suffer from fistula in order to facilitate their participation in social activities.

We need to encourage the woman to know that she is healed and she can approach the community and act like a normal woman. (Matron, Kissidougou)

Host families suggested counseling for women so that they recognize they are now able to participate in social ceremonies.

Encouraging women to get rid of their stress, to feel healed as normal women. (Woman, Host family, Kissidougou)

Host families also suggested teaching women small trades, extending the length of stay of women with host families, and awareness raising at the community level to accommodate women with fistula.

We ask the program to increase public and community awareness so that other families could host these women. By doing so, women will know that they are loved. (Woman, Host family, Labé)

Host families also suggested support for small businesses when women are back home, and a better financial involvement of the authorities in the management of these women as ways to sustain the program. Finally, they advised that the program should encourage host families by accompanying measures such as food supply and taking into account the issue of the long-term reintegration of these women.

27.5 Improving the Reproductive Health of Women After Fistula Repair

Women who benefit from fistula repair in sub-Saharan Africa still face many challenges in exercising their reproductive autonomy. Most women who undergo fistula repair are of reproductive age. Returning to a "normal life" with successful reintegration means fulfilling personal desires and social norms, which most often includes resuming marital life and sexual activity, becoming pregnant and giving birth again. Having a live baby can heal some of the loss women experienced during the delivery that led to the fistula and temper the infertility-related stigma they have suffered. However, access and quality of reproductive health services remain low in many contexts and women repaired for fistula face similar challenges to care as when they developed the fistula initially. Together, these three studies point out important considerations pertaining to social and reproductive health after fistula repair.

First, health-related challenges for women who experience obstetric fistula do not end after successful repair. Limiting the assessment of a fistula program's performance to point of hospital discharge prevents programs from using their potential (human, material, and financial resources) to sustain their performance beyond surgery. Therefore, it is paramount to rethink the assessment of fistula management programs in Guinea. Currently, most fistula care programs are assessed on the number of fistula repairs performed and the outcomes after surgery and at hospital discharge in terms of fistula closure and continence. Based on the findings from these studies, it is clear there is a need to go beyond repair so that women can benefit from reintegration programs to sustain the gains of the surgery.

Second, current and future programs should integrate postrepair follow-up into fistula management programs for at least 12 months to mitigate the vulnerabilities. Despite the fact that three-quarters of women who became pregnant postrepair achieved at least one antenatal care visit, findings reveal that fistula recurrence and maternal and neonatal complications during postrepair pregnancies and deliveries were more frequent among women in Guinea than what has been reported from other settings in Africa, such as Malawi and Ethiopia. This is possibly due to the high proportion of vaginal deliveries or emergency C-sections in a context characterized by negative impacts of epidemics (such as Ebola), poverty, and geographical barriers. Therefore, postrepair follow-up must be achieved through strategies that include training of healthcare workers at health center and health post levels, the use of mobile phones for follow-up and community-based follow-up. Community health workers could conduct outreach for follow-up for women who do not have cell phones and link women to the nearest health facility. This is of importance as many women are repaired far from their residence or sent from one repair hospital to another, depending on the availability of the surgeon.

Third, the findings also emphasize the need to provide social support to women postrepair. In fact, women who benefit from a strong social support network after repair and have easy access to and use of health services are likely to be more protected against adverse health outcomes than those who do not. In the studies analyzed here, fistula recurrence largely occurred in women who engaged in heavy physical activities such as farming. In addition, adverse health outcomes such as stillbirth and fistula recurrence were more likely to occur with vaginal delivery and emergency C-section than with an elective C-section. Therefore, social support should build on strategies that address women's emotional, physical, and economic vulnerabilities. This can include counseling and psychological support initiatives for women repaired from OF, placement of women in host families after surgery (social immersion), and community involvement in maternal and child health. In addition, as mentioned above, involving healthcare workers and community health workers in postrepair follow-up for at least 12 months is crucial. Finally, implementing economic empowerment activities to support women repaired through income-generating activities would improve women's contribution to healthcare decision-making, increase their income and value in their families, and address any medical or other social needs.

Finally, improving social and reproductive health of women after obstetric fistula repair will require both preventing fistula from recurring and ensuring that women are less vulnerable socioemotionally, physically, and economically. To this end, helping women develop new opportunities for resuming work and gaining economic autonomy is extremely important for restoring their dignity. Reducing social and economic vulnerabilities will preserve their physical health and reduce the likelihood of fistula recurrence, which will protect them from entering into a negative spiral of physical, psychosocial, and economic adversity.

27.6 Conclusions

Women who experience obstetric fistula in sub-Saharan African countries such as Guinea encounter many challenges related to their physical, socioeconomic, and reproductive health. If unaddressed, these challenges might impede their successful reintegration postfistula repair. For example, despite their desire to have children, many women may be reluctant to become pregnant after fistula repair due to fear of fistula reoccurrence or fetal demise and lack of appropriate social and medical support. To improve this situation, it is important to ensure free access to quality maternity care and transportation, including elective cesarean deliveries for all women who have experienced fistula. In addition, close monitoring of women who have specific clinical characteristics that put them at high-risk of surgical failure or fistula recurrence in the postrepair period is needed.

Achieving the goal of eliminating obstetric fistula in sub-Saharan Africa will require targeted prevention of obstetric fistula, increased accessibility of emergency obstetric care, and education, and consistent follow-up of women postrepair to prevent fistula re-occurrence. Rethinking of the performance of fistula management programs by integrating postrepair indicators, decentralizing quality fistula care, and implementing interventions to improve reproductive health of women after fistula repair will help us finally end fistula.

Acknowledgments The author thanks Alison El Ayadi (University of California, San Francisco, USA), Moussa Soka DOUNO and Delphin Kolié (Africa Center of Excellence, University Gamal Abdel Nasser, Conakry, Guinea), Vandana Tripathi (EngenderHealth, New-York, USA), Moustapha Diallo (Engenderhealth, Guinea), Thérèse Delvaux (Institute of Tropical Medicine, Antwerp, Belgium), Bonnie Ruder (Terrewode Women's Fund, USA), and Vincent De Brouwere (Professor Emiritus), for their significant contributions to the studies used in this chapter and their useful guidance and advice.

References

Ahmed, S., Anastasi, E., & Laski, L. (2016). Double burden of tragedy: Stillbirth and obstetric fistula. *The Lancet Global Health, 4*(2), e80–e82. https://doi.org/10.1016/S2214-109X(15)00290-9

Arrowsmith, S. D., Barone, M. A., & Ruminjo, J. (2013). Outcomes in obstetric fistula care: A literature review. *Current Opinion in Obstetrics and Gynecology, 25*, 399–403. https://doi.org/10.1097/GCO.0b013e3283648d60

Arrowsmith, S. D., Ruminjo, J., & Landry, E. G. (2010). Current practices in treatment of female genital fistula: A cross sectional study. *BMC Pregnancy and Childbirth, 10*(1), 73. https://doi.org/10.1186/1471-2393-10-73

Arrowsmith, S., Hamlin, E. C., & Wall, L. L. (1996). Obstructed labor injury complex: Obstetric fistula formation and the multifaceted morbidity of maternal birth trauma in the developing world. *Obstetrical and Gynecological Survey, 51*, 568–574. https://doi.org/10.1097/00006254-199609000-00024

Barone, M. A., Frajzyngier, V., Ruminjo, J., Asiimwe, F., Barry, T. H., Bello, A., Danladi, D., Ganda, S. O., Idris, S., Inoussa, M., Lynch, M., Mussell, F., & Podder, D. C. (2012). Determinants of postoperative outcomes of female genital fistula repair surgery. *Obstetrics and Gynecology, 120*, 524–531. https://doi.org/10.1097/AOG.0b013e31826579e8

Browning, A. (2009). Pregnancy following obstetric fistula repair, the management of delivery. *BJOG: An International Journal of Obstetrics and Gynaecology, 116*(9), 1265–1267. https://doi.org/10.1111/j.1471-0528.2009.02182.x

Browning, A., & Menber, B. (2008). Women with obstetric fistula in Ethiopia: A 6-month follow-up after surgical treatment. *BJOG: An International Journal of Obstetrics & Gynaecology, 115*(12), 1564–1569. https://doi.org/10.1111/j.1471-0528.2008.01900.x

Delamou A. (2018). *Towards a fistula-free generation: Lessons learned from long-term follow-up of women after obstetric fistula repair in Guinea. PhD thesis (Unpublished)*. Université Libre de Bruxelles.

Delamou, A., Delvaux, T., El Ayadi, A. M., Tripathi, V., Camara, B. S., Beavogui, A. H., Romanzi, L., Cole, B., Bouedouno, P., Diallo, M., Barry, T. H., Camara, M., Diallo, K., Leveque, A., Zhang, W. H., & De Brouwere, V. (2017). Fistula recurrence, pregnancy, and childbirth following successful closure of female genital fistula in Guinea: A longitudinal study. *The Lancet Global Health, 5*(11), e1152–e1160. https://doi.org/10.1016/S2214-109X(17)30366-2

Donnelly, K., Oliveras, E., Tilahun, Y., Belachew, M., & Asnake, M. (2015). Quality of life of Ethiopian women after fistula repair: Implications on rehabilitation and social reintegration policy and programming. *Culture, Health and Sexuality, 17*(2), 150–164. https://doi.org/10.1080/13691058.2014.964320

Drew, L. B., Wilkinson, J. P., Nundwe, W., Moyo, M., Mataya, R., Mwale, M., & Tang, J. H. (2016). Long-term outcomes for women after obstetric fistula repair in Lilongwe. Malawi: A qualitative study. *BMC Pregnancy and Childbirth., 16*(1), 2. https://doi.org/10.1186/s12884-015-0755-1

Epiu, I., Alia, G., Mukisa, J., Tavrow, P., Lamorde, M., & Kuznik, A. (2018). Estimating the cost and cost-effectiveness for obstetric fistula repair in hospitals in Uganda: A low income country. *Health Policy and Planning, 33*(9), 999–1008. https://doi.org/10.1093/heapol/czy078

Frajzyngier, V., Ruminjo, J., & Barone, M. A. (2012). Factors influencing urinary fistula repair outcomes in developing countries: A systematic review. *American Journal of Obstetrics and Gynecology, 207*, 248–258. https://doi.org/10.1016/j.ajog.2012.02.006

Gupta, N. P., Mishra, S., Mishra, A., Seth, A., & Anand, A. (2012). Outcome of repeat supratrigonal obstetric vesicovaginal fistula repair after previous failed repair—Abstract. *Urologia Internationalis, 88*(3), 259–262. Retrieved October 3, 2020, from https://www.karger.com/Article/Abstract/331503

Kerber, K. J., de Graft-Johnson, J. E., Bhutta, Z. A., Okong, P., Starrs, A., & Lawn, J. E. (2007). Continuum of care for maternal, newborn, and child health: From slogan to service delivery. *The Lancet, 370*, 1358–1369. https://doi.org/10.1016/S0140-6736(07)61578-5

Kopp, D. M., Wilkinson, J., Bengtson, A., Chipungu, E., Pope, R. J., Moyo, M., & Tang, J. H. (2017). Fertility outcomes following obstetric fistula repair: A prospective cohort study. *Reproductive Health, 14*(1), 159. https://doi.org/10.1186/s12978-017-0415-1

Landry, E., Frajzyngier, V., Ruminjo, J., Asiimwe, F., Barry, T. H., Bello, A., Danladi, D., Ganda, S. O., Idris, S., Inoussa, M., Kanoma, B., Lynch, M., Mussell, F., Podder, D. C., Wali, A., Mielke, E., & Barone, M. A. (2013). Profiles and experiences of women undergoing genital fistula repair: Findings from five countries. *Global Public Health, 8*(8), 926–942. https://doi.org/10.1080/17441692.2013.824018

Lombard, L., de St, J. J., Geddes, R., El Ayadi, A. M., & Grant, L. (2015). Rehabilitation experiences after obstetric fistula repair: Systematic review of qualitative studies. *Tropical Medicine & International Health, 20*(5), 554–568. https://doi.org/10.1111/tmi.12469

Lozano, R., Wang, H., Foreman, K. J., Rajaratnam, J. K., Naghavi, M., Marcus, J. R., Dwyer-Lindgren, L., Lofgren, K. T., Phillips, D., Atkinson, C., Lopez, A. D., & Murray, C. J. (2011). Progress towards millennium development goals 4 and 5 on maternal and child mortality: An updated systematic analysis. *The Lancet, 378*(9797), 1139–1165. https://doi.org/10.1016/S0140-6736(11)61337-8

Mafo Degge, H., Hayter, M., & Laurenson, M. (2017). An integrative review on women living with obstetric fistula and after treatment experiences. *Journal of Clinical Nursing, 26*, 1445–1457. https://doi.org/10.1111/jocn.13590

Mattison, C., & Fiorentino, R. (2011). *Strengthening health systems through the levels of fistula care framework—A literature review.* Engenderhealth.

Maulet, N., Keita, M., & Macq, J. (2013). Medico-social pathways of obstetric fistula patients in Mali and Niger: An 18-month cohort follow-up. *Tropical Medicine & International Health, 18*(5), 524–533. https://doi.org/10.1111/tmi.12086

McCarthy, J., & Maine, D. (1992). A framework for analyzing the determinants of maternal mortality. *Studies in Family Planning, 23*(1), 23–33. https://doi.org/10.2307/1966825

Nielsen, H. S., Lindberg, L., Nygaard, U., Aytenfisu, H., Johnston, O. L., Sørensen, B., Rudnicki, M., Crangle, M., Lawson, R., & Duffy, S. (2009). A community-based long-term follow-up of women undergoing obstetric fistula repair in rural Ethiopia. *BJOG: An International Journal of Obstetrics and Gynaecology, 116*(9), 1258–1264. https://doi.org/10.1111/j.1471-0528.2009.02200.x

Osotimehin, B. (2013). Obstetric fistula: Ending the health and human rights tragedy. *The Lancet, 381*, 1702–1703. https://doi.org/10.1016/S0140-6736(13)61001-6

Osotimehin, B. D. (2015). *Message on the occasion of international day to end obstetric fistula by Dr. Babatunde Osotimehin.* United Nations Under-Secretary-General and Executive Director of UNFPA, the United Nations Population Fund. Retrieved October 3, 2020, from https://www.unfpa.org/press/statement-international-day-end-obstetric-fistula-dr-babatunde-osotimehin-united-nations-under

USAID and EngenderHealth. (2014). *Fistula care associate cooperative agreement, GHS-A-OO-07-00021-00. Final project report October 2007 to December 2013. Part II: Country accomplishments.* USAID and EngenderHealth.

Wall, L. L. (2012a). Obstetric fistula is a "neglected tropical disease". *PLoS Neglected Tropical Diseases., 6*(8), e1769. https://doi.org/10.1371/journal.pntd.0001769

Wall, L. L. (2012b). A framework for analyzing the determinants of obstetric fistula formation. *Studies in Family Planning., 43*(4), 255–272. https://doi.org/10.1111/j.1728-4465.2012.00325.x

Wegner, M. N., Ruminjo, J., Sinclair, E., Pesso, L., & Mehta, M. (2007). Improving community knowledge of obstetric fistula prevention and treatment. *International Journal of Gynecology & Obstetrics, 99*(S1), S108–S111. https://doi.org/10.1016/j.ijgo.2007.06.030

Wilson, A. L., Chipeta, E., Kalilani-Phiri, L., Taulo, F., & Tsui, A. O. (2011). Fertility and pregnancy outcomes among women with obstetric fistula in rural Malawi. *International Journal of Gynecology & Obstetrics, 113*(3), 196–198. https://doi.org/10.1016/j.ijgo.2011.01.006

World Health Organization. (2014). *WHO | 10 facts on obstetric fistula.* WHO. Retrieved October 3, 2020, from https://www.who.int/features/factfiles/obstetric_fistula/facts/en/

Urinary Incontinence Following Obstetric Fistula Surgery

Hannah G. Krause and Judith Goh

28.1 Definitions and Prevalence of Urinary Incontinence

Ongoing urinary incontinence following the successful closure of obstetric fistula (OF) has been a longstanding problem with limited understanding of the aetiology of such urinary symptoms, and with treatment options lacking. In contrast to the numerous studies documenting the success rates of surgical closure of fistulas, follow-up of patients with urinary incontinence has been limited, and there has been little attention given as to whether these women with successful fistula closure have ongoing troublesome urinary symptoms including incontinence.

In general, urinary incontinence is a common condition affecting women worldwide. The Continence Foundation of Australia has defined urinary incontinence as follows: 'Incontinence is a term that describes any accidental or involuntary loss of urine from the bladder. Incontinence is a widespread condition that ranges in severity from 'just a small leak' to complete loss of bladder control' (Continence Foundation of Australia, 2018).

Overall prevalence rates of urinary incontinence are difficult to define as definitions of urinary incontinence often vary between studies. The total number of cases of urinary incontinence in the population at a specific time are between 15.7% (Nygaard et al., 2008) and 49.6% in the USA (Dooley et al., 2008). Studies which subdivide urinary incontinence document the prevalence of urinary stress incontinence between 12% and 25% (Dooley et al., 2008; Peyrat et al., 2002), urge incontinence 1.6–9.9% (Minassian et al., 2008; Peyrat et al., 2002) and mixed urinary incontinence between 9% and 17% (Dooley et al., 2008; Hannestad et al., 2000). Large population-based studies of prevalence of lower urinary tract symptoms by Coyne et al. (2009), Irwin et al. (2006) and Milsom et al. (2001) demonstrated an overall prevalence from 59.2% to 76.3%; however, the prevalence of urinary incontinence was 9.3% – 14.8%. More recently, Markland et al. (2011) analysed data in the United States

H. G. Krause
Greenslopes Hospital, QEII Hospital, Brisbane, QLD, Australia

J. Goh (✉)
Griffith University, Gold Coast, QLD, Australia

Greenslopes Hospital, QEII Hospital, Brisbane, QLD, Australia
e-mail: judith@qpfs.com.au

© Springer Nature Switzerland AG 2022
L. B. Drew et al. (eds.), *A Multidisciplinary Approach to Obstetric Fistula in Africa*, Global Maternal and Child Health, https://doi.org/10.1007/978-3-031-06314-5_28

from 2001 through to 2008, and age standardised prevalence estimates and prevalence odds ratios using urinary incontinence trends were determined. The age standardised prevalence of urinary incontinence increased in women from 2001 through to 2008, from 49.5% in 2001/2002 to 53.4% in 2007/2008.

The causes of urinary incontinence include stress urinary incontinence, urgency urinary incontinence, voiding difficulty with overflow incontinence, urinary tract infection or bladder pathology and urogenital fistula. A combined International Continence Society (ICS)/International Urogynecological Association (IUGA) paper has proposed definitions for abnormal urinary symptoms including urinary incontinence and diagnoses and is stated below (Haylen et al., 2010).

Stress urinary incontinence (SUI) is activity-related incontinence and is the complaint of involuntary loss of urine on effort or physical exertion, or with sneezing or coughing. Urgency urinary incontinence (UUI) is the complaint of involuntary loss of urine associated with urgency. Overactive bladder (OAB) is a symptom complex of urinary urgency, usually accompanied by frequency and nocturia, with or without urinary incontinence, in the absence of urinary tract infection or other obvious pathology. The term voiding difficulty includes numerous voiding symptoms such as hesitancy, slow stream, intermittency, straining to void and feeling of incomplete voiding. The complete inability to pass urine despite persistent effort is urinary retention. Acute urinary retention is defined as a generally painful, palpable or percussible bladder, when urine cannot be passed despite the bladder being full. Chronic urinary retention is defined as a non-painful bladder, where there is a chronic high post-void residual volume. Overflow incontinence is involuntary incontinence when there is no associated urge to urinate.

Because urinary incontinence affects greater than 50% of women overall (Markland et al., 2011), it is therefore not unexpected that women who have experienced an obstetric fistula would also be at risk of post-fistula closure urinary incontinence.

28.2   Assessment of Women with Post-Fistula Surgery Urinary Incontinence

In women who have developed urinary incontinence following surgery for fistula, we suggest that the following protocol be followed in evaluating and diagnosing the cause(s) of the condition.

1. Check for urinary tract infection.
   - Obtain mid-stream urine sample and assess microscopy/culture.
2. Assess for failed fistula repair.
   - Speculum examination and dye test; if required perform examination under anaesthesia of vagina and cystoscopy.
3. Assess for ureteric fistula.
   - Speculum examination; renal tract imaging, e.g. ultrasound scan, CT scan, intravenous urogram.
4. Check for bladder stones or bladder/urinary tract pathology.
   - Imaging, e.g. ultrasound; metal catheter—can feel stone; cystoscopy.
5. Urodynamics studies assessment.
   - Validated urodynamics test.
   - Simplified clinical urodynamics test.
6. Bladder diary.
   - Simple tool to accurately assess urinary frequency and voided volumes.

28.2.1 Urinary Tract Infection

Urinary tract infection is a common cause of urinary frequency, urgency, dysuria and also incontinence. Treatment with antibiotics is usually effective. If recurrent urinary tract infections occur, further assessment may be indicated to check for renal tract stones or foreign material in the bladder secondary to previous surgery, voiding dysfunction or other bladder pathology.

28.2.2 Persistent Urogenital Tract Fistula

Careful assessment for persistent urogenital tract fistula is important. This involves a vaginal examination in combination with a dye test. In cases where there is significant scarring and vaginal restriction or where the examination is limited by pain, then an examination under anaesthesia of the vagina with dye test and cystoscopy if available is recommended.

28.2.3 Ureteric Fistula

In those cases where urine is observed in the vagina with speculum examination, but the dye test is negative, then evaluation for ureteric fistula is performed with imaging. Renal ultrasound, CT scan or intravenous urogram will usually indicate the side and site of ureteric fistula.

28.2.4 Bladder Stones

Bladder stones are frequently seen following fistula surgery. Insertion of a metal catheter may be adequate to identify stones in the bladder. Alternatively, radiological imaging such as a plain X-ray or renal tract ultrasound scan is useful. Cystoscopy gives a very accurate assessment of any intra-vesical pathology.

28.2.5 Urodynamics Assessment, Uroflowmetry and Cystometry

Ideally a validated urodynamics assessment should be performed to give an accurate diagnosis of urodynamic stress incontinence, detrusor overactivity and voiding dysfunction. Urodynamics testing is the functional study of the lower urinary tract (Walters & Karram, 2015). It is designed to provide information regarding bladder filling, storage of urine and voiding. Urodynamics testing includes assessment with free uroflowmetry with check of post-void residual urine volume, and filling and voiding cystometry.

Free uroflowmetry is the voluntary passing of urine over a uroflowmetre. This then measures the flow rate, voided volume, maximum urine flow rate, flow time, average flow rate, voiding time, time to maximum flow and interpretation of the normality of free uroflowmetry. The post-void residual urine volume is the volume of urine which is left in the bladder at completion of micturition. It can be assessed using an ultrasound to measure the volume retained or by emptying the residual urine volume with a catheter. Cystometry is the measurement of the pressure/volume relationship of the bladder during filling and/or pressure flow study during voiding. To achieve this, catheter tubing is placed into the bladder (to obtain intra-vesical pressure = p ves) and either into the vagina or rectum (to obtain abdominal pressure = p abd). The detrusor pressure (p det) is the measurement obtained when the pressures in the bladder and vagina/rectum are subtracted. Filling cystometry assesses bladder sensation, bladder capacity, detrusor activity and bladder compliance during filling. Detrusor function is considered normal when there is little or no change in detrusor pressure with filling. In contrast, detrusor overactivity may be diagnosed with the occurrence of involuntary detrusor contractions, either spontaneous or provoked, during filling cystometry (Haylen et al., 2010). A cystometrogram (CMG) is a graphical recording of the bladder pressures and volumes over time.

There are several different techniques available to assess urethral function. Urethral pressure and urethral closure pressure are concepts which represent the ability of the urethra to prevent incontinence. The urethral pressure profile (UPP) at rest measures the pressure within the length of the urethra. Maximum urethral closure pressure (MUCP), which is the maximum difference between the urethral pressure and intra-vesical pressure, is commonly used. The indirect techniques of leak point pressures can also be used. The abdominal leak point pressure can be defined as the vesical pressure at leakage during abdominal stress (in the absence of any detrusor contraction). A cough or valsalva maneuver can be used to acquire the abdominal stress.

Urodynamic stress incontinence is assessed by coughing during the test to assess for involuntary leakage of urine in the absence of a detrusor rise. Voiding cystometry is measured during micturition, and is the pressure/volume relationship of the bladder. The measurements recorded include the intra-vesical, intra-abdominal and detrusor pressures and urine flow rate. The detrusor function during voiding is considered to be normal when urethral relaxation followed by a continuous detrusor contraction leads to complete bladder emptying within a normal time span.

The terminologies used for urodynamic diagnoses have been documented in a joint report by the ICS/IUGA (Haylen et al., 2010). Urodynamic stress incontinence is a diagnosis by symptom, sign and urodynamic investigations and involves the finding of involuntary urinary leakage during filling cystometry, associated with increased intra-abdominal pressure, in the absence of detrusor contractions. The diagnosis of detrusor overactivity is by symptoms and urodynamic investigations, when involuntary detrusor muscle contractions occur during filling cystometry. Voiding dysfunction is defined as abnormally slow urine flow rates and abnormally high post-void residuals and is a diagnosis by symptoms and urodynamics investigations.

In resource poor settings where standardised equipment for formal validated urodynamics assessment is not available, then a simplified clinical urodynamics test (Krause et al. 2013) can be used. An initial dye test should be performed to exclude any undiagnosed residual fistula. The patient first voids and is then catheterised to measure post-void residual urine volume. The normal post-void residual urine volume is less than 100 ml. The bladder is then filled via the catheter with saline to at least 300 ml if tolerated, while the patient is asked for their bladder sensation during filling. To estimate the vesical pressure, the catheter is held vertically approximately 15 cm above the pubic symphysis and the level of fluid in the catheter identified. The detrusor is considered to be stable when there are no urge symptoms and no elevation of the fluid in the catheter (i.e. normal vesical pressure). When the fluid level rises above 15 cm in height above the symphysis pubis with associated urge symptoms, then detrusor overactivity may be diagnosed. If leakage occurs with coughing in the absence of detrusor overactivity, then stress incontinence is diagnosed.

28.2.6 Bladder Diary

A bladder diary is a useful tool assessing urinary dysfunction to accurately identify urinary frequency, nocturia, episodes of urinary incontinence, voided volumes and fluid intake. The bladder diary can be documented over 1–2 days. Each void is measured and times recorded. Each episode of urgency and/ or incontinence is recorded. Intake and volume of consumed fluids are also recorded. Normal daytime frequency is ≤7 and nocturia should be ≤1 per night. Voided volumes usually range between 250 and 500 ml. Appropriate fluid intake is variable and is dependent on gastrointestinal tract absorption and overall activity level and loss of fluids via sweat, etc.; however, urine should not be excessively concentrated. Bladder diaries have been successfully introduced and utilised in low-resource areas in Africa and Asia (by the authors).

28.3   Prevalence and Diagnosis of Post-Fistula Incontinence

Despite successful closure of the fistula, many women still remain incontinent or have other troublesome urinary symptoms. Persisting urinary incontinence despite successful fistula closure has been reported in between 16% and 24% of women (Goh et al., 2008, Roenneburg et al., 2006, Wall et al., 2004). Stress urinary incontinence, symptoms of overactive bladder and incomplete bladder emptying all occur commonly following successful OF repair.

Browning and Menber (2008) reported on a 6-month follow-up of women following obstetric fistula repair in Ethiopia with 61.5% returning for review. Among a total cohort of 390 cases, 24.3% complained of ongoing urethral urinary incontinence at discharge. Patients with residual urinary symptoms at discharge were twice as likely to return for their follow-up appointment as those discharged with no significant incontinence. Overall, continence status at discharge was largely maintained.

There are few studies documenting the urodynamics assessments of women with urinary dysfunction following successful repair of OF. Schleicher et al. (1993) reviewed 16 women following successful fistula repair. One-half had no urinary incontinence and the remaining eight complained of stress urinary incontinence. These eight women underwent urodynamic testing. Urodynamic stress incontinence was diagnosed in 62.5% (five women), no abnormalities in 25% (two women) and mixed incontinence in 12.5% (one woman). In 2002, Murray et al. (2002) published their review of 55 women following fistula repair in Ethiopia and identified 30 women with urinary incontinence. The 30 women with residual urinary incontinence underwent urodynamic studies. Urodynamic stress incontinence only was diagnosed in 56.7% (17 women). Detrusor overactivity only was diagnosed in 6.7% (two women), and mixed incontinence was present in 36.7% (11 women).

In 2013, Goh et al. published their findings of urodynamic assessments on 149 Ethiopian women following successful fistula closure but with persisting urinary dysfunction. The majority of these women complained of being 'wet all the time' or having continuous incontinence. Validated urodynamic assessments were performed; however, some modifications were required to accommodate specific post-fistula issues. Most of the women were not accustomed to voiding on a commode with catheters in-situ, and hence they were only able to void in the squatting position which did not allow for the use of the uroflowmetry equipment. Therefore, voiding studies and monitoring detrusor pressure during voiding were not obtained. Post-void residual urine volumes were checked with the passage of a catheter following voiding. In addition, digital para-urethral compression was often required during cystometry filling as one in three women leaked per urethra without a detrusor rise or provocation. Goh et al. also found that 92% (139) of the women had urodynamic stress incontinence, with 49% (73) having urodynamic stress incontinence only. About 46% (69 women) had detrusor overactivity, 43% (64 women) had both detrusor overactivity and urodynamic stress incontinence, seven women had neither detrusor overactivity nor urodynamic stress incontinence with two of the seven women having high post-void residual volumes (>200 ml), one had bladder hypersensitivity and four women had no abnormalities detected. There was a total of 6% (nine women) with residual urine volumes of 150 ml or greater (range 150–500 ml).

In summary, greater than 90% of the women presenting with urinary dysfunction following successful closure of OF had urodynamic stress incontinence and 46% had detrusor overactivity, with the rate of mixed urinary incontinence 42.7% (Goh et al., 2013).

In areas where OF is common, post-operative follow-up of women after successful fistula closure after they are discharged can be difficult. The issues which prevent women from returning for review include low income/poverty with a lack of funds available for their transportation to return to the hospital, the financial cost of taking time off work to attend follow-up and regional or political instability with resultant dangers including personal safety especially when women travel alone. In addition, the lack of postal services, and limited or no access to a reliable phone (cost to maintain air-time or cost and availability of electricity to charge phone) limit other forms of effective follow-up and communication. Following fistula surgery with documented closure of the fistula (usually after 2–3 weeks), women will be discharged home to continue with their post-surgical recovery. When a woman is discharged with ongoing urinary leakage or if urinary incontinence recurs after discharge, she may not have the resources to return to the hospital. Even when women do re-present with urinary incontinence in the absence of OF, many hospitals performing fistula surgery do not have the funds nor expertise to manage post-fistula closure bladder dysfunction.

There is a paucity of published data regarding post-fistula closure bladder dysfunction with limited evidence on assessment and management options available. Often clinicians have resorted to surgical options to treat women with urinary incontinence with no prior investigations, and therefore outcomes have not been satisfactory. Both standard stress incontinence surgeries and unproven novel surgical approaches have been used to treat women with urinary incontinence following successful OF repair with minimal data on outcomes reported.

28.4   Treatment Options for Women with Stress Urinary Incontinence Following Repair of Obstetric Fistula

Stress urinary incontinence (SUI) following successful OF closure is a common and challenging problem. Various treatment options have been utilised over many decades; however, the effective management of post-fistula stress urinary incontinence remains unresolved. As there is often significant tissue loss and scarring of the genital tract and lower urinary tract with the development of OF and its subsequent surgical closure, it is not surprising that these women are at a high risk of post-fistula closure bladder dysfunction including stress urinary incontinence. Unfortunately, many women have been subjected to invasive surgery without adequate evaluation.

Treatment options for SUI following repair of OF include pelvic floor rehabilitation, continence devices/urethral plugs and continence surgery. There is limited literature available regarding success rates of supervised pelvic floor rehabilitation including pelvic floor exercises following OF closure. The International Continence Society (ICS) Physiotherapy Committee (Brook and The ICS Physiotherapy Committee 2019) has advised that patient outcomes can be improved if physiotherapy is provided as a part of the multidisciplinary team management for women with OF. In the non-OF population of women with SUI, the Cochrane database reports that supervised pelvic floor rehabilitation can cure or improve symptoms of SUI and all other types of UI (Dumoulin et al., 2018).

Other non-surgical options for treatment of USI include continence devices and urethral plugs. A few fistula units have utilised urethral plugs where the women are taught to use and self-manage the plugs (Goh & Browning, 2005). The possible complications of using urethral plugs include urinary tract infections as well as losing the plug into the bladder which then requires retrieval. The size of the urethral plug often needs to be increased over time and this may be due to stretching of the urethra. Brook and Tessema (2013) reviewed outcomes from urethral plug use for incontinence following successful OF surgery, and concluded that the urethral plug was an effective means of improving continence although long-term data on outcomes were not available.

Documented continence surgery options following OF closure include bulking agents, abdominal sling procedures using fascia lata, rectus fascia or synthetics and vaginal pubococcygeal or fibromuscular slings. Urinary diversion is also an established alternative.

For over a century, peri-urethral injections of bulking agents have been used in the treatment of stress urinary incontinence in women with SUI unrelated to OF (Meyer, 1904). More recently, there has been significant improvement in safety and success rates with the development of material technologies. Peri-urethral injections of autologous fat for the treatment of 'sphincter insufficiency' following successful closure of obstetric urogenital fistula were first described by Hilton et al., 1998. There were six women with stress urinary incontinence following OF closure included in that series which demonstrated a 66% cure/improvement rate with short-term follow-up. Another study which assessed 189 women with stress urinary incontinence without a history of OF (Lee et al., 2001) compared peri-urethral injection of fat with peri-urethral injection of saline (control) at a follow-up of three months. The success rate for both groups was 20–22%, with no benefit of the fat injection compared to the saline injection. There was one death due to pulmonary fat embolism.

There are currently several bulking agents in use for women with SUI without a history of OF, including bovine collagen, porcine collagen, carbon-coated zirconium beads, silicon particles, calcium hydroxylapatite and polyacrylamide hydrogel. A review in 2014 (Kirchin et al., 2012) included 2004 women without a history of OF, participating in 14 trials. The conclusions were that the evidence available was insufficient to guide clinical practice. One potential benefit of peri-urethral bulking agents is that it is minimally invasive surgery. Polyacrylamide hydrogel (Lose et al., 2006) has been demonstrated to have a good safety profile and useful success rates in women with symptomatic stress urinary incontinence. There was a 66% subjective response rate in 135 women with symptomatic stress or mixed urinary incontinence at 12-month follow-up, with no injection site or product-specific adverse events identified (Lose et al., 2006). Eighty-two women were studied following peri-urethral bulking by Maggiore et al. (2013) with a 12-month follow-up, with a subjective success rate of over 74%. No intra-operative complications were noted in this group and the women were discharged on the same day. In another study with a 24-month follow-up of peri-urethral injection of polyacrylamide hydrogel for women with stress and stress predominant mixed urinary incontinence, the subjective responder rate was 64% (Toozs-Hobson et al., 2012). A 12-month follow-up of elderly women with stress urinary incontinence treated with one of four types of injection therapy was published by Mohr et al. (2013). This study included 44 women receiving polyacrylamide hydrogel. After bulking therapy, pad tests were negative in over 73% of women. There was a low overall complication rate for all agents, and no complications at all were documented for the group who received polyacrylamide hydrogel.

In general, the overall success of peri-urethral injection of polyacrylamide hydrogel ranges from 64% to 74% depending on outcome measures (Lose et al., 2006, 2010; Maggiore et al., 2013; Mohr et al., 2013; Toozs-Hobson et al., 2012). However, the success rates in women with serious anatomical dysfunction or loss of tissue secondary to OF trauma would be expected to be lower.

In a more recent study by Krause et al. (2013), peri-urethral injections of polyacrylamide hydrogel (Bulkamid, Ethicon, Johnson & Johnson Medical Pty, Ltd., North Ryde, Australia) were used in a series of four women with residual stress urinary incontinence following successful closure of their OF. Bulkamid hydrogel is a transparent polyacrylamide gel consisting of 97.5% non-pyrogenic water and 2.5% cross-linked polyacrylamide (Ethicon, Johnson & Johnson). As validated urodynamics testing was not available in Democratic Republic of the Congo at that time, simplified clinical urodynamics testing was utilised as described above. Following voiding, the bladder was catheterised to check the residual urine volume. The bladder was then filled via the catheter with ≥300 ml of saline, and the catheter was held vertically. The level of fluid in the catheter above the plane of the symphysis pubis was identified. Where there was no significant elevation of the fluid (i.e. less than 15 cm) and no urge symptoms, then the detrusor was considered to be stable. A positive cough test when the bladder was stable was given a diagnosis of stress urinary incontinence. Post-void residual urine volumes of >100 ml provided a diagnosis of voiding dysfunction. Only women with a diagnosis of stress urinary incontinence with a stable bladder and normal voiding were offered treatment with a bulking agent.

The injection of the bulking agent was performed under general anaesthetic, and as no cystoscopic equipment was available, cystoscopy was not used. The surgical technique involved measuring the urethral length, identifying the urethrovesical junction (using a Foley catheter) and establishing the direction and path of the urethra using a metal catheter. One millilitre of Bulkamid was injected with a long 23G needle through the peri-urethral skin and vaginal epithelium in three sites—at 3, 6 and 9 o'clock. The bladder was emptied and subsequent post-void residual volumes were checked. All four women in this study had significant improvement of their SUI with three out of four reporting no incontinence between 5 and 12 days post-operatively before discharge. Prior to the surgery, all women had described continuous urinary leakage. Larger studies are required to determine outcomes and success rates for this form of treatment. The authors have treated further patients in Uganda with peri-urethral Bulkamid with equally good outcomes.

Other surgical options used for post-OF closure stress urinary incontinence include abdominal and vaginal sling procedures. Ascher-Walsh et al. (2010) reviewed 140 women who had undergone treatment with a sling procedure for stress urinary incontinence following successful fistula closure. These included 96 fascia lata, 16 rectus sheath and 15 synthetic slings. The outcomes were assessed clinically with a median follow-up time of just over 2 months, with overall only 24.4% being identified as dry. There was a 17.3% rate of de novo fistula formation, and in the synthetic mesh sling group the mesh erosion rate was 20% (Ascher-Walsh et al., 2010). Carey et al. (2002) used validated urodynamic assessment to identify a group of nine women with urodynamic stress incontinence only following OF closure. They performed continence surgery which included abdominal retropubic urethrolysis, and insertion of a rectus sheath fascial sling and retropubic omental graft. The immediate subjective success rate at 4-weeks follow-up was 78%. At 16-months follow-up the success rate (subjective and objective with repeat urodynamic studies) was 67%. This series demonstrated abdominal urethrolysis with rectus sheath fascial sling resulting in good success rates; however, it does require an abdominal approach which often includes complicated dissections as the space of Retzius is usually obliterated and therefore does increase the risk of significant complications. Local muscle sling procedures were first described for the treatment of post-fistula stress urinary incontinence by McConnachie, 1958. A similar technique was re-introduced in 2004 (Browning, 2004) which did result in good success rates of 67% immediately post-operatively (Browning, 2006). However, it is not always possible to fashion an adequate pubococcygeal/fibro-muscular sling in many women who have suffered serious injury with loss of tissue. To date, long-term follow-up results of this technique are not available and the benefit of the local tissue sling would be expected to decline over time.

The external genitalia anatomy is often distorted following previous injuries and OF surgery. The bladder neck can be reliably identified with a Foley catheter thus usually allowing accurate placement of a bulking agent. When placing a sling either in the mid-urethral position or at the bladder neck, anatomical distortion and scarring can make the placement difficult. The retropubic dissection and dissection to create a tunnel for sling placement can also be complicated by urethral injury or cystotomy due to the scarring and poor tissue quality, resulting in iatrogenic injuries which may be difficult to repair.

28.5   Treatment for Women with Overactive Bladder

The treatments for women with overactive bladder (OAB) symptoms following successful OF closure include most of the options which are recommended for any women with idiopathic OAB. Continence surgery may worsen the symptoms of OAB.

The bladder diary is a useful tool to identify daytime frequency, nocturia, episodes of urgency or incontinence and voided volumes, together with intake of fluid volumes. The diary also identifies likely bladder irritants such as caffeine which may aggravate overactive bladder symptoms.

28.5.1 Pelvic Floor Rehabilitation

Initial therapy is supervised pelvic floor rehabilitation, in particular bladder retraining. The goal of bladder retraining is to modify bladder function, reduce voiding frequency, increase bladder capacity and eliminate detrusor overactivity by using scheduled voiding rather than voiding in response to urgency (Arnold et al., 2012).

28.5.2 Medications

In addition to pelvic floor rehabilitation or when conservative measures alone are unsuccessful, then medications may be indicated. The two main groups of medications include the anticholinergic options and beta3-adrenoreceptor agonists. Other medications including low-dose tri-cyclic antidepressants may also be effective. The costs, side-effects and availability of medications often determine which are used. The evolving evidence on risk of dementia associated with the use of anticholinergic medications needs to be monitored and women advised accordingly.

Anticholinergic medications include:

1. Oxybutynin.
2. Tolterodine.
3. Solifenacin.
4. Darifenacin.
5. Trospium.
6. Propantheline.

Beta3-adrenoreceptor agonists include:

1. Mirabegron

Tri-cyclic antidepressants include:

1. Amitriptyline.
2. Imipramine.

The authors have used short-term oral oxybutynin with pelvic floor muscle rehabilitation with success in remote central Africa in women following fistula repair with symptoms of OAB.

28.5.3 Nerve Modulation

These treatments include posterior tibial nerve stimulation (PTNS) and sacral nerve stimulation (SNS).

28.5.4 Surgery

Surgical options include intra-vesical injection of Botox® and bladder augmentation.

28.6 Treatment for Women with Voiding Dysfunction

There exists much variation in the types and severity of voiding dysfunction. In those cases where the post-void residual urine volumes are not excessive, then management with voiding techniques and double voiding may be adequate. When the post-void residual urine volumes are high or a patient has urinary retention, then catheterisation is necessary.

The options for catheterisation include:

1. Clean intermittent self-catheterisation (CISC).
2. Indwelling catheter (IDC).
3. Suprapubic catheter.

28.7 Conclusion

It is important that women with ongoing urinary symptoms following closure of OF receive a thorough clinical examination and assessment to exclude any persisting fistulas or bladder pathology. Urodynamic studies are then required to diagnose the cause of their urinary symptoms, with stress urinary incontinence, detrusor overactivity and voiding dysfunction all common sequelae following OF. Conservative management options including pelvic floor rehabilitation need to be provided. Importantly, the women must have access to treatment options following OF closure. Suitable medications for detrusor overactivity are often unavailable to this group of women due to limited resources. Surgical management options for treatment of SUI following OF closure need further research to establish techniques which provide good outcomes despite the significant surgical challenges of anatomical distortion and low-resource surgical venues.

References

Arnold, J., McLeod, N., Thani-Gasalam, R., & Rashid, P. (2012). Overactive bladder syndrome. Management and treatment options. *Australian Family Physician, 41*(11), 878–883.

Ascher-Walsh, C. J., Capes, T. L., Lo, Y., Idrissa, A., Wilkinson, J., Echols, K., Crawford, B., & Genadry, R. (2010). Sling procedures after repair of obstetric vesicovaginal fistula in Niamey, Niger. *International Urogynecology Journal, 21*(11), 1385–1390. https://doi.org/10.1007/s00192-010-1202-5

Brook, G., & The ICS Physiotherapy Committee. (2019). Obstetric fistula: The role of physiotherapy: A report from the Physiotherapy Committee of the International Continence Society. *Neurourology Urodynamics, 38*(1), 407–416. https://doi.org/10.1002/nau.23851

Brook, G., & Tessema, A. B. (2013). Obstetric fistula: The use of urethral plugs for the management of persistent urinary incontinence following successful repair. *International Urogynecology Journal, 24*(3), 479–484. https://doi.org/10.1007/s00192-012-1887-8

Browning, A. (2004). Presentation of residual urinary incontinence following successful repair of obstetric vesicovaginal fistula using a fibro-muscular sling. *BJOG: An International Journal of Obstetrics and Gynaecology, 111*(4), 357–361. https://doi.org/10.1111/j.1471-0528.2004.00080.x

Browning, A. (2006). A new technique for the surgical management of urinary incontinence after obstetric fistula repair. *BJOG: An International Journal of Obstetrics and Gynaecology, 113*, 475–478. https://doi.org/10.1111/j.1471-0528.2006.00847.x

Browning, A., & Menber, B. (2008). Women with obstetric fistula in Ethiopia: a 6-month follow-up after surgical treatment. *BJOG: An International Journal of Obstetrics and Gynaecology, 115*, 1564–1569. https://doi.org/10.1111/j.1471-0528.2008.01900.x

Carey, M. P., Goh, J. T., Fynes, M. M., & Murray, C. J. (2002). Stress urinary incontinence after delayed primary closure of genitourinary fistula: A technique for surgical management. *American Journal of Obstetrics and Gynecology, 186*, 948–953. https://doi.org/10.1067/mob.2002.122247

Continence Foundation of Australia. (2018). Retrieved from https://www.continence.org.au/

Coyne, K. S., Sexton, C. C., Thompson, C. L., Milsom, I., Irwin, D., Kopp, Z. S., et al. (2009). The prevalence of lower urinary tract symptoms (LUTS) in the USA, the UK and Sweden: Results from the epidemiology of LUTS (EpiLUTS) study. *BJU International, 104*, 352–360. https://doi.org/10.1111/j.1464-410X.2009.08427.x

Dooley, Y., Kenton, K., Cao, G., Luke, A., Durazo-Arvizu, R., Kramer, H., et al. (2008). Urinary incontinence prevalence: Results from the National Health and nutrition examination survey. *Journal of Urology, 179*(2), 656–661. https://doi.org/10.1016/j.juro.2007.09.081

Dumoulin, C., Cacciari, L., & Hay-Smith, E. C. (2018). Pelvic floor muscle training versus no treatment, or inactive control treatments, for urinary incontinence in women. *Cochrane Database of Systematic Reviews, 10*(10), CD005654. https://doi.org/10.1002/14651858.CD005654.pub4

Goh, J. T. W., & Browning, A. (2005). Use of urethral plugs for urinary incontinence following fistula repair. *Australian and New Zealand Journal of Obstetrics and Gynaecology, 45*, 237–238. https://doi.org/10.1111/j.1479-828X.2005.00395.x

Goh, J. T. W., Browning, A., Berhan, B., & Chang, A. (2008). Predicting the risk of failure of closure of obstetric fistula and residual urinary incontinence using a classification system. *International Urogynecology Journal, 19*, 1659–1662. https://doi.org/10.1007/s00192-008-0693-9

Goh, J. T. W., Krause, H., Tessema, A. B., & Abraha, G. (2013). Urinary symptoms and urodynamics following obstetric genitourinary fistula repair. *International Urogynecology Journal, 24*, 947–951. https://doi.org/10.1007/s00192-012-1948-z

Hannestad, Y. S., Rortveit, G., Sandvik, H., & Hunskaar, S. (2000). A community –based epidemiological survey of female urinary incontinence: The Norwegian EPINCONT study. *Journal of Clinical Epidemiology, 53*(11), 1150–1157. https://doi.org/10.1016/S0895-4356(00)00232-8

Haylen, B. T., de Ridder, D., Freeman, R. M., Swift, S. E., Berghmans, B., Lee, J., et al. (2010). An International Urogynecological Association (IUGA)/International Continence Society (ICS) joint report on the terminology for female pelvic floor dysfunction. *International Urogynecology Journal, 2010*(21), 5–26. https://doi.org/10.1007/s00192-009-0976-9

Hilton, P., Ward, A., Molloy, M., & Umana, O. (1998). Periurethral injection of autologous fat for the treatment of post-fistula repair stress incontinence: A preliminary report. *International Urogynecology Journal, 9*, 118–121. https://doi.org/10.1007/BF01982221

Irwin, D. E., Milsom, I., Hunskaar, S., Reilly, K., Kopp, Z., Herschorn, S., et al. (2006). Population-based survey of urinary incontinence, overactive bladder, and other lower urinary tract symptoms in five countries: Results of the EPIC study. *European Urology, 50*, 1306–1314. https://doi.org/10.1016/j.eururo.2006.09.019

Kirchin, V., Page, T., Keegan, P. E., Atiemo, K., Cody, J. D., & McClinton, S. (2012). Urethral injection therapy for urinary incontinence in women. *Cochrane Database of Systematic Reviews*, (2), CD003881. https://doi.org/10.1002/14651858.CD003881.pub3

Krause, H. G., Lussy, J. P., & Goh, J. T. W. (2013). The use of periurethral injections of polyacrylamide hydrogel for treating post-vesicovaginal fistula closure urinary stress incontinence. *Journal of Obstetrics and Gynaecology Research, 40*, 521–525. https://doi.org/10.1111/jog.12176

Lee, P. E., Kung, R. C., & Drutz, H. P. (2001). Periurethral autologous fat injection as treatment for female stress urinary incontinence: A randomized double-blind controlled trial. *Journal of Urology, 165*, 153–158. https://doi.org/10.1097/00005392-200101000-00037

Lose, G., Mouritsen, L., & Nielsen, J. B. (2006). A new bulking agent (polyacrylamide hydrogel) for treating stress urinary incontinence in women. *BJU International, 98*(1), 100–104. https://doi.org/10.1111/j.1464-410X.2006.06205.x

Lose, G., Sorensen, H. C., Axelsen, S. M., Falconer, C., Lobodasch, K., & Safwat, T. (2010). An open multicenter study of polyacrylamide hydrogel (Bulkamid) for female stress and mixed urinary incontinence. *International Urogynecology Journal, 21*, 1471–1477. https://doi.org/10.1007/s00192-010-1214-1

Maggiore, L. R., Alessandri, F., Medica, M., Gabelli, M., Venturini, P. L., & Ferrero, S. (2013). Outpatient periurethral injections of polyacrylamide hydrogel for the treatment of female stress urinary incontinence: Effectiveness and safety. *Archives of Gynecology and Obstetrics, 288*, 131–137. https://doi.org/10.1007/s00404-013-2718-y

Markland, A. D., Richter, H. E., Few, C., Eggers, P., & Kusek, J. W. (2011). Prevalence and trends of urinary incontinence in adults in the United States, 2001 to 2008. *Journal of Urology, 186*(2), 589–593. https://doi.org/10.1016/j.juro.2011.03.114

McConnachie, E. (1958). Fistulae of the urinary tract in the female; a proposed classification. *South African Medical Journal, 32*(20), 524–527. https://doi.org/10.1097/00006254-195812000-00053

Meyer, L. (1904). 2 tilfaeide af incontinentia urinae helbredede ved parafininjektioner. *Ugeskrift for Laeger, 104*, 5.

Milsom, I., Abrams, P., Cardozo, L., Roberts, R. G., Thüroff, J., & Wein, A. J. (2001). How widespread are the symptoms of an overactive bladder and how are they managed? A population-based prevalence study. *BJU International, 87*, 760–766. https://doi.org/10.1046/j.1464-410x.2001.02228.x

Minassian, V. A., Stewart, W. F., & Wood, G. C. (2008). Urinary incontinence in women: Variation in prevalence estimates and risk factors. *Obstetrics & Gynecology, 111*, 324–331. https://doi.org/10.1097/01.AOG.0000267220.48987.17

Mohr, S., Siegenthaler, M., Mueller, M. D., & Kuhn, A. (2013). Bulking agents: An analysis of 500 cases and review of the literature. *International Urogynecology Journal, 24*, 241–247. https://doi.org/10.1007/s00192-012-1834-8

Murray, C., Goh, J. T., Fynes, M., & Carey, M. P. (2002). Urinary and faecal incontinence following delayed primary repair of obstetric genital fistula. *BJOG: An International Journal of Obstetrics and Gynaecology, 109*, 828–832. https://doi.org/10.1111/j.1471-0528.2002.00124.x. Retrieved July 10, 2019, from obgyn.onlinelibrary.wiley.com

Nygaard, I., Barber, M. D., Burgio, K. L., Kenton, K., Meikle, S., Schaffer, J., et al. (2008). Prevalence of symptomatic pelvic floor disorders in US women. *Journal of the American Medical Association, 300*, 1311–1316. https://doi.org/10.1001/jama.300.11.1311

Peyrat, L., Haillot, O., Bruyere, F., Boutin, J. M., Bertrand, P., & Lanson, Y. (2002). Prevalence and risk factors of urinary incontinence in young and middle-aged women. *BJU International, 89*, 61–66. https://doi.org/10.1046/j.1464-410X.2002.02546.x

Roenneburg, M. L., Genadry, R., & Wheeless, C. R. (2006). Repair of vesicovaginal fistulas in Africa. *American Journal of Obstetrical Gynecology, 195*, 1748–1752. https://doi.org/10.1016/j.ajog.2006.07.031

Schleicher, D. J., Ojengbede, O. H. A., & Elkins, T. E. (1993). Urological evaluation after closure of vesicovaginal fistulas. *International Urogynecology Journal, 4*, 262–265. https://doi.org/10.1007/BF00372732

Toozs-Hobson, P., Al-Singary, W., Fynes, M., Tegerstedt, G., & Lose, G. (2012). Two-year follow-up of an open-label multicenter study of polyacrylamide hydrogel (Bulkamid) for female stress and stress-predominant mixed incontinence. *International Urogynecology Journal, 23*, 1373–1378. https://doi.org/10.1007/s00192-012-1761-8

Wall, L. L., Karshima, J. A., Kirschner, C., & Arrowsmith, S. D. (2004). The obstetric vesicovaginal fistula: Characteristics of 899 patients from Jos, Nigeria. *American Journal of Obstetrics & Gynecology, 190*, 1011–1019. https://doi.org/10.1016/j.ajog.2004.02.007

Walters, M. D., & Karram, M. M. (2015). *Urogynecology and reconstructive pelvic surgery* (4th ed.). Elsevier Saunders.

A Multidisciplinary Approach to Obstetric Fistula in Northern Ghana: "Not Counted Among Women"

29

Kimberly Jarvis, Helen Vallianatos, Solina Richter, and Priscilla N. Boakye

29.1 Introduction

The Ghanaian maxim *"there is no wealth where there are no children"* underlines the importance placed on the birth of a child in Ghanaian society (Gyekye, 2003, p. 84). Traditionally, Ghanaian women establish their status in society after giving birth (Jansen, 2006). Currently over one-half (55%) of births in rural Ghana are unattended by skilled birth attendants (Nakua et al., 2015). Skilled birth attendants can include midwives as well as individuals who have received some training on basic childbirth care from doctors and/or nurses. When there is no skilled birth attendant present, the risks for unrecognized complications that can impact the birth as well as the long-term well-being of the mother and her infant are significantly increased.

Obstetric fistula (OF) is one of the most serious and tragic childbirth injuries associated with prolonged, obstructed labor unrelieved by timely intervention. OF is an abnormal opening or openings between the vagina and the bladder and/or rectum that frequently leaves women incontinent of urine and/or feces (Lewis & de Bernis, 2006). Although the exact prevalence of OF is difficult to determine,

---

The material used in this chapter was adapted from the dissertation Jarvis, K. (2016). *An exploration of a culture of reintegration with women who have experienced obstetrical fistula repair in northern* Ghana, *West Africa*. [Doctoral dissertation, University of Alberta]. ProQuest Dissertations.

K. Jarvis (✉)
Faculty of Nursing, Memorial University, St. John's, NL, Canada

University of Alberta, Edmonton Clinic Health Academy, Edmonton, AB, Canada
e-mail: kimberly.jarvis@mun.ca

H. Vallianatos
Department of Anthropology, University of Alberta, Edmonton, AB, Canada

S. Richter
College of Nursing, University of Saskatchewan, Saskatoon, SK, Canada

P. N. Boakye
Lawrence S. Bloomberg Faculty of Nursing, University of Toronto, Toronto, ON, Canada

in Asia and sub-Saharan Africa, it is generally believed that between 2 to 3 million women live with untreated OF (Kalembo & Zgambo, 2012; World Health Organization [WHO], 2018). In Ghana between the years 2011 and 2014, 1538 OF patients had been assessed and 616 had received a surgical repair (Ghana Health Services, 2015). The highest number of OF cases are reported in the northern part of the country; however, the true number of cases are difficult to calculate because case-finding is challenging because the condition is highly stigmatized. Estimates of the incidence in Ghana suggest that from 500 to 1000 new cases of OF occur annually (Danso et al., 2007), affecting women's physical, psychological, and sexual health, and their social and economic status (Pacagnella et al., 2010). The culmination of effects on women is evident in the quotation in our title; these words were repeatedly shared, and succinctly capture the experiences of many women who had experienced OF as they spoke of the trauma, stigmatization, and ostracization experienced because of OF (and which will be elaborated upon below).

The approach to care of women with OF is threefold and includes educational awareness, treatment (surgery), and community reintegration. Although there is much documentation concerning awareness and treatment, little is known regarding how women reintegrate after their OF repair (Mselle et al., 2011). This may primarily be because follow-up in low- and middle-income countries (LMIC) can be challenging and time consuming, but also because of the stigmatization and negative effects of OF on Ghanaian women's status.

The needs and the challenges affecting women in northern Ghana as they resume the cultural, social, familial, spousal, and economic day-to-day lives following their OF repair are critically explored in this chapter. Insight into the experiences of women within their cultural context to generate emancipatory knowledge concerning reintegration following an OF repair is organized around Habermas' critical theory[1] (Edgar, 2006; Habermas, 1991a, 1991b; Mill et al., 2001; Singh, 1999). Emancipatory knowledge recognizes social and political "injustices or inequity, to realize that things could be different, and to piece together complex elements of experience and context to change a situation as it is to a situation that improves people's lives" (Chinn & Kramer, 2011, p. 64). Through dialectic communication with women and reflection upon their needs and challenges experienced after OF repair, it is anticipated that the knowledge generated in this study will inform public policy to maximize the health and well-being of women returning home after an OF repair.

29.2 Methods

29.2.1 Research Design and Setting

An ethnographic design framework was employed using a social justice/health equity lens to critically explore underlying historical, economic, psychosocial, and political issues related to reintegration, after OF repair in northern Ghana. The design allowed engagement with participants that challenged dominant societal views and exposed the hidden structures that were oppressive or potentially oppres-

---

[1] Jürgen Habermas (b. 1929) is a German sociologist and philosopher whose academic work has focused on foundations of social theory, epistemology, the rule of law in the social-evolutionary context, and critical analysis of democracy and advanced capitalism. The roots of his postulates lie in the traditions of German philosophy from Kant to Marx, and he has been associated with the Frankfurt school of critical theorists. Habermas' Critical Theory has some features in common with the beliefs of Karl Marx; however, they differ in other opinions.

sive. The aim of implementing this design was to consciously strengthen participants so that they were more able to reflect on actions that could be taken to change oppressive forces. Additionally, the design provided a view beyond the metaphors typically used in Ghanaian society, to aid in understanding the hidden meaning behind the importance of socio-economic reintegration after OF repair. Metaphors are often used in Ghanaian culture to speak the unspeakable because Ghanaians often dislike verbal confrontation, which threatens social harmony and their own physical well-being and public image (Galyan, 1999). For example, this statement, "*Baandɔyu ku di naanzua ka di waligu puhi pololi*" translated to "the lizard does not eat pepper for the frog to sweat" can signify how a woman who has experienced an OF repair is responsible for her own health actions and well-being.

This study was conducted in Upper East, Upper West, and Northern regions within northern Ghana (see Fig. 29.1). Northern Ghana is known to be exceedingly rural as well as economically and socially disadvantaged (Tsikata & Seini, 2004). Figures 29.2 and 29.3 illustrate typical village housing and streetscapes. These deficiencies may be best seen in the lack of responsiveness to the social determinants of health (SDOH) contributing to higher rates of OF (and other health conditions) in northern Ghana. The SDOH are defined as "*the conditions in which people live, work and play*" (WHO, 2019, para.1). These conditions are shaped by the allocation of money, power, and resources at all levels of government and are believed to be in large part responsible for health equities and/or inequities (WHO, 2019).

Fig. 29.1 Ghana map. (Source: Ghana map showing major cities as well as parts of surrounding countries and the Gulf of Guinea. The World Factbook 2021. Washington, DC: Central Intelligence Agency, 2021. https://www.cia.gov/the-world-factbook/)

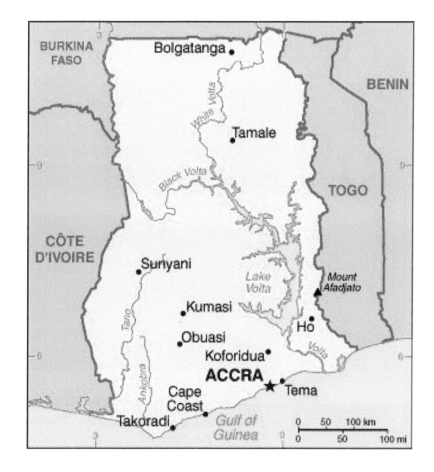

Fig. 29.2 Typical housing in rural communities in Northern Ghana. (Published with permission from © Kimberly Jarvis. All Rights Reserved)

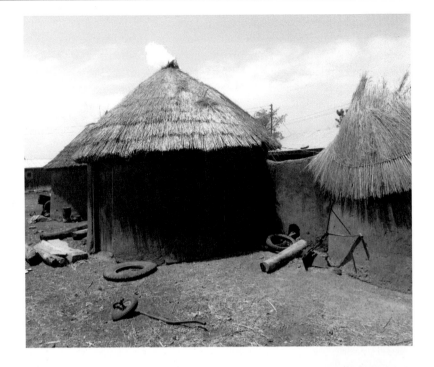

Fig. 29.3 Common streetscape in rural communities in Northern Ghana. (Published with permission from © Kimberly Jarvis. All Rights Reserved)

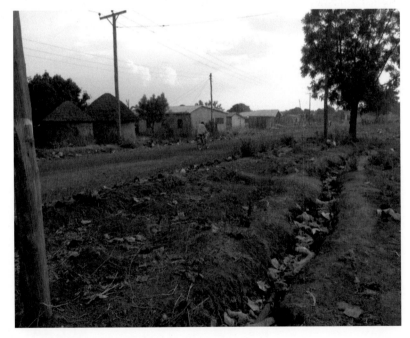

Northern Ghana has been arguably the most challenging region in the country when considering underdevelopment—access to health facilities/medical resources, schools/education, transportation, employment, infrastructure, food, and water security. These difficulties are grounded in colonial histories, where southern Ghana (predominantly the Ashanti region[2]) was known for its natural resources—the deposit of gold in the soil. Portuguese, British, and Dutch colonizers were attracted to southern Ghana and exploited and exported their gold as well as other resources such as cocoa. The colonizers contributed to the social, economic, educational, and the healthcare system in the south, which it occupied, but neglected the north that possessed few resources (Akologo & van Klinken, 2008). Colonial policy biases continued postindependence, as government policies continued to ignore the needs of the Northern Ghana, neglecting the fundamental issues underpinning social and economic deprivation (Oteng-Ababio et al., 2017). These events set the stage for Ghana's current North-South divide.

Poverty is the main issue affecting all aspects of health and well-being. While Ghana has been reclassified from a low-income to a low-middle-income country following the discovery of crude oil in 2007, the economic boom has been short-lived, as oil prices fell on the world market shortly thereafter (Institute for Fiscal Studies, 2015). This has altered Ghana's ability to meet their development goals of accelerated growth and poverty reduction (Institute for Fiscal Studies, 2015). The shift in economic climate has been of great concern in northern Ghana where the rate of poverty is 50.4% and the depth of poverty, those living on less than $1.25 U.S per day, is the highest in the country (Cooke et al., 2016). Furthermore, in northern Ghana where the economic livelihood is chiefly agriculture, the dry savannah climate can have a devastating economic impact.

Many communities in northern Ghana are isolated, scattered along the countryside. Major roads within northern Ghana are tarred; however, secondary and feeder roads are unpaved and inadequately maintained. During the rainy season, many roads are not usable due to flooding, preventing women from accessing maternal health services despite it being covered under the National Health Insurance Scheme (NHIS). Reports of maternal health care being inappropriate due to the lack of skilled physicians and/or nurse midwives are also common. Women frequently conveyed stories of traveling to a Community-based Health Planning Services (CHPS) clinic, a national health initiative designed to provide public health services and programs within communities including maternity care, to find no healthcare provider to address their health concern. Similar stories were narrated about other healthcare clinics and regional hospitals in northern Ghana. Fistula stakeholders' comments on the difficulties of attracting healthcare providers to the north reinforced the stories that other women had shared. Stakeholders related that the factors which deterred healthcare providers from working in this region included the lack of infrastructure such as running water, reliable electricity, internet, and mobile cell service, the inaccessibility of both personal and medical provisions, and the geographical remoteness and isolation which create struggles for educational and advancements in employment opportunities.

The main site for the study was the Tamale Fistula Center (TFC) located in the Northern Region, the only state-run fistula center in the country. This Center is housed on the hospital grounds, in a building donated by the Northern Regional Health Directorate and refurbished by Pathfinder-Ghana and the United Nations Population Fund (UNFPA)-Ghana.

The facility is composed of a gynecological operating theater and ten inpatient beds. Women congregated outside in an area off to the side of the fistula clinic. This area was sheltered from the sun with metal roofing held up by seven wooden planks. Inside this shelter, a fire pit made of small stones

---

[2]The Ashanti region is located in south Ghana and is the third largest of the country's ten administrative regions. The Ashanti people are a matrilineal ethnic group native to the Asante region of Ghana. Their ethnic language, *Twi*, is a common name for two former mutually unintelligible dialects, *Asante* and *Akuapem*, and is spoken by approximately nine million persons as either a first or second language.

Fig. 29.4 Shelter outside the Tamale Fistula Center, located in northern Ghana, where women who experience fistula congregated. (Published with permission from © Kimberly Jarvis. All Rights Reserved)

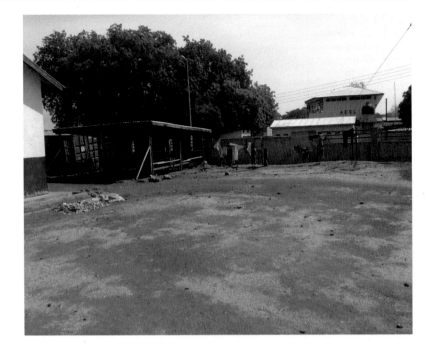

could be seen, surrounded by wooden benches where women sat and can be seen in Fig. 29.4. This is where women could cook their traditional meals—those who could afford to do so. Women were observed preparing *fufu*, a meal where they first boil and then mix and pound equal portions of a starchy food like cassava, yams, cocoyams or green plantain thoroughly with water until it has a dough-like consistency. *Fufu* is eaten with fingers; a small amount is rolled into a ball with one's right hand, and then dipped into a traditional soup such as groundnut, palm nut or light soup. *Tuo Zaafi* (TZ) is another delicacy, especially in the north, prepared similarly to *fufu* but from corn or millet flour and served with a green vegetable soup made from hibiscus (*bra* or *bito*) or jute (*ayoyo*) leaves as is illustrated in Fig. 29.5. Jollof rice, is also a popular meal eaten daily by most Ghanaians, a rice dish prepared with tomato sauce.

Women washed their rags or clothes used to absorb the leakage of urine in a back room of the fistula clinic where running water was available. They hung their clothes on the clotheslines just outside the clinic where they sat interacting and engaging in conversation. They appear to be relaxed and to enjoy mingling, as though it is something they yearned for since being inflicted with OF. Ghanaian culture is characteristically friendly and hospitable where individuals frequently congregate at a common place within the community to socialize. OF hinders a women's ability to mingle among her peers for fear of being ridiculed because of the stench of human waste, a consequence of her condition. These women at the Center, however, appeared to be bonded by OF, for they each carried a bucket connected to a tube known as a urinary catheter. This tube allows urine to drain freely into the bucket from their bladder which they disposed of in a bathroom located in the fistula clinic. Many women for example shared similar stories of perinatal loss/miscarriage, rejection, and stigmatization from their husband, families, and communities, as well as the tribulations of seeking OF treatment and care.

The women were observed welcoming each other and the staff at the fistula clinic. Women often bowed their bodies either greeting or responding "*nnaaah- nnaaah*" when other women approach, signifying a respectful greeting. Some women choose not to join the daily conversations, opting to sit

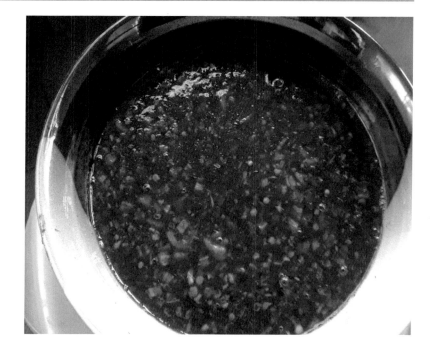

Fig. 29.5 Green vegetable soup. A traditional meal in northern Ghana. (Published with permission from © Priscilla N. Boakye. All Rights Reserved)

alone or lay on their hospital bed. Women continued to come throughout the week, and by week's end on Sunday the fistula clinic has doubled its normal 10-bed capacity. Women lay on mattress on the floor and in the courtyard by the clinic's entrance.

The clinic was staffed mainly by two gynecologists, two "in charge" nurse-midwives who oversaw the nursing care, and several other nurses-midwives who provided direct patient care and health teaching over a 24-h period. While the "in charge" nurse-midwives were specifically assigned to the fistula clinic, other nurses-midwives could be expected to "float" to the obstetrical unit. Additional surgical expertize came from a nearby teaching hospital when required. This Center was additionally supported with the regular visits of physicians from other countries, who spend a short amount of time in the clinic, perform surgeries, and worked with local staff. Although there are qualified urogynecologists in the country, many women waited for foreign physicians, often from the West, to come to their aid believing they possessed better surgical techniques. A nurse at the clinic noted:

> most of them [women with OF] we book them in the mass cases and when [the American doctor] comes, he does them as mass cases and goes back. Three months he comes and then goes back… but of course it depends on his schedule.

Twenty-four northern communities were visited for the purpose of data collection on women's reintegration experiences post-OF repair. These communities differed considerably, especially between a metropolitan area such as Tamale, municipalities like Bolga or Yendi, and districts like Kpandai. For example, Tamale is the largest city in the north and the fourth largest city in Ghana, and has significantly better services compared to municipalities and /or districts in more remote northern communities. Tamale is the hub of the north and its infrastructure is much more developed, thus individuals have access to resources such as a teaching hospital, OF clinic, and airport, as well as various businesses, shops, financial institutions, and schools. In the remote district communities, families typically lived in thatch houses, fetched water from the borehole, gathered firewood to cook their meals because they have limited or no electricity, and used outdoor bathroom facilities. Individuals in remote communities have correspondingly fewer healthcare services and are observed seeking more traditional forms of medicine from traditional healers such as herbalists, spiritualists, diviners, and

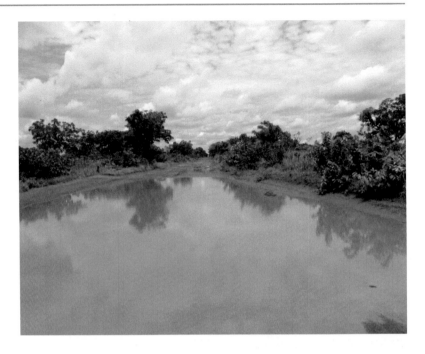

faith healers. In these regions, children actively participate in domestic chores and selling goods instead of attending school—which also speaks to the economic needs of families. Livestock, mainly goats and foul, often roamed freely. In the rainy season, these communities are green, lush, and smell fresh; however, motorways are often flooded making them dangerous for travel as can be seen in Fig. 29.6.

29.2.2 Sample

Ninety-nine participants were recruited using purposive, convenience, and snowball sampling techniques. Participants consisted of 41 women who had experienced an OF repair, 24 family members who identified themselves as the primary caregiver for affected women, 17 healthcare providers (HCPs) including nurses and physicians at the TFC, community health nurses (CHN), nurse-midwives and skilled birth attendants, and 17 stakeholders who were involved in OF care, specifically reintegration. The stakeholders included community, political, and religious leaders, both men and women. A list of potential participants (women) was retrieved from the TFC. Women who met the inclusion criteria were contacted by a staff nurse at the TFC and invited to participate. A family member, if present, was also invited to participate in a separate interview. Women frequently knew of other women who had experienced an OF repair and referred them to the study as potential participants. HCPs and stakeholders were selected on the grounds of potential knowledge they had about OF care. They were initially recruited from the TFC, Ghana Health Service, Ghanaian Government Ministries, and later by word of mouth.

29.2.3 Data Collection Methods

Fieldwork occurred over two-time intervals: March to June 2014 and April to May 2015. Although observation and the review of government, nongovernment, and TFC documents were used in data collection, semi-structured interviews with each participant were the main method utilized. Interviews, which were audio-recorded, varied from 30 to 90 min in length. Participants responded in seven different languages which were translated with the support of a translator(s). Interviews took a dialogical approach which allowed for stimulating questions to conceptualize the hidden meanings, historical, economic, social, cultural, and political aspects behind the needs and challenges of reintegration post-OF repair.

Ethics approval was received from the Ethics Review Board at the University of Alberta, Canada and the Navrongo Health Research Center, Ghana. The risks and benefits of participation were explained in the local language to participants who were not fluent in English. Participation was voluntary and consent was obtained by signature or thumbprint. Data collected were stored in the Health Research Data Repository (HRDR), a secure and confidential virtual research environment, at the University of Alberta, Canada.

29.2.4 Data Analysis

Interviews were transcribed verbatim. Data were analyzed according to Hammersley and Atkinson's (2007) approach to ethnographic analysis. A subset of the data was randomly selected and read line-by-line to capture key ideas. Memos and reflections were placed in the margins to assist with generating concepts that were then organized into larger categories. Ten categories were used to construct a coding framework, which was then tested on other randomly selected interviews from the four groupings of participants (women, family members, HCPs, and stakeholders). Adjustments to the framework were made before being applied to the remaining data for critical analysis. Nvivo 10.0 software was used for data management. Trustworthiness was maintained by employing forward and backward translation and a stepwise replication procedure, where two members of the research team analyzed a subset of the data separately and compared the results to ensure accuracy with how the data were understood.

29.3 Women's Stories of Obstetric Fistula

Prior experiences shape who we are, influencing how we perceive and manage future events. All women discussed the economic and psychosocial impacts of living with OF, and how those experiences continued to affect their lives after OF repair. Understanding the needs of women after OF repair is complex since it is deeply embedded into the historical, economic, social, and cultural fabric of Ghanaian society. To highlight how these aspects interplay in the lives of individual women, we begin by highlighting the stories of three women. The first woman, whom we call Anna (a pseudonym), illustrates particularly the interplay of social and cultural factors on her experiences of OF, and reintegration efforts. This is followed by the story of Zelda (a pseudonym), who had lived with OF for a much longer time, experiencing unsuccessful treatments and post-OF repair, struggling financially, physically, and socially. The final story provides a counterpoint to some of the experiences of Anna and Zelda, for Mary (a pseudonym) who was an educated woman employed in a career of her choosing, and had the emotional support of her husband. She articulated the need for greater awareness and education about OF and its care. As we share the findings below, which incorporate multiple participants' views and experiences, Anna's, Zelda's, and Mary's stories become touchstones to highlight the complexity of women's experiences.

29.3.1 Anna's Story

She has lived with obstetric fistula for two months before receiving a surgical repair. By some accounts, she is considered lucky because most women who acquire the condition live with it for years. She developed the condition after laboring for more than 24 h. It was her father-in-law, head of the family clan, who gave permission for her to go to the hospital but when she arrived, it was too late to save her baby. As a result, she was left grieving the loss of her child and her ability to have future children because doctors had to remove her uterus. In Ghana, barrenness is considered a great calamity, and women who are unable to bear children are often ridiculed. Anna was ridiculed for more than barrenness—she was mocked for having an obstetric fistula. She recalls that unfortunate day:

> I was getting wet and I tried to look maybe I sat on water and then I moved to a different seat which is virtual dry and then I realized that this seat again is wet so I was standing up to see urine there, water trickling down.

When people in her community learned of her condition, she remembers "*they use to spit when they see me.*" A woman is supposed to be clean and smelling nice and the stench of urine was repulsive. For months, she retreated to her room to weep for she was not permitted to partake in cooking family meals, attending community programs (i.e., outdoorings,[3] weddings) or praying at the mosque because she had the "urine sickness". She questioned the cause of her condition, was it from the delivery, from God, or from a fellow human being who had cursed her?

Her husband and extended family were supportive in helping her to find a cure and to return home to the life she lived before obstetric fistula. She remarks:

> [it was all] joy when I came home [post-surgical repair] they [her family] were beating a drum.

Her husband explained:

> in this compound [family home] we do everything communally. So when [my wife] came home we discussed all the things she shouldn't do so all the women were aware. The things men can help with, we did but if it's something related to women's work then the other women would help with that.

29.3.2 Zelda's Story

She lived in a remote community in northern Ghana, which could only be accessed by motorbike. Zelda had delayed seeking obstetric care and by the time she presented herself at the health clinic, no nurse or midwife was available to attend to her obstetric crises. She was forced to make her way to Tamale, the capital city of the Northern Region of Ghana, to seek medical care. She had labored for 2 days. Her baby was now deceased, and she was left with an obstetric fistula and damage to her peroneal nerve, a frequent consequence of fistula, resulting in numbness/weakness in her foot (foot drop). She lived with a fistula for 6 years. In the years that followed, she had three unsuccessful fistula surgeries and was starting to lose hope that a cure was possible. She noted that her "*life was meaningless.*" Her husband was committed to her, but his family believed he was wasting his money looking for a cure because in some sub-Saharan African communities "*the condition is seen as a punishment or a curse for an assumed wrongdoing, rather than as a medical condition*" (United Nations Population Fund [UNFPA] (n.d.), What is Fistula, para.5). Her fourth surgery, performed by a visiting doctor from the United States, was successful. She notes her feelings the day she left the hospital after having her fistula repair:

---

[3] In Ghana, an outdooring is a celebration in which a baby is brought outside for the first time, typically around eight days after birth.

I was so happy… knowing that I'm coming back into my community and having the mind that well I can now go and do whatever I want to do.

However, doing whatever she wanted was not that simple because the surgery placed restrictions on her ability to lift heavy objects, fetching water and firewood, walking long distances, or to being intimate with her husband for several months. She had no means to financially support herself and to assist her family. A local nongovernmental organization (NGO) offered her skills training to make dough loaves and the startup funds to be sell the baked goods in her community. Unfortunately, this would require her to walk around the community carrying the heavy dough loaves. Although she was grateful for the opportunity, she indicated it was not realistic given her postsurgical limits for she stated:

I can't carry the things [dough loaves] and the walking and distance. For six years, I've been bedridden. I don't do anything, and it was becoming difficult to carry the things [dough loafs]. I had to stop it because I think it's not good for me.

She was apprehensive about her decision to stop selling the dough loaves believing that the NGO would follow up and condemn her for not doing the skill she was taught; however, no follow-up was provided.

29.3.3 Mary's Story

Mary was an educated woman, a school teacher. She developed a fistula more than 20 years ago but recalls the details as though it was yesterday, an indication of how profound the illness can be. She recalls she was just a young girl starting a career and a family with her husband when she developed a recto-vaginal fistula, a hole between her vagina and her rectum. She noted:

I began to experience uncontrolled feces or some abnormalities with discharge [from] my bowels. I was made to understand from my interaction with elders and experienced women with children that what I was experiencing was a result of not sitting on hot water after childbirth.

She continued to seep feces and became pregnant a year later. This time during labor she followed the instructions of the elders, but her delivery resulted in a second stillbirth and "*sitting on hot water after childbirth*" did little to relieve the fecal discharge. Shortly thereafter, her husband began working with the health authority and learned his wife needed to see a gynecologist. He was told his wife's condition could be corrected. Mary stated, "*because of my husband's work I knew where to go for help*" which she did with the support of her husband. She questions if there is enough awareness about how to prevent fistula and if women know how to access care. Mary stated:

creating awareness is one important factor… Nurses and healthcare providers should be trained to limit the disease. I want the government to pay attention to training healthcare providers.

Following her fistula surgery, a nurse told her that for future pregnancies she would need to deliver by cesarean section and the importance of not doing strenuous work. She was fortunate to be able to take an "excused duty to heal" from her workplace but recognizes this is not the reality of most Ghanaian women who experience the illness and work as farmers or market women trading and selling their goods. Mary is now a fistula advocate having a sense of responsibility to help other women with similar experiences for she remarks:

I know the illness is not a pleasant thing to have. I sometimes think even I who has had some education and my experience with this illness before my repair. I should educate those without education because some [women] would see no need to visit the hospital [for care].

29.4   Demographics of the Participants

Most of the 41 women who were interviewed for this study were less than one-year post-OF repair. The vast majority of these women indicated having experienced one to four previous fistula surgeries before being "cured," or where they could define their physical health as restored. Although women noted being "cured," some women did describe experiencing residual incontinence, which negatively impacted their return to their family and community. The majority of women, however, were welcomed home but there were many challenges related to their post-OF care such as their economic roles and other traditional role as Ghanaian women. Many of these women worked in the fields or traded in the marketplace, both physically intensive activities. Many of these women also participated in traditional practices of "women's work," which included gathering firewood and water, preparing and cooking meals, and caring for children and elders (See Fig. 29.7).

Women's work was also physically laborious, where gathering firewood and water would equate to walking on average 4 h per day with heavy loads on their heads (Porter et al., 2013); preparing meals entailed pounding starches for approximately 1–2 h per day for a family of seven; and caring for family members could involve physically lifting or supporting individuals with mobility needs. Additionally, women in the north lived in a patriarchal society, where women did not typically participate in decision-making, illustrated by their inability to refuse their husbands' advances for sexual intercourse. The sociocultural context greatly impacted the majority of women in this study, whose post-OF care included no heavy lifting, no walking long distances, and no sexual intercourse for 3–6 months—activities that were all part of women's everyday lives. Women were also supposed to return to the fistula clinic when or should they become pregnant, but this was also impacted by women's decision-making role (or lack thereof) within the family. It was observed that OF affected some of the most impoverished and illiterate women in northern Ghana, but in the few cases where women

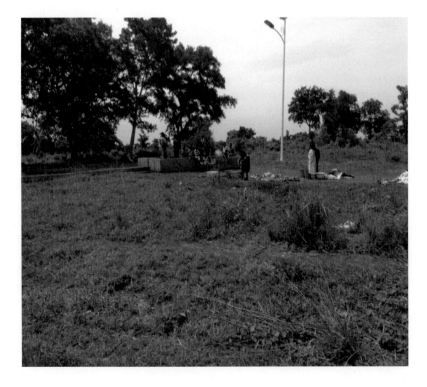

Fig. 29.7 Women's work: washing clothes at the borehole. (Published with permission from © Kimberly Jarvis. All Rights Reserved)

had some education or lived in a family where their roles differed from the typical description just given, their ability to seek treatment and reintegrate back to the life they once lived was enhanced as in Mary's story.

29.5   Sociocultural Contexts of Obstetric Fistula

Individuals living in northern Ghana have fewer opportunities to access the social and economic determinants required for maternal and reproductive health related to inequalities in services. The Human Development Index (HDI) is a tool that measures well-being on three dimensions: income, education, and health (United Nations Development Program [UNDP], 2015). Ghana's HDI is 0.579, giving the country a ranking of 140 out of 187 countries with comparable data and placing Ghana slightly above the regional average for sub-Saharan Africa (Index of Economic Freedom, 2015). While the overall poverty rate in Ghana has declined, in the north it is two to three times the national average (Cooke et al., 2016). According to one government stakeholder:

> Northern Ghana has the highest rates of poverty, illiteracy, malnutrition, and maternal mortality and morbidity in the country. It is underdeveloped in terms of infrastructure; the roads going from community to community are very bad. Sometimes you can't get to a community because of flooding in the rainy season. It is extremely hard to get doctors and nurses to go to these areas and so many times communities are left without services but we are working to make changes but those changes can't happen overnight.

The women in this study who experienced OF repair all lived in the north. All of them were engaged in farming or petty trades except for two who held professional positions. Many women alluded to their troubling economic status that was further influenced by the inequalities between the north and south and the harsh climatic and geographical conditions such as drought, floods, pest infestation, and the resultant low crop production. An NGO Administrator and stakeholder commented:

> We are an NGO… to help women be self-employed so that they [women] won't move to the South. But in the South, in urban areas, there is a lot of work. In northern villages, most of the schools are not effective and there are certain places where there are no schools. Where there are schools they mostly deny [the] girl child from attending school. By so doing she idles and joins women carrying people's goods for money "kayayo" [head porters]…If you ask where woman are, they [the community] would say they [women] have gone to the South to do 'kayayo'. Then you ask why do you allow them to do that? There is nothing we [northern community/family] can do, we don't have money and the farming we do is just a little. It cannot take us to the next season. Women go to 'kayayo' even though the work is tedious and difficult but they are able to work…buy cheap food and send to us. So don't you think that if they have something here [in the north] which can bring daily income, it would be good?

As well, because northern women live in a patrilineal society, women traditionally are unable to inherit or own property, perpetuating gender inequality and hindering economic prosperity. This is exemplified with Anna's story, where her treatment path required the permission and support of her father-in-law. A nurse and community stakeholder stated:

> Here in the north, we are a patrilineal society… men lower the importance of women traditionally-speaking but all families are different. Women have not been able to own or inherit land in the north. This one woman I know when the husband died the family took everything even the cloths she worn.

Many women also noted that they were unable to make healthcare decisions, such as whether to seek prenatal or maternity care when in labor, which could have an effect on their maternal/reproductive health. These decisions were often those of their husbands, fathers or other influential males as was the case for Anna. An elder male family member stated:

> They [the family] tell me when someone is sick and if it is troubling, I tell them to go [seek medical treatment]. Here in this family, I tell them to go to the hospital especially when someone is pregnant now that we see what can happen when you don't go. But as head of this family they [the family] will always come and tell me first.

29.6   Economic Effects of Obstetric Fistula

A condition such as OF impacts both the woman and the family unit and can have devastating and long-lasting effects. Women in this study recalled that working while having a fistula was challenging if not impossible. A woman stated:

> when you are leaking urine, and you are smelling you are not trading. You are not working, there is nothing that you will sell, and they will buy. So already you are in a cash trap.

Another woman stated:

> I couldn't go to the farm [be]cause it was hard to get water and soap to regularly clean myself. You can't be staying wet like that; the urine burns the skin and the smell, so I had to be sitting at home while my husband was doing the work in the farm.

Accounts such as these illustrate the economic burden OF can have in a society where financial security is dependent on the productivity of all family members. Family members frequently had to take on an additional workload or forgo the income of the family member who was unable to work because of the stigma or ill health of OF. A husband stated:

> When [his wife] came home ... it was still big money problems [be]cause she was unable to work for some time. I [husband] had to leave the farm when she was sick and the weeds destroyed almost everything… My small boy would come assist me in the farm…I [husband] had to go to the bush, cut firewood and burn charcoal to sell to make some small money to buy foodstuff.

Many women in this study also described the financial cost of seeking treatment. Women sought treatment from traditional and spiritual healers. Traditional Ghanaian medicine includes herbal remedies for specific diseases such as OF, as well as folk knowledge, traditions, and health practices, costing the family money or valuable assets such as livestock (Tabi et al., 2006). One woman stated:

> I paid the juju man[4] 100 Ghana [cedis], and he demanded one goat, one sheep and one fowl to sacrifice for pacification to the gods…if you are sick whatever it takes you have to do it… but nothing was helping me.

While OF surgery is publicly funded in Ghana through the National Health Insurance Scheme (NHIS), women reported selling everything to pay for hidden costs, such as transportation, accommodation, and medical supplies associated with seeking conventional health care. A woman recalls:

> I sold all my belongings. My husband even sold the roofing sheets so we could get fuel to be going up and down [to the city] visiting doctors.

Another woman commented:

> when it was time to go home I had no money for lorry fare, if it wasn't for the nurses who paid I would still be waiting there.

After OF repair, women are instructed not to perform strenuous work. This threatens their ability to earn money since in rural Ghana most work requires physical labor. While men work to provide for major cash expenditures (Harley, 2007), women's work provides for the family's basic needs. A woman's livelihood has implications not only for herself but also for the livelihood of her family as is highlighted in Zelda's story. In Ghana, the economic role of women is important since it is positively associated with well-being by way of more spending allocated to food in the home (Women's Economic Empowerment, 2013). A woman noted:

---

[4]In West Africa, the juju man is a practitioner of juju (from the French, joujou, or plaything). JuJu is a traditional spiritual belief system that incorporates religious spells and objects, such as amulets, as part of witchcraft. They also have a knowledge of the medicinal use of local plants and herbs.

I need capital [economic] to buy food stuff and to provide for my children. That was my biggest worry coming home, finding capital to care for my children and my family

Being able to work and provide for one's family is also a source of pride and intrinsic self-worth, as can be observed when women greet each other on the farm or in the market "*adwuma, adwuma*" meaning "work, work". A woman noted:

It is not easy for me to be sitting down, not to be going to the farm. Women can't be sitting like that, they will call you lazy and if you need something you can't buy it. You can't expect your husband to buy for you.

Recognizing the importance that economics plays in the lives of women after OF repair, the United Nations Population Fund (UNFPA) Ghana and the Ministry of Gender, Children, and Social Protection assist in providing skills training to northern women who have experienced an OF repair. One government stakeholder commented:

The training is aimed toward economic empowerment to support women with fistula... To build their self-esteem and also their advocacy skills so that they can go back to their communities and be doing something. Economically they have not been engaged for some time so what we are doing is giving them something to make a small business.

Skills training was offered in soap or pomade making, confectionary, or batik tie-dying. Figure 29.8 displays a woman's baking supplies she received after participating in skills training activities. More than one-half of the women in this study found the program to be beneficial, while those remaining women found it to be unfavorable to their economic plight. As one woman stated:

It is good and not good. They taught me to make soap. It gives me something to be doing and I get soap to wash my things but the chemicals to make the soap are too expensive. I have to get the chemicals from Tamale, it is too expensive and you have to sell it, gather the money and then buy the chemicals. Sometimes I even have to sell some of my own property to add to go buy so it is not profitable.

Fig. 29.8 A woman's baking supplies, which were received after partaking in UNFPA training. (Published with permission from © Kimberly Jarvis. All Rights Reserved)

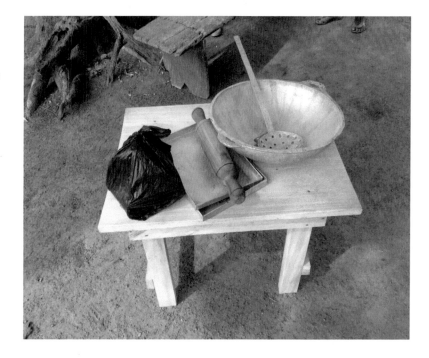

Other women voiced similar concerns. Although they believed skills training was a good idea, they noted that the type of skills taught had to complement the economic climate and their physical ability to carry out their work. One woman stated:

> they trained me to make batik but here in my village, they don't buy. So I took the little capital I had to buy slippers, to be selling in the villages over there

Similarly, another woman like Zelda indicated that she was trained to make dough loaves, but she was physically unable to walk long distances to market and sell the loaves. This was because of foot drop, an abnormal gait caused by nerve damage, and paralysis of muscles in the lower leg; often a side effect of fistula. She notes:

> I made these dough loaves [pointing to them] to sell but I can't walk these long distances selling with my leg dragging like that. I had this small girl [daughter] helping me but she is not selling well and you can't keep the dough loafs two or three days, they will not buy.

The types of work supported by the skills training was also deemed by some women to be foreign to the social nature of work that they were used to and preferred. Many of the women in this study were farmers. A woman stated:

> I stopped doing the trade I was taught as they [community] were not buying. Now I go to the farm and work small. I sit with the others [other women] picking groundnut... I like this better [farming] than soap making; it is more profitable for me. We all go to the farm, even the children and if there is something I can't be doing someone will help me...its better than sitting home.

This woman noted that she tells women at the farm and in her community about her experience with OF and how they should not delay seeking medical assistance once they are in active labor:

> I tell them. I go around this community and when I see they are pregnant, I tell them not to delay. Even at the farm when we are sitting, I tell them don't delay that they don't want to be suffering like that...to go to the health clinic when they are in labour [be]cause having this condition really hurts you. It affects your capital, relationships, health, and mind.

Similar to our story about Mary, this woman took on the role of an active OF advocate. She educates women about OF, that there is a place to receive care and treatment as well as the importance of prenatal care and not delaying in seeking maternal/obstetrical care when in labor.

The health of women is a necessary precondition to a woman's economic strength. A woman who has OF is often unable to effectively obtain productive resources or take advantage of any opportunities from economic activities occurring around her. Equally important is the impact of economic empowerment on a woman's health after OF repair. Increases in a woman's income allow her to make more of an investment in her and her family's health and well-being, and government stakeholders can be encouraged to consider this a priority need for women reintegrating post-OF repair.

29.7 Psychosocial Consequences

After OF repair, women return to an environment where there are strong cultural values and beliefs about being a mother, a wife, and a productive member of society, as well as deeply ingrained beliefs about illnesses and their causes. Similar to Anna, another woman with fistula questioned the cause of the sickness, even suspecting another human being had the power to curse her—creating havoc and turmoil in her life. She stated:

> I believed the sickness was bewitched on me by my husband's brother since we had been arguing with him before the delivery. It was not until after I went to the hospital that the nurses told me it was because I delayed in the house.

Additionally, many women and families believe that OF cannot be cured, especially when they had sought traditional treatments which were ineffective. As a result, after an OF repair, many women are stigmatized because of their community's perception of the condition. One woman stated that she became:

...less than human,... not to be counted among women, it is traumatizing. When you have this condition [OF], they [the community] see you as dead

In contrast to, Anna, Zelda, and Mary whose husbands supportive, some women reported that their husbands had divorced them and they did not have a home to return to, necessitating that they move back with their natal family. For many Ghanaian tribes, particularly the Dagaaba,[5] to be unmarried or divorced is a stain on the clan or family's name (Abdul-Korah, 2014). One woman reported that she was forced to move to another community when her husband would not accept her nor did her natal family or her community accept her. She stated, *"my friend had to rent me this room to isolate myself from the shame I brought to my family and community"*. The majority of women like Anna, Zelda, and Mary in this study, however, stated they were welcomed back into their families and communities:

They accepted me very nicely. When I came, it was in the night. The next morning when I woke they could not believe it was me...I had become fat. People from the community passed through [the house] all day to greet me. They danced and sang with joy.

Another woman recalled:

it was all joy when I came home. They even organized some drumming and dancing in my house. Everybody including my husband and children and the whole family was full of happiness

The feelings of acceptance that comes from being acknowledged as someone who is worthwhile after experiencing OF is extremely important for these women. Being accepted in a communal society where individuals depend on and support each other is important for survival and well-being. Women who return home after OF repair do everything they can to reconnect with family and community. One participant talked about how community members visited when she was washing clothes:

They come to see if I am washing rags, the rags I used when I had the sickness. When they see it is only my panties I am washing they go away...now I hang my panties out for them to see.

Another described proving herself to the community after her OF repair:

I had to strip my clothes and expose my body to show them [the community] I was not leaking

A common problem after fistula repair, however, is that women may be left with some degree of urinary incontinence, making acceptance into the community more challenging. One woman comments:

they see the urine is still coming when I sit and then stand up. They tell me I have wasted my husband's money looking for a cure...the sickness is a curse that can't be cured

Additionally, a healthcare provider noted:

women who continue to suffer from incontinence after surgery have a difficult time being accepted. Ghanaian women are supposed to be gentle, clean, and smelling nice...when her colleagues [peers] smell her stench they will still stigmatize her

Women who reported experiencing mild urinary incontinence following OF repair hid that fact from others. One woman stated:

---

[5]The Dagaaba ethnic group are a people residing at the convergence of the countries of Ghana, Burkina Faso, and Côte d'Ivoire. They speak a Gur language, termed Dagaare.

when I get out of bed it is a little wet...the doctor told me it is okay and I should do my pelvic exercises. I am worried my colleagues [peers] will see I am still leaking small small

This woman continued sharing why she feared others knowing. She stated:

...if others know they will say I am not cured and I will not be welcomed to community programs. They will not say directly to me but they whisper and they will leave me when I sit. ...it is important for women to be doing in the community like preparing food for outdoorings [baptism/ naming ceremony] and wedding if not they will be saying you are lazy and you cannot [be] cooking if you are leaking urine ...even church they will not let you go, Muslims and urine, doesn't go, it is seen as dirty.

Women also noted challenges connected with marital intimacy during the illness:

we lived like brother and sister when the urine was flowing. I was not allowed to cook and you know the wife who cooks is the one who he [the husband] meets in the night

This participant continued that her husband told her:

it was worrying to him. It wasn't an easy thing to have his wife with this kind of condition. Even now, he is worried, because he wants to have children but he is worried about the sickness coming back

A woman's ability to have children was not only important for social status (Gyekye, 2003) but also for economic reasons in a country where social programs and old age security are limited. Furthermore, since some Ghanaian men pay a bride wealth (also termed bride price)—money, property or goods given to the family of a bride by the bridegroom—it is expected that his wife will bear him many children. One woman described her need to become pregnant soon after having her fistula repair as well as her desire to have a male child:

I hope to have a boy soon but the doctor says no sex for six months. I ask God why he has only given me girls because, in our tribe, it's boys who are valued because when you grow old it is the boy who will stay, take up the farming activity and provide for you but girls will marry and go... my husband's family is telling him I must have a boy child.

Overall, women in this study suggested that being culturally accepted back into their community after OF repair was central to reintegration. However, acceptance came only when women could *"be counted among women"*. This points to an increased need for OF awareness within northern Ghanaian communities as Mary articulated in her story.

29.8   Political and Emancipatory Issues

Many women in this study acknowledged feeling powerless during various stages of OF and OF care. One woman stated she had suicidal ideations at her lowest point while experiencing OF. However, the desire to protect her reputation in the community combined with the fear of leaving her child without a mother gave her the strength to live and find a cure. She stated:

I use to think of committing suicide, but then I thought they [the community] will know I have the sickness. They will say I have gone somewhere to develop that condition. You know blacks they will say I have gone to sleep with a different man or something. Who would care for my little boy? I needed to live, to find a cure to this sickness. It has not been easy but I am better now and look at my happy boy, he has his mother.

Women like Mary in this study verbalized a call to action to advocate for themselves and for others. While Mary was well-informed about OF care, many other women spoke about persevering with little education to find their way through a health system. Women demonstrated remarkable resilience in how to seek for care. A woman stated:

You know, you become powerless to the system when you don't have knowledge. But you see, and then you don't have words to say it. I found somebody to direct me... show me that there is a place where they help people like me. But if I had a daughter like you, counseling me, who is educated, she'll be able to tell me this is how you do this, this is the information, and this is where you go.

Women were able to access the resources they needed to seek treatment for their condition despite many not having the ability to read and write. Through this process, they learned to be advocates for other women experiencing OF in their communities and provided emotional support for others who had returned home after OF repair. A community stakeholder and women's leader noted:

I am the magajia [plays a traditional role, as a woman leader, in northern communities] of this community. I am chief of the women and I organize them [women] on their issues. I get the information that they need... Knowing women with the sickness [OF] in this community...whenever there is a program [meeting] we try to talk about it [OF] to educate women on it. Smaller groupings like outdooring [baptism/naming ceremony] we [women] also try to reach out and chat among ourselves as women so that we will know about it... We tell women it is not a curse but problems with labor.

Similarly, a community health nurse [CHN][6] in a rural Ghanaian community initiated an OF awareness campaign to educate the community, including men and school children, about OF. She also stated that in the community, a play about OF was performed by school children as part of the awareness campaign:

Education is the key... When you educate the children, girls, and boys, about seeing the dangers they will tell their mothers who are still of childbearing age. They will want to find out, Mama have you gone to the clinic, let me see your card... young boys learn not to refuse their wives from going to the hospital for whatever reason.

Women in this community who had returned home after their OF repair verbalized that the creation of awareness and the support from this nurse had assisted them to be accepted in the community and had encouraged them to push forward as valued human beings striving to reach their full potential. A woman stated:

If it was not for Mama [CHN] I would be nothing. She helped me to be someone, to believe in myself when I came home [post-OF]. She let me work in the health clinic doing small things. Now I am learning to read and to type.

Many women also expressed feelings of obligation to have their plight heard, and in the process received a sense of authority and power over their situation.

The white people come, wanting to know how it was [having OF] and so I tell them. I am responsible to tell them [be]cause they know the book [educated] and they know how to write about fistula for others to know.

Anna, Zelda, and Mary's participation in telling their stories about living with OF, seeking OF care, and returning home to their families and communities post-OF provides a voice for other women as well as demonstrates great strength and resilience—advocating for improved OF awareness and care.

29.9 Discussion

The majority of women in this study noted they were welcomed home post-OF repair. However, they did indicate that possessing economic capital and having social acceptance were essential to successful reintegration. These two factors are intertwined and historically and culturally rooted.

The "north-south divide" in Ghana places the northern people at an economic disadvantage, the result of unequal and uneven development inherited from British colonialism (Akologo & van

---

[6]CHNs were introduced in Ghana to deliver health care in deprived rural areas. CHNs in Ghana are professionally trained in a two-year certificate or three-year nursing diploma and are responsible for such activities as health promotion, community mobilization, advocacy, and disease prevention. They typically work in health clinics and *Community-Based* Health Planning and Services [CHPS].

Klinken, 2008). This underdevelopment and lack of adequate resources have increased the risk of maternal morbidities partially because of inadequate access to healthcare services in remote rural areas of the north. Cultural practices in northern Ghana regarding a woman's lack of autonomy over her maternal/reproductive health, the lack of skilled birth attendants, and the knowledge and preparation of those responsible for maternal healthcare delivery also contribute to the occurrence of OF.

An individual's prior experiences can greatly affect their perception of future events. Much of our knowledge about the external world is based on inferences that arise from our assumptions about the past. For example, in this study, a woman's account about her illness-treatment trajectory while experiencing OF and the financial difficulties incurred potentially shape her views about returning home after her repair. It is important to first understand and then acknowledge these assumptions, assess their impact, and challenge current practices to move toward a way of reintegrating, which includes emancipatory knowledge. Habermas noted that emancipatory knowledge *"involves interest in the way one's history and biography has expressed itself in the way one sees oneself, one's roles and social expectations"* (Haneef et al., 2014, p. 504). Engaging women in reflecting on their underlying needs and challenges following OF repair leads to deeper understanding of a culture of reintegration in northern Ghana and can help to bring about improved public policy in women's maternal and reproductive health.

Economic capital is a concern for women returning home since the ability to earn money ensures the basic livelihood and safety of the family (Opoku-Ware, 2014). Many of these women invested their life savings in seeking a cure thus placing them in a position of impoverishment upon their return home after their repair. Training programs offer women skills in soap making, confectionery, or batik tie-dye. Many women in this study found these skills to be inappropriate in remote Ghanaian communities where a limited market for such products exists. Women value the opportunity to take part in skills training programs but need to be involved in deciding the types of skills required for practical employment postrepair. Employment also offers women a sense of self-worth and dignity and defines the quality of the community. For example, suitable skills training assists women postrepair to move into progressively higher paying and more satisfying work with suitable remuneration, and gender equality (Somavia, 2014).

Many women in this study recounted how their social experiences were associated with the stigma of having OF. OF can bring great humiliation (Semere & Nour, 2008) and can have a lasting social impact for women even after having an OF repair. Ghanaian cultural values, beliefs, and practices affected the reintegration process, in particular regarding how many of the communities viewed OF not as a medical condition but as a curse or a punishment for some wrongdoing (Nuertey, 2013). Acceptance into the community and family life as a wife and as a mother holds great cultural status (Gyekye, 2003), and the women in this study recognized that it is the responsibility of a woman returning home postrepair to verify that she is "cured" and worthy of acceptance back into the community. However, women who continued to have urinary incontinence after their OF repair reported a more challenging reintegration experience as their condition reaffirmed the community and family's belief that OF is untreatable.

Many of those who experienced OF, together with women leaders, have initiated awareness campaigns about OF in their communities with the aim of improving the reintegration experiences of others who have had OF repair. Serving as fistula advocates, these women promote improved maternal, reproductive, and fistula care within their communities. However, these grassroots movements are only the beginning. Political influence at the national level is necessary to initiate and sustain change. This can only be acquired by embracing the *"wider range of historical and contextual considerations…emphasizes the fundamental intent to seek freedom from conditions largely hidden that restricts the realization of full human potential"* (Chinn & Kramer, 2011, pp. 87–88). Developing awareness of these factors is an important step forward in creating social and political change in OF care and reintegration.

29.10 Lessons for Clinical Practice

In exploring the needs and challenges of women reintegrating following OF repair, several recommendations for OF clinical practice are indicated. Health education about OF as a medical condition, its causes, and treatment/care options must be available to all women. This education must also be extended to families and communities because of the role women play in Ghanaian society. Creating community awareness about the reintegration process and the limitations placed on women post-OF repair will aid to reduce the economic and psychosocial stigma of the condition and to improve a woman's self-esteem and acceptance back into her family and community.

More educated nurses and nurse-midwives are needed in the north to provide maternal and reproductive care to help reduce the incidence of OF. Health professionals need an acceptable level of knowledge and skill to practice and care for women with OF and their families. In order to accomplish this, healthcare providers must be supported to partake in continuing education courses and be mentored by leaders in the field of maternal and reproductive health.

Additionally, there is a need for collaborative partnerships. OF care does not happen in isolation. It requires a collaborative effort on the part of all stakeholders such as women, families, communities, government, nongovernmental, health professionals, academics/researchers, and OF advocates to hear and address the clinical needs of women who require OF care. Only through collaborative teams can innovative ideas for improvement in OF care flourish.

29.11 Limitations to Research

Being an outsider to Ghanaian cultures and to the country provided a unique perspective, but it also created challenges regarding language comprehension, cultural interpretation, and access to participants. This research employed several community partnerships to assist with overcoming the anticipated cross-cultural challenges. Training was provided to translators and transcriptionists. Additionally, this study provides an overview of the post-OF needs and challenges of women in northern Ghana and not specific northern communities. Conducting further in-depth research into remote northern Ghanaian communities (municipalities/districts) could provide greater insight into a woman's needs after an OF repair.

29.12 Conclusion

Northern Ghana was overlooked during colonial times when government structures such as hospitals, schools, and roads were being built in the south, creating what has come to be known as the north-south economic divide. These effects are still experienced today, with the north being grossly underdeveloped in comparison to many areas in its southern counterpart. This contributes to a high rate of OF in the north in comparison to other regions of the country. The needs and challenges experienced by women who are reintegrating into their families and communities after OF repair are important. This knowledge can be developed to inform public policy about the reintegration process and to make recommendations where national priorities could focus. Many women's needs and challenges following OF repair are historically and culturally rooted. Economic and psychosocial factors contribute to determining how successful women reintegrate after their repair. Securing capital is a huge concern for women who return home since most have spent their life savings seeking a cure. Skill-training activities have helped to offset the financial hardship for some but not all women postrepair. A closer look at the types and suitability of trades for women is necessary to strengthen a woman's economic capability.

Acceptance is a fundamental human need that brings about a sense of belonging or "being home". For many women, the need to prove themselves worthy postrepair to be accepted back into their communities is humiliating and demonstrates the need for more community awareness of the causes and treatment of OF. Many women, family members, and those working with women post-OF repair acknowledge the importance of being able to fully participate in day-to-day life without fear of rejection. Despite the challenges faced by women following their OF repair, they demonstrated great resilience to seek out OF services and to educate themselves in order to reach their full potential. Additionally, many women post-OF experienced a sense of obligation to have their plight heard, which in the process gave them a sense of control over their situation.

References

Abdul-Korah, G. B. (2014). If it's your money, I will pay and go: Shifting and contested significance of brideprice payment among the Dagaaba of Northwest Ghana. *Journal of Asian and Africa Studies, 49*(3), 332–346. https://doi.org/10.1177/0021909613486088

Akologo, S. Z., & van Klinken, R. (2008). *Ghana: Why the north matters.* Retrieved February 15, 2019, from www.pambazuka.org/governance/ghana-why-the-north-matters

Chinn, P. L., & Kramer, M. K. (2011). *Integrated theory and knowledge development in nursing* (8th ed.). Mosby.

Cooke, E., Hague, S., & McKay, A. (2016). *The Ghana poverty and inequality report: Using the 6th Ghana living standards survey.* Retrieved February 15, 2019, from www.unicef.org/ghana/Ghana_Poverty_and_Inequality_Analysis_FINAL_Match_2016(1).pdf

Danso, K. A., Opare-Addo, H. S., & Turpin, C. A. (2007). Obstetric fistula admissions at Komfo Anokye Teaching Hospital, Kumasi, Ghana. *International Journal of Gynecology & Obstetrics, 1*, S69–S70. https://doi.org/10.1016/j.ijgo.2007.06.029

Edgar, A. (2006). *Habermas: The key concepts.* Taylor & Francis Group.

Galyan, D. (1999). Speaking the "unspeakable". *Research & Creative Activity, 11*(3). Retrieved April 3, 2016, from www.indiana.edu/~rcapub/v21n3/p10.html

Ghana Health Service. (2015). *Report on the assessment of obstetric fistula in Ghana.* Retrieved February 15, 2019, from: http://unfpaghana.org/assets/user/file/Report%20on%20Fistula%20Report%20Burden%20in%20Ghana_Final_1_1_compressed.pdf

Gyekye, K. (2003). *African cultural values: An introduction.* Sankofa Publishing.

Habermas, J. (1991a). *The theory of communicative action, volume two: Lifeworld and systems: The critique of functionalist reason,* T. McCarthy, Trans. Beacon Press.

Habermas, J. (1991b). *The theory of communicative action, volume one: Reason and the rationalization of society,* T. McCarthy, Trans. Beacon Press.

Hammersley, M., & Atkinson, P. (2007). The process of analysis. In M. Hammersley & P. Atkinson (Eds.), *Ethnography: Principles in practice* (3rd ed., pp. 158–190). Routledge.

Haneef, M., Zulfiqar, M., Alvi, A. K., & Faisal, A. (2014). Jurgon Habermas: A critical prologue. *Science International (Lahore), 26*(1), 503–506.

Harley, S. (2007). *Women's labor in the global economy: Speaking in multiple voices.* Rutgers University Press.

Index of Economic Freedom. (2015). *Ghana.* Retrieved February 15, 2019, from www.heritage.org/index/country/Ghana

Institute for Fiscal Studies. (2015, August). *Ghana: Impact of the falling crude oil prices.* Retrieved January 22, 2019, from http://www.ifsghana.org/wp-content/uploads/2015/12/Fiscal-Alert-No.-2-Ghana-Impact-of-the-Falling-Crude-Oil-Prices-Sept-2015.pdf

Jansen, I. (2006). Decision making in childbirth: The influence of tradition structures in a Ghanaian village. *International Nursing Review, 53*(1), 41–46. https://doi.org/10.1111/j.1466-7657.2006.00448.x

Kalembo, F., & Zgambo, M. (2012). Obstetric fistula: A hidden public health problem in sub-Saharan Africa. *Arts and Social Sciences Journal.* Retrieved January 22, 2019, from www.astonjournals.com/manuscripts/Vol2012/ASSJ-41_Vol2012.pdf

Lewis, G., & de Bernis, L. (2006). Obstetric fistula: Guiding principles for clinical management and programme development. World Health Organization: . Retrieved from www.who.int/reproductivehealth/publications/maternal_perinatal_health/9241593679/en/

Mill, J., Allen, N., & Morrow, R. A. (2001). Critical theory: Critical methodology to disciplinary foundations in nursing. *Canadian Journal of Nursing Research, 33*(2), 109–127. Retrieved January 31, 2019, from http://cjnr.archive.mcgill.ca/article/view/1638/1638

Mselle, L. T., Moland, K. M., Evjen-Olsen, B., Mvungi, A., & Kohi, T. W. (2011). "I am nothing": Experience of loss among women suffering from severe birth injuries in Tanzania. *BMC Women's Health, 11*, 49. https://doi. org/10.1186/1472-6874-11-49. Retrieved February, 1 2019, from https://bmcwomenshealth.biomedcentral.com/ articles/10.1186/1472-6874-11-49

Nakua, E. K., Sevugu, J. S., Dzomeku, V. M., Otuoiri, E., Lipkovich, H. R., & Owusu-Dabo, E. (2015). Home birth without skilled attendants despite millennium villages project intervention in Ghana: Insight from a survey of women's perceptions of skilled obstetric care. *BMC Pregnancy and Childbirth, 15*(243). https://doi.org/10.1186/s12884-015-0674-1. Retrieved February 2, 2019, from https://www.ncbi.nlm.nih.gov/pmc/articles/PMC4597447/

Nuertey, B. D. (2013). *Risk factors for obstetric fistula among women seeking care in the Tamale Metropolis*. University of Ghana.

Opoku-Ware, J. (2014). Women's productive and economic roles towards household poverty reduction in Ghana. A survey of Bongo District in Northern Ghana. *Research on Humanities and Social Sciences, 4*(19), 148–155. Retrieved February 2, 2019, from https://www.google.com/url?sa=t&rct=j&q=&esrc=s&source=web&cd=2&cad= rja&uact=8&ved=2ahUKEwiFw46uqJ7gAhUJmuAKHSxHBYoQFjABegQICBAC&url=https%3A%2F%2Fiiste. org%2FJournals%2Findex.php%2FRHSS%2Farticle%2Fdownload%2F15775%2F16569&usg=AOvVaw0cPZ4lB 2QuBeh-qf4gGxMH

Oteng-Ababio, M., Mariwah, S., & Kusi, L. (2017). Is the underdevelopment of northern Ghana a case of environmental determinism or governance crisis? *Ghana Journal of Geography, 9*(2 Special Issue), 5–39.

Pacagnella, R. C., Cecatti, J. G., Camargo, R. P., Silveira, C., Zanardi, D. T., Souza, J. P., et al. (2010). Rationale for a long-term evaluation of the consequences of potentially life-threatening maternal conditions and maternal "near-miss" incidents using a multidimensional approach. *Journal of Obstetrics and Gynaecology Canada, 32*(8), 730–738. Retrieved February 2, 2019, from https://www.jogc.com/article/S1701-2163(16)34612-6/pdf

Porter, G., Hampshire, K., Dunn, C., Hall, R., Levesley, M., Burton, K., et al. (2013). Health impacts of pedestrian head-loading: A review of the evidence with particular reference to women and children in sub-Saharan Africa. *Social Science & Medicine, 88*, 90–97. https://doi.org/10.1016/j.socscimed.2013.04.010

Semere, L., & Nour, N. (2008). Obstetric fistula: Living with incontinence and shame. *Review of Obstetrics & Gynecology, 1*(4), 193–197. Retrieved February 3, 2019, from http://medreviews.com/journal/reviews-in-obstetrics-gynecology/ vol/1/no/4/obstetric-fistula-living-incontinence-and-shame

Singh, R. P. (1999). Critical theory of Jurgen Habermas: critique of enlightenment rationality. *Indian Philosophical Quarterly, 26*(3), 381–394.

Somavia, J. (2014). Valuing the dignity of work. *2014 Human development report*. Retrieved September 2, 2016, from: www.hdr.undp.org/en/content/valuing-dignity-work-0

Tabi, M. M., Powell, M., & Hodnicki, D. (2006). Use of traditional healers and modern medicine in Ghana. *International Nursing Review, 53*(1), 52–58. Retrieved February 3, 2019, from: http://www.urbanlab.org/articles/Ghana_%20 Use%20of%20Traditional%20healers.pdf

The World Factbook 2021. (2021). *Washington, DC: Central Intelligence Agency, 2021*. Retrieved September 24, 2021, from https://www.cia.gov/the-world-factbook/

Tsikata, D., & Seini, W. (2004). *Identities, inequalities and conflicts in Ghana*. University of Oxford: Center for Research on Inequality, Human Security and Ethnicity. Retrieved February 15, 2019, from: https://www.research-gate.net/publication/228917698_Identities_Inequalities_and_Conflicts_in_Ghana/download

United Nations Development Programme. (2015). *Human development indicators*. Retrieved February 26, 2019, from www.hdr.undp.org/en/countries/profiles/GHA

United Nations Population Fund [UNFPA]. (n.d.), *What is fistula*. Retrieved February 14, 2019, from http://www. endfistula.org/what-fistula

Women's Economic Empowerment. (2013). *Women's economic empowerment: A CESO perspective*. Canadian International Development Agency: Canada. Retrieved February 15, 2019, from www.ceso-saco.com/app/ uploads/2016/03/Women-s_Economic_Empowerment_FINAL-ENGLISH_online-version.pdf

World Health Organization. (2018). *10 facts on obstetric fistula*. Retrieved January 22, 2019, from https://www.who. int/features/factfiles/obstetric_fistula/en/

World Health Organization. (2019). *Social determinants of health*. Retrieved February 15, 2019, from www.who.int/ topics/social_determinants/en/

Making the Case for Holistic Fistula Care: Implementation of a Model Reintegration Program in Uganda

30

Bonnie Ruder and Alice Emasu

30.1 Introduction

Obstetric fistula is a debilitating childbirth injury with severe physical, social, and psychological consequences. Women with fistula experience continuous leakage of urine and/or feces, along with co-morbidities which may include secondary infections, neurological damage, genital ulcerations, and secondary infertility (Arrowsmith et al., 1996). The psychosocial consequences are also extreme, as the odor from the continuous incontinence commonly leads to discrimination, social shaming, stigma, and ostracization from family, friends, and community members. As a result, women with fistula report high rates of depression and a range of negative emotions, including feeling humiliated, lonely, sad, and angry (Barageine et al., 2015; Mselle et al., 2011; Pope et al., 2011; Weston et al., 2011). Many women turn to self-isolation as a means to cope with feelings of shame and the stigma they experience in their communities (El Ayadi et al., 2017; Hamed et al., 2017). Marital discord, divorce, and abandonment are common, though not universal, experiences for women with fistula (Ahmed & Holtz, 2007; Barageine et al., 2015; Mwini-Nyaledzigbor et al., 2013).

Most obstetric fistulas can be repaired with reconstructive surgery. And while significant barriers to treatment remain, including a shortage of qualified surgeons and health facilities, insufficient funding, and the lack of awareness of the availability of treatment, access to treatment has improved in recent years (Bellows et al., 2015). After surgery, many women report increased quality of life, decreased rates of depression, and relief from the constant worry and stress they experienced while living with fistula (Browning et al., 2007; Drew et al., 2016). Many women also report reconciliation with their husbands and family members, and overall improvement in interpersonal relationships and social life (Yeakey et al., 2009). However, several studies report that some women continue to experience psychosocial distress, depression, and anxiety even after successful treatment (Khisa & Nyamongo, 2012; Muleta et al., 2008). Acceptance back into their community post-treatment is not

B. Ruder (✉)
Terrewode Women's Fund, Eugene, OR, USA

International Fistula Alliance, Sydney, Australia

A. Emasu
TERREWODE and Terrewode Women's Community Hospital, Soroti, Uganda

© Springer Nature Switzerland AG 2022
L. B. Drew et al. (eds.), *A Multidisciplinary Approach to Obstetric Fistula in Africa*, Global Maternal and Child Health, https://doi.org/10.1007/978-3-031-06314-5_30

immediate or universal, and many women experience on going stigma and discrimination. Women experience varying levels of isolation due to this and to the fact that some were uninterested in reconciliation with their husbands or remarriage after their traumatic experience of living with fistula (Khisa et al., 2016). Others report anxiety and confusion regarding infertility and their fears of fistula recurrence (Donnelly et al., 2015; Pope et al., 2011).

Even following successful surgery to close a fistula, as many as 16–55% of women may experience persistent residual incontinence post-repair in the form of stress incontinence, urge incontinence, and increased urinary urgency and frequency (Murray et al., 2002; Wall et al., 2004). A minority of obstetric fistula survivors will have such extensive tissue damage that the fistulas are irreparable or require complicated urinary diversions that transplant the ureters into the colon (Wall et al., 2008). Continued mental health concerns and reintegration challenges are especially pronounced for these women (Nielsen et al., 2009; Wilson et al., 2016).

Financially, women with fistula experience increased poverty and hardship. Many women deplete their savings or borrow money from relatives to cover increased costs in health and hygiene needs and to access treatment. Additionally, women report high rates of workplace discrimination and are rarely employable outside of the home, and thus are often pushed deeper into poverty as a result of their injury (Bangser, 2007; El Ayadi et al., 2019). Even after successful repair, women may continue to experience stigma and workforce discrimination, especially in communities that do not understand the cause of fistula. This economic precarity contributes to poor mental health due to the additional stress in meeting one's needs and decreased ability to care for others, especially children. In Burkina Faso, even one year after surgery many women had not regained their former financial status (Desalliers et al., 2017). In Uganda, the economic impact of fistula was devastating to young women, who reported high rates of unemployment and economic abuse (Emasu et al., 2019).

Taken together, these findings reveal the complex and multifaceted toll fistula has on women. All aspects of their lives are profoundly impacted, and this impact is greater the longer women live with fistula. Despite these findings, most fistula treatment programs remain focused on surgical repair, as the majority of funders often prefer to fund treatment, but not holistic or comprehensive services. However, a recent review by El Ayadi et al. (2020) found a growing number of treatment programs that provide various intervention components, including health education combined with physical therapy (Castille et al., 2014; Keyser et al., 2014), psychosocial counseling (Johnson et al., 2010; Ojengbede et al., 2014; Watt et al., 2015), and economic training (Jarvis et al., 2017). While this is an encouraging development, fistula programs that provide holistic multicomponent reintegration programs continue to be rare (El Ayadi et al., 2020).

The Association for the Rehabilitation and Re-orientation of Women for Development (TERREWODE), a Ugandan nongovernmental organization established in 1999 and dedicated to eradicating obstetric fistula, found this to be the case in their early work helping women access fistula treatment in Uganda. In response, they developed a holistic reintegration program which they continue to refine through an on going iterative process designed to meet the needs of fistula survivors with whom they work. This chapter draws on years of ethnographic fieldwork, program implementation and delivery experience, and narratives collected from TERREWODE's Reintegration Program participants. Our purpose is to share TERREWODE's experience of creating a holistic reintegration program in Uganda and the key components that we have found most impactful for women recovering from fistula.

30.1.1 Obstetric Fistula Treatment in Uganda

Obstetric fistulas are both preventable and treatable. They are virtually unknown in high-resource nations and occur almost exclusively in low-resource countries with poor investment in reproductive health care and restricted access to quality emergency obstetric care. Uganda, with its chronically underfunded healthcare system, has both a tragically high maternal mortality rate, 336 maternal deaths per 100,000 live births, and one of the highest fistula prevalence rates in the world—an estimated 114,000 women suffer from fistula (UBOS, 2018), though exact prevalence is difficult to measure (Chap. 1, this volume).

In Uganda, routine fistula treatment at public hospitals has long been a stated goal, yet financial, workforce, and infrastructure constraints have delayed progress. Instead, fistula treatment is fragmented and typically occurs sporadically during temporary surgical "camps" staged at public and missionary hospitals throughout the country. Fistula camps are designed to treat large numbers of women in a short-time period, yet the camps are often overcrowded, provide poor follow-up care, and create multiple treatment barriers for women. Patient education on the cause of fistula and post-surgical care recommendations are often provided during camps and at public hospitals in Uganda; however, comprehensive reintegration programming is not included. This is true despite the World Health Organization (WHO) and Uganda Ministry of Health's guidelines for fistula care, both of which include recommendations for social reintegration and rehabilitation (Ministry of Health 2010/2011–2015/2016; WHO, 2006).

30.2 TERREWODE's Reintegration Program

30.2.1 Development of a Holistic Reintegration Program

On August 16, 2019, TERREWODE opened the Terrewode Women's Community Hospital (TWCH). Located in Soroti, a rural eastern town seven hours from the capital, TWCH is the first specialized fistula hospital in the country. A key component of the hospital is the 30-bed Reintegration Center, which sits at the northeast corner of the hospital grounds, slightly elevated and overlooking the other buildings. This location is fitting, for TERREWODE's Reintegration Program has long been their centerpiece of care for fistula patients. While the reintegration needs of women post-fistula repair have been brought to greater attention recently, TERREWODE's Reintegration Program was developed 18 years ago and for years faced a tremendous struggle to secure funding for the program and to have reintegration needs of women recognized as a critical component of care.

TERREWODE was founded in 1999 by second author, Alice Emasu. A journalist at the time, she responded to a contest to increase rural women's participation in community development. Originally Emasu planned to focus on rural women's human rights and development projects in eastern Uganda. However, after realizing that maternal mortality rates in the country had stagnated for 10 years without improvement, with an accompanying high rate of maternal morbidities, she turned her attention and focus of TERREWODE to women suffering from obstetric fistula. Today Emasu uses obstetric fistula as a "wedge issue" to address the broader maternal health tragedy and lack of women's rights and sexual and reproductive health rights in Uganda.

In the early 2000s, obstetric fistula was just beginning to draw attention internationally among development agencies. In Uganda, fistula was still largely unknown, as women with fistula often isolated and attempted to conceal their incontinence. Most women and communities were unaware that obstetric fistulas are treatable and preventable. Women who sought medical attention were often given misinformation or an inaccurate diagnosis, leading to further confusion and distress about their condition (Ruder et al., 2018). At that time, fistula camps were relatively new in Uganda and carried out with the assistance of international fistula surgeons who worked alongside and provided training to Ugandan surgeons.

It was in this context that Emasu focused TERREWODE's efforts on increasing women's access to fistula treatment, along with awareness and advocacy for fistula prevention. TERREWODE's role within Uganda's treatment model at that time was to identify women with fistula in rural communities, mobilize them to attend a fistula camp, and provide patient support during the camp. In order to facilitate treatment, TERREWODE sought funding for patient transportation and upkeep at the hospitals, supplies for the surgery itself, and even top-up funds for the government-employed local surgeons. Emasu and her team, most of whom had backgrounds in social work and counseling, quickly realized the women turning up for the fistula camps were quite traumatized after living with fistula for years. They began educating the women on the cause and prevention of fistula and providing counseling pre- and post-surgery at the partner hospitals. Through these counseling sessions, Emasu and her team discovered that many of the women were suffering with profound mental health issues, including depression and suicidal ideation.

The TERREWODE team also followed up with patients after their surgery, a rarity in obstetric fistula care, for although follow-up care is recommended, it is not prioritized and remains largely unfunded (Ruder & Emasu, 2021). They found that the effects of the trauma of living with fistula do not easily disappear after surgery. They became increasingly aware that many women continued to face challenges reintegrating into their communities after treatment. Even women who were successfully treated (fistula closed and continent) reported strained relationships, ongoing discrimination, isolation, and continued to live in extreme poverty. TERREWODE found that women with supportive partners and families usually cope the best and with time are able to successfully reintegrate back into their community. However, women who experienced withdrawal of support, abandonment, and other forms of abuse, often struggle to reintegrate. This is more pronounced for extremely impoverished women, and women who continue to experience physical co-morbidities from fistula, such as stress incontinence, secondary infertility, sexual dysfunction, or pain. Young women and girls are particularly at-risk for on going reintegration difficulties. In our study on the reintegration needs of young women and girls with fistula, we found almost half of the women reported ongoing health issues, one third desired additional personal or family counseling, and virtually all were struggling economically (Emasu et al., 2019). These experiences mobilized Emasu and the TERREWODE team to design a holistic program to address the multifaceted psychosocial and economic needs of fistula survivors (see Box 30.1).

Box 30.1 TERREWODE's Reintegration Program Goals and Objectives
The main goal of TERREWODE's Reintegration Program is to provide the comprehensive care women need to fully heal from the trauma of fistula and successfully reintegrate into communities post-fistula repair surgery.

Objectives
- Improve mental health outcomes and family reunification/marital satisfaction among women through the provision of psychosocial and family counseling.
- Improve women's long-term health outcomes and prevent fistula recurrence through the provision of education on obstetric fistula, safe motherhood, and family planning.

- Improve the economic well-being of women and their ability to meet their basic needs through the provision of microfinance, entrepreneurship, and income-generating skills training.
- Create on going reintegration support networks for women through the formation of Fistula Solidarity Groups and Music, Drama, and Dance groups.
- Increase women's awareness and understanding of their sexual reproductive health rights.
- Empower women as change agents for increased advocacy efforts toward improved sexual reproductive health and rights at local and national levels.

30.2.2 TERREWODE Reintegration Program Components

TERREWODE defines reintegration as the ability to resume previous responsibilities, roles, and relationships after treatment. A successfully reintegrated woman is accepted back into her community and treated with respect, or, when conditions and attitudes prevent this, she is able to reintegrate into a new community, establish new relationships, and live with dignity and agency.

TERREWODE's holistic residential two-week Reintegration Program consists of five key components, described in detail in Box 30.2. Women are invited to participate in the program based on a needs assessment completed during surgical treatment, which identifies patients who are experiencing psychological distress and lack of family and community support. These vulnerable patients are invited back after treatment to participate in the reintegration program. Women who experience residual incontinence after repair are also identified, as they often have difficulty with reintegration and can benefit from additional rehabilitation support. Women who have retained strong family support and have accessed treatment promptly are less likely to require intensive reintegration support. For these women, the counseling and education they receive during fistula treatment are sufficient support to facilitate successful reintegration.

TERREWODE's Reintegration Program begins with completing a detailed needs assessment intake form, which allows TERREWODE to individualize specific aspects of the program to meet each woman's needs. For example, some women may need marital counseling while other women may need legal aid in order to establish her rights, especially property rights after the breakup of her marriage or widowhood. Intake needs assessments are conducted by one of TERREWODE's trained fistula counselors; as women first tell their fistula story, this is also the beginning of their individual therapy. For many women, this may be the first time they have shared their complete story. Individual and group counseling sessions then continue throughout the two-week program, helping women move from understanding what happened to them and why, to self-acceptance, forgiveness, coping strategies, and positive living. TERREWODE's counseling program was developed by trained social workers who adopted best practices that are aligned with the Uganda Ministry of Health standards used to guide HIV/AIDS counseling. The program was adapted over time, based on program delivery experience and informed by fistula survivors to create the unique TERREWODE counseling program that is in place today.

Each day includes both individual components working one-on-one with a fistula counselor (see Fig. 30.1) and group classes in the various program modalities. For many women, the health and safe motherhood education is the first time they truly understand why they experienced fistula. Critically, they also learn how to prevent fistula in future pregnancies. Women are provided free time to socialize with each other, sharing their stories with other women who understand the difficulties they have

Fig. 30.1 TERRE-
WODE fistula counselor
Mary Adiedo provides
counseling and
education to a patient
prior to surgery at a
public hospital. Photo by
Lynne Dobson

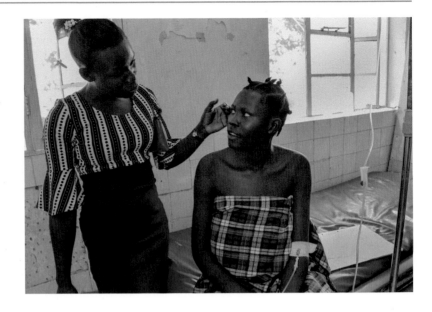

faced. Outside of treatment, for many women this is the first time they have met other women suffering from fistula and feel understood in their experience. Many create life-long bonds and
friendships.

Box 30.2 TERREWODE's Reintegration Program Key Components

1. *Health Education*: Nutrition and health education, including post-surgical care and personal
   hygiene. Safe motherhood education, with a focus on the cause and prevention of obstetric
   fistula. Family planning education and referrals.
2. *Counseling*: Individual and group psychosocial counseling. Family and marital counseling
   as needed. Women suffering from severe depression or suicidal ideation receive additional
   longer-term support.
3. *Economic Empowerment*: Training in community-based savings groups, business management, and skills training in income-generating activities with five different modules based on
   interest and community feasibility. Women are encouraged to join savings groups when they
   return to their communities.
4. *Advocacy, Rights, and Leadership Training*: Women's rights, legal rights, sexual and reproductive health rights, and advocacy training. TERREWODE staff equip women and girls
   with the tools and knowledge needed to enable them to advocate for their rights, to share
   their knowledge with their community, and to serve in leadership roles.
5. *Social Reintegration Support, Solidarity Groups, and Music, Drama, and Dance Groups:*
   Following program completion, TERREWODE staff provide follow-up reintegration support and encourage women to join Solidarity Groups and/or Music, Drama, and Dance
   groups for on going community-based support as well as to contribute to advocacy and fistula awareness efforts.

Fig. 30.2 After completing TERREWODE's Reintegration program, Immaculate perfected her newly acquired skills as a tailor. Today she is employed by TERREWODE as a trainer in the reintegration program. Photo by Lynne Dobson

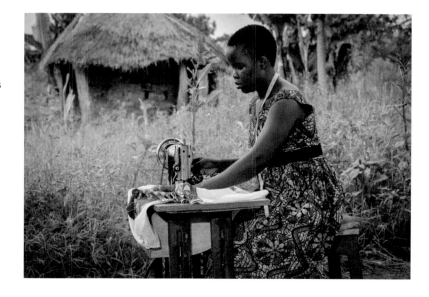

The effects of fistula are economically devastating to both women and their families. Thus, TERREWODE's Reintegration Program views economic empowerment and training as a critical component to helping women successfully reintegrate and attain financial security after treatment. Women receive training in financial literacy and savings groups, and business management. They also receive skills training in income-generating activities with five different modules based on individual interest and community feasibility and need. Accessing community feasibility is an important component to ensure income-generating activities will be successful and financially viable long term. After graduating from the program, women have developed businesses in soap making, beading, jewelry, tailoring, knitting, baking, and agribusiness, among others (see Fig. 30.2).

During the Advocacy, Rights, and Leadership training modules, women receive education on their sexual and reproductive health rights and gain an understanding of how poor maternal healthcare services are a violation of their rights. Women are provided knowledge, tools, and mentoring to advocate for their rights and for improved maternal healthcare provision.

A fundamental component of TERREWODE's Reintegration Program stems from the understanding that social reintegration is a process and many women will require additional support after the two-week intensive program. To support this process, TERREWODE staff provide long-term follow-up for the women, utilizing both in-person visits and check-in via mobile phones. These follow-up visits allow women to share any physical symptoms they are experiencing, yet also psychological, relationship, and economic struggles. TERREWODE staff continue to provide individual and family counseling as needed for fistula survivors, viewing their support as a long-term process when necessary to help a woman successfully reintegrate and live an empowered life with dignity.

Additionally, TERREWODE facilitates the formation of Solidarity Groups. Composed of fistula survivors, women's group leaders, and community members, Solidarity Groups provide critical on going support, co-counseling, and self-reliance skills for women. Solidarity Groups serve as referral points for women with obstetric fistula or childbirth injuries; group leaders refer women suspected of suffering from fistula to TERREWODE for treatment and assist with reintegration post-treatment. Solidarity Groups also serve the wider community need by providing safe motherhood and sexual and reproductive health rights education and advocacy, and women-to-women support systems. Many

Fig. 30.3 Three members from one of TERREWODE's Music, Drama, and Dance groups. The groups perform songs on fistula prevention and safe motherhood for the community. Photo by Joni Kabana

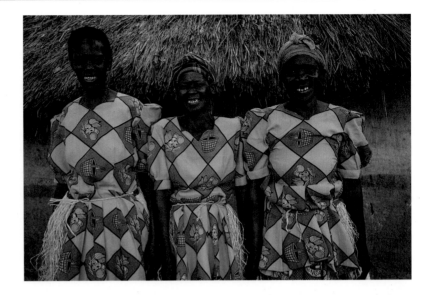

women form microsavings groups and assist one another with business strategies. TERREWODE staff provide on going support visits and field-based training to all Solidarity Groups. Currently, there are 27 TERREWODE Solidarity Groups with close to 800 members.

Another innovative component of the program is TERREWODE's Music, Drama, and Dance program (Fig. 30.3). During training, women use music, drama, and dance as part of their healing journey—singing, dancing, writing, and acting out skits are all deeply therapeutic. Later, women have the option to join Music, Drama, and Dance groups and perform for local secondary schools, community groups, and during advocacy events, such as the International Day to End Fistula. The Music, Drama, and Dance program is a powerful, culturally resonate method to deliver messages about fistula awareness, ending child-marriage, and gender-based violence, among others. It provides an on going support network for women and a source of income. Music, Drama, and Dance groups are also open to male community members, and provide an opportunity for participation and training of men in sexual and reproductive health rights and as allies in the movement.

The two-week residential program now takes place at Terrewode Women's Community Hospital. The dedicated Reintegration Center at the hospital was specifically constructed to accommodate the needs of this program. Transportation, meals and upkeep, supplies and family planning are all provided free of cost. Additionally, TERREWODE is able to offer the first physical therapy program for fistula and related childbirth injuries in Uganda. Physical therapy is provided pre- and post-operatively, along with education on strengthening exercises and postures to protect the pelvic floor once women return to normal demands of life. The Reintegration Program provides an opportunity for women to receive additional physical therapy care and education post-treatment.

Each of these components was developed through an iterative, grassroots process of working closely with fistula survivors, refining and updating the program to meet their needs and stated desires. Reintegration Program modules also compliment and overlap with TERREWODE's other program components, which include prevention, treatment, awareness and advocacy, and research. For instance, Music, Drama, and Dance are components of the Reintegration Program yet also contribute to prevention and fistula awareness and advocacy. Music, Drama, and Dance activities have a beneficial effect on the wider community as these groups perform for community events or partner with local radio stations to broadcast announcements and songs in the local languages on sexual and reproductive health rights, women's experiences with obstetric fistula, and gender-based violence. Music, Drama, and Dance groups also perform for secondary schools and community events, spreading their safe motherhood and sexual and reproductive health rights message. Similarly, through the Awareness and Advocacy Program, TERREWODE has been successful in bringing national attention to obstetric fistula through participation and amplification of events such as the International Day to End Fistula. This attention has led to greater awareness of the risks of fistula, increased demand for treatment from women suffering from fistula, and resulted in increases in resources devoted to ending obstetric fistula in Uganda.

30.2.3 Women's Experiences with TERREWODE's Reintegration Program

TERREWODE's Reintegration Program has been highly successful in helping women to make positive change in their lives and successfully reintegrate in their communities. Here women shared their experiences with the program:

> What helped me a lot was the counseling. TERREWODE taught me not to worry a lot about my life. That alone helped me because I have accepted myself. It helped me a lot. (Woman successfully treated for fistula).

> My husband got counseling. I also personally counseled him because I got training from TERREWODE—there was a lot of counseling and advice. So when I went back home, I shared with him. And he accepted. And that's why he's now with me. (Woman successfully treated for fistula).

Reintegration is remarkably more difficult for women with residual incontinence or failed fistula repair. TERREWODE has developed additional resources and counseling to support these patients.

> I tell you for me it is TERREWODE that helped. The business that I am doing, we were trained by TERREWODE. They told us that we can also still do something, we are still important. This business, the one that I'm doing, it is the result of the training that I started doing this—because I used to do nothing. But now I'm able to go out to the marketplace and take care of myself.
> (Woman with residual incontinence after fistula repair)

> TERREWODE also gave me counseling, which has helped me a lot. Even right now, I still have fistula. But because of that counseling, I have hope that one day I will be okay. I am even here because of that counseling. At least I am now somehow strong. (Woman with failed fistula repair).

Understandably, women with incurable fistula often continue to struggle with depression and have a very difficult time reintegrating. TERREWODE provides on going staff support for these women and connects them to community support through Solidarity Groups, as this woman shares:

> My relationship with TERREWODE has helped me a lot to live up to this time. One, the counseling I got from TERREWODE has helped me to understand myself and accept myself the way I am now. Secondly, it has given me that chance to join the group. Right now, I am in the number seven Solidarity Group. When I don't have anything, I go to the group and borrow money from there. Up to now, if it was not for TERREWODE, I don't know how I would have managed.
> (Woman with incurable fistula)

30.3 Conclusion

Women with obstetric fistula experience a myriad of physical, psychosocial, and economic challenges. Some women recover quickly post-fistula repair and successfully reintegrate into their families and communities. Yet for many women, the journey to wellness is more complex. For these women to fully reintegrate post-treatment and participate in family and community life with positive emotional and mental health, additional services and support are needed.

TERREWODE's Reintegration Program offers a successful model for providing comprehensive reintegration and rehabilitation care to meet women's needs post-treatment. In our experience, we have found that holistic reintegration programming should include counseling, including marital and family counseling as needed, health and safe motherhood education, economic empowerment, physical therapy, long-term follow-up care, and income generation training for the most vulnerable women. Exact services provided to each woman should be based on each individual woman's specific needs, determined with a detailed needs assessment conducted by a skilled counselor. In this chapter, we have reported outcomes based on program interviews, evaluations, and ethnographic research. Additional research is needed to further understand the reintegration process and program priorities. A longitudinal study on TERREWODE's Reintegration Program is now in the early stages; results will be disseminated widely within the global fistula community in order to share best practices and facilitate coordination.

The goal of fistula treatment is to restore women's health and well-being. It is increasingly clear that for many women who suffer from obstetric fistula, treatment that includes reintegration programming as an integral component of fistula care is necessary to achieve this well-being. In sharing this model, we hope that more fistula treatment programs adopt a holistic approach to care that extends beyond surgery to include social and psychological well-being and successful reintegration.

References

Ahmed, S., & Holtz, S. A. (2007). Social and economic consequences of obstetric fistula: Life changed forever? (Article). *International Journal of Gynecology & Obstetrics, 99*, S10–S15. https://doi.org/10.1016/j.ijgo.2007.06.011

Arrowsmith, S., Hamlin, E. C., & Wall, L. L. (1996). Obstructed labor injury complex: Obstetric fistula formation and the multifaceted morbidity of maternal birth trauma in the developing world. *Obstetrical Gynecological Survey, 51*(9), 568–574.

Bangser, M. (2007). Strengthening public health priority-setting through research on fistula, maternal health, and health inequities. *International Journal of Gynecology & Obstetrics, 99*, 16–20. https://doi.org/10.1016/j.ijgo.2007.06.016

Barageine, J. K., Beyeza-Kashesya, J., Byamugisha, J. K., Tumwesigye, N. M., Almroth, L., & Faxelid, E. (2015). "I am alone and isolated": A qualitative study of experiences of women living with genital fistula in Uganda. *BMC Womens Health, 15*(1), 73. https://doi.org/10.1186/s12905-015-0232-z

Bellows, B., Bach, R., Baker, Z., & Warren, C. (2015). *Barriers to obstetric fistula treatment in low-income countries: A systematic review (review)*. Population Council.

Browning, A., Fentahun, W., & Goh, J. T. (2007). The impact of surgical treatment on the mental health of women with obstetric fistula. *BJOG: An International Journal of Obstetrics & Gynaecology, 114*(11), 1439–1441. https://doi.org/10.1111/j.1471-0528.2007.01419.x

Castille, Y.-J., Avocetien, C., Zaongo, D., Colas, J.-M., Peabody, J. O., & Rochat, C.-H. (2014). Impact of a program of physiotherapy and health education on the outcome of obstetric fistula surgery. *International Journal of Gynecology & Obstetrics, 124*(1), 77–80.

Desalliers, J., Pare, M. E., Kouraogo, S., & Corcos, J. (2017). Impact of surgery on quality of life of women with obstetrical fistula: A qualitative study in Burkina Faso. *International Urogynecology Journal, 28*(7), 1091–1100. https://doi.org/10.1007/s00192-016-3235-x

Donnelly, K., Oliveras, E., Tilahun, Y., Belachew, M., & Asnake, M. (2015). Quality of life of Ethiopian women after fistula repair: Implications on rehabilitation and social reintegration policy and programming. *Culture Health & Sexuality, 17*(2), 150–164. https://doi.org/10.1080/13691058.2014.964320

Drew, L. B., Wilkinson, J. P., Nundwe, W., Moyo, M., Mataya, R., Mwale, M., et al. (2016). Long-term outcomes for women after obstetric fistula repair in Lilongwe, Malawi: A qualitative study. *BMC Pregnancy and Childbirth, 16*, 2–2. https://doi.org/10.1186/s12884-015-0755-1

El Ayadi, A., Nalubwama, H., Barageine, J., Neilands, T. B., Obore, S., Byamugisha, J., et al. (2017). Development and preliminary validation of a post-fistula repair reintegration instrument among Ugandan women. *Reproductive Health, 14*(1), 1–13.

El Ayadi, A. M., Barageine, J., Korn, A., Kakaire, O., Turan, J., Obore, S., et al. (2019). Trajectories of women's physical and psychosocial health following obstetric fistula repair in Uganda: A longitudinal study. *Tropical Medicine & International Health, 24*(1), 53–64.

El Ayadi, A. M., Painter, C. E., Delamou, A., Barr-Walker, J., Korn, A., Obore, S., et al. (2020). Rehabilitation and reintegration programming adjunct to female genital fistula surgery: A systematic scoping review. *International Journal of Gynecology & Obstetrics, 148*, 42–58.

Emasu, A., Ruder, B., Wall, L. L., Matovu, A., Alia, G., & Barageine, J. K. (2019). Reintegration needs of young women following genitourinary fistula surgery in Uganda. *International Urogynecology Journal, 30*(7), 1101–1110.

Hamed, S., Ahlberg, B.-M., & Trenholm, J. (2017). Powerlessness, normalization, and resistance: A Foucauldian discourse analysis of women's narratives on obstetric fistula in eastern Sudan. *Qualitative Health Research, 27*(12), 1828–1841. https://doi.org/10.1177/1049732317720423

Jarvis, K., Richter, S., & Vallianatos, H. (2017). Exploring the needs and challenges of women reintegrating after obstetric fistula repair in northern Ghana. *Midwifery, 50*, 55–61.

Johnson, K., Turan, J., Hailemariam, L., Mengsteab, E., Jena, D., & Polan, M. (2010). The role of counseling for obstetric fistula patients: Lessons learned from Eritrea. *Patient Education and Counseling, 80*(2), 262–265.

Keyser, L., McKinney, J., Salmon, C., Furaha, C., Kinsindja, R., & Benfield, N. (2014). Analysis of a pilot program to implement physical therapy for women with gynecologic fistula in the Democratic Republic of Congo. *International Journal of Gynecology & Obstetrics, 127*(2), 127–131.

Khisa, A. M., & Nyamongo, I. K. (2012). Still living with fistula: An exploratory study of the experience of women with obstetric fistula following corrective surgery in west Pokot, Kenya. *Reproductive Health Matters, 20*(40), 59–66. https://doi.org/10.1016/s0968-8080(12)40661-9

Khisa, W., Wakasiaka, S., McGowan, L., Campbell, M., & Lavender, T. (2016). Understanding the lived experience of women before and after fistula repair: A qualitative study in Kenya (journal article). *BJOG: An International Journal of Obstetrics & Gynaecology, 124*(3), 503–510. https://doi.org/10.1111/1471-0528.13902

Ministry of Health Uganda (2010/2011–2015/2016). National obstetric fistula strategy.

Mselle, L. T., Moland, K. M., Evjen-Olsen, B., Mvungi, A., & Kohi, T. W. (2011). "I am nothing": Experiences of loss among women suffering from severe birth injuries in Tanzania. *BMC Womens Health, 11*(1), 49. https://doi.org/10.1186/1472-6874-11-49

Muleta, M., Hamlin, E. C., Fantahun, M., Kennedy, R. C., & Tafesse, B. (2008). Health and social problems encountered by treated and untreated obstetric fistula patients in rural Ethiopia. *Journal of Obstetrics and Gynaecology Canada, 30*(1), 44–50.

Murray, C., Goh, J. T., Fynes, M., & Carey, M. P. (2002). Urinary and faecal incontinence following delayed primary repair of obstetric genital fistula. *BJOG: An International Journal of Obstetrics & Gynaecology, 109*(7), 828–832.

Mwini-Nyaledzigbor, P. P., Agana, A. A., & Pilkington, F. B. (2013). Lived experiences of Ghanaian women with obstetric fistula. *Health Care Women International, 34*(6), 440–460. https://doi.org/10.1080/07399332.2012.755981

Nielsen, H. S., Lindberg, L., Nygaard, U., Aytenfisu, H., Johnston, O. L., Sorensen, B., et al. (2009). A community-based long-term follow-up of women undergoing obstetric fistula repair in rural Ethiopia. *BJOG: An International Journal of Obstetrics & Gynaecology, 116*(9), 1258–1264. https://doi.org/10.1111/j.1471-0528.2009.02200.x

Ojengbede, O. A., Baba, Y., Morhason-Bello, I. O., Armah, M., Dimiti, A., Buwa, D., et al. (2014). Group psychological therapy in obstetric fistula care: A complementary recipe for the accompanying mental ill health morbidities? *African Journal of Reproductive Health, 18*(1), 156–160.

Pope, R., Bangser, M., & Requejo, J. H. (2011). Restoring dignity: Social reintegration after obstetric fistula repair in Ukerewe, Tanzania (research support, non-U.S. Gov't). *Global Public Health, 6*(8), 859–873. https://doi.org/10.1080/17441692.2010.551519

Ruder, B., Cheyney, M., & Emasu, A. A. (2018). Too long to wait: Obstetric fistula and the sociopolitical dynamics of the fourth delay in Soroti, Uganda. *Qualitative Health Research, 28*(5), 721–732.

Ruder, B., & Emasu, A. (2021). The promise and neglect of follow-up care in obstetric fistula treatment in Uganda. In L. J. Wallace, M. E. MacDonald, & K. T. Storeng (Eds.), *Anthropologies of global maternal and reproductive health: From policy spaces to sites of practice*. Springer.

UBOS. (2018). *Uganda demographic and health survey 2016*. Uganda Bureau of Statistics and The DHS Program, ICF.

Wall, L. L., Arrowsmith, S. D., & Hancock, B. D. (2008). Ethical aspects of urinary diversion for women with irreparable obstetric fistulas in developing countries. *International Urogynecology Journal of Pelvic Floor Dysfunction, 19*(7), 1027–1030. https://doi.org/10.1007/s00192-008-0559-1

Wall, L. L., Karshima, J. A., Kirschner, C., & Arrowsmith, S. D. (2004). The obstetric vesicovaginal fistula: Characteristics of 899 patients from Jos, Nigeria. *American Journal of Obstetrics and Gynecology, 190*(4), 1011–1016.

Watt, M. H., Wilson, S. M., Sikkema, K. J., Velloza, J., Mosha, M. V., Masenga, G. G., et al. (2015). Development of an intervention to improve mental health for obstetric fistula patients in Tanzania (article). *Evaluation and Program Planning, 50*, 1–9. https://doi.org/10.1016/j.evalprogplan.2015.01.007

Weston, K., Mutiso, S., Mwangi, J. W., Qureshi, Z., Beard, J., & Venkat, P. (2011). Depression among women with obstetric fistula in Kenya. *International Journal of Gynaecology and Obstetrics, 115*(1), 31–33. https://doi.org/10.1016/j.ijgo.2011.04.015

WHO. (2006). *Obstetric fistula: Guiding principles for clinical management and programme development; making pregnancy safer.* Lewis, G. & de Bernis, L. World Health Organization, Geneva, Switzerland.

Wilson, S., Sikkema, K., Watt, M., Masenga, G., & Mosha, M. (2016). Psychological symptoms and social functioning following repair of obstetric fistula in a low-income setting. *Maternal & Child Health Journal, 20*(5), 941–945. https://doi.org/10.1007/s10995-016-1950-z

Yeakey, M. P., Chipeta, E., Taulo, F., & Tsui, A. O. (2009). The lived experience of Malawian women with obstetric fistula. *Culture, Health & Sexuality, 11*(5), 499–513. https://doi.org/10.1080/13691050902874777

Addressing Mental Health in Obstetric Fistula Patients: Filling the Void

Meghan Beddow and Mary J. Stokes

31.1 Introduction: Unmet Need and Prevalence

The current number of women in Asia and sub-Saharan Africa who are living with obstetric fistula today are estimated to be two million, with 50,000 to 100,000 new cases each year (WHO, 2018). In Malawi alone, the site of these authors' work, the prevalence is estimated to be 1.6 per 1000 women (Kalilani-Phiri et al., 2010). While the physical stigma and the social stigma of obstetric fistula are well documented, the mental health impact has more recently become a topic of discussion in the global health community. Women with obstetric fistula suffer from higher rates of depression (Duko et al., 2020). The prevalence of depression and other mental health disorders in this population varies in different settings, likely due to cultural and societal differences among the locations studied, and/ or different research methods that were employed in the research. Browning et al. found that 100% of women in a cohort in Ethiopia screened positive for depressive symptoms (Browning et al., 2007). Another study of women in Ethiopia with obstetric fistula similarly demonstrated that 97.3% of women who had any type of obstetric fistula experienced depression, and 100% of those who had both vesicovaginal and rectovaginal fistulae were depressed (Zeleke et al., 2013). Likewise, 97% of women in Goh's 2005 study in Ethiopia and Bangladesh screened positive for mental health dysfunction, although only 23.3–38.8% were estimated to have major depression (Goh et al., 2005). Researchers in Kenya found that 72% of fistula patients were depressed, with 14.3% in the "mild" range, 25.7% "severe," 2.9% with self-reported history of psychiatric illness, and 17.1% reporting suicidal ideation (Weston et al., 2011). A study comparing obstetric fistula patients to outpatient gynecological patients found that fistula patients have significantly higher symptoms of depression, post-traumatic stress disorder, somatic complaints, and maladaptive coping compared to women without fistula (Wilson et al., 2015). Further supporting such findings, a qualitative study gave voice to women who expressed feelings of depression, shame, and anger – but also, of hope for the future (Kay et al., 2015).

M. Beddow (✉)
Southcentral Foundation, Alaska Native Medical Center, Anchorage, AK, USA
e-mail: meghan.beddow@gmail.com

M. J. Stokes
Department of Global Women's Health, Obstetrics and Gynecology, Baylor College of Medicine, Houston, TX, USA

The importance of addressing mental health in patients with obstetric fistula cannot be overstated. The acknowledgment of psychiatric morbidity in a patient population has been directly linked to improved health outcomes (Patel et al., 1998). The unnoticed illness is the untreated illness. Psychiatric disorders, when left untreated, are second only to cardiovascular disease as the leading noncommunicable cause of disability in both low- and high-resource settings (Abas et al., 1994). Disability of any sort is defined as the "social implication to the individual's physical condition or impairment" (Mselle et al., 2011). A physical impairment is viewed by society as disabling, and therefore may significantly alter or destroy one's identity (Goffman, 1963).

31.2   Fistula Mental Health Complex and Social Implications

The obstructed labor that leads to fistula causes much more than physical injury; it results in a cascade of consequences that Arrowsmith called the "obstructed labor injury complex" (Arrowsmith et al., 1996). Obstetric fistula affects a woman's social identity, and can often leave her isolated (Barageine et al., 2015), divorced, and childless, suffering from worsened poverty and/or malnutrition, excluded from religious activities, and emotionally devastated (Ahmed & Holtz, 2007).

The social stigma related to fistula arises from the appearance and odor of urine leaking, and also from a poor understanding of the condition and its causes (Bashah et al., 2018). Affected women can develop puddles of urine that surround their feet while standing in one place that result from constant dribbling of urine and may also have odiferous fecal incontinence (Semere & Nour, 2008). Sometimes, fistula may incorrectly be considered a sexually transmitted disease and a "punishment from God" (Ahmed & Holtz, 2007). A recent study in Tanzania described the pervasive belief that fistula is caused by association with witchcraft or an ancestor's curse, and that the shame-imposed lack of discourse on the subject resulted in decreased awareness regarding cause and treatment (Lyimo & Mosha, 2019).

In West Pokot, women with fistula are labeled "unclean," "socially polluted," and unfit to take part in traditional roles of women in the community, even when fully healed and "dry" (Khisa & Nyamongo, 2012). These women are often unable to fulfill social obligations such as attending funerals, religious ceremonies, community gatherings, and even family meals (Mselle et al., 2011). In qualitative studies, women have shared the damaging and disparaging comments they have received from within their community (Bashah et al., 2018), leading to more social isolation and exclusion. Such social deprivation and discrimination are associated with low quality of life (Holzemer et al., 2009), reduced self-esteem (Markowitz, 1998), and worsened health outcomes (Schwatzmann, 2009). Women living with fistula describe feeling constant sadness and hopelessness, and their husbands and female family members shared these feelings when interviewed (Yeakey et al., 2009). While such social exclusion and ostracism is experienced by many, it is not universal. In a qualitative study in Malawi, many women and their families reported high levels of support from a few close individuals (Yeakey et al., 2009).

Additionally, the smell and leakage of urine due to obstetric fistula can impact a woman's ability to work outside the home. This inability to earn an income and be financially independent can cause many challenges. Women with fistula have described feeling dependent upon their husbands, "similar to that of a child," "useless," and grappling with "self-contempt" (Mselle et al., 2011).

A woman's roles and interpersonal relations within both the nuclear as well as extended family can also be impacted by obstetric fistula. When a woman has a fistula, she can feel that her role as wife and mother have been taken from her, resulting in high rates of psychosocial morbidity including lack of confidence, isolation, shame, depression, and in some cases, suicidal ideation. In the absence of timely fistula repair surgery, divorce or abandonment by the husband may follow the fistula injury, especially when coupled with infertility, inability to work or perform household tasks, or the inability to have sexual intercourse due to severe vaginal scarring. During interviews of 21 women living with obstetric fistula in Somalia, Mohamed et al. (2018)[1] found the majority of women suffered social consequences of their fistulas. According to one woman,

> *My husband left me when I got this problem. I lived without partner for 18 years. My husband said that he cannot cope with the smell and decided to leave me alone. I used to stay at home like a paralyzed person because I cannot go to the community meetings. They abuse me. When our neighbours see me, they say 'the urinator' is coming, and they ask their friends 'can you smell urine, what is smelling, where is it coming from.' I feel ashamed and talk to my self "self-mumbling" and say: yes they are talking about you. They are gossiping about you. Sometimes, some of them turn their lips up. Yes I hear. I never feel good. I don't have interest in people to seeing me.* (Dhubado, 39-years old, lived with obstetric fistula for 18 years) (Mohamed et al., 2018)

Another woman, aged 18 years, said,

> *My husband said: 'I can't stay with a woman urinating every minute' and he decided to leave me and seek a new life. Yes that Sheikh 'the husband' was not happy to live with me. Even me, I was feeling ashamed to face my husband. I can't carry out my daily duty.* (Aisha, 18-years old, lived with obstetric fistula for three years) (Mohamed et al., 2018)

A study in Bangladesh demonstrated that 33.3% of women with fistula had difficulty maintaining a sexual relationship, 50% had decreased libido, 59% had reduction in frequency of coitus, 45% had delay in orgasm, and 37.9% had dyspareunia (Islam & Begum, 1992). In some cases, women with fistula reported being forced into sex though it was painful, and described the experience as rape (Barageine et al., 2015). In some cases, husbands leave their wives who have fistulas, and some may marry again. As Mohamed et al. (2018) found,

> *Since I developed this problem, my husband limited his visiting to us because he has married another woman. Although I'm ok with it he shouldn't have abandoned us. I live with my four children and always I'm confined to the house. Yes he doesn't visit us. Yes we are not hearing his voice for up to six months.* (Safi, 40-years old, lived with obstetric fistula for eight years)

> *Yes, he didn't support me when my injury came. It was only my mother and siblings that supported me. He was the person I was getting the least support from before he lastly divorced me.* (Shukri, 22-years old, lived with fistula for one year)

While disruption of marriages and sexual relationships is significant (Yeakey et al., 2009), some marriages are maintained. A full 47% of women in a Ugandan study were abandoned or separated from their partner, and 23% reported emotional or physical abuse from that partner (Emasu et al., 2019).

For a majority of women with fistula, the obstructed labor that caused the injury also resulted in a stillbirth or neonatal death. In from 83% to 90% of pregnancies complicated by obstetric fistula, the infant is stillborn or dies within weeks of delivery (Tebeu 2009 & Ahmed 2007). Many women perceive their fistula and infertility issues to be intimately linked (Yeakey et al., 2009). In those settings where fistula frequently occurs, the sustainability of a marriage is often directly related to a woman's ability to bear children (Yeakey et al., 2009). The link between childlessness and depression is unclear, with some studies showing an association (Stokes et al., 2019) and others none (Weston et al., 2011), whether predominantly due to social concerns or personal psychological well-being, various focus groups have identified future fertility as an important concern for many women with fistula (Yeakey et al., 2009).

---

[1] Adam A. Mohamed, Abiodun O. Ilesanmi, M. David Dairo. (2018). The Experience of Women with Obstetric Fistula following Corrective Surgery: A Qualitative Study in Benadir and Mudug Regions, Somalia. *Obstetrics and Gynecology International*, Vol. 2018, Article ID 5250843, 10 pages. https://doi.org/10.1155/2018/5250843, licensed under the terms of the Creative Commons Attribution License (https://creativecommons.org/licenses/by/4.0/).

The cascading effects of the obstructive labor injury complex profoundly disturb a women's sense of well-being. Women with fistula often feel that they have brought shame to their families (Gharoro & Agholor, 2009), and they report feeling bitter, depressed, and unhappy (Gharoro & Agholor, 2009). They also report experiencing stress, anxiety, and low self-esteem (Ojanuga, 1991). Mselle et al. (2011) describe their

> deep sense of loss… loss of body control, loss of the social roles as women and wives, loss of integration in social life, and loss of dignity and self-worth.

As a result, many women with fistula find it difficult to engage in activities of daily living. In one study, 78.6% of patients with fistula reported difficulty with daily tasks and social interactions (Weston et al., 2011). Additionally, many women plagued by these circumstances report contemplation of suicide (Barageine et al., 2015 & Gharoro & Agholor, 2009). In Somalia, Muno was dismissed from her job as a local clothes washer due to the bad odors emanating from her fistula:

> I was domestic worker, I used to wash clothes of the neighbouring families. Some of the families heard that I'm a urinating woman and they chased me. Yes they said: we don't want you, you are not clean (you are dirty). I was really stigmatized by the neighbouring families. You lose your job because of this condition. The worst consequence of the OBF is the isolation. (Muno, 27-years old, lived with obstetric fistula for eight years) (Mohamed et al., 2018)

31.3 Tools for Study/Assessment of Mental Health Among Women with Fistula

Evaluating mental health can be difficult in a cross-cultural context. The presentation of mental illness or mood disorders, as well as the terminology used to describe related symptoms, differs throughout the world. Several authors have emphasized the importance of assessing mood in those with multiple somatic complaints. Depression and anxiety may present with somatic symptoms, especially in low- and middle-income countries (Abas et al., 1994). A study from Zimbabwe described labels such as "*shenjing shuairuo*" (neurasthenia) in China, "*ghabrahat*" (anxiety) in India, "*pelo y tata*" (heart too much) in Botswana, and "*nerves*" throughout Latin America and some places in South Africa, as aliases for or comparisons to conditions that overlap with depression (Patel et al., 2001). Terminology for mental health conditions can also vary across cultures. A Nigerian study reports that 33% of women with fistulas were psychologically depressed, but an additional 51% were "bitter about life" (Angioli et al., 2000). Traditional healers, local community leaders, and other individuals who are familiar with the cultural context should be enlisted to help translate and interpret local terminology for depressive symptoms (Abas et al., 1994).

Several qualitative studies have provided insight into the mental health of fistula patients (Kay et al., 2015; Yeakey et al., 2009), with findings that can help identify particular needs within the fistula community to guide interventions. These studies also serve as a reminder that each patient's experience is distinct (Kay et al., 2015). For these reasons, additional research is needed to better understand the breadth of mental health outcomes among fistula patients.

Several quantitative tools have been used to evaluate mental health among fistula patients, including Beck's Depression Inventory (Zeleke et al., 2013), the General Health Questionnaire or GHQ-28 (Browning & Menber, 2008; Goh et al., 2005), the Center for Epidemiologic Studies Depression Scale (Wilson et al., 2016), the PTSD Checklist-Civilian Version (Wilson et al., 2016), and the Patient Health Questionnaire 9 (PHQ-9) (Gelaye et al., 2013; Hanlon et al., 2015; Kroenke et al., 2001; Manea et al., 2012; Stokes et al., 2019). The PHQ-9 has been studied in low-resource countries to validate and identify the optimal cut-off score for depression screening (Bitew et al., 2017; Hanlon et al., 2015; Kroenke et al., 2001; Manea et al., 2012; Weobong et al., 2014). Based on DSM-IV criteria for major depressive disorder, the PHQ-9 was evaluated in Ethiopia in 2010 by Gelaye et al., and was found to have excellent reliability and validity for diagnosis of major depression in that context (Gelaye et al., 2013), using a cut-off score of 5 (in contrast, the cut-off score in higher-income countries is 10) (Gelaye et al., 2013).

The Perceived Quality of Life Scale (PQoL) and Reintegration to Normal Living Index (RNLI) have also been used to evaluate fistula patients (Pope et al., 2011). The PQoL tool is a ten-point scale, converted to picture format and adapted to a rural Tanzanian context, to assess their population's mental health, alongside other facets of well-being (Pope et al., 2011). Both Pope et al. and El Ayadi et al. modified the RNLI to fit their contexts, in Tanzania and Uganda, respectively, and El Ayadi found that the reintegration score correlated significantly with quality of life, depression, self-esteem, stigma, and social support (El Ayadi et al., 2017).

In a recent Ugandan study, amongst several other tools to evaluate quality of life and mental health, the HIV/AIDS Stigma Instrument—PLWA (HASI-P) was modified for use in fistula patients to quantify the level of stigma they experienced (El Ayadi et al., 2019).

Although more research is needed to have a better understanding of mental health among women with fistula, the tools described above can provide an objective framework through which to assess mental health over time, even in a cross-cultural context, to ensure change and improvement after therapy and interventions.

31.4 Persistent Urinary Incontinence and Mental Health

The effects of a fistula reach far beyond the physical injury. But can simple repair of the fistula also repair the social damage that the obstructed labor injury complex has caused? Browning et al. performed a prospective study in Ethiopia in which 100% of participants (51) screened positive for mental health disorders prior to surgery, and 2 weeks after repair only 36% screened positive, including all six of those without cure of incontinence. There were no formal psychological interventions (Browning et al., 2007). Wilson et al. performed a similar study in Tanzania, in which 28 patients were followed and evaluated for symptoms of depression and PTSD symptoms. Prior to surgery, all participants demonstrated high baseline psychological distress. Following surgery, women who were "dry" showed significantly improved mental health on assessment. Women with persistent incontinence continued to have high rates of PTSD and depression, and the severity of leaking was directly correlated to the level of psychological distress (Wilson et al., 2016).

Mental health may correlate with a patient's ability to reintegrate into her community following repair. Pope et al. studied the relationship between surgical outcomes of fistula patients and their perceived quality of life and ability to reintegrate into society postoperatively using the previously described PQoL and RNLI tools. Women in this study described their transition back home as "easy," and were more apt to respond this way if they were "dry" and had a family support system. Forty-eight percent of women reported persistent physical problems, including pain and weakness while working. However, by 1 year after the repair, those who described themselves as "healed" or "mostly healed" reported feeling "themselves again." The degree of perceived surgical success was directly correlated with quality of life and with ability to reintegrate into their communities (Pope et al., 2011).

Gharoro and Agholor had similar findings in their 2009 study, in which over one-half of patients experienced a positive change in societal attitudes toward them following successful repair; however, women who continued to leak urine found reintegration difficult (Gharoro & Agholor, 2009). El Ayadi et al. (2019) found a correlation between lower psychological health and persistent self-reported physical symptoms following repair, though improvement in all areas of psychological well-being was demonstrated over time, with the exception of negative self-perception which had a slight increase at 12 months postrepair (El Ayadi et al., 2019). A retrospective study in Malawi found that persistent depression after repair was associated with persistent incontinence, but depression improved for all patients who continued to return for follow-up at 3 and 6 months, even when incontinence persisted (Stokes et al., 2019). In a cohort of 290 women following VVF repair, only ten (3.5%) met criteria for major depressive disorder using the PHQ-9 criteria, all of whom had residual incontinence, though a full 19.3% of women reported some degree of continued leakage (Kopp et al., 2019). These studies suggest that "wet vs. dry" is not the ultimate determinant of a fistula patient's mental well-being, but that community support and counseling regarding postrepair outcomes may help improve mental health without formal mental health interventions.

31.5   Task Shifting to Improve Mental Health Care

The scarcity of mental health professionals in low-resource settings creates an obstacle for addressing mental health needs once identified. Significant time and resources are necessary for the implementation of psychosocial interventions and for the training of staff. A researcher in Zimbabwe noted that the country had only ten psychiatrists for ten million people (Abas et al., 1994). A "training of trainers" (Abas et al., 1994) is necessary for the dissemination of applicable knowledge and skills to reach nonpsychiatric providers—the "task shifting" (Watt et al., 2015) that allows more patients to have access to psychiatric care.

Specialized training, organization of services, and supervision are necessary for the successful integration of skilled providers into the mental healthcare system. Patel et al. (2009) proposed a District Mental Health Program in India to shadow the National Mental Health Program of India, which organizes the delivery of health services by the health district manager, the program leader, the health counselor, and finally by volunteers and users of the services themselves. The proposed mental health program distributes responsibilities and roles in a similar fashion, including a Mental Health Program Leader (MHPL) and health counselors (Patel et al., 2009). It has been demonstrated that trained nurse-level facilitators have been successful in delivering effective interventions related to mental health (Araya et al., 2003; Watt et al., 2017). In Zimbabwe, the "Multiple Symptoms Card" was created to lead primary health workers through an algorithm to diagnose probable depression, and then through a seven-step management plan (Abas et al., 1994).

Psychological health must be a responsibility and priority for the entire health system—not just the handful of psychiatrists who are generally absent from low-resource populations at the periphery—to ensure that the tools for mental well-being reach a larger portion of the population in need.

31.6   Successful Programs for Mental Health Needs of Women with Fistula

A successful strategy to address the psychosocial health of fistula patients must consider all components of their mental well-being, as well as their reintegration with family and community after repair. Several fistula center programs offer examples of effective interventions that can begin to address the need gap.

The WHO asserts that "at the very least, basic counseling for all women with fistula should include information on what fistula is" (WHO 2006), including its etiology, risk factors, and prevention. This should include family planning counseling and discussion of accessing obstetric care in any subsequent pregnancies. As described above, in many places in the world, a fistula is attributed to a "curse" or sexually transmitted infection—and therefore a certain stigma is attached. Educating a woman about obstetric fistula empowers her to seek appropriate medical care for herself and other women when it is needed, and may also allow her to begin to heal psychologically. In a Nigerian fistula hospital, a simple educational brochure was created for this purpose (Gerten et al., 2009). In Eritrea, the primary goal of the first formal counseling program for fistula patients was education (Johnson et al., 2010), with secondary goals of building self-esteem and introducing social reintegration topics.

Even after repair or "cure," women may continue to face discrimination back home (Mehta & Bangser, 2006), and in certain places, may need to present a certificate of good health to re-enter their community (Okoye et al., 2014). Some women report relocating from their original community, even after successful repair, so that they were not surrounded by those who knew their history (Bomboka et al., 2019). Support from individuals in the community, such as family members, husband, friend, or other survivors of fistula, can facilitate a smoother reintegration. Individuals who lack a support network during recovery had poor emotional well-being, and scored lowest on PQoL and RNLI tools (Pope et al., 2011). Given the extreme distances that some women must travel to seek fistula care, one group uses mobile phones to contact supportive individuals back home to engage them in the recovery process (Watt et al., 2015). Finally, educating the woman's community can assist greatly in healthy reintegration, and some programs provide a nurse or social worker to escort the woman home to have conversations with her family and community about the etiology and prevention of obstetric fistula causes.

Beyond social challenges, women recovering from obstetric fistula also face economic challenges. Emasu et al. (2019) point out that overall, this is a group that already had been economically vulnerable prior to development of a fistula, and many reported economic abuse by their partner (26%) or exploitation by parents, community groups, other relatives, or employers (Emasu et al., 2019). Several fistula centers now offer educational and skills-training programs (Mselle et al., 2011), including tangible means of maintaining an income. Such skills and educational training can enable women to become more financially independent, which may boost self-esteem, their sense of self-worth, and improve their mental health.

To directly address the mental health of fistula patients, individual counseling and group therapy both have important roles. Counselling should prepare women for the possibility of incomplete cure, and help develop coping strategies in case they continue to suffer from incontinence after repair (Watt et al., 2017 & Wilson et al., 2016). Ojengbede et al. implemented group interpersonal psychotherapy (GIPT) in a South Sudan fistula population, grouping patients with similar mental health disorders together for therapy. A trained professional facilitated sessions with particular focus on depression, self-esteem, and risk of self-harm. The patients shared information, experiences, and coping strategies with each other. Mental health assessments were performed before and after surgical repair, and the researchers found significantly lower levels of poor mental health in the group who had GIPT, although only patients with successful surgical repairs and no subsequent incontinence were included in the analysis. Benefits of GIPT include building confidence and hope prior to surgery, discussing concerns and misconceptions, and the availability of this method to use in large-scale settings with minimal resources—making it an ideal tool for many fistula hospital settings (Ojengbede et al., 2014). In contrast, Watt et al. chose an individual model of cognitive behavioral therapy (CBT) in order to allow the patient to fully share her story and progress through topics in an organized manner (Watt et al., 2015). A community health nurse led a series of six-hour-long, topic-driven sessions—two prior to surgery and four afterwards. The sessions began with a recounting of the individual fistula story, and then flowed toward creating a new story about the fistula, validating her story but reframing it with medical information. Subsequent sessions included discussion of associated thoughts and emotions, creation and development of coping mechanisms, consideration of social relationships, and planning for the future (Watt et al., 2015). A future randomized controlled trial is planned, but initial results of the pilot program were positive; all patients said that they would be willing to participate again. However, the mental health facilitator did recognize several challenges, most relating to helping the woman identify the changeable nature of her thoughts and her social relationships, and to generating solutions to the stressor of poverty (Watt et al., 2015).

Even without a formal mental health program, a "sisterhood of suffering" (Arrowsmith et al., 1996) develops at fistula hospitals and provides a supportive community that may outperform many formal mental health interventions (Browning et al., 2007). A recent study in Malawi demonstrated that a fistula care community that provides long-term follow-up and support—even in the absence of a formal mental health service structure—can improve symptoms of depression (Stokes et al., 2019). Nearly one-half of the obstetric fistula patients in the study screened positive for depression on the PHQ-9 assessment prior to repair, and all 96 patients who completed a PHQ-9 assessment six-months postoperatively were negative for depression. Established fistula hospitals provide a setting for the development of a supportive fistula community and space for mental health screening and long-term follow-up; however, such community and structure may be lacking at short-term surgical camps.

Ideally, obstetric fistula patients would have access to trained clinical psychologists and counselors, but this simply is not the reality or feasible in most low-resource settings. However, fistula patients often stay in the hospital for several weeks, and this provides a window of opportunity to address both mental health concerns and the social factors that will greatly impact their psychosocial well-being once they return home.

31.7   Areas for Future Research to Address Mental Health Needs of Women with Fistula

There is ample opportunity for continued mental health research in the obstetric fistula population, which will identify specific needs as well as effective and feasible mental health interventions for women with fistula. Identifying which characteristics put patients most at risk for adverse mental health outcomes should be a priority (Wilson et al., 2016), as should identifying protective factors that promote resilience (Wilson et al., 2015), given the many factors that affect the outcomes of these women, "*preventative strategies for depression should include social policies aimed at increasing sex equality, eliminating poverty, and strengthening social support networks for populations at risk*" (Patel et al., 2001). Future studies should additionally look beyond the walls of the fistula center, assessing the long-term psychosocial outcomes of recovering fistula patients after they re-entered their families and communities. A significant barrier to such follow-up is accessing the patients since many women travel great distances for access to fistula care. However, similar to other pregnancy-related complications, it is those mothers who are most remote from care that are at greatest risk of poor outcomes, and thus identifying ways to address their needs should be a priority.

References

Abas, M., & Broadhead, J. (1994). Mental disorders in the developing world. *BMJ, 308*, 1052.

Ahmed, S., & Holtz, S. (2007). Social and economic consequences of obstetric fistula: Life changed forever? *International Journal of Gynaecology and Obstetrics, 99*(Suppl 1), 10–15.

Angioli, R., Gomez-Marin, O., Cantuaria, G., & O'sullivan, M. (2000). Severe perineal lacerations during vaginal delivery: The University of Miami experience. *American Journal of Obstetrics and Gynecology, 182*(5), 1083–1085.

Araya, R., Rojas, G., Fritsch, R., Gaete, J., Rojas, M., Simon, G., & Peters, T. (2003). Treating depression in primary care in low-income women in Santiago, Chile: A randomized controlled trial. *The Lancet, 361*, 995–1000.

Arrowsmith, S., Hamlin, E., & Wall, L. (1996). Obstructed labor injury complex: Obstetric fistula formation and the multifaceted morbidity of maternal birth trauma in the developing world. *Obstetrical & Gynecological Survey, 51*(9), 568–574.

Barageine, J., Beyeza-Kashesya, J., Byamugisha, J., Tumwesigye, N., Almroth, L., & Faxelid, E. (2015). "I am alone and isolated": A qualitative study of experiences of women living with genital fistula in Uganda. *BMC Women's Health, 15*, 73. https://doi.org/10.1186/s12905-015-0232-z

Bashah, D., Worku, A., & Mengisu, M. (2018). Consequences of obstetric fistula in sub Sahara African countries, from patients' perspective: A systematic review of qualitative studies. *BMC Women's Health, 18*(1), 106. https://doi.org/10.1186/s12905-018-0605-1

Bitew, T., Hanlon, C., Kebede, E., Honikman, S., Onah, M., & Fekadu, A. (2017). Antenatal depressive symptoms and utilization of delivery and postnatal care: A prospective study in rural Ethiopia. *BMC Pregnancy and Childbirth, 17*, 206.

Bomboka, J. B., N-Mboowa, M. G., & Nakilembe, J. (2019). Post - effects of obstetric fistula in Uganda; a case study of fistula survivors in KITOVU mission hospital (MASAKA), Uganda. *BMC Public Health, 19*(1), 696. https://doi.org/10.1186/s12889-019-7023-7

Browning, A., Fentahun, W., & Goh, J. (2007). The impact of surgical treatment on the mental health of women with obstetric fistula. *BJOG: An International Journal of Obstetrics & Gynaecology, 114*, 1439–1441. https://doi.org/10.1111/j.1471-0528.2007.01419.x

Browning, A., & Menber, B. (2008). Women with obstetric fistula in Ethiopia: a 6-month follow-up after surgical treatment. *BJOG: An International Journal of Obstetrics & Gynaecology, 115*, 1564–1569.

Duko, B., Wolka, S., Seyoum, M., & Tantu, T. (2020). Prevalence of depression among women with obstetric fistula in low-income African countries: A systematic review and meta-analysis. *Archives of Women's Mental Health, 24*(1), 1–9. https://doi.org/10.1007/s00737-020-01028-w

El Ayadi, A., Nalubwama, H., Barageine, J., et al. (2017). Development and preliminary validation of a post-fistula repair reintegration instrument among Ugandan women. *Reproductive Health, 14*, 109. https://doi.org/10.1186/s12978-017-0372-8

El Ayadi, A. M., Barageine, J., Korn, A., Kakaire, O., Turan, J., Obore, S., Byamugisha, J., Lester, F., Nalubwama, H., Mwanje, H., Tripathi, V., & Miller, S. (2019). Trajectories of women's physical and psychosocial health following obstetric fistula repair in Uganda: A longitudinal study. *Tropical Medicine & International Health: TM & IH, 24*(1), 53–64. https://doi.org/10.1111/tmi.13178

Emasu, A., Ruder, B., Wall, L. L., Matovu, A., Alia, G., & Barageine, J. K. (2019). Reintegration needs of young women following genitourinary fistula surgery in Uganda. *International Urogynecology Journal, 30*(7), 1101–1110. https://doi.org/10.1007/s00192-019-03896-y

Gelaye, B., Williams, M. A., Lemma, S., Deyessa, N., Bahretibeb, Y., Shibre, T., Wondimagegn, D., Lemenhe, A., Fann, J. R., Stoep, A. V., & Zhou, X. A. (2013). Validity of the patient health questionnaire-9 for depression screening and diagnosis in East Africa. *Psychiatry Research, 210*(2), 653–661.

Gerten, K., Venkatesh, S., Norman, A., & Shu'aibu, J., Richter, H. (2009). Pilot study utilizing a patient educational brochure at a vesicovaginal fistula hospital in Nigeria, Africa. *International Urogynecology Journal and Pelvic Floor Dysfunction, 20*, 33–37.

Gharoro, E., & Agholor, K. (2009). Aspects of psychosocial problems of patients with vesicovaginal fistula. *Journal of Obstetrics & Gynaecology, 29*(7), 644–647.

Goffman, E. (1963). *Stigma: Notes on the management of spoiled identity*. Prentice-Hall.

Goh, J., Sloane, K., Krause, H., Browning, A., & Akhter, S. (2005). Mental health screening in women with genital tract fistulae. *BJOG: An International Journal of Obstetrics & Gynaecology, 112*(9), 1328–1330.

Hanlon, C., Medhin, G., Selamu, M., Breuer, E., Worku, B., Hailemariam, M., Lund, C., Prince, M., & Fekau, A. (2015). Validity of brief screening questionnaires to detect depression in primary care in Ethiopia. *Journal of Affective Disorders, 186*, 32–39.

Holzemer, W., Human, S., Arudo, J., Rosa, M., Hamilton, M., Corless, I., & Maryland, M. (2009). Exploring HIV stigma and quality of life for persons living with HIV infection. *Journal of the Association of Nurses in AIDS Care, 20*, 161–168. https://doi.org/10.1016/J.JANA.2009.02.002

Islam, A., & Begum, A. (1992). A psycho-social study on genito-urinary fistula. *Bangladesh Medical Research Council Bulletin, 18*(2), 82–94.

Johnson, K., Turan, J., Hailemariam, L., Mengsteab, E., Jena, D., & Polan, M. (2010). The role of counseling for obstetric fistula patients: Lessons learned from Eritrea. *Patient Education and Counseling, 80*, 262–265.

Kalilani-Phiri, L., Umar, E., Lazaro, D., Lunguzi, J., & Chilungo, A. (2010). Prevalence of obstetric fistula in Malawi. *International Journal of Gynaecology and Obstetrics, 109*(3), 204–208.

Kay, A., Nishimwe, A., & Hampton, B. (2015). Giving voice to the experiences of Rwandan women with urogenital fistula. *Annals of Global Health, 81*(5), 636–644.

Khisa, A., & Nyamongo, I. (2012). Still living with fistula, an exploratory study of the experience of women with obstetric fistula following corrective surgery in West Pokot Kenya. *Reproductive Health Matters, 20*(40), 59–66.

Kopp, D. M., Tang, J. H., Bengtson, A. M., Chi, B. H., Chipungu, E., Moyo, M., & Wilkinson, J. (2019). Continence, quality of life and depression following surgical repair of obstetric vesicovaginal fistula: A cohort study. *BJOG: An International Journal of Obstetrics and Gynaecology, 126*(7), 926–934. https://doi.org/10.1111/1471-0528.15546

Kroenke, K., Spitzer, R., & Williams, J. (2001). The PHQ-9: Validity of a brief depression severity measure. *Journal of General Internal Medicine, 16*(9), 606–613.

Lyimo, M. A., & Mosha, I. H. (2019). Reasons for delay in seeking treatment among women with obstetric fistula in Tanzania: A qualitative study. *BMC Women's Health, 19*(1), 93. https://doi.org/10.1186/s12905-019-0799-x

Manea, L., Gilbody, S., & McMillan, D. (2012). Optimal cut-off score for diagnosing depression with the patient health questionnaire (PHQ-9): A meta-analysis. *Canadian Medical Association Journal, 184*(3), E191–E196.

Markowitz, F. (1998). The effects of stigma on the psychological Well-being and life satisfaction of persons with mental illness. *Journal of Health and Social Behaviour, 39*(4), 335–347. https://doi.org/10.2307/2676342

Mehta, M., Bangser, M. (2006). *Risks and resilience: Obstetric fistula in Tanzania.* Dar es Salaam: Women's Dignity Project and Engender Health. Retrieved February 19, 2019, from https://www.engenderhealth.org/pubs/maternal/risk-resilience-fistula/

Mohamed, A. A., Ilesanmi, A. O., & Dairo, M. D. (2018). The experience of women with obstetric fistula following corrective surgery: A qualitative study in Benadir and Mudug regions, Somalia. *Obstetrics and Gynecology International, 2018*, 5250843. https://doi.org/10.1155/2018/5250843

Mselle, L., Moland, K., Evjen-Olsen, B., Mvungi, A., & Kohi, T. (2011). "I am nothing": Experiences of loss among women suffering from severe birth injuries in Tanzania. *BMC Women's Health, 11*, 49. https://doi.org/10.1186/1472-6874-11-49

Ojanuga, D. (1991). Preventing birth injury among women in Africa: Case studies in northern Nigeria. *American Journal of Orthopsychiatry, 61*(4), 533–539.

Ojengbede, O., Baba, Y., Morhason-Bello, I., Armah, M., Dimiti, A., Buwa, D., & Kariom, M. (2014). Group psychological therapy in obstetric fistula care: A complementary récipe for the accompanying mental ill health morbidities? *African Journal of Reproductive Health, 18*, 155–159.

Okoye, U., Emma-Echiegu, N., & Tanyi, P. (2014). Living with vesico-vaginal fistula: Experiences of women awaiting repairs in Ebonyi State. *Tanzania Journal of Health Research, 16*(4), 1–9.

Patel, V., Abas, M., Broadhead, J., Todd, C., & Reeler, A. (2001). Depression in developing countries: Lessons from Zimbabwe. *BMJ, 322*(7284), 482–484. https://doi.org/10.1136/bmj.322.7284.482

Patel, V., Todd, C., Winston, M., Gwanzura, F., Simunyu, E., Acuda, S., et al. (1998). The outcome of common mental disorders in Harare, Zimbabwe. *The British Journal of Psychiatry, 172*, 53–57.

Patel, V., Singh Goel, D., Desai, R. (2009). Scaling up services for mental and neurological disorders in low-resource settings. *International Health, 1*(1), 37–44.

Pope, R., Bangser, M., & Requejo, J. (2011). Restoring dignity: Social reintegration after obstetric fistula repair in Ukerewe, Tanzania. *Global Public Health, 6*(8), 859–873.

Schwatzmann, L. (2009). Research and action: Toward good quality of life and equity in health. *Expert Review of Pharmacoeconomics & Outcomes Research, 9*(2), 143–147. https://doi.org/10.1586/erp.09.3

Semere, L., & Nour, N. M. (2008). Obstetric fistula: Living with incontinence and shame. *Reviews in Obstetrics & Gynecology, 1*(4), 193–197.

Stokes, M. J., Wilkinson, J. P., Ganesh, P., Nundwe, W., & Pope, R. (2019). Persistent depression after obstetric fistula repair. *International Journal of Obstetrics and Gynaecology., 147*(2), 205–211.

Watt, M., Mosha, M., Platt, A., Sikkema, K., Wilson, S., Turner, E., & Masenga, G. (2017). A nurse-delivered mental health intervention for obstetric fistula patients in Tanzania: Results of a pilot randomized controlled trial. *Pilot Feasibility Study, 3*, 35. https://doi.org/10.1186/s40814-017-0178-z

Watt, M., Wilson, S., Sikkema, K., Velloza, J., Mosha, M., Masenga, G., Bangser, M., Browning, A., & Nyindo, P. (2015). Development of an intervention to improve mental health for obstetric fistula patients in Tanzania. *Evaluation and Program Planning, 50*, 1–9.

Weobong, B., ten Asbroek, A., Soremekun, S., Manu, A., Owusu-Agyei, S., Prince, M., & Kirkwood, B. (2014). Association of antenatal depression with adverse consequences for the mother and newborn in rural Ghana: Findings from the DON population-based cohort study. *PLoS One, 9*, 12.

Weston, K., Mutiso, S., Mwangi, J., Qureshi, Z., Beard, J., & Venkat, P. (2011). Depression among women with obstetric fistula in Kenya. *International Journal of Gynecology and Obstetrics, 115*, 31–33.

WHO. (2018). *Obstetric fistula.* World Health Organization Newsroom 19 February 2018. Retrieved from https://www.who.int/news-room/facts-in-pictures/detail/10-facts-on-obstetric-fistula

Wilson, S., Sikkema, K., Watt, M., & Masenga, G. (2015). Psychological symptoms among obstetric fistula patients compared to gynecology outpatients in Tanzania. *International Journal of Behavioral Medicine, 22*(5), 605–613. https://doi.org/10.1007/s12529-015-9466-2

Wilson, S., Sikkema, K., Watt, M., Masenga, G., & Mosha, M. (2016). Psychological symptoms and social functioning following repair of obstetric fistula in low-income setting. *Maternal and Child Health Journal, 20*(5), 941–945.

Yeakey, M., Chipeta, E., Taulo, F., & Tsui, A. (2009). The lived experience of Malawian women with obstetric fistula. *Culture, Health, and Sexuality, 11*(5), 499–513. https://doi.org/10.1080/13691050902874777

Zeleke, B., Ayele, T., Woldetsadik, M., Bisetegn, T., & Adane, A. (2013). Depression among women with obstetric fistula and pelvic organ prolapse in Northwest Ethiopia. *BMC Psychiatry, 13*, 236.

Theresa Spitznagle

32.1 Introduction

The inclusion of physical therapy in the care of women with obstetric fistula has the potential to greatly improve treatment outcomes. Currently up to 40% of women treated for obstetric fistula continue to experience residual urinary incontinence postsurgical repair, and as many as 10% of women continue to have lower extremity weakness and range of motion loss that affects their ability to function (Emasu et al., 2019; Nardos, Ayenachew, et al., 2020; Wall, 2016). In addition, many women report on-going pain and generalized weakness following fistula repair (El Ayadi et al., 2019). Postsurgical pain commonly is expected to improve as the tissues heal; however, nearly half of all women experience postpartum pelvic girdle or low back pain (Gutke et al., 2018; Manyozo et al., 2019), and thus, women with postfistula repair may also have pain due to the physical changes of pregnancy. In many regions of the world, fistula treatment is primarily focused on surgery and there is little attention paid or few resources devoted to treating ongoing physical issues women commonly experience after surgical repair. Incorporating physical therapy as an essential element to fistula treatment is a relatively low-cost method to greatly mitigate the lingering physical morbidities associated with obstetric fistula.

Physical therapy is a profession that identifies impairments within the movement system and provides individualized interventions with the goal of improving the way women move. Physical therapy interventions improve continence, physical function, and pain. Though high-resourced countries are likely to provide care for the physical impairments that arise from pregnancy and childbirth, there are continued gaps in this continuum. For example, despite endorsement by the American College of Gynecology (2018) to include physical therapy in the postpartum team, many medical professionals are still unaware of the benefits of physical therapy for women during pregnancy and postpartum

T. Spitznagle (✉)
Program in Physical Therapy, Department of Obstetrics and Gynecology, Washington University School of Medicine in St. Louis, St. Louis, MO, USA

Global Women's Health Initiative, Millis, MA, USA

Worldwide Fistula Fund, Schaumburg, IL, USA
e-mail: spitznaglet@wustl.edu

© Springer Nature Switzerland AG 2022
L. B. Drew et al. (eds.), *A Multidisciplinary Approach to Obstetric Fistula in Africa*, Global Maternal and Child Health, https://doi.org/10.1007/978-3-031-06314-5_32

phase of the childbearing year (Nielsen, 2010). In the case of obstetric fistula, this lack of awareness can be even more profound for several reasons. First, consider that the surgical training needed to care for women with obstetric fistula arises from multiple surgical perspectives, urology, gynecology, and colorectal surgery. During medical school training, each discipline will likely be exposed to physical therapy at varying levels, ranging from no exposure at all, a single lecture, or an integrated educational program that is interprofessional in nature. Combine this with the fact that many under-resourced countries have a limited number of physical therapists (Ago & John, 2017) and one can appreciate the difficulty of developing a physical therapy program for women with obstetric fistula. It should not go without recognition that physical therapy care for women is a relatively new specialty and thus many programs do not include the education for pregnancy and postpartum impairment's in entry level curriculums. Due to both the limited awareness of the benefits of physical therapy combined with the potential lack of infrastructure to sustain a program, finding an individual who can adequately deliver the care can be challenging. To establish a physical therapy program in conjunction with surgical treatment for obstetric fistula, supplemental education and mentoring is required. Programs that include physical therapy as part of the team caring for women with obstetric fistula have an overarching altruistic belief that women need support for their physical impairments both pre- and postsurgery as these impairments have a significant impact on their ability to fully reintegrate into society. Those who cannot engage in their communities due to limitations in walking, carrying, and sustaining a livelihood can greatly benefit from physical therapy services. The purpose of this chapter is to outline the spectrum of musculoskeletal issues that women with obstructed birth experience and to highlight the need and benefits of physical therapy for women with obstetric fistula. Current models of fistula care that include physical therapy are described with the hope of inspiring others to engage in developing programs for all women who suffer from obstetric fistula.

32.2   History of Physical Therapy for Childbirth Injuries

In 435 BC, Hippocrates was the first advocate for physical techniques to reduce pain or increase strength. However, it was not until 1916 during the polio epidemic that the profession of physical therapy or physiotherapy (European perspective) was birthed (Klinteberg, 1992). The scope of practice for physical therapy has since grown from a specialty trained technician who provided activities to reduce pain and improve strength to a doctoral prepared professional who has a full command of the human movement system. The care for women during pregnancy, labor and delivery, and postpartum has been an ongoing theme across the development of the profession (Bastiaanssen, de Bie, Bastiaenen, Essed, & van den Brandt, 2005; Bastiaanssen, de Bie, Bastiaenen, Heuts, et al., 2005). In the 1940s, with the recognition that assisted birth had several undesirable outcomes, there was a surge of avocation for natural childbirth. Both Britain and France lead this practice and included physical therapy as part of the labor and delivery team. The Lamaze technique, based on principles of Pavlovian Psychology, was originally developed in France and included a physical therapist as part of the antepartum preparation as well as labor and delivery (Tanzer, 1972). The engagement of physical therapists during antepartum and immediately postpartum care is still common in Europe, yet the same is not true for physical therapists educated in the United States (Boissonnault et al., 2020). In addition, physical therapy educational programs in high-resource countries typically provide basic information about pregnancy and childbirth. However, pelvic floor muscle examination and treatment (critical to obstetric fistula care) is rarely included in these curriculums (Boissonnault et al., 2020; Dockter et al., 2008). Physical therapists who choose to specialize in pelvic floor care in high-resource countries must seek training beyond their entry level education. Unfortunately, low-resource countries that have educational programs for physical therapy typically do not include education related to pregnancy or pelvic floor muscle impairments. For example, in Ethiopia there are several physical therapy educational programs that have both Bachelor's and Master's Degree Programs. However, only one program currently provides education on pregnancy (Mekelle University) and none provide specific pelvic floor muscle education. Thus, worldwide the numbers of physical therapists who are adequately educated about pelvic health remain stunted. The multifactorial needs of women with obstetric fistula require an understanding of the mechanism of the injury and the physical impairments that occur to both external and internal pelvic structures. Educational programs in physical therapy worldwide adequately prepare physical therapists with the skills needed to treat external impairments associated with obstetric fistula. There is a need however, to bridge the knowledge gap related to the internal impairments associated with physical therapy for obstetric fistula.

32.3   Etiology of Physical Impairments Associated with Obstetric Fistula

The loss of bladder control is well documented in women with obstetric fistula. The mechanical pressure of the child unable to successfully navigate the birth canal causes vascular, neural, and connective tissue compromise. There is a spectrum of changes that occurs in the pelvic region due to a physical stress of a vaginal birth. On one end of the spectrum, prolonged labor can result in birth-related neural compression, pelvic muscle weakness with associated pelvic organ prolapse, or incontinence disorders. On the other end of the spectrum, full compromise of the tissue occurs to the point of necrosis (Wall, 2012). The sustained compression of an obstructed birth results in injury to the internal iliac artery and vein causing secondary damage to the lumbosacral neural plexus and muscles of the pelvis and lower limb. The resulting pelvic and limb weakness is most consistently reported to be on the right leg. The vascular supply to the limbs typically is not arranged at the mid line of the body but is shifted to the right side of the spine, thus, pressure on the right internal vessels as they enter the pelvis sustains a greater amount of physical stress. Foot drop during gait is the most common reported impairment that results (Arrowsmith et al., 1996). This gait pattern illustrates a sparing of the hip flexors as the patient is commonly able to lift the leg; however, distal limb weakness prevents control of the ankle and thus the foot slaps or drops once the heel hits the ground. Less commonly recognized, simply due to the limb being obscured by clothing, is atrophy that presents in the thigh and buttock. Due to the ischemia occurring at the level of the pelvis, it is logical that the more proximal muscles would also be compromised. Other less commonly reported symptoms in women who present with obstetric fistula include poor tolerance to limb dependency in the initial phases of recovery and neuropathic pain.

32.4   Physical Therapy for Obstetric Fistula

Surgical repair of an obstetric fistula can successfully reverse a tragic situation. Even though there may be underlying persistent leg weakness and functional activity loss due to pain, many women recover physically enough to return to their communities. Unfortunately, as many as 40% of all obstetric fistula repairs result in a surgically closed fistula but a "wet" patient, meaning they have postfistula repair incontinence (Nardos, 2020; Wall, 2016). This can be utterly devastating as the social stigma of being wet is why they mustered the moral courage to initially seek care. Physical therapy for urinary and fecal incontinence due to an underlying postpartum pelvic muscle weakness has been demonstrated to be quite successful (Ptak et al., 2019; Wein, 2012). Pelvic floor muscle impairments in women who have incurred an obstetric fistula have not been fully studied but are believed to be present (Brook, 2019; Castille et al., 2015; Keyser et al., 2014). The scope of the physical therapy care needed for women who have suffered obstetric fistula requires an understanding of the state of the tissues, the status of the women's presenting movement impairments, and the ability to provide culturally competent care. Table 32.1 provides a comprehensive list of interventions that may be warranted for women who have sustained an obstetric fistula. In addition, consideration of a comprehensive

Table 32.1 Physical therapy interventions for obstetric fistula

Intervention	Description	Rationale
Strengthening/stretching exercises	Abdominal muscles Hip extensors/hip lateral rotator Knee extensors and flexors Ankle Dorsi and plantar flexion, toe intrinsic strengthening Coordination exercises for the pelvic floor muscles: exhale draw in abdomen and contract your pelvic floor muscles, inhale relax both	Postpartum abdominal weakness and L5-sacral dermatomal/peripheral nerve weakness Vascular compromise due to compression of the internal and external iliac vessels Loss of coordination occurs commonly postpartum
Aerobic exercises	Group classes: dance class, mat classes for general exercise Bike or walking in the parallel bars if too weak to walk without devices	Especially needed if have been immobile due to fear of worsening fistula but also for self-efficacy/well-being
Gait training	Walker, crutches, heel lift, brace for foot drop or Functional electrical stimulation for foot drop	Possible postpartum pelvic girdle instability, LE weakness due to vascular compromise
Use of supports	Abdominal binders and SIJ belts as needed for pain and gait instability	Abdominal wall lengthening due to pregnancy or pelvic instability due to pregnancy and vaginal delivery
Pelvic floor-specific modalities	Electrical stimulation for pelvic floor muscle strengthening grades 100 Hz or greater (200 Hz or higher is typically more comfortable) Biofeedback for pelvic floor muscle activation: perianal electrodes can be used preoperatively	Electric stimulation requires a muscle grade range from a flicker to 2/5. (nerve has to be intact for success) Biofeedback requires a muscle grade of 2/5–4/5
Vaginal dilators	Used for stenosis of the vagina, pelvic muscle stretching or passive relaxation with dilator in place	Common postoperative complication due to fibrosis
Diaphragmatic breathing exercises	Inhale, abdomen lifts Exhale, abdomen lowers Inhale, pelvic floor relaxes Exhale, pelvic floor contracts	Used for overactive pelvic floor and abdominal muscles as well as used for sympathetic nervous system quieting
Soft tissue mobilization of the pelvic floor	Manually or with a wand	Indications are muscle spasm, vaginal stenosis or scars
Functional activity training	Emphasis on avoiding breath holding and improving coordination of the abdominals, pelvic floor during specific functional activities	Practice with supine to sit, sit to stand, rolling, and lifting, cough, mechanics of bowel movement, squat, culturally specific activities
Urologic/vagina-specific patient education	Patient education for: 1. Self-catheterization 2. Use of urethral plugs 3. Use of pessaries 4. Stoma care	Commonly performed by continence nurses, this is a cross over skill that a physical therapist can be trained to perform

clinical pathway is needed to provide insight as to when physical therapy should be considered for women with obstetric fistula. There are acute needs immediately after the development of the fistula as the tissue changes can be quite rapid (Labbe et al., 1987). Early mobilization is paramount to avoiding secondary weakness, fibrosis, and connective tissue changes (Morris et al., 2010). Thus, preoperative care should be implemented even though the fistula itself has not yet been repaired. Postoperative care in the acute phase is needed to prevent effects of bed rest and postsurgical complications including pneumonia, constipation, and muscle weakness. Finally, ongoing outpatient care postsurgery is warranted for those with presenting weakness, gait instabilities, pain, and lower urinary tract symptoms, including urgency and stress urinary or fecal incontinence.

Understanding the mechanisms of injury and state of the tissues will help guide physical therapists in the future. Thus, careful documentation of the physical therapy examination, including parameters that capture changes in muscle strength (dynamometry, manual muscle testing, or circumferential measurements of the limbs), muscle length (hip, knee, and ankle range of motion), sensation loss (light touch, joint position sense, and balance), and functional movement impairments (bending, lifting, squatting, walking, child care) combined with an objective report on the response to care is desperately needed to inform future clinical decision-making. There are very few population-specific outcome measures that have been validated for women with obstetric fistula. One such measure was developed at the Hamlin Fistula Hospital specifically for incontinence postsurgical repair (Keyser et al., 2014). In addition, pain and endurance outcome measures should be considered. Due to the high prevalence of pelvic girdle pain during the childbearing year (Albert et al., 2006) (see following discussion), the Pelvic Girdle Pain Questionnaire is a logical measure to consider. It has been validated in pregnancy and postpartum women in both high- and low-resource countries (Ogollah et al., 2019). The Oswestry Low Back Disability Scale (Elden et al., 2016) has been found to be reliable in multiple languages, thus could be considered for demonstrating change when low back pain is present. A ten-minute walk test (Evensen et al., 2015, 2016), a timed up and go (Christensen, Vollestad, et al., 2019), or a sit to stand test (Yenisehir et al. 2020) could all be utilized for documentation of endurance, these measures are simple to execute and will likely be feasible in low-resourced countries. Lastly, for an ongoing pain measure one should consider the use of visual face chart for pain so that spoken language barriers can be minimized (Kim et al., 2017).

32.4.1 Physical Therapy Treatment of Postfistula Repair Incontinence

One aspect of pelvic floor muscle interventions that has been consistently deployed postfistula repair is exercises, specifically Kegel exercises. Women are commonly instructed to begin Kegel exercises, or contracting their pelvic floor muscles, in the acute postsurgical phase of care while the catheter is still placed. Classically pelvic floor muscle exercises are prescribed for stress urinary incontinence; there is an underlying assumption that the pelvic floor muscles are weak and not able to contract adequately to retain urine when the trunk is pressurized. However, there is emerging evidence that focusing on the contraction of the muscle without regard to the state of the muscle performance can be deleterious to those presenting with pelvic floor-related issues like urinary incontinence or constipation. Focusing on strengthening may be aggravating to the patient if they are presenting with a non-relaxing pelvic floor muscle (Spitznagle et al., 2017). To address this, coordination of the pelvic floor muscle is emerging as an intervention for bowel, bladder, and intercourse-related pelvic floor muscle impairments. Interventions are now focused on regaining control over the ability to relax the pelvic floor muscle instead of the ability to contract the muscle, thus improving functional activities like voiding or intercourse. This shift in knowledge should also be considered when treating women with an obstetric fistula. Interestingly, there are limited studies that actually indicate that in women with obstetric fistula, the pelvic floor muscle truly has a force production deficit warranting strengthening. There have been only three published studies that have documented the physical therapy care of women with fistula (Castille et al., 2014, 2015; Keyser et al., 2014). All three studies had a multimodal approach including patient education on body mechanics and active exercises that included a strengthening program for the pelvic floor muscle. All three studies reported positive outcomes for postsurgical stress incontinence; however, these limited number of studies make it quite difficult to provide evidence-based recommendation for what to expect when examining the pelvic floor muscles of women who have sustained an obstetric fistula.

In my personal observations, examining women who presented with postfistula repair incontinence at the Hamlin Fistula Hospital in Addis Ababa in 2011, several themes emerged. All of the cases I observed were greater than a year from their original obstructed birth and all had either a bladder or urethral compliance issue requiring the use of a urethral plug or a "believed stress urinary incontinence". First, I was taken aback by the rigidity of the patients' tissues when palpated with a transvaginal examination; not only were there several patients with an exceptionally narrowed introitus, barely being able to place an index finger into the vagina, but also there was no palpable contraction. It is very difficult to ascertain all the reasons for the rigidity; the tissues felt similar to tissues that have undergone radiation and fibrosis of the connective tissue have occurred. The effect of surgery in the region could cause scarring, but one cannot discount that the tissue rigidity may be due to the obstructed birth itself as this would cause prolonged compression or loss of blood supply for an extended period of time. My observations are well supported by descriptive reports related to obstetric fistula. Vaginal scarring is considered a common finding in obstetric fistula patients and has been reported as one of the factors that influence the outcome of surgeries (Carey et al., 2002; Schleicher et al., 1993). Tissue fibrosis, vaginal narrowing, and dyspareunia have been reported postrepair (Arrowsmith et al., 1996). For the cases I observed at the Hamlin Fistula Hospital, the focus of care was on strengthening the pelvic floor muscle with no soft tissue management of the ridged scared vaginal tissues. Thus, future considerations for care should include a protocol for early intervention to affect the scarring, as myofascial mobilization of the soft tissues in the vaginal and rectal region may mitigate some of the tissue stiffness. Soft tissue mobilization has been found to improve tissues in patient who have undergone pelvic radiation (Bruner et al., 1993; Robinson et al., 1999), thus it is reasonable that postfistula repair, women with ridged pelvic floor muscles would benefit from being taught self-soft tissue mobilization, either stretching manually with their own thumb or with a dilator to reduce rigidity in the tissues. This observation highlights a key point for those who aspire to treat pelvic floor muscle impairments in women with fistula, do not assume the pelvic floor muscles are weak, but instead do a physical examination and determine the presence of scar tissue, the stiffness of the tissues and the ability to contract and relax the pelvic floor muscle. Treatment should be based on what is found on examination. More research is needed to objectively identify pelvic muscle stiffness, strength, and coordination in women with fistula. Consideration of the length of time since injury and the state of the tissues are critical for success.

Finally, I believe it important to mention that a physical therapist should understand the type and method of repair of an obstetric fistula. This information allows the ability to correlate the functional impairments of the women with state of the pelvic musculature. For example, several surgeries have been described for postfistula repair incontinence that utilize muscle flaps from remnants of pelvic muscles (bulbospongiousus and pubococcygeus) or use of hip muscles (gracilis) or a fascial graft from either fibrotic vaginal tissue or the tensor fascia lata (Arrowsmith et al., 1996). Communication with the surgical team is paramount to successful understanding of the functional implications of the loss of these tissues.

32.5   Musculoskeletal Changes Due to Pregnancy and Obstructed Birth

All women who develop an obstetric fistula were once pregnant, and an appreciation of the state of the female musculoskeletal system during pregnancy and postpartum is needed to better understand the scope of the physical impairments women with obstetric fistula may face. When a woman becomes pregnant, her physical status undergoes an amazing transformation. Postural adjustments, muscle length, and strength changes as well as bony adaptions occur to accommodate the growth of the fetus and prepare the mother for delivery. Because of the physical changes of pregnancy, all women are at risk for back and pelvic girdle pain (Albert et al., 2006; Bastiaanssen, de Bie, Bastiaenen, Essed, & van den Brandt, 2005; Bastiaanssen, de Bie, Bastiaenen, Heuts, et al., 2005), and other musculoskeletal impairments associated with weight gain and hormonally mediated connective tissue laxities (Casagrande et al., 2015; Prather et al., 2012).

32.5.1   Postural Changes

Normal weight gain during pregnancy will cause an increased mechanical stress on the lower extremities and spine. As the uterus enlarges, there is a consequential postural shift to accommodate the center of mass changes. Thus, women will commonly present with progressive increase in lumbar lordosis, posterior trunk sway, subsequent knee hyperextension, and plantarflexion across their pregnancy.[1] Increased motion into flexion in the thoracic region of the spine can be observed as the enlarged uterus causes a reduction of lumbar spine motion, women will tend to flex in the thoracic region at the pivot point where the uterus stopped growing. Mid-pregnancy, the lumbar spine becomes more stable and the thoracic region tends to be the site of too much mobility. These motion and postural changes happen gradually; however, they are superimposed during a time when the connective tissues that support the limbs and pelvis are hormonally undergoing relaxation to allow for the delivery of the fetus. Thus, without specific education on exercises for trunk alignment, postural changes can persist beyond pregnancy into the postpartum phase of the childbearing year. Awareness of these changes so that one can screen for them is an important starting point when performing a physical therapy examination for women with obstetric fistula.

32.5.2   Bone Changes

Typical bony changes associated with pregnancy should also be considered when examining women with obstetric fistula. For example, widening of the ribcage to accommodate the enlarging uterus occurs prior to delivery. The rib angle can widen up to 30 degrees from a standard of a 70- to 80-degree angle in nonpregnant women (LoMauro & Aliverti, 2015). This widening creates an unstable base for both the diaphragm and the abdominal muscles, contributing to postpartum abdominal and trunk muscle weakness. Not only does the ribcage widen in pregnancy but also typically does the pelvis in order to prepare the mother for delivery, pelvic ring widening most typically occurs due to relaxation of the ligamentous structure. The second bony change that should be considered also occurs within the pelvic ring. Due to the mechanics of a vaginal delivery, pubic bone bruising has been reported (Brandon et al., 2012). In obstetric fistula, due to the potential that the pelvic outlet has not widened

---

[1]Lumbar lordosis is an exaggeration of the arch in the low back, trunk sway is typically described as a posterior shift of the upper trunk backward, knee hyper extension is a position of the knees beyond the normal straight position, and plantar flexion is a term used to describe the position of the foot beyond the normal 90° needed to stand upright.

sufficiently to accommodate the fetal head, it should be considered that pubic bone bruising has occurred. Lastly, due to the need to sustain appropriate nutrition for the mother, some women incur osteopenia[2] during pregnancy (Boissonnault & Boissonnault, 2001) and are at risk for stress fractures of the femoral neck or pubic rim. Though each of the changes to bone is transient, if a woman with obstetric fistula presents with pain with walking over the pubic arch, deep in the groin or along the sacrum and they have a high physical demand and/or poor nutrition, a bone bruise or fracture should be considered as the source of the pain.

32.5.3 Gait Changes in Pregnancy

Gait instabilities can occur during pregnancy due to both weight gain and ligamentous laxity. Specifically, difficulty with load transfer of the weight of the trunk onto a limb during walking occurs due to instability of the sacroiliac joints or pubis (Vleeming et al., 2008). Increased trunk motion and reduce speed of walking have been reported in normal pregnancy (Christensen, Veierod, et al., 2019; Christensen, Vollestad, et al., 2019; Wu et al., 2008). Combine the normal changes in gait during pregnancy with the potential bruising of the pubic bone (as noted previously) and the coinciding vascular trauma that induces lower extremity muscle weakness in women with obstetric fistula and one can better understand why these women can present with profound gait abnormalities. Unfortunately, self-imposed bed rest is commonly reported among women with fistula who live in remote regions, both as a response to the emotional devastation of fistula and the hope that if they "stay still" the fistula will heal on its own. Pain with walking or complaints of gait instability have not been well documented; however, in Ethiopia it is not uncommon to have a family member physically carry the women to the hospital for care. It is feasible that this lack of ability to walk is due to the physical trauma induced during the obstructed birth. Lower limb contractures due to this self-imposed bed rest are an unfortunate side effect of the self-imposed bed rest and require adequate physical therapy interventions to address.

32.5.4 Muscle Changes Associated with Pregnancy

Lastly, there are several muscular changes associated with pregnancy that warrant discussion. Abdominal muscle weakness is common postpartum due to the mechanical lengthening incurred while the uterus is enlarging. The relative mechanical strain of the abdominal muscle presents with changes that are associated with denervation, including fatty infiltrate and loss of fascial integrity. Postpartum, the return to normal function of the abdominal muscles does not always occur. Binding of the abdomen postpartum may be needed to act as a stimulus to support the abdominal wall and encourage muscle activity with the hope of improving muscle length over time. Development of a diastasis recti abdominis (DRA), a split in the rectus abdominis muscle due to the internal pressure of the growing uterus, is commonly reported pregnancy-related muscle impairment. Regardless if a woman has had an uncomplicated delivery or an obstructed delivery and is now suffering from a fistula, this muscle impairment will likely be present. It is important to screen for DRA in women with fistula as it has been associated with not only abdominal muscle weakness but also support related impairments such as urinary and fecal incontinence or pelvic organ prolapse (Spitznagle et al., 2007). Thus, persistent abdominal wall weakness may be one possible factor why women present with stress urinary incontinence postfistula repair.

---

[2]Low bone mineral density.

Finally, the most commonly occurring musculoskeletal change associated with pregnancy is in the pelvic floor muscles. During an uncomplicated vaginal birth, there are several impairments that will occur. Immediately postpartum, there are acute pain and edema that occur due to the compression on the vasculature and soft tissues. There is the possibility of perineal tissue tearing or intentional cutting (episiotomy) to assist the passage of the baby's head. There is lengthening of the connective tissues and thinning of the pelvic floor muscles. These changes have been suggested to occur due to the mechanics of childbirth, muscle lengthening, and compression from the head of infant.

32.5.5 Postpartum Incontinence

Pelvic muscle lengthening and weakness are associated with postpartum incontinence—not only are the supportive structures of the organs compromised but also the mechanism of the urethra is also affected (Brincat et al., 2011). There is strong evidence to support the use of pelvic floor muscle training to improve stress urinary incontinence (Bo & Herbert, 2013). However, postpartum urinary incontinence continues to be poorly understood; the benefits of the pelvic floor muscle exercise may have more to do with the secondary improvement in neurological control and less to do with the improvements in pelvic muscle performance. Unfortunately, there is a percentage of women who deliver vaginally, who develop postpartum incontinence, and do not respond to pelvic floor muscle training. Thus, in the case of obstetric fistula, the relative sparing of the urethra after the trauma of the birth is critical for successful resolution of continence regardless of the performance of the pelvic muscles. Just to reiterate, in the case of obstructed birth, the compression injury to the tissues is prolonged and thus the extent of the tissue damage is more profound. Women with obstetric fistulas will present with varying degrees of pelvic muscle impairment based on the severity of the presenting fistula (Dietz & Williams, 2012).

32.5.6 Postpartum Pelvic Girdle Pain

Due to the ligamentous laxity of pregnancy and the mechanical trauma of an obstructed birth, pain will likely be present. Physical therapy for pregnancy-related pelvic girdle pain has been found to be effective in reducing pain and improving function (Shiri et al., 2018). Thus, due to precipitating events that cause obstetric fistula, women should be examined with the intent of ruling out pelvic girdle pain as a moderator to their care. Key exam items to determine the presence of load transfer impairment are needed. Specifically the following should be considered: palpation of the posterior SIJ and pubic symphysis; pelvic alignment: single leg stance for movement and then the Stork test (Hungerford et al., 2007) for pelvic-specific mechanical assessment; FABER test to assess pelvic versus hip pain; posterior pelvic thrust test (Vleeming et al., 2008) specific for the sacroiliac joint; forward bending and return and trunk rotation to rule out spine-mediated pain (Van Dillen et al., 2003); pelvic compression in standing supine and with leg motions (Vleeming et al., 2008) to determine the need for belting. In the presence of pelvic girdle pain, stabilization exercises should be started and if not tolerated then a gentle joint mobilization to correct the presenting positional impairment can be utilized. Long-term use of mobilization is not warranted in a postpartum population; however, one or two bouts may be needed prior to tolerating the stabilization exercises. Gait instabilities in women with obstetric fistula may be greatly improved if the clinician recognizes the pelvic girdle load transfer impairment is the driver in this impairment.

32.6   Strategies for Successful Implementation of a Physical Therapy Program

A purposeful introduction of physical therapy to the existing medical staff is critical for the successful implementation of a physical therapy program. Interprofessional engagement is emerging in high-resourced countries as a core criterium for ongoing programmatic quality improvement and patient-specific care plan management. Due to lack of exposure to the discipline of physical therapy during training, many healthcare providers do not know the scope of the practice of a physical therapist. Thus, regular contact of the team in patient-specific settings will allow the opportunity to exchange ideas and educate the care team. Surgeons, nurses, and counseling staff benefit from the engagement and this can facilitate communication in the future. Allowing time for the physical therapist to observe the processes of the hospital, intake, preop screening, surgery, postop care as provided across all disciplines will provide each team member the ability to highlight what they do and provide an opportunity for learning about physical therapy. Creating a culture such that the physical therapist is comfortable communicating with each team member is paramount to successful integration of the service and will improve quality of patient care over time.

Ongoing engagement once the basic observations have occurred can include participation of the physical therapist in postop patient rounds, team care planning meetings, and discharge planning. Though the fistula patient may be surgically ready to go home, additional time may be needed to finalize the home exercise program and provide patient education related to modifying functional activities that increase abdominal pressure. Learning these motor control strategies are critical for protecting the surgical site. Allowing the physical therapist to be present for discharge planning will aide in understanding if the patient is physically ready for return to her home environment. Thus, common patient outcomes can more easily be managed as a team. For example, it is becoming widely accepted that pain is the fifth vital sign and should be monitored by all team members. Standardizing a pain rating scale for monitoring pain either by way of a body diagram or face rating scale (Kim et al., 2017) may be helpful not only because the population served may not be literate but also so that each team member provides a consistent assessment of pain. Other hospital system-wide educational contributions that the physical therapist can provide to the staff as a whole include: body mechanic education, safe strategies for moving patients including rolling, bed mobility, and postoperative ambulation, and supportive coughing and chest wall percussion education for nursing staff.

32.7   Models of Care for Physical Therapy Services

The first documented hospital system that provided comprehensive care for women with obstetric fistula is in Ethiopia. Designed by Reginald and Catherine Hamlin in the 1950s, the Hamlin Fistula Hospital System (HFH, 2020) employs a holistic approach to the care of the women, including surgical care, pre- and postoperative physical therapy, counseling, and community reintegration (Nardos, Ayenachew, et al., 2020). Critically, the Hamlin Fistula Hospital was the first to provide both aspects of physical therapy care needed for women with obstetric fistula: (1) physical rehabilitation program for extra pelvic/lower limb impairments and (2) continence program for intrapelvic impairments to address the postsurgical incontinence. Since the Hamlin's groundbreaking work, fistula treatment programs have developed in other parts of the world, yet the inclusion of physical therapy is rare and continues to be dependent on the awareness of the surgical team of the benefits of physical therapy. Several models of care that include physical therapy for women with obstetric fistula have since developed, with differing implementation considerations for each.

32.7.1 Fistula Hospital System

A fistula hospital system is a model of care that includes a central or main hospital with several peripheral centers within one region or country. The Hamlin Fistula Hospital system, as noted above, is an example of an established countrywide hospital system. This fistula hospital system has a centralized hospital designed for more complicated cases and several regional centers strategically built in varied regions of Ethiopia. The surgical care is coordinated by a lead surgeon who oversees the program as a whole, and local surgeons who work at the region centers. Similarly, a locally bachelors trained physical therapist who has obtained specialty education related to pelvic health manages the physical therapy services across the entire system. The peripheral centers relay on physical therapy extenders to provide basic exercises and postsurgical ambulation. (See below for more detail on physical therapy extenders). One benefit to this model of care is that protocols for care standardization can be developed and implemented across the entire system. In an attempt to improve educational gaps in knowledge, there are ongoing exchanges with visiting physical therapy educators from a variety of countries (Australia, England, Germany, New Zealand, United States, etc.). One challenge to this, however, is that physical therapy practice is based on the standards of the country of origin and thus there are differences in professional opinion which can create confusion on treatment strategies. For the Hamlin Fistula Hospital system, the use of a bachelors trained physical therapist as the manager of the physical therapy program is a shift from their prior model where a nurse was recruited and trained to lead the physical therapy program. Many low-resourced countries now have or are starting physical therapy educational programs, thus, hiring a medical professional specific to the discipline will likely be more common in the future.

32.7.2 Physical Therapy Extenders

A physical therapy extender is a trained aide who can execute basic treatments that are designed by the supervising physical therapist. For the Hamlin Fistula Hospital system, physical therapy extenders are utilized both at the central hospital as well as in the regional settings. The training of the physical therapy extender is the responsibility of the managing physical therapist who does yearly site visits to all of the regional centers. At the regional sites, the head nurse is responsible for supervision of the physical therapy extender when the physical therapist is not onsite. Thus, documentation of the skills taught and proper communication to the management team at the center regarding scope of the training are paramount to program efficacy and safety. A full understanding by the supervisory nurse of the scope of the physical therapy extender education is required for safe application of this model. It is important to emphasize that, treatment techniques are learned but only administered after the supervising nurse or physical therapist has evaluated the patient and has determined the initial plan of care. One benefit from this model is that the personnel recruited to fill these roles may provide employment for someone from the region who is fluent in local dialects and could potentially assist with translation during care. A second benefit as mentioned earlier is related to the consistent message shared on the methods of physical therapy skill delivery for all who work within the system. With a consistent message, institutional knowledge can be retained and culturally competent care can be more consistently delivered. A challenge to this system is that if a woman needs more skilled physical therapy care, she is required to either wait for the managing physical therapist to visit or travel to the main fistula care center.

Implementation of a program that utilizes physical therapy extenders requires the identification of an individual who has the following characteristics: (1) the capacity to communicate well with the women being served, (2) has ties to the region so to improve the likelihood that they would remain engaged at the center, and (3) has the ability to understand, retain, and demonstrate safe execution of the skills taught prior to being able to independently work with the women. Box 32.1 provides a suggested modified pelvic floor muscle assessment for pelvic floor muscle treatment executed by a physical therapy extender. It is important to note that in many regions of the world, a male caregiver will not be culturally accepted due to the nature of the conditions that the women are being treated; women will not want a male extender to do vaginal examinations and treatment. Training a female nurse to provide the care has been utilized successfully in several remote centers. Another potential physical therapy extender is an obstetric fistula survivor who has been through physical rehabilitation.

Box 32.1 Modified Pelvic Muscle Examination: Designed To Use When Training an Extender
Will need a private room/screen for privacy, appropriate table, light, and drape

1. Explain rationale for exam and obtain patient consent.
2. Use a lubricated glove for the exam.
3. Place gloved finger into vaginal with the pad of the finger down: ask the following.
4. Do you feel my finger?
5. Does it hurt? Require the examiner to inquire about openness to report pain,
    i.e., Will you honestly report pain to me? Please share if pain is present it help me understand how to help you
6. Touch all regions of vaginal area sweeping first from the top right side of the vaginal vault to the midline and then top left of vaginal vault to midline using your finger as a guide for depth of palpation. (First layer at the first bend in finger, second layer at second bend in finger, and third layer at third bend in finger).
    (a) Feel for scars or "rings of tissue", nodules or tender bumps, or area's that do not feel smooth.
    (b) Record what you feel on a paper image of the pelvic muscles.
7. Ask patient to squeeze on your finger: Record number of contractions up to at best performance level that can be done in 10 s.
    0: no contraction.
    1: contraction present no lift.
    2: contraction present and lift present.

32.7.3 Stand-Alone Regional Fistula Centers

A regional fistula center is a treatment center that may exist as a stand-alone center or as an outpost of a hospital system dedicated to the care of women with birth-related injuries. The Danja Fistula Center in Niger (Worldwide Fistula Fund, 2020) is an example of a dedicated regional obstetric fistula care center that stands alone and is not associated with a system of hospitals. Construction of this fistula center was funded by the Worldwide Fistula Fund (WFF) in partnership with SIM International (SIM, 2020) in 2012. The surgical center was designed to support an onsite surgeon, nursing staff for pre- and postoperative cases, rehabilitation (Physical Therapy), reintegration, and social services. Since opening, the WFF has provided ongoing funding while the SIM organization has been the on-the-ground management and operations partner. SIM provides daily oversight and staffing (local and missionary staff) by leveraging local relationships developed over their 70-year presence in Niger.

SIM has an extensive history as an international missionary organization working with underserved populations in Africa since 1902. The SIM organization has a tremendous ability to: (1) recruit medically trained personnel to work in this remote area of the world, (2) provide language training for assistance in local language development for those recruited, and (3) ensure long term commitments to the center that allow for program development over time. Upon opening this fistula center, the physical therapy services were initially provided by an orthopedic physical therapist from Canada, also a dedicated SIM missionary, who trained in the specialty of pelvic health in order to serve at the center. There are some significant challenges to consider in relationship to a stand-alone treatment center like the Danja Fistula Center: (1) centers may be located in remote areas, thus transportation of supportive resources and personnel can be difficult, (2) without connection to a system of hospitals for referrals, patient recruitment must be done solely based on the personnel resources of the hospital, and finally, (3) there can be a loss of institutional knowledge when any one missionary completes their time of service and returns home. To balance these issues and create a more sustainable program, The Danja Fistula Center has informally partnered with the adjacent Leprosy Center staff with an attempt to utilize a locally trained physical therapist to work with the lower extremity impairments that commonly occur as a result of arrested birth. The managemant at the Danja Fistula cetner has also been successful with developing a partnership with a Physical Therapy School in Niger to host "students" at the center so that others may learn about the care of women with obstetric fistula. Finally, they have attempted to recruit more than one missionary physical therapist at a time, in order to provide an overlap in services and stabilize institutional knowledge.

32.8 Conclusion

Despite considerable challenges, several physical therapy programs for women with obstetric fistula have been successfully implemented in low-resourced regions of the world. There is a full spectrum of movement impairments that persist in women with obstetric fistula not only due to the obstructed birth but also due to the fact that they were once pregnant. Thus, the scope of the physical therapy care needed for women who have suffered obstetric fistula requires understanding of the state of the tissues, the status of the women's presenting movement impairments, and the need to provide culturally competent care in the region that one is working. I hope this chapter increases awareness for the need for physical therapy for women with obstetric fistula and inspires others to engage in developing programs for all women who suffer from childbirth injuries.

References

Ago, A. O., & John, E. B. (2017). Occupational therapy and physiotherapy education and workforce in Anglophone sub-Sahara African countries. *Human Resources for Health, 15*(1), 37.

Albert, H. B., Godskesen, M., Korsholm, L., & Wetergarrd, J. G. (2006). Risk factors in developing pregnancy-related pelvic girdle pain. *Acta Obstetricia Gynecologia Scandinavia, 85*(5), 539–544.

American College of Gynecology. (2018). Committee on obstetric practice: Optimizing postpartum care. *ACOG, 151*, 140–150.

Arrowsmith, S., Hamlin, E. C., & Wall, L. L. (1996). Obstructed labor injury complex: Obstetric fistula formation and the multifaceted morbidity of maternal birth trauma in the developing world. *Obstetric Gynecology Survey, 51*(9), 568–574.

Bastiaanssen, J. M., de Bie, R. A., Bastiaenen, C. H., Essed, G. G., & van den Brandt, P. A. (2005). A historical perspective on pregnancy-related low back and/or pelvic girdle pain. *European Journal of Obstetric and Gynecology Reproductive Biology, 120*(1), 3–14.

Bastiaanssen, J. M., de Bie, R. A., Bastiaenen, C. H., Heuts, A., Kroese, M. E., Essed, G. G., & van den Brandt, P. A. (2005). Etiology and prognosis of pregnancy-related pelvic girdle pain; design of a longitudinal study. *British Medical Central Public Health, 5,* 1.

Bo, K., & Herbert, R. D. (2013). There is not yet strong evidence that exercise regimens other than pelvic floor muscle training can reduce stress urinary incontinence in women: A systematic review. *Journal of Physiotherapy, 59*(3), 159–168.

Boissonnault, J. S., Kuhn, A., Meeker, M., Strong, S., & Stephenson, R. G. (2020). An international survey of women's and pelvic health physical therapy organizational practice. *Journal of Women's Health Physical Therapy, 44*(4), 160–175.

Boissonnault, W. G., & Boissonnault, J. S. (2001). Transient osteoporosis of the hip associated with pregancy. *The Journal of Orthopaedic and Sports Physical Therapy, 31*(7), 359–367.

Brandon, C., Low, J. J., Park, L. K., DeLancey, J. O., & Miller, J. (2012). Pubic bone injuries in primiparous women: Magnetic resonance imaging in detection and differential diagnosis of structural injury. *Ultrasound Obstetrics Gynecology, 39*(4), 441–451.

Brincat, C. A., Delancey, J. O., & Miller, J. M. (2011). Urethral closure pressures among primiparous women with and without levator ani muscle defects. *International Urogynecology Journal, 22*(12), 1491–1495.

Brook, G. (2019). Obstetric fistula: The role of physiotherapy: A report from the physiotherapy Committee of the International Continence Society. *Neurourology and Urodynamics, 38*(1), 407–416.

Bruner, D. W., Keegan, L. R., Corn, M., Martin, B., & Hanks, G. E. (1993). Vaginal stenosis and sexual function following intracavitary radiation for the treatment of cervical and endometrial carcinoma. *International Journal of Radiation Oncology Biology Physics, 27*(4), 825–830.

Carey, M. P., Goh, J. T., Fynes, M. M., & Murray, C. J. (2002). Stress urinary incontinence after delayed primary closure of genitourinary fistula: A technique for surgical management. *American Journal of Obstetrics and Gynecology, 186*(5), 948–953.

Casagrande, D., Gugala, Z. C., & S. M. and Lindsey R. W. (2015). Low back pain and pelvic girdle pain in pregnancy. *Journal of the American Academy of Orthopedic Surgery, 23*(9), 539–549.

Castille, Y. J., Avocetien, C., Zaongo, D., Colas, J. M., Peabody, J. O., & Rochat, C. H. (2014). Impact of a program of physiotherapy and health education on the outcome of obstetric fistula surgery. *International Jounal of Gynaecology and Obstetrics, 124*(1), 77–80.

Castille, Y. J., Avocetien, C., Zaongo, D., Colas, J. M., Peabody, J. O., & Rochat, C. H. (2015). One-year follow-up of women who participated in a physiotherapy and health education program before and after obstetric fistula surgery. *International Jounal of Gynaecology and Obstetrics, 128*(3), 264–266.

Christensen, L., Veierod, M. B., Vollestad, N. K., Jakobsen, V. E., Stuge, B., Cabri, J., & Robinson, H. S. (2019). Kinematic and spatiotemporal gait characteristics in pregnant women with pelvic girdle pain, asymptomatic pregnant and non-pregnant women. *Clinical Biomechanics, 68,* 45–52.

Christensen, L., Vollestad, N. K., Veierod, M. B., Stuge, B., Cabri, J., & Robinson, H. S. (2019). The timed up & go test in pregnant women with pelvic girdle pain compared to asymptomatic pregnant and non-pregnant women. *Musculoskeletal Science and Practice, 43,* 110–116.

Dietz, H. P., & Williams, G. (2012). Pelvic floor structure and function in women with vesicovaginal fistula. *Journal of Urology, 188*(5), 1772–1777.

Dockter, M. P., Abraham, K., Coe, J. B., & Boissonnault, J. S. (2008). Technical report of specialty practice in Women's health physical therapy. *Journal of Women's Health Physical Therapy, 32*(1), 12–25.

El Ayadi, A. M., Painter, C. E., Delamou, A., Barr-Walker, S., Obore, J., Byamugisha, J., Korn, A., & Barageine, J. K. (2019). Rehabilitation and reintegration programming adjunct to female genital fistula surgery: A scoping review protocol. *British Medical Journal Open, 9*(10), e027991.

Elden, H., Gutke, A., Kjellby-Wendt, G., Fagevik-Olsen, M., & Ostgaard, H. C. (2016). Predictors and consequences of long-term pregnancy-related pelvic girdle pain: A longitudinal follow-up study. *Biomedical Cenral Musculoskeletal Disorders, 17,* 276.

Emasu, A., Ruder, B., Wall, L. L., Matovu, A., Alia, G., & Barageine, J. K. (2019). Reintegration needs of young women following genitourinary fistula surgery in Uganda. *International Urogynecology Journal, 30*(7), 1101–1110.

Evensen, N. M., Kvale, A., & Braekken, I. H. (2015). Reliability of the timed up and go test and ten-metre timed walk test in pregnant women with pelvic girdle pain. *Physiotherapy Research International, 20*(3), 158–165.

Evensen, N. M., Kvale, A., & Braekken, I. H. (2016). Convergent validity of the timed up and go test and ten-metre timed walk test in pregnant women with pelvic girdle pain. *Manual Therapy, 21,* 94–99.

Gutke, A., Boissonnault, J., Brook, G., & Stuge, B. (2018). The severity and impact of pelvic girdle pain and Low-Back pain in pregnancy: A multinational study. *Journal of Womens Health (Larchmt), 27*(4), 510–517.

Hamlin Fistula Hospital. (2020). Retrieved September 6, 2020, from https://hamlinfistula.org

Hungerford, B. A., Gilleard, W., Moran, M., & Emmerson, C. (2007). Evaluation of the ability of physical therapists to palpate intrapelvic motion with the stork test on the support side. *Physical Therapy, 87*(7), 879–887.

Keyser, L., McKinney, J., Salmon, C., Furaha, C., Kinsindja, R., & Benfield, N. (2014). Analysis of a pilot program to implement physical therapy for women with gynecologic fistula in the Democratic Republic of Congo. *Interntional Journal of Gynaecology and Obstetrics, 127*(2), 127–131.

Kim, S. H., Jo, M. W., Ock, M., & Lee, S. I. (2017). Exploratory study of dimensions of health-related quality of life in the general population of South Korea. *Journal of Prevenative Medicine and Public Health, 50*(6), 361–368.

Klinteberg, M. (1992). The history and present scope of physical therapy. *International Journal of Technology Assess Health Care, 8*(1), 4–9.

Labbe, R., Lindsay, T., & Walker, P. (1987). The extent and distribution of skeletal muscle necrosis after graded periods of complete ischemia. *Journal of Vascular Surgery, 6*(2), 152–157.

LoMauro, A., & Aliverti, A. (2015). Respiratory physiology of pregnancy: Physiology masterclass. *Breathe, 11*(4), 297–301.

Manyozo, S. D., Nesto, T., Bonongwe, P., & Muula, A. S. (2019). Low back pain during pregnancy: Prevalence, risk factors and association with daily activities among pregnant women in urban Blantyre, Malawi. *Malawi Medicine Journal, 31*(1), 71–76.

Morris, B. A., Benetti, M., Marro, H., & Rosenthal, C. K. (2010). Clinical practice guidelines for early mobilization hours after surgery. *Orthopaedic Nursing, 29*(5), 290–316.

Nardos, R., Ayenachew, F., Roentgen, R., Abreha, M., Jacobson, L., Haile, A., Berhe, Y., Gold, K., Gregory, W. T., Spitznagle, T., Payne, C. K., & Wall, L. L. (2020). Capacity building in female pelvic medicine and reconstructive surgery: Global Health Partnership beyond fistula care in Ethiopia. *International Urogynecology Journal, 31*(2), 227–235.

Nardos, R., Phoutrides, E. K., Jacobson, L., Knapper, A., Payne, C. K., Wall, L. L., Garg, B., Tarekegn, S., Teamir, A., & Marye, M. A. (2020). Characteristics of persistent urinary incontinence after successful fistula closure in Ethiopian women. *International Urogynecology Journal, 31*(11), 2277–2283.

Nielsen, L. L. (2010). Clinical findings, pain descriptions and physical complaints reported by women with post-natal pregnancy-related pelvic girdle pain. *Acta Obstetricia et Gynecologia Scandinavia, 89*(9), 1187–1191.

Ogollah, R., Bishop, A., Lewis, M., Grotle, M., & Foster, N. E. (2019). Responsiveness and minimal important change for pain and disability outcome measures in pregnancy-related low back and pelvic girdle pain. *Physical Therapy, 99*(11), 1551–1561.

Prather, H., Spitznagle, T., & Hunt, D. (2012). Benefits of exercise during pregnancy. *Physical Medicicne and Rehabilitation, 4*(11), 845–850; quiz 850.

Ptak, M., Ciecwiez, S., Brodowska, A., Starczewski, A., Nawrocka-Rutkowska, J., Diaz-Mohedo, E., & Rotter, I. (2019). The effect of pelvic floor muscles exercise on quality of life in women with stress urinary incontinence and its relationship with vaginal deliveries: A randomized trial. *Biomedical Research International, 2019*, 5321864.

Robinson, J. W., Faris, P. D., & Scott, C. B. (1999). Psychoeducational group increases vaginal dilation for younger women and reduces sexual fears for women of all ages with gynecological carcinoma treated with radiotherapy. *International Journal of Radiation Oncology Biology Physics, 44*(3), 497–506.

Schleicher, D. J., Ojengbede, O. H. A., & Elkins, T. E. (1993). Urologic evaluation after closure of vesicovaginal fistulas. *Interntional Urogynecology Journal, 4*, 262–265.

Shiri, R., Coggon, D., & Falah-Hassani, K. (2018). Exercise for the prevention of low back and pelvic girdle pain in pregnancy: A meta-analysis of randomized controlled trials. *European Journal of Pain, 22*(1), 19–27.

SIM Interntional. (2020). Retrieved September 4, 2020, from https://www.sim.org/web/secondary-landing

Spitznagle, T. M., Cabelka, C., Clinton, S., Abraham, K., & Norton, B. (2017). Diagnosis dialog for women's health conditions: The process and proposed pelvic floor muscle diagnoses. *Journal of Women's Health Physical Therapy, 41*(3), 154–162.

Spitznagle, T. M., Leong, F. C., & Van Dillen, L. R. (2007). Prevalence of diastasis recti abdominis in a urogynecological patient population. *International Journal of Urogynecology and Pelvic Floor Dysfunction, 18*(3), 321–328.

Tanzer, D. (1972). *Why natural childbirth? A psychologist's report on the benefits to mothers, fathers and babies.* Schocken Books.

Van Dillen, L. R., Sahrmann, S. A., Norton, B. J., Caldwell, C. A., McDonnell, M. K., & Bloom, N. (2003). The effect of modifying patient-preferred spinal movement and alignment during symptom testing in patients with low back pain: A preliminary report. *Archives of Physical Medicine and Rehabilitation, 84*(3), 313–322.

Vleeming, A., Albert, H. B., Ostgaard, H. C., Sturesson, B., & Stuge, B. (2008). European guidelines for the diagnosis and treatment of pelvic girdle pain. *European Spine Journal, 17*(6), 794–819.

Wall, L. L. (2012). Obstetric fistula is a "neglected tropical disease". *PLoS Neglected Tropical Diseases, 6*(8), e1769.

Wall, L. L. (2016). Residual incontinence after obstetric fistula repair. *Obstetrics and Gynecology, 128*(5), 943–944.

Wein, A. J. (2012). Re: Pelvic floor exercise for urinary incontinence: A systematic literature review. *Journal of Urology, 187*(4), 1353–1354.

Worldwide Fistula Fund. (2020). *Danja Fistula Center.* Retrieved September 6, 2020, from https://worldwidefistula-fund.org/who-we-are/our-programs/danja-fistula-center.aspx

Wu, W. H., Meijer, O. G., Bruijn, S. M., Hu, H., van Dieen, J. H., Lamoth, C. J., van Royen, B. J., & Beek, P. J. (2008). Gait in pregnancy-related pelvic girdle pain: Amplitudes, timing, and coordination of horizontal trunk rotations. *European Spine Journal, 17*(9), 1160–1169.

Yenişehir S, Çıtak Karakaya İ, Sivaslıoğlu AA, Özen Oruk D, Karakaya MG. Reliability and validity of Five Times Sit to Stand Test in pregnancy-related pelvic girdle pain. Musculoskelet Sci Pract. 2020;48:102157. https://doi.org/10.1016/j.msksp.2020.102157. Epub 2020 May 5. PMID: 32560864.

Comprehensive Pelvic Floor Health: Beyond the "Hole" in the Wall

33

Rahel Nardos and Laura Jacobson

33.1 Introduction

Obstetric fistula is a devastating condition that almost exclusively affects women in low- and middle-income countries (LMICs) and deserves widespread international attention. Obstetric fistula, however, is only one of many pelvic floor disorders related to childbirth. Many of the circumstances that predispose women to obstetric fistula in LMICs also predispose them to other chronic and devastating pelvic floor conditions. The aim of this chapter is to encourage readers, particularly the international humanitarian community, to take a step back and re-focus their attention to the larger unattended crisis of chronic childbirth-related pelvic floor disorders that affect women in low-resource countries. These include, among others, pelvic organ prolapse, persistent urinary incontinence after successful repair of obstetric fistula, nonfistula-related urinary and anal incontinence, and musculoskeletal disorders of the pelvic floor.

The epidemiology of pelvic floor disorders is complex. Researchers have used a chronic disease model that categorizes risk factors into three categories: predisposing (e.g., genetic predisposition and race); inciting (e.g., vaginal delivery, parity); and intervening (e.g., age) (Hallock & Handa, 2016). Although these pelvic floor conditions are much more prevalent than obstetric fistula and severely impact the quality of life and productivity of women, they currently receive little or no attention in LMICs. Although nonfistula-related pelvic floor disorders affect large numbers of women worldwide, women in low-resource settings carry a heavier burden due to their particular risk factors related to childbirth such as prolonged and sometimes obstructed labor and multiple vaginal deliveries in the absence of adequate and timely obstetric and reproductive health care. Once women develop these

R. Nardos (✉)
Division of Female Pelvic Medicine and Reconstructive Surgery, Department of Ob/Gyn & Women's Health, Center for Global Health and Social Responsibility, University of Minnesota, Minneapolis, MN, USA
e-mail: nardosr@umn.edu

L. Jacobson
Oregon Health & Science University-Portland State University, School of Public Health, Portland, OR, USA

© Springer Nature Switzerland AG 2022
L. B. Drew et al. (eds.), *A Multidisciplinary Approach to Obstetric Fistula in Africa*, Global Maternal and Child Health, https://doi.org/10.1007/978-3-031-06314-5_33

disorders, they also lack access to trained healthcare providers who can provide appropriate and timely diagnosis and treatment. In this chapter, we urge readers to look "beyond the hole in the wall" when it comes to women's pelvic floor health in LMICs. We call for reframing the approach from one focused on providing relatively short term, heavily surgical mission-based interventions for a single disorder (obstetric fistula) to building in-country healthcare capacity that provides ongoing comprehensive pelvic floor care to all women affected by childbirth injuries. This includes women with obstetric fistula who continue to suffer from persistent pelvic floor disorders long after their fistula is deemed "cured." In this chapter, we share our experience with one model of pelvic floor care involving a multi-institutional partnership that is expanding care beyond the obstetric fistula.

33.2 Pelvic Floor Disorders Beyond Fistula

One major inciting factor that contributes to pelvic floor disorders is childbirth. In LMICs, where access to family planning and timely obstetric care is often lacking, repeated trauma from multiple deliveries, prolonged obstructed labor, and lack of access to timely care for pelvic floor injuries can have a severe impact. Although childbirth is thought to be a key player in development of pelvic floor disorders, multiple factors play a role offering opportunities for risk reduction and intervention (Fig. 33.1).

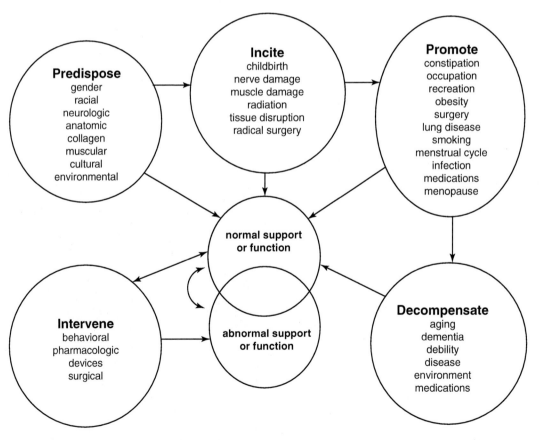

Fig. 33.1 Model for the development of pelvic floor dysfunction in women (Reprinted from *Obstetrics and Gynecology Clinics of North America*, 25(4), R.C. Bump & P.A. Norton, Epidemiology and Natural History of Pelvic Floor Dysfunction, pp. 723–746, Copyright © 1998 W. B. Saunders Company, with permission from Elsevier)

33.2.1 Pelvic Organ Prolapse

Pelvic organ prolapse (POP) is caused by loss of pelvic floor support, resulting in descent of the vaginal wall with its eventual protrusion together with adjacent organs such as uterus, bladder, or bowel (Fig. 33.2). This may result in various dysfunctions such as difficulty in emptying the bladder and/or bowel; irritative bladder symptoms; urinary and fecal incontinence; sexual dysfunction; and pelvic pain and discomfort. This condition, which afflicts millions of women worldwide, can negatively impact a woman's quality of life and is increasingly recognized as a significant burden on women's health (Akmel & Segni, 2012; Ballard et al., 2016; Kenton & Mueller, 2006; Wu et al., 2014). In high-resource nations, the prevalence of pelvic organ prolapse is estimated anywhere between 3% and 50%

Fig. 33.2 Pelvic organ prolapse (Illustrated by Robin M. Jensen. Courtesy of the artist)

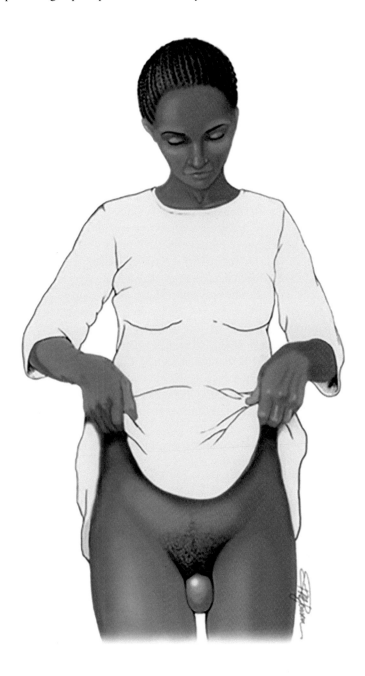

depending on the definition of prolapse used (Maher et al., 2008; Nygaard et al., 2008; Samuelsson et al., 1999; Swift et al., 2003). In general, it is estimated that up to 50% of women will develop some form of prolapse, and between 10% and 20% will seek care for their condition (Maher et al., 2013). Estimates of the prevalence of POP in low-resource countries are limited and vary substantially (3.4–56.4%) (Zeleke et al., 2013). According to a cross-sectional community-based study in three rural zones in Ethiopia of $n = 23,023$ women, the prevalence of symptomatic POP was much higher (100:10,000) compared with prevalence of clinically confirmed obstetric fistula (6:10,000) (Ballard et al., 2016). The etiology of POP is complex and multifactorial; possible risk factors for primary and recurrent POP include advanced age, parity, vaginal delivery, high body mass index, diabetes, low educational status, family history, and pelvic floor muscle defects secondary to childbirth-related trauma. For patients who have already developed POP, having advanced stage prolapse (stage 3 or 4) is a significant risk factor for recurrence after repair (Friedman et al., 2018; Vergeldt et al., 2015; Whiteside et al., 2004). In low-income countries, women may have increased risk factors due to high number of pregnancies starting at a younger age; less access to timely obstetric care; and a resulting risk of multiple and sometimes severe trauma to the pelvic floor as a result. These women also have significantly more exposure to strenuous activities, especially in rural communities where women often fetch water or fire wood from long distances, carry their children on their back while tending to field and home chores among other tasks. In a community-based cross-sectional study of 395 women in Ethiopia, researchers found that carrying heavy objects for five or more hours a day, a history of prolonged labor, and highland rural residence were associated with anatomical pelvic organ prolapse (Megabiaw et al., 2013). Additionally, women in low-income countries often have poor nutrition which may compromise their tissue quality, although there is scant to absent data available on the impact of poor nutrition on pelvic floor support. Women in LMICs also have limited timely access to appropriate pelvic floor care when symptoms initially develop. This means that they are more likely to have advanced stage prolapse by the time they seek care, increasing their risk of recurrence—even if they receive care. The risk of recurrence is also likely much higher than in low-resource countries given that the surgical interventions available are typically suboptimal due to few or no trained pelvic floor specialists. It is therefore possible that pelvic floor disorders such as POP are more common and more severe than suggested by reports from high-income settings (Zeleke et al., 2013). Studies have demonstrated that POP has significant impact on quality of life and psychological well-being (Krause et al., 2017; Zeleke et al., 2013). It is often associated with urinary, bowel, and sexual dysfunctions (Caruso et al., 2010; Hefni et al., 2013; Vitale et al., 2016). Pelvic organ prolapse is also associated with reduced functional status in older women (Sanses et al., 2016) with recovery of baseline functional status with treatment (Oliphant et al., 2014). Pelvic organ prolapse can be effectively managed with both nonsurgical interventions such as pessary (a prosthetic device that provides support to vaginal tissues) and pelvic floor muscle training (Culligan, 2012; Poma, 2000) as well as surgery (Nygaard et al., 2013). Lack of access to these interventions in LMICs is therefore a great disservice to women and to society in general.

33.2.2 Urinary Incontinence

Urinary incontinence (UI) is the loss of bladder control defined by the International Continence Society as "*the complaint of any involuntary leakage of urine*" (Abrams et al., 2003). The most common types of incontinence are stress incontinence (leakage with triggers that increase intraabdominal pressure such as coughing, sneezing, or physical exertion) and urgency incontinence (leakage of urine associated with urgency). These conditions can range in severity from occasional leakage to daily incontinence that restricts day-to-day social or physical functions. Common risk factors for UI include vaginal delivery (Blomquist et al., 2018), age, gender (women) (Linde et al., 2017), obesity (Hunskaar, 2008), and smoking (Hannestad et al., 2003).

In a review of population studies from numerous countries, the prevalence of UI varied greatly from ~5% up to 70%, with most studies reporting a prevalence of any UI in the range of 25–45% (Milsom & Gyhagen, 2019). This variation in prevalence is largely due to the discordance in the definition of incontinence used in data and is seen both within and between countries. The WHO reports that the prevalence of UI is twice as high in older women as compared to older men. Pregnancy, childbirth, menopause, and female anatomy are thought to account for this difference (The World Health Organization, 2017). In a systematic review of 49 studies, Islam et al. (2019) found the overall prevalence of UI in LMICs to be 30% (95% CI 25–35%) (Islam et al., 2019). As life expectancy increases in low-resource countries, the global prevalence of UI is also expected to increase given the association between incontinence and age (Irwin et al., 2011; Sexton et al., 2011).

In addition to advancing age, risk factors for UI that are more commonly observed in LMICs include high parity and greater risk of prolonged labor in the setting of poor or unavailable obstetric care. Additional risk factors include suboptimal nutrition that may compromise tissue integrity, and heavy physical strain from manual labor and daily life (Islam et al., 2017; Walker & Gunasekera, 2011). Incontinence is associated with depression, anxiety, and social isolation; it brings on a substantial economic burden; and can drastically impact quality of life (Coyne et al., 2009; Hagan et al., 2018; Hu & Wagner, 2005; Irwin et al., 2009, 2011). A review of 23 studies of perceptions of female UI showed that women across different racial and ethnic groups shared similar stories in which they experienced fear, stigmatization, and shame. This review did illuminate some differences in experiences where non-White women, for example, expressed more self-blame for incontinence, Hispanic women displayed more secrecy, and Muslim women referenced additional disruption because of cleanliness requirements for prayer (Siddiqui et al., 2014). The impact of incontinence can therefore be disproportionately great on women in LMICs given the lack of recognition of this condition, stigmatization, cultural factors, lack of access to sanitary and hygiene products, the demand for heavy physical labor, and lack of access to healthcare providers who can provide timely counseling and treatment.

33.2.3 Residual Incontinence After Obstetric Fistula

Women with a history of obstetric fistula have endured significant injuries to their pelvic floor and therefore may be at a higher risk for pelvic floor dysfunctions (Goh et al., 2013; Murray et al., 2002; Wall, 2016). A common but neglected problem following fistula repair is persistent urinary incontinence. An estimated 19–40% of women with obstetric fistula suffer from this debilitating persistent incontinence even after "successful" closure of their fistula (Browning, 2006; Kopp et al., 2018; Siddle et al., 2014). Residual urinary incontinence following repair can damage a women's social and family relationships, lower income-earning abilities, impact mental health and well-being, and limit her coping capabilities particularly given her history of fistula-related trauma and incontinence (Arrowsmith et al., 1996; Bashah et al., 2018; Drew et al., 2016; Kopp et al., 2018). Women often do not understand why they are not healed after fistula repair, and this is particularly traumatic when they see others with similar surgeries doing better. Postrepair urinary incontinence may be due to neurological compromise resulting in abnormalities in sensory and motor functions, loss of urethra or urethral support or a reduction in the size or compliance of the bladder (Dolan et al., 2008; Wall, 2016). The ability to maintain continence depends on whether the mechanisms for bladder storage and voiding are intact. The location of the fistula (e.g., whether or not the urethra and bladder neck are involved) and the extent and severity of the injury, and scarring to the bladder and surrounding structures can influence continence outcomes (Browning, 2006; Dolan et al., 2008; Hilton & Dolan, 2004; Williams et al., 2018).

In a prospective cohort study of 401 women undergoing obstetric vesicovaginal fistula repair in Malawi, researchers found that although 93% of women had successful closure of their fistula, 24% had persistent urinary incontinence within 120 days postrepair (Bengtson et al., 2016). They found that predictors of residual incontinence included age, number of years with fistula, prior fistula repair, fistula size, circumferential fistula, vaginal scarring, bladder size, and urethral length. Using these predictors, they generated a predictive model with reasonable sensitivity and specificity. Despite the high prevalence of residual incontinence in this population, very little research has been undertaken to characterize the type of residual incontinence and its impact on the quality of life of those who are affected.

Our team conducted a cross-sectional cohort study in Ethiopia where we enrolled women (ages 18–80 years) with a history of obstetric fistula repair ($n = 51$) and a control group of women with history of obstetric fistula without persistent incontinence ($n = 50$). We assessed severity of incontinence and impact on quality of life using the International Consultation on Incontinence Questionnaire short form (ICIQ-SF) (Avery et al., 2004) and ICIQ-QOL (Kelleher et al., 1997). Additionally, clinical evaluation of cases captured indicators of stress urinary incontinence and ruled out current vesicovaginal fistula. We found that 80.4% of cases reported moderate/severe incontinence; 19.6% reported very severe incontinence; and almost all cases reported both stress (98%) and urgency (94%) incontinence; and half reported leaking all the time (49%). Women with more severe incontinence reported more negative impact on their quality of life (ICIQ-QoL scores; 67.8 ± 6.3 vs. 57.8 ± 15.9; $p = 0.008$). Although there was no significant difference between the groups on thoughts of suicidal ideation, of the cases ($n = 23$) and controls ($n = 16$) who responded to the question "do you have plans for suicide," more cases admitted to having plans as compared to controls (39% vs. 12%; $p = 0.003$) (Nardos, Phoutrides, et al., 2020). In a parallel crosssectional study study in Uganda by our team, we found that 53% of women with persistent incontinence after successful fistula closure rated their incontinence as very severe and reported high negative impact on their quality of life (ICIQ-QoL scores; $62.8+12.8$). This population also has a high mental health burden with 36% reporting having had suicidal ideation at some point after their fistula (Nardos et al., 2022).

These findings show that women with history of obstetric fistula who are considered "cured" may continue to have persistent urinary incontinence and are severely impacted both physically and psychologically. Understanding the type of persistent incontinence and its impact on women's quality of life will encourage local healthcare providers and charitable organizations to provide a more long-term and holistic approach to care of women with childbirth injuries that extends beyond the "hole in the wall."

33.2.4 Anal Incontinence

Anal incontinence (AI) is the involuntary loss of gas, mucous, liquid or solid stool. The sense of shame and stigma associated with this disorder has led many women to hide their symptoms leading to difficulty in properly identifying those who are affected (Bharucha et al., 2015). As such, reported estimates of AI prevalence rates must be interpreted cautiously and viewed within their respective context. An analysis of 14,759 participants in the United States National Health and Nutrition Examination Survey revealed a fecal incontinence prevalence of 8.4% among adults in the US (Ditah et al., 2014). International population-based studies suggested a fecal incontinence prevalence ranging from 0.4% to 18% (Roslani et al., 2014; Saldana Ruiz & Kaiser, 2017).

Causes of AI can include muscle or nerve damage that may be associated with childbirth or aging; chronic constipation; diarrhea; hemorrhoids; loss of storage capacity in the rectum; surgery; rectal prolapse; and rectocele (Boreham et al., 2005; Whitehead et al., 2009). A number of factors may increase the risk of developing AI, including age, gender, increasing parity, operative vaginal delivery, and medical comorbidities such as long-standing diabetes or multiple sclerosis that can damage nerves, dementia, irritable bowel syndrome, and some physical disabilities. A major risk factor for AI is vaginal delivery with obstetric anal sphincter injuries (OASIS) (Jangö et al., 2018). Sphincter tears occur in approximately 18% of deliveries and may not be recognized by examination at the time of delivery in 23–35% of women even in high-resource countries (Fenner et al., 2003). Risk factors for sphincter tears include nullipartity, primiparity, high infant birthweight, prolonged second-stage labor, epidural anesthesia, midline episiotomy, operative vaginal delivery, and fetal position (occiput posterior) (Angioli et al., 2000; Combs et al., 1990; de Leeuw et al., 2001; FitzGerald et al., 2007; Handa et al., 2001; Hudelist et al., 2005; Jandér & Lyrenäs, 2001; Richter et al., 2002; Robinson et al., 1999). In LMICs, some of these risk factors and their consequences could be more burdensome given poor access to trained obstetric services to manage labor and delivery and to provide timely and effective diagnosis and repairs when anal sphincter injuries do happen. The World Health Organization estimates that 99% of childbirth takes place in LMICs (World Health Organization, 2018) where the majority of women deliver with untrained birth attendants (UNICEF, 2009). For women who deliver at home, there is a real concern that perineal injuries may go unrecognized and unattended. In those who deliver at medical facilities, there is concern for high rates of routine episiotomies that predispose women to anal sphincter or other pelvic floor injuries. In a systematic review and meta-analysis looking at birth-related perineal trauma (BPT) in LMICs, researchers found that BPTs affect up to 70% of women having vaginal birth with overall episiotomy rates at medical facilities as high as 46% (Aguiar et al., 2019). The World Health Organization recommends an episiotomy rate of 10% (World Health Organization, 1997), and it is generally recommended that routine episiotomy be avoided and the decision to perform episiotomy should be based on clinical indications (American College of Obstetricians and Gynecologists' Committee on Practice Bulletins—Obstetrics, 2016). This is based on findings showing that routine episiotomy is not associated with maternal benefits (Hartmann et al., 2005) and in fact may have worse outcomes such as increased risk of blood loss, pain, and severe lacerations (Carroli & Mignini, 2009). In high-resource countries, there has been a major shift in this practice. In one large US hospital where 1,658,327 spontaneous vaginal deliveries were evaluated, the episiotomy rates dropped from 54% in 1994 to 13% in 2010 (Howard & Hockenberry, 2019).

Since AI is strongly associated with age, its incidence will likely increase as the global population ages. Left unaddressed, this will continue to play a significant role in disability of women. The emotional consequences of AI often exceed the physical challenges where many women report withdrawing from society to hide the problem from their families, friends, and even healthcare providers (Bartlett et al., 2009; Meyer & Richter, 2015). It is critical that we increase awareness of this debilitating condition and support programs that strengthen health systems in LMICs working toward prevention and treatment.

33.3 The Way Forward: Pelvic Floor Care Beyond Fistula

The current model of pelvic floor care for obstetric fistula overlooks the larger set of pelvic floor disorders that affect women. Despite the high prevalence and risk factors for pelvic floor disorders in LMICs, there is a huge shortage of appropriately trained pelvic floor specialists who can provide optimal treatment. Adequate care for pelvic floor disorders in LMICs goes beyond general gyneco-logic surgery or obstetric fistula care, and requires educating a multidisciplinary team that includes nurses, pelvic floor physical therapists, mental health counselors, and physicians trained in advanced medical and surgical management of pelvic floor disorders. Treatment options need to integrate both conservative (first line) and surgical management under the direction of specialists trained in female pelvic medicine and reconstructive surgery. In the following discussion, we share our experience with pelvic floor care capacity-building work in Ethiopia.

33.3.1 Pelvic Floor Care Capacity in Ethiopia

As of 2015, there was no formal training in pelvic medicine and reconstructive surgery in Ethiopia, a country with the second largest population in Africa. Most Ob-Gyn residents who receive training in Ethiopia, similar to other LMICs, do not have access to expert mentors in the surgical and medical management of pelvic floor disorders, and their training leaves them ill equipped to manage the full range of complexities seen in these conditions. As a result, women with POP or persistent inconti-nence suffer in silence while their condition worsens. Those who do receive care do so when their clinical condition is severely advanced. They are often treated by gynecologists who are not trained to provide optimal surgical treatment leaving patients at even higher risk for recurrence or complications (Gjerde et al., 2018). In our own experience in Ethiopia, we compared surgical outcomes of women who underwent traditional vaginal repairs of stage 4 uterovaginal prolapse before and after proper pelvic floor medicine and reconstructive surgery (FPMRS or also known as urogynecology) training was instituted. We found that women who were repaired prior to the launching of the training program ($n = 40$) had significantly lower subjective ($p = 0.013$) and objective ($p = 0.05$) cure compared to those who received surgical care by trained surgeons ($n = 40$) (unpublished data).

The international medical community, including scientific societies in high-resource nations dedi-cated to pelvic floor health, can and should play a critical role in elevating pelvic floor care in LMICs. Although many pelvic floor specialists from high-resource nations currently provide evaluation and surgical treatment through humanitarian missions, most of the health services are delivered through short-term surgical missions and are not designed to leave a system in place to provide long-term and comprehensive care by local providers. This is further complicated by the fact that most pelvic floor specialists from high-resource countries seem to favor providing care for obstetric fistula patients (rather than for patients with prolapse or nonfistula incontinence) for a variety of reasons: availability of funds earmarked to treat fistulas, familiarity with the devastating stories of women affected by obstetric fistulas, and the fact that these conditions are restricted primarily to LMICs making them attractive opportunities for Western medical teams to be involved in unique global surgical learning and experience (Wall et al., 2006). Unfortunately, this restricted service model ignores the need to address the larger and more global burden of pelvic floor disorders that continue to debilitate women disproportionately, including those who are successfully "cured" of their fistulas.

To address this gap in the provision of care, a paradigm shift is needed. We need to first acknowl-edge: (1) that women are disproportionately affected by chronic and devastating pelvic floor condi-tions due to childbearing and these disorders extend beyond fistula; (2) that obstetric fistula patients continue to be severely impacted by incontinence and other pelvic floor disorders after they are deemed cured of their fistulas; and (3) that an investment in partnerships that prioritizes building local healthcare capacity will provide much more comprehensive and sustainable results.

In 2015, obstetric fistula surgeons at the internationally known Hamlin Fistula Ethiopia recognized that as the number of obstetric fistula patients decreased (Wright et al., 2016) with improving obstetric care, they were increasingly ill equipped to care for women with persistent urinary incontinence after fistula and for the large number of women who did not have fistula but suffered from pelvic floor disorders such as prolapse and urinary and anal incontinence. They urged their existing international and local academic and nonprofit partners to go beyond supporting fistula work and join hands to creating a formal urogynecology fellowship training program for Hamlin fistula surgeons and others who are interested in expanding these services in academic centers. This resulted in a multi-institutional partnership between Hamlin Fistula Ethiopia, Mekelle University College of Health and Sciences, Worldwide Fistula fund, Maternal Health Fund, and US-based academic global health programs such as Footsteps to Healing at Oregon Health & Science University and now Center for Global Health and Social Responsibility at the University of Minnesota (Nardos, Ayenachew, et al., 2020). This partnership also worked closely with community-based women's health outreach organizations and local health bureaus to reach patients needing clinical care and to help coordinate relevant clinical research needed to inform and improve upon the care model.

In this partnership model, core faculty from the United States, Latin America, and Europe helped provide program oversight, curriculum updates, and ongoing mentorship. Nongovernmental organization (NGO) partners provided financial and human resource support and participate in the fellowship oversight committee. The local academic partner serves as the academic home of the program including covering the cost of care for patients and formal acknowledgment of successful completion of fellowship training.

The curriculum for the fellowship training program was developed by the partners and required careful modification of existing urogynecology training models from developed countries to fit the Ethiopian context. For example, high-technology-based procedures were replaced with conservative management options and surgical interventions that can be achieved effectively yet safely with more limited resources. Additional in-depth training was also provided in urologic and colorectal conditions that overlap with pelvic floor conditions given the shortage of subspecialists in these areas. Furthermore, given that trainees have other competing patient care and leadership responsibilities, the curriculum was structured in such a way that trainings were provided in brief but high-intensity blocks of 1–2 weeks every 1–2 months by core faculty. The fellowship curriculum, which incorporates both clinical and research training, was approved by the Ethiopian Ministry of Education in 2015. In conjunction with the fellowship training, the partnership works on capacity building efforts in nursing, perioperative services, critical care, and quality improvement in health systems to strengthen the overall resiliency of the healthcare environment.

Since the launching of this fellowship program, hundreds of women have received comprehensive pelvic floor care year-round, care that is provided by local surgeons and goes beyond fistula care. Fellows have completed and presented impactful studies on pelvic floor care and outcomes. Traditional, less-effective treatments for prolapse have been replaced by evidence-based and effective surgical approaches. The program has graduated four fellows to date with more in training. These graduates have now joined the ranks of urogynecology faculty and play a vital role in training the junior fellows in the program as well as obstetrics and gynecology residents from partner academic centers that rotate with them. Graduates have also assumed more leadership roles including taking over the role of directing the fellowship. The fellowship program is also creating opportunities for other healthcare providers (nurses, midwives, physical therapists, etc.) to receive training in conservative management techniques for pelvic floor disorders, such as the use of pessaries, behavioral interventions, and pelvic muscle rehabilitation.

This program has relied heavily on creating sustainable partnerships geared toward local provider training, context-specific curriculum, and building health systems. This model of care is undoubtedly challenging and requires strong, well-aligned partnerships, and committed champions. Yet it is one which endures way after the visiting surgeons have gone home and ensures that women will receive ongoing and dependable quality care by their own locally trained providers. The long-term success of this type of program depends on the commitment of local institutions and partners, the ability and willingness of trained pelvic floor specialists to be advocates and leaders, and the willingness of national health institutions and academic centers to improve access to resources and scale this care model across the country. Success also depends on building the capacity of providers such as nurses, midwives, general practitioners, and physical therapists who can partner with physicians and can be trained to provide first-line conservative treatment options and education. This is particularly important in low-resource settings where patients do not have readily available access to physicians trained in pelvic medicine and reconstructive surgery. Furthermore, existing primary care and community health outreach infrastructures should be leveraged to develop population-level pelvic floor health awareness and facilitate early conservative interventions for pelvic floor disorders.

33.4   A Call for Action

There is a massive shortage in trained health workforce to address the large unmet need of pelvic floor disorders in LMICs. This is particularly true in Africa which bears over one-third of the world's maternal, newborn, and childhood diseases but has less than 3% of the world's health workforce. We have a moral obligation to respond. Strong academic, NGO, and government partnerships that aim to build sustainable health systems can transform the care of women everywhere. We call upon humanitarian groups, charity organizations, ministries of health, and national and international scientific societies to leverage their expertise and responsibilities as advocates for women's pelvic floor health so women can live healthy and productive lives. We also urge global health funders to re-prioritize to support initiatives that build skilled healthcare workforce and resilient health systems. This type of investment will have far-reaching impact that goes beyond serving women with specific pelvic floor dysfunction.

References

Abrams, P., Cardozo, L., Fall, M., Griffiths, D., Rosier, P., Ulmsten, U., et al. (2003). The standardisation of terminology in lower urinary tract function: Report from the standardisation sub-committee of the International Continence Society. *Urology, 61*(1), 37–49. https://doi.org/10.1016/s0090-4295(02)02243-4

Aguiar, M., Farley, A., Hope, L., Amin, A., Shah, P., & Manaseki-Holland, S. (2019). Birth-related perineal trauma in low- and middle-income countries: A systematic review and meta-analysis. *Maternal and Child Health Journal, 23*(8), 1048–1070. https://doi.org/10.1007/s10995-019-02732-5

Akmel, M., & Segni, H. (2012). Pelvic organ prolapse in Jimma university specialized hospital, Southwest Ethiopia. *Ethiopian Journal of Health Sciences, 22*(2), 85–92. Retrieved August 20, 2019, from http://www.ncbi.nlm.nih.gov/pubmed/22876071

American College of Obstetricians and Gynecologists' Committee on Practice Bulletins—Obstetrics. (2016). Practice bulletin no. 165: Prevention and management of obstetric lacerations at vaginal delivery. *Obstetrics & Gynecology, 128*(1), e1–e15. https://doi.org/10.1097/AOG.0000000000001523

Angioli, R., Gómez-Marín, O., Cantuaria, G., & O'Sullivan, M. J. (2000). Severe perineal lacerations during vaginal delivery: The University of Miami experience. *American Journal of Obstetrics and Gynecology, 182*(5), 1083–1085. https://doi.org/10.1067/mob.2000.105403

Arrowsmith, S., Hamlin, E. C., & Wall, L. L. (1996). Obstructed labor injury complex: Obstetric fistula formation and the multifaceted morbidity of maternal birth trauma in the developing world. *Obstetrical & Gynecological Survey, 51*(9), 568–574. Retrieved January 15, 2019, from http://www.ncbi.nlm.nih.gov/pubmed/8873157

Avery, K., Donovan, J., Peters, T. J., Shaw, C., Gotoh, M., & Abrams, P. (2004). ICIQ: A brief and robust measure for evaluating the symptoms and impact of urinary incontinence. *Neurourology and Urodynamics, 330*(May), 322–330. https://doi.org/10.1002/nau.20041

Ballard, K., Ayenachew, F., Wright, J., & Atnafu, H. (2016). Prevalence of obstetric fistula and symptomatic pelvic organ prolapse in rural Ethiopia. *International Urogynecology Journal, 27*(7), 1063–1067. https://doi.org/10.1007/s00192-015-2933-0

Bartlett, L., Nowak, M., & Ho, Y.-H. (2009). Impact of fecal incontinence on quality of life. *World Journal of Gastroenterology: WJG, 15*(26), 3276. https://doi.org/10.3748/WJG.15.3276

Bashah, D. T., Worku, A. G., & Mengistu, M. Y. (2018). Consequences of obstetric fistula in sub Sahara African countries, from patients' perspective: A systematic review of qualitative studies. *BMC Women's Health, 18*(1), 106. https://doi.org/10.1186/s12905-018-0605-1

Bengtson, A. M., Kopp, D., Tang, J. H., Chipungu, E., Moyo, M., & Wilkinson, J. (2016). Identifying patients with vesicovaginal fistula at high risk of urinary incontinence after surgery. *Obstetrics & Gynecology, 128*(5), 945–953. https://doi.org/10.1097/AOG.0000000000001687

Bharucha, A. E., Dunivan, G., Goode, P. S., Lukacz, E. S., Markland, A. D., Matthews, C. A., et al. (2015). Epidemiology, pathophysiology, and classification of fecal incontinence: State of the science summary for the National Institute of Diabetes and Digestive and Kidney Diseases (NIDDK) workshop. *The American Journal of Gastroenterology, 110*(1), 127–136. https://doi.org/10.1038/ajg.2014.396

Blomquist, J. L., Muñoz, A., Carroll, M., & Handa, V. L. (2018). Association of delivery mode with pelvic floor disorders after childbirth. *JAMA, 320*(23), 2438–2447. https://doi.org/10.1001/jama.2018.18315

Boreham, M. K., Richter, H. E., Kenton, K. S., Nager, C. W., Gregory, W. T., Aronson, M. P., et al. (2005). Anal incontinence in women presenting for gynecologic care: Prevalence, risk factors, and impact upon quality of life. *American Journal of Obstetrics and Gynecology, 192*(5), 1637–1642. https://doi.org/10.1016/j.ajog.2004.11.030

Browning, A. (2006). Risk factors for developing residual urinary incontinence after obstetric fistula repair. *BJOG: An International Journal of Obstetrics and Gynaecology, 113*(4), 482–485. https://doi.org/10.1111/j.1471-0528.2006.00875.x

Bump, R. C., & Norton, P. A. (1998). Epidemiology and natural history of pelvic floor dysfunction. *Obstetrics and Gynecology Clinics of North America, 25*(4), 723–746. https://doi.org/10.1016/S0889-8545(05)70039-5

Carroli, G., & Mignini, L. (2009). Episiotomy for vaginal birth. *Cochrane Database of Systematic Reviews,* (1), CD000081. https://doi.org/10.1002/14651858.CD000081.pub2

Caruso, S., Bandiera, S., Cavallaro, A., Cianci, S., Vitale, S. G., & Rugolo, S. (2010). Quality of life and sexual changes after double transobturator tension-free approach to treat severe cystocele. *European Journal of Obstetrics & Gynecology and Reproductive Biology, 151*(1), 106–109. https://doi.org/10.1016/j.ejogrb.2010.03.016

Combs, C. A., Robertson, P. A., & Laros, R. K. (1990). Risk factors for third-degree and fourth-degree perineal lacerations in forceps and vacuum deliveries. *American Journal of Obstetrics and Gynecology, 163*(1 Pt 1), 100–104. https://doi.org/10.1016/s0002-9378(11)90678-4

Coyne, K. S., Wein, A. J., Tubaro, A., Sexton, C. C., Thompson, C. L., Kopp, Z. S., & Aiyer, L. P. (2009). Evaluating the effect of LUTS on health-related quality of life, anxiety and depression: EpiLUTS. *BJU International, 103*(Supp 3), 4–11.

Culligan, P. J. (2012). Nonsurgical management of pelvic organ prolapse. *Obstetrics & Gynecology, 119*(4), 852–860. https://doi.org/10.1097/AOG.0b013e31824c0806

de Leeuw, J. W., Struijk, P. C., Vierhout, M. E., & Wallenburg, H. C. (2001). Risk factors for third degree perineal ruptures during delivery. *BJOG : An International Journal of Obstetrics and Gynaecology, 108*(4), 383–387. Retrieved August 21, 2019, from http://www.ncbi.nlm.nih.gov/pubmed/11305545

Ditah, I., Devaki, P., Luma, H. N., Ditah, C., Njei, B., Jaiyeoba, C., et al. (2014). Prevalence, trends, and risk factors for fecal incontinence in United States adults, 2005–2010. *Clinical Gastroenterology and Hepatology, 12*(4), 636–643.e2. https://doi.org/10.1016/j.cgh.2013.07.020

Dolan, L., Dixon, W., & Hilton, P. (2008). Urinary symptoms and quality of life in women following urogenital fistula repair: A long-term follow-up study. *BJOG: An International Journal of Obstetrics & Gynaecology, 115*(12), 1570–1574. https://doi.org/10.1111/j.1471-0528.2008.01927.x

Drew, L. B., Wilkinson, J. P., Nundwe, W., Moyo, M., Mataya, R., Mwale, M., & Tang, J. H. (2016). Long-term outcomes for women after obstetric fistula repair in Lilongwe, Malawi: A qualitative study. *BMC Pregnancy and Childbirth, 16*, 2. https://doi.org/10.1186/s12884-015-0755-1

Fenner, D. E., Genberg, B., Brahma, P., Marek, L., & DeLancey, J. O. (2003). Fecal and urinary incontinence after vaginal delivery with anal sphincter disruption in an obstetrics unit in the United States. *American Journal of Obstetrics and Gynecology, 189*(6), 1543–1549. https://doi.org/10.1016/j.ajog.2003.09.030

FitzGerald, M. P., Weber, A. M., Howden, N., Cundiff, G. W., Brown, M. B., & Pelvic Floor Disorders Network. (2007). Risk factors for anal sphincter tear during vaginal delivery. *Obstetrics & Gynecology, 109*(1), 29–34. https://doi.org/10.1097/01.AOG.0000242616.56617.ff

Friedman, T., Eslick, G. D., & Dietz, H. P. (2018). Risk factors for prolapse recurrence: Systematic review and meta-analysis. *International Urogynecology Journal, 29*(1), 13–21. https://doi.org/10.1007/s00192-017-3475-4

Gjerde, J. L., Rortveit, G., Adefris, M., Belayneh, T., & Blystad, A. (2018). Life after pelvic organ prolapse surgery: A qualitative study in Amhara region, Ethiopia. *BMC Women's Health, 18*(1), 74. https://doi.org/10.1186/s12905-018-0568-2

Goh, J. T. W., Krause, H., Tessema, A. B., & Abraha, G. (2013). Urinary symptoms and urodynamics following obstetric genitourinary fistula repair. *International Urogynecology Journal, 24*(6), 947–951. https://doi.org/10.1007/s00192-012-1948-z

Hagan, K. A., Erekson, E., Austin, A., Minassian, V. A., Townsend, M. K., Bynum, J. P. W., & Grodstein, F. (2018). A prospective study of the natural history of urinary incontinence in women. *American Journal of Obstetrics and Gynecology, 218*(5), 502.e1–502.e8. https://doi.org/10.1016/j.ajog.2018.01.045

Hallock, J. L., & Handa, V. L. (2016). The epidemiology of pelvic floor disorders and childbirth: An update. *Obstetrics and Gynecology Clinics of North America, 43*(1), 1. https://doi.org/10.1016/J.OGC.2015.10.008

Handa, V. L., Danielsen, B. H., & Gilbert, W. M. (2001). Obstetric anal sphincter lacerations. *Obstetrics and Gynecology, 98*(2), 225–230. https://doi.org/10.1016/s0029-7844(01)01445-4

Hannestad, Y. S., Rortveit, G., Daltveit, A. K., & Hunskaar, S. (2003). Are smoking and other lifestyle factors associated with female urinary incontinence? The Norwegian EPINCONT study. *BJOG : An International Journal of Obstetrics and Gynaecology, 110*(3), 247–254. Retrieved August 20, 2019, from http://www.ncbi.nlm.nih.gov/pubmed/12628262

Hartmann, K., Viswanathan, M., Palmieri, R., Gartlehner, G., Thorp, J., & Lohr, K. N. (2005). Outcomes of routine episiotomy: A systematic review. *JAMA, 293*(17), 2141. https://doi.org/10.1001/jama.293.17.2141

Hefni, M., Barry, J. A., Koukoura, O., Meredith, J., Mossa, M., & Edmonds, S. (2013). Long-term quality of life and patient satisfaction following anterior vaginal mesh repair for cystocele. *Archives of Gynecology and Obstetrics, 287*(3), 441–446. https://doi.org/10.1007/s00404-012-2583-0

Hilton, P., & Dolan, L. M. (2004). Pathophysiology of urinary incontinence and pelvic organ prolapse. *BJOG: An International Journal of Obstetrics & Gynaecology, 111*, 5–9. https://doi.org/10.1111/j.1471-0528.2004.00458.x

Howard, D. H., & Hockenberry, J. (2019). Physician age and the abandonment of episiotomy. *Health Services Research, 54*(3), 650–657. https://doi.org/10.1111/1475-6773.13132

Hu, T.-W., & Wagner, T. H. (2005). Health-related consequences of overactive bladder: An economic perspective. *BJU International, 96*(s1), 43–45. https://doi.org/10.1111/j.1464-410X.2005.05654.x

Hudelist, G., Gelle'n, J., Singer, C., Rueckinger, E., Czerwenka, K., Kandolf, O., & Keckstein, J. (2005). Factors predicting severe perineal trauma during childbirth: Role of forceps delivery routinely combined with mediolateral episiotomy. *American Journal of Obstetrics and Gynecology, 192*(3), 875–881. https://doi.org/10.1016/j.ajog.2004.09.035

Hunskaar, S. (2008). A systematic review of overweight and obesity as risk factors and targets for clinical intervention for urinary incontinence in women. *Neurourology and Urodynamics, 27*(8), 749–757. https://doi.org/10.1002/nau.20635

Irwin, D. E., Kopp, Z. S., Agatep, B., Milsom, I., & Abrams, P. (2011). Worldwide prevalence estimates of lower urinary tract symptoms, overactive bladder, urinary incontinence and bladder outlet obstruction. *BJU International, 108*, 1132–1139. https://doi.org/10.1111/j.1464-410X.2010.09993

Irwin, D. E., Mungapen, L., Milsom, I., Kopp, Z., Reeves, P., & Kelleher, C. (2009). The economic impact of overactive bladder syndrome in six Western countries. *BJU International, 103*(2), 202–209. https://doi.org/10.1111/j.1464-410X.2008.08036.x

Islam, R. M., Oldroyd, J., Karim, M. N., Hossain, S. M., Md Emdadul Hoque, D., Romero, L., & Fisher, J. (2017). Systematic review and meta-analysis of prevalence of, and risk factors for, pelvic floor disorders in community-dwelling women in low- and middle-income countries: A protocol study. *BMJ Open, 7*(6), 1–6. https://doi.org/10.1136/bmjopen-2016-015626

Islam, R. M., Oldroyd, J., Rana, J., Romero, L., & Karim, M. N. (2019). Prevalence of symptomatic pelvic floor disorders in community-dwelling women in low- and middle-income countries: A systematic review and meta-analysis. *International Urogynecology Journal, 30*(12), 2001–2011. https://doi.org/10.1007/s00192-019-03992-z

Jandér, C., & Lyrenäs, S. (2001). Third and fourth degree perineal tears. Predictor factors in a referral hospital. *Acta Obstetricia et Gynecologica Scandinavica, 80*(3), 229–234. Retrieved August 21, 2019, from http://www.ncbi.nlm.nih.gov/pubmed/11207488

Jangö, H., Langhoff-Roos, J., Rosthøj, S., & Saske, A. (2018). Long-term anal incontinence after obstetric anal sphincter injury—Does grade of tear matter? *American Journal of Obstetrics and Gynecology, 218*(2), 232.e1–232.e10. https://doi.org/10.1016/j.ajog.2017.11.569

Kelleher, C. J., Cardozo, L. D., Khullar, V., & Salvatore, S. (1997). A new questionnaire to assess the quality of life of urinary incontinent women. *British Journal of Obstetrics and Gynaecology, 104*(12), 1374–1379. Retrieved March 19, 2019, from http://www.ncbi.nlm.nih.gov/pubmed/9422015

Kenton, K., & Mueller, E. R. (2006). The global burden of female pelvic floor disorders. *BJU International, 98*(SUPPL. 1), 1–5. https://doi.org/10.1111/j.1464-410X.2006.06299.x

Kopp, D., Tang, J., Bengtson, A., Chi, B., Chipungu, E., Moyo, M., & Wilkinson, J. (2018). Continence, quality of life, and depression following surgical repair of obstetric vesicovaginal fistula: A cohort study. *BJOG: An International Journal of Obstetrics & Gynaecology*. https://doi.org/10.1111/1471-0528.15546

Krause, H. G., Hall, B. A., Ng, S.-K., Natukunda, H., Singasi, I., & Goh, J. T. W. (2017). Mental health screening in women with severe pelvic organ prolapse, chronic fourth-degree obstetric tear and genital tract fistula in western Uganda. *International Urogynecology Journal, 28*(6), 893–897. https://doi.org/10.1007/s00192-016-3177-3

Linde, J. M., Nijman, R. J. M., Trzpis, M., & Broens, P. M. A. (2017). Urinary incontinence in the Netherlands: Prevalence and associated risk factors in adults. *Neurourology and Urodynamics, 36*(6), 1519–1528. https://doi.org/10.1002/nau.23121

Maher, C., Baessler, K., Glazener, C. M. A., Adams, E. J., & Hagen, S. (2008). Surgical management of pelvic organ prolapse in women: A short version Cochrane review. *Neurourology and Urodynamics, 27*(1), 3–12. https://doi.org/10.1002/nau.20542

Maher, C., Feiner, B., Baessler, K., & Schmid, C. (2013). Surgical management of pelvic organ prolapse in women. *Cochrane Database of Systematic Reviews*, (4), CD004014. https://doi.org/10.1002/14651858.CD004014.pub5.

Megabiaw, B., Adefris, M., Rortveit, G., Degu, G., Muleta, M., Blystad, A., et al. (2013). Pelvic floor disorders among women in Dabat district, Northwest Ethiopia: A pilot study. *International Urogynecology Journal, 24*(7), 1135–1143. https://doi.org/10.1007/s00192-012-1981-y

Meyer, I., & Richter, H. E. (2015). Impact of fecal incontinence and its treatment on quality of life in women. *Women's health (London, England), 11*(2), 225. https://doi.org/10.2217/WHE.14.66

Milsom, I., & Gyhagen, M. (2019). The prevalence of urinary incontinence. *Climacteric, 22*(3), 217–222. https://doi.org/10.1080/13697137.2018.1543263

Murray, C., Goh, J. T., Fynes, M., & Carey, M. P. (2002). Urinary and faecal incontinence following delayed primary repair of obstetric genital fistula. *BJOG: An International Journal of Obstetrics and Gynaecology, 109*(7), 828–832. https://doi.org/10.1016/S1470-0328(02)00124-6

Nardos, R., Ayenachew, F., Roentgen, R., Abreha, M., Jacobson, L., Haile, A., et al. (2020). Capacity building in female pelvic medicine and reconstructive surgery: Global Health Partnership beyond fistula care in Ethiopia. *International Urogynecology Journal, 31*(2), 227–235. https://doi.org/10.1007/s00192-019-04197-0

Nardos, R., Phoutrides, E. K., Jacobson, L., Knapper, A., Payne, C. K., Wall, L. L., et al. (2020). Characteristics of persistent urinary incontinence after successful fistula closure in Ethiopian women. *International Urogynecology Journal, 31*(11), 2277–2283. https://doi.org/10.1007/s00192-020-04265-w

Nardos, R., Jacobson, L., Garg, B., Wall, L. L., Emasu, A., Ruder, B. (2022). Characterizing persistent urinary incontinence after successful fistula closure: the Uganda experience. *American Journal of Obstetrics and Gynecology*, S0002-9378(22)00178-8. https://doi.org/10.1016/j.ajog.2022.03.008. Epub ahead of print. PMID: 35283092

Nygaard, I., Barber, M. D., Burgio, K. L., Kenton, K., Meikle, S., Schaffer, J., et al. (2008). Prevalence of symptomatic pelvic floor disorders in US women. *JAMA, 300*(11), 1311. https://doi.org/10.1001/jama.300.11.1311

Nygaard, I., Brubaker, L., Zyczynski, H. M., Cundiff, G., Richter, H., Gantz, M., et al. (2013). Long-term outcomes following abdominal sacrocolpopexy for pelvic organ prolapse. *JAMA, 309*(19), 2016. https://doi.org/10.1001/jama.2013.4919

Oliphant, S. S., Lowder, J. L., Lee, M., & Ghetti, C. (2014). Most older women recover baseline functional status following pelvic organ prolapse surgery. *International Urogynecology Journal, 25*(10), 1425–1432. https://doi.org/10.1007/s00192-014-2394-x

Poma, P. A. (2000). Nonsurgical management of genital prolapse. A review and recommendations for clinical practice. *The Journal of Reproductive Medicine, 45*(10), 789–797. Retrieved August 20, 2019, from http://www.ncbi.nlm.nih.gov/pubmed/11077625

Richter, H. E., Brumfield, C. G., Cliver, S. P., Burgio, K. L., Neely, C. L., & Varner, R. E. (2002). Risk factors associated with anal sphincter tear: A comparison of primiparous patients, vaginal births after cesarean deliveries, and patients with previous vaginal delivery. *American Journal of Obstetrics and Gynecology, 187*(5), 1194–1198. https://doi.org/10.1067/mob.2002.126977

Robinson, J. N., Norwitz, E. R., Cohen, A. P., McElrath, T. F., & Lieberman, E. S. (1999). Episiotomy, operative vaginal delivery, and significant perinatal trauma in nulliparous women. *American Journal of Obstetrics and Gynecology, 181*(5 Pt 1), 1180–1184. https://doi.org/10.1016/s0002-9378(99)70104-3

Roslani, A. C., Ramakrishnan, R., Azmi, S., Arapoc, D. J., & Goh, A. (2014). Prevalence of faecal incontinence and its related factors among patients in a Malaysian academic setting. *BMC Gastroenterology, 14*, 95. https://doi.org/10.1186/1471-230X-14-95

Saldana Ruiz, N., & Kaiser, A. M. (2017). Fecal incontinence - challenges and solutions. *World Journal of Gastroenterology, 23*(1), 11–24. https://doi.org/10.3748/wjg.v23.i1.11

Samuelsson, E. C., Victor, F. T., Tibblin, G., & Svärdsudd, K. F. (1999). Signs of genital prolapse in a Swedish population of women 20 to 59 years of age and possible related factors. *American Journal of Obstetrics and Gynecology, 180*(2 Pt 1), 299–305. https://doi.org/10.1016/s0002-9378(99)70203-6

Sanses, T. V. D., Schiltz, N. K., Couri, B. M., Mahajan, S. T., Richter, H. E., Warner, D. F., et al. (2016). Functional status in older women diagnosed with pelvic organ prolapse. *American Journal of Obstetrics and Gynecology, 214*(5), 613.e1–613.e7. https://doi.org/10.1016/j.ajog.2015.11.038

Sexton, C. C., Coyne, K. S., Thompson, C., Bavendam, T., Chen, C. I., & Markland, A. (2011). Prevalence and effect on health-related quality of life of overactive bladder in older americans: Results from the epidemiology of lower urinary tract symptoms study. *Journal of the American Geriatrics Society, 59*(8), 1465–1470. https://doi.org/10.1111/j.1532-5415.2011.03492.x

Siddiqui, N. Y., Levin, P. J., Phadtare, A., Pietrobon, R., & Ammarell, N. (2014). Perceptions about female urinary incontinence: A systematic review. *International Urogynecology Journal, 25*(7), 863–871. https://doi.org/10.1007/s00192-013-2276-7

Siddle, K., Vieren, L., & Fiander, A. (2014). Characterising women with obstetric fistula and urogenital tract injuries in Tanzania. *International Urogynecology Journal, 25*(2), 249–255. https://doi.org/10.1007/s00192-013-2185-9

Swift, S. E., Tate, S. B., & Nicholas, J. (2003). Correlation of symptoms with degree of pelvic organ support in a general population of women: What is pelvic organ prolapse? *American Journal of Obstetrics and Gynecology, 189*(2), 372–377; discussion 377-9. https://doi.org/10.1067/s0002-9378(03)00698-7

The World Health Organization. (1997). Care in normal birth: A practical guide. Technical working group, World Health Organization. *Birth (Berkeley, Calif.), 24*(2), 121–123. Retrieved September 2, 2019, from http://www.ncbi.nlm.nih.gov/pubmed/9271979

The World Health Organization. (2017). *Integrated care for older people (ICOPE) Guidelines on community-level interventions to manage declines in intrinsic capacity.* Retrieved August 6, 2019, from https://www.who.int/ageing/health-systems/icope/evidence-centre/ICOPE-evidence-profile-urinary-incont.pdf

The World Health Organization. (2018). *Maternal Mortality Fact Sheet.* Retrieved August 21, 2019, from http://www.who.int/news-room/fact-sheets/detail/maternal-mortality

UNICEF. (2009). *The state of the World's children.*

Vergeldt, T. F. M., Weemhoff, M., IntHout, J., & Kluivers, K. B. (2015). Risk factors for pelvic organ prolapse and its recurrence: A systematic review. *International Urogynecology Journal, 26*(11), 1559–1573. https://doi.org/10.1007/s00192-015-2695-8

Vitale, S. G., Caruso, S., Rapisarda, A. M. C., Valenti, G., Rossetti, D., Cianci, S., & Cianci, A. (2016). Biocompatible porcine dermis graft to treat severe cystocele: Impact on quality of life and sexuality. *Archives of Gynecology and Obstetrics, 293*(1), 125–131. https://doi.org/10.1007/s00404-015-3820-0

Walker, G. J. A., & Gunasekera, P. (2011). Pelvic organ prolapse and incontinence in developing countries: Review of prevalence and risk factors. *International Urogynecology Journal, 22*(2), 127–135. https://doi.org/10.1007/s00192-010-1215-0

Wall, L. L. (2016). Residual incontinence after obstetric fistula repair. *Obstetrics & Gynecology, 128*(5), 943–944. https://doi.org/10.1097/AOG.0000000000001734

Wall, L. L., Arrowsmith, S. D., Lassey, A. T., & Danso, K. (2006). Humanitarian ventures or "fistula tourism?": The ethical perils of pelvic surgery in the developing world. *International Urogynecology Journal, 17*(6), 559–562. https://doi.org/10.1007/s00192-005-0056-8

Whitehead, W. E., Borrud, L., Goode, P. S., Meikle, S., Mueller, E. R., Tuteja, A., et al. (2009). Fecal incontinence in US adults: Epidemiology and risk factors. *Gastroenterology, 137*(2), 512–517, 517.e1–2. https://doi.org/10.1053/j.gastro.2009.04.054

Whiteside, J. L., Weber, A. M., Meyn, L. A., & Walters, M. D. (2004). Risk factors for prolapse recurrence after vaginal repair. *American Journal of Obstetrics and Gynecology, 191*(5), 1533–1538. https://doi.org/10.1016/j.ajog.2004.06.109

Williams, G., Browning, A., & Petros, P. E. (2018). The integral theory and its tethered vagina syndrome revisited: Vaginal scarring may cause massive urinary incontinence. *BJU International, 122*(4), 532–534. https://doi.org/10.1111/bju.14218

Wright, J., Ayenachew, F., & Ballard, K. (2016). The changing face of obstetric fistula surgery in Ethiopia. *International Journal of Women's Health, 8*, 243–248. https://doi.org/10.2147/IJWH.S106645

Wu, J. M., Matthews, C. A., Conover, M. M., Pate, V., & Funk, M. J. (2014). Lifetime risk of stress incontinence or pelvic organ prolapse surgery. *Obstetrics and Gynecology, 123*(6), 1201–1206. https://doi.org/10.1097/AOG.0000000000000286

Zeleke, B. M., Ayele, T. A., Woldetsadik, M. A., Bisetegn, T. A., & Adane, A. A. (2013). Depression among women with obstetric fistula, and pelvic organ prolapse in Northwest Ethiopia. *BMC Psychiatry, 13*(1), 236. https://doi.org/10.1186/1471-244X-13-236

Index

A
Aberdeen women's centre (AWC), 283, 284, 337, 338
    fistula prevalence, 286
    fistula programme, 338–340
    fistula services, 285
    freetown, 337, 338
    inadequate resources, 284
    incontinence, 283
    infrastructure, 285
    interhospital care coordination, 285
    interhospital consultation, 287
    maintaining medical equipment, 285
    maternal mortality, 337
    maternity services, 284
    poor post surgical follow up, 286
    procuring, 285
    recurrent fistula, 287
    stress incontinence, 286, 287
Acceptability, 329
Acute obstetric injury, 42
Anal incontinence (AI), 472, 473
Ancillary needs, 299
Antenatal, 298
Antenatal clinic (ANC), 196
Anthropometric characteristics, 309
Anthropometry, 346
Appropriateness, 320
Assets-based approach, 331
Avicenna, 34, 35

B
Basic emergency obstetric care (BEmOC), 198, 213
Basic emergency obstetric service (BEmOS), 94–95
Basic routine care
    awareness and access barriers, 294, 295
    structure and process, 292–294
Basic routine care model, 292
Bladder diary, 396
Bladder stones, 395
Body mass index (BMI), 346
Boromo health district, 356
Burkina Faso, 356, 359–363

C
Capacity building, 475
Central Africa, 256
Centre for Scientific and Technological Research
    (CNRST), 359
Cephalopelvic disproportion (CPD), 108, 129, 198, 199,
    345, 346, 351
Cervical injuries, 248
Cervical menstrual cup, 326
Challenges, 406, 422, 425
Childbirth, 283
    experiences, 123–125
    experiences living with obstetric fistula, 125–128
    gender disparities in health, 130–131
    lifespan view, 131–132
    policy recommendations, 132–133
    politico-economic conditions, 130–131
    research methodology, 123
    socio-cultural and politico-economic conditions, 128
    socio-cultural conditions, 131
    tracing obstetric fistula pathway, 129–130
    treatment for women with fistula, 128
Circumferential fistula, 206
Clean intermittent self-catheterization (CISC), 244, 402
Cognitive behavioral therapy (CBT), 447
Community-based health planning services (CHPS), 409
Competency-based training, 269
Community health nurses (CHN), 412
Community health workers (CHWs), 383
Community outreach, 294
Comprehensive community based rehabilitation tanzania
    (CCBRT), 189
Comprehensive emergency obstetric care
    (CEmOC), 95, 198
Computed tomodensitometry (CT), 346
Cystometrogram (CMG), 396

D
Darifenacin, 401
Data analysis, 191, 192, 413
Data collection methods, 292, 413
Delivery, 298

© Springer Nature Switzerland AG 2022
L. B. Drew et al. (eds.), *A Multidisciplinary Approach to Obstetric Fistula in Africa*, Global
Maternal and Child Health, https://doi.org/10.1007/978-3-031-06314-5

Printed by Printforce, the Netherlands